Health Today

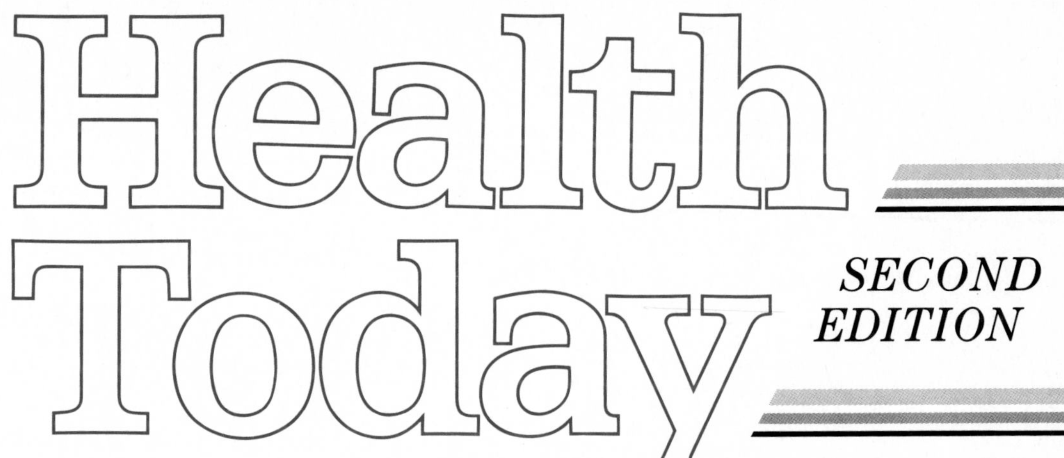

Health Today

SECOND EDITION

Larry K. Olsen
Arizona State University

Kerry J. Redican
Virginia Polytechnic Institute and State University

Charles R. Baffi
Virginia Polytechnic Institute and State University

Macmillan Publishing Company
NEW YORK

Printed in the United States of America

Macmillan Publishing Company
866 Third Avenue, New York, New York 10022

Collier Macmillan Canada, Inc.

Library of Congress Cataloging in Publication Data

Olsen, Larry K.
Health today.

Rev. ed. of: Health today / consultants, Larry K. Olsen . . . [et al.]. ©1983.
Includes bibliographies and index.
1. Health. 2. Health—Examinations, questions, etc.
I. Redican, Kerry J. II. Baffi, Charles R.
III. Title. [DNLM: 1. Health. 2. Hygiene.
QT 180 052h]
RA776.H449 1986 613
ISBN 0-02-389260-9

Printing: 1 2 3 4 5 6 7 8 Year: 6 7 8 9 0 1 2 3 4 5

Chapter opening photograph credits:
Page 1: © Photo Fournier Schelga/Rapho-Photo Researchers, Inc.; *page 12:* Frederick D. Bodin/Stock, Boston; *page 38:* Paul Waldman; *page 68:* Jim Pozarik/Liason Agency; *page 104:* © Marc Anderson; *page 128:* © Ellis Herwig/The Picture Cube; *page 156:* Laurel Eisenberg; *page 184:* Joan Lifton 1981/Archive Pictures, Inc.; *page 206:* Paul S. Conklin/Monkmeyer; *page 232:* Bonnie Freer/Photo Researchers, Inc.; *page 264:* Omikron/Photo Researchers, Inc.; *page 296:* © David Burnett 1981/Woodfin Camp & Associates; *page 322:* Paul Waldman; *page 354:* Marc P. Anderson; *page 380:* Cathy Cheney/EKM-Nepenthe; *page 416:* University of Michigan Health Sciences Information Services; *page 444:* Camera Press/Photo Trends; *page 474:* © Christopher Morrow/ Stock, Boston; *page 500:* © 1976 Dick Hanley/Photo Researchers, Inc.; *page 534:* Marc P. Anderson; *page 568:* Arkansas Dept. of Parks and Tourism.

ISBN 0-02-389260-9

Preface

MANY PEOPLE take health for granted until they experience some sort of health problem. Fortunately, medical science has made numerous breakthroughs to solve many of the problems confronting humankind. But, even though we know how to prevent many health problems, merely knowing what is best or what is available does not mean that we will put this knowledge into practice. This is especially true for college students, who are often too young to have experienced any major difficulties with their health.

You are constantly confronted by choices about your health. The choices you make can either enhance or detract from your inherited potential and can affect your well-being for the rest of your life. As medical knowledge increases, the number of available choices concerning health products, information, and services also increases. Thus, it is necessary that you know as much as possible about these things in order to make the personal decisions that will help you to achieve and maintain optimal health.

This second edition of *Health Today* is not designed as a mere compendium of health facts, however. It is meant, in addition, to help students to gain insight into their own attitudes and behavior regarding health and health practices. To help you to examine your own personal health knowledge, attitudes, and practices, several important features have been incorporated into this second edition.

Features

- Every chapter contains one or more self-assessment exercises designed to give you insight about yourself and how you approach health. A list of these exercises can be found at the end of the contents section.

- At the beginning of each chapter, key points are included that highlight the major emphases within the chapter.
- Each chapter contains boxed inserts entitled "Your Health Today" that deal with important contemporary personal health issues.
- At the conclusion of a chapter, a detailed summary and a number of thought-provoking review questions are presented. The review questions are designed to help you to apply the concepts and facts contained in the chapter.
- If you wish more detail about any given topic, a series of annotated suggested readings are presented.
- To ensure that you understand the terminology that is used within the chapter, glossary terms are included in the margin. A comprehensive glossary also appears at the end of the book.

Conceptually divided into six major sections, the text explores health from both the personal and the social aspects, from the mental and emotional to the environmental aspects, and from birth through death. Part I, "Knowing Yourself," includes an examination of many psychological factors that influence physical and emotional health, and it concentrates on attaining a positive mental outlook and on effective ways of dealing with stress. Part II, "Life Cycles," covers reproduction and birth control, sexuality, relationships, aging, and dying and death. "Drugs: Use and Abuse" is the title of Part III. Included are discussions of alcohol; tobacco; and prescription, over-the-counter, and illicit drugs. In Part IV, "Personal Health," the shift from a nation of spectators to a nation of participants who are concerned about health is explored. Basic concepts of fitness, nutrition, and weight control are included, and you have the opportunity to assess your status in each of these areas so that you can develop a personal plan for health promotion. In Part V, "Disease," a practical approach for dealing with cardiovascular diseases, cancer, and communicable and noncommunicable diseases of particular importance to the college population, along with ways to reduce the risk of getting these diseases, are presented. The final section, "Community Well-Being," contains a discussion of pertinent consumer issues, safety and accident prevention, and the need for protecting the environment and conserving natural resources.

Just as there is no best way to teach a course, there is no best way to organize a textbook. Thus, we have tried to order the various sections in such a manner that the instructor can adapt the sequence to suit his or her style and the needs of the students in the class. To further aid the instructor, a comprehensive Test Item File and an Instructor's Manual have been developed.

Acknowledgments

We would like to acknowledge the consultants who contributed to the first edition of *Health Today:* Terry Adcock (Human Sexuality), Loren Bensley (Death and Dying), Lee Burkett (Nutrition, Weight Control), James Eddy (Alcohol, Tobacco, Drugs), Robert Buthmann (Safety and Accident Prevention), Joan McMahon (Mental Health), Richard St. Pierre (Alcohol, Tobacco, Drugs), William Stone (Physical Fitness, Nutrition), Alyson Taub (Aging), and Molly Wantz (Stress) —for it was their diligent efforts in the first edition that laid the groundwork for the second edition.

We would also like to acknowledge the useful reviews and comments made by many of the instructors and students who used the first edition of the text, and those who did a detailed review of the manuscript before and after this revision was completed:

Cory Bates, *Ohio State University*
Betty Bennison, *Texas Christian University*
Bryan Cooke, *University of Northern Colorado*
David deJoy, *University of Georgia*
Judy Drolet, *Southern Illinois University*
Ray Goldberg, *State University of New York–Cortland*
Mark Kittleson, *Youngstown State University*
Philip Marty, *University of Arkansas*
Robert McDermott, *Southern Illinois University*
John Murray, *Catonsville Community College*
Robert Nye, *West Chester University*
Leslie Ramsdale, *Eastern Kentucky University*
Barbara Rienzo, *University of Florida*
Steve Roberts, *University of Toledo*
Sally Rudmann, *Ohio State University*
Loretta Taylor, *Southwestern College*

Finally, we wish to thank James D. Anker, Senior Editor, at Macmillan Publishing Company for overseeing the project and offering invaluable support; Anne Pietropinto, Development Editor, who kept us on target, asking probing and often difficult questions so that we became better communicators of what we had to say, Robert Hunter and Aliza Greenblatt, Production Supervisors, for directing the copyediting and production stages of the project; Dubose McLane, Production Manager, for directing the manufacturing stages of the project; Andrew Zutis, Design Manager, for creating the design and supervising page layout; and Charlotte Green, Photo Researcher, for providing pertinent and lively photographs for this edition. We would also like to thank Editorial Assistants Katherine Evancie and Britt Buckwald for their diligent work in the reviewing, permissions, and photo-acquiring processes. Special thanks go to Lynne Greenberg for overseeing the final stages of the project and to Chris Cardone for her able supervision of the marketing process.

Larry K. Olsen
Kerry J. Redican
Charles R. Baffi

Contents

Part IV Personal Health

Part VI Community Well-Being

Self-Assessment Exercises

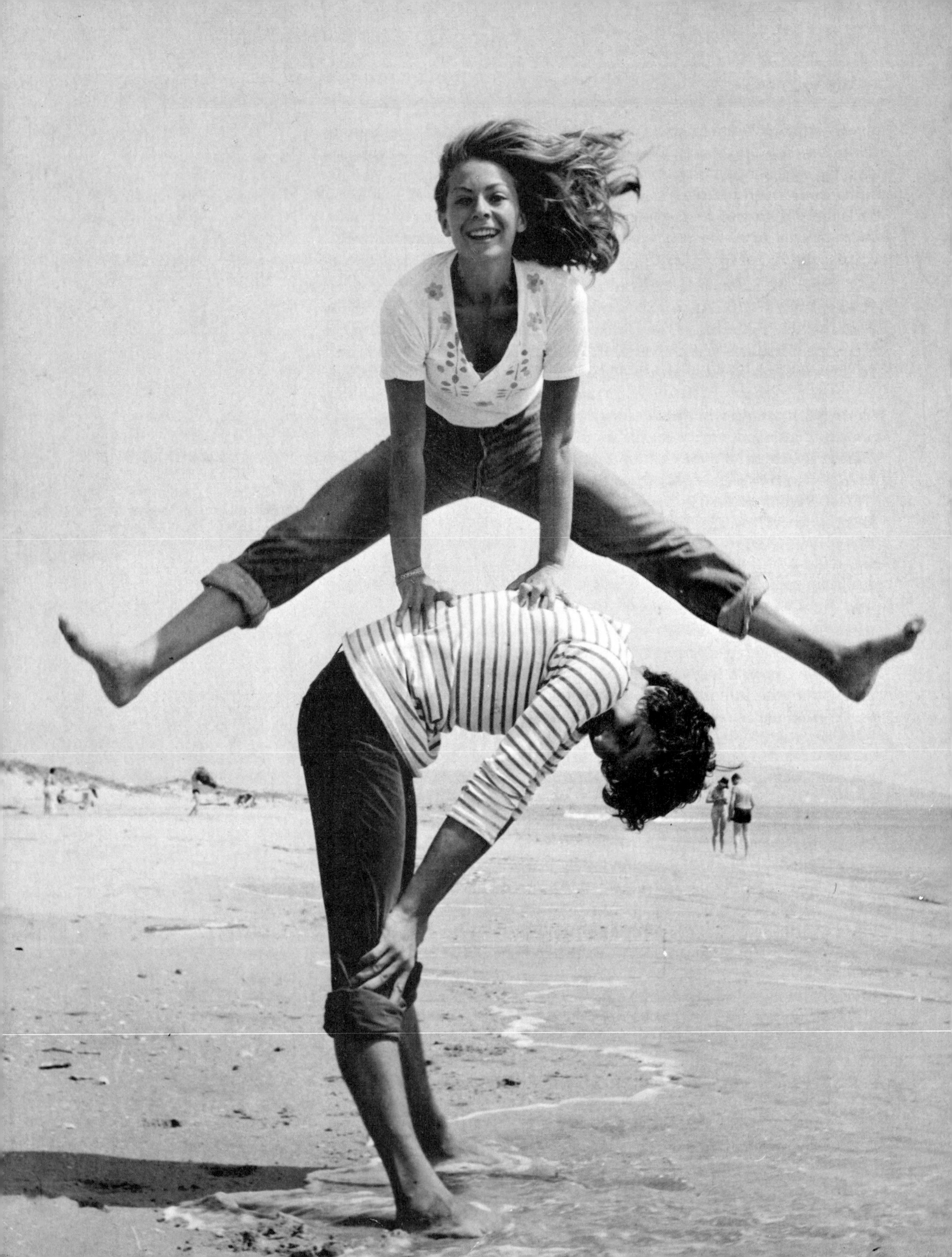

Chapter 1
A Healthy Life

KEY POINTS

- ☐ Although good health has always been a central human concern, Americans today are more interested than ever before in living a healthy life.
- ☐ Health and illness form a continuum, ranging from total well-being to death.
- ☐ The concept of well-being through the life span can serve as a guide to understanding health as part of human development and growth.
- ☐ There is increased emphasis today on individual responsibility for establishing good health practices and thereby avoiding illness.
- ☐ Awareness of health issues is an important part of achieving well-being.

IF YOU were to ask children, "What is health?" they might answer, "You aren't sick" or "You feel good, so you don't have to go to the doctor." If you asked the same question of college students, the sophistication of the response would be greater, but the emphasis on the absence of disease would probably remain. In 1947, however, the World Health Organization described health as "a state of complete physical, mental, and social well-being, not merely the absence of disease or infirmity." This understanding of human potential and growth allows us to see a positive range of health values beyond the absence of sickness. In this view of health, there is a continuum of sickness and health ranging from death as the total absence of health to optimal or total well-being. (See Figure 1-1, which describes the Illness/Wellness Continuum.) Every individual is born with a certain potential, and if this potential is fulfilled, the individual will have found optimal well-being.

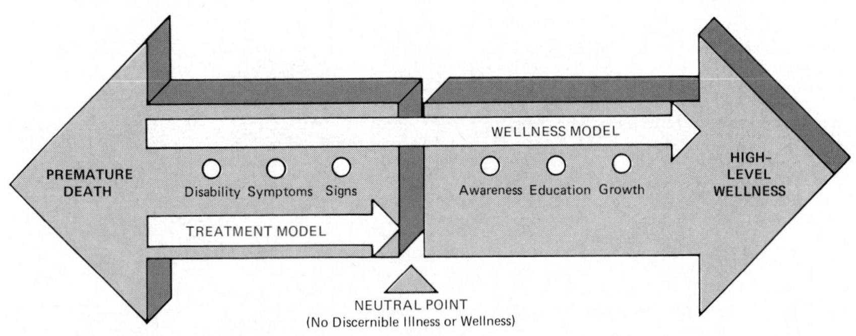

Figure 1-1. The Illness/Wellness Continuum. Health may be considered a continuum from premature death at one end of the scale to high-level wellness at the other. Traditional medicine helps us reach a neutral, or zero, point where there is no defined illness, but this is not wellness. Wellness is what we attain through individual efforts to integrate physical, mental, and social dimensions of life. (Source: The Illness/Wellness Continuum, used with permission. Copyright © 1972, 1981, John W. Travis, M.D., Wellness Associates, Box 5433, Mill Valley, CA 94942. From Ryan and Travis, *Wellness Workbook* [Berkeley: Ten Speed Press, 1981.])

This approach to health presents an idealistic goal, and no one has defined a state of complete physical, mental, and social well-being—or **wellness,** as it is often referred to—that would apply to everyone. Nevertheless, total health remains a goal all of us would like to achieve. As we live and grow, each of us will find different approaches to fulfillment, but in all cases the physical, mental, and social dimensions will be involved.

Wellness A potentially ever-expanding experience of healthful, enjoyable living.

Life-Style and Health

In the past the emphasis in health care was curative. When you were ill you went to be cured; when you were well, you presumed that everything was fine. Recently, however, the idea of illness as related to **life-style factors** and illness prevention has received much attention. This is partly because the diseases that had killed millions of people in the late nineteenth and early twentieth centuries were found to have specific causes—certain bacteria or viruses, for exam-

Life-style factors The day-to-day practices, habits, and activities that influence the health of the individual.

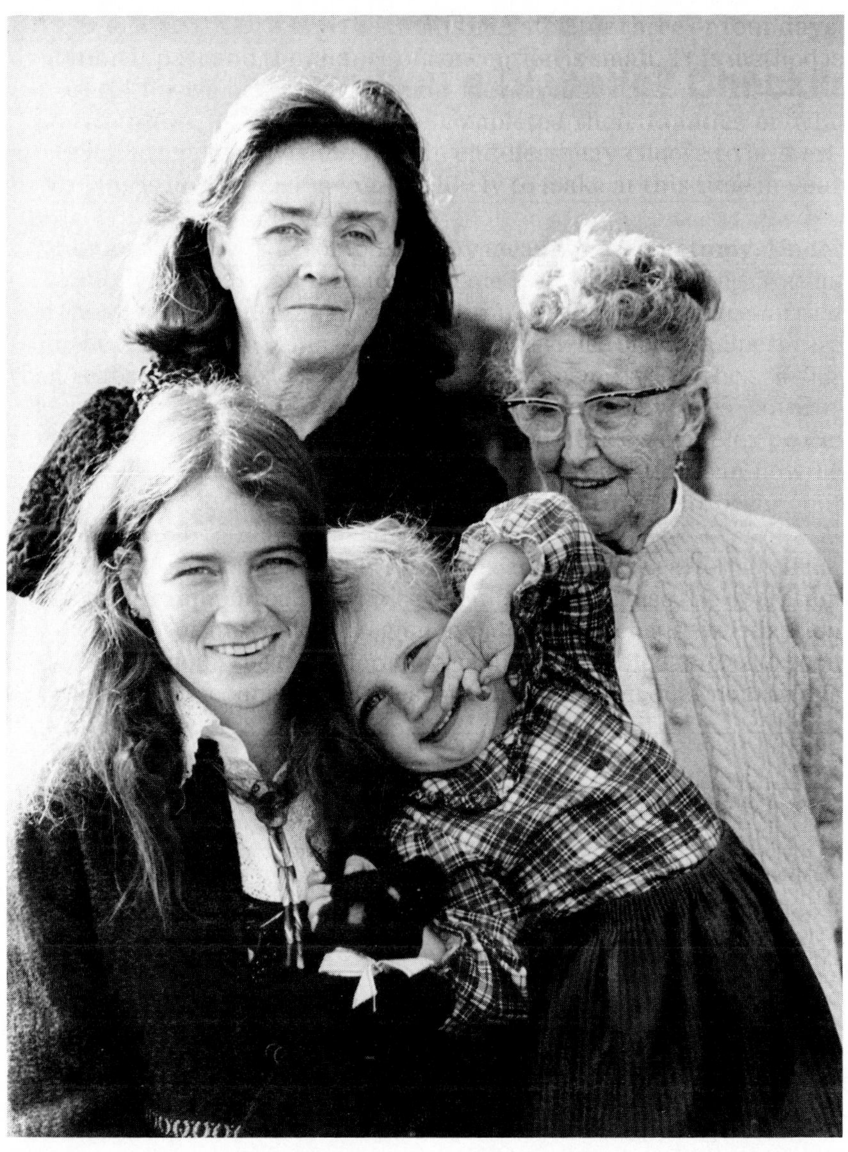

Four generations. Although different challenges exist throughout the lifespan, growth and development and the need for a healthy life-style continue. (Photo by Peter Simon/Stock, Boston)

ple. These diseases were brought under control and even eliminated through education, immunization, or drug therapy.

Today, however, the four leading causes of death in the United States are heart disease, cancer, stroke, and accidents (see Figure 1–2). No one has developed a cure for heart disease, and there is no inoculation that will prevent fatal automobile accidents. But much is known about the risk factors that lead to these forms of death. Although some of the factors are hereditary and thus presently are beyond our control, others are the result of *life-style* factors — that is, day-to-day health practices — and can be prevented.

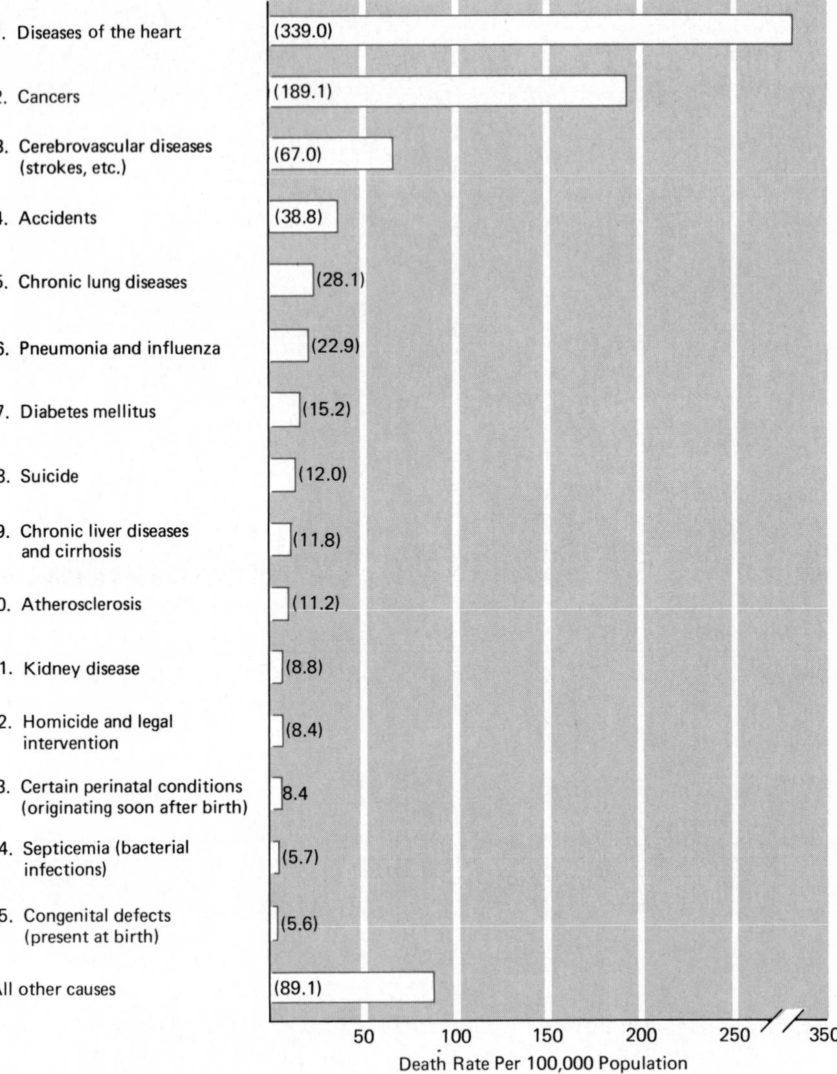

Figure 1-2. Death Rate per 100,000 Population for the 15 Leading Causes of Death in the United States, 1983. Many of these causes of death could be controlled through life-style alteration on the part of individuals. (Source: Adapted from National Center for Health Statistic, *Monthly Vital Statistics Report,* 32:12 [March 26, 1984]: 6–7.)

The *Prevention Profile* prepared by the U.S. Department of Health and Human Services lists eight life-style factors that have a major effect on health. These eight factors are—

- smoking
- weight control
- nutrition
- risky driving
- stress and hazards on the job
- misuse of alcohol and drugs
- exercise and fitness
- strong relationships with other people.[1]

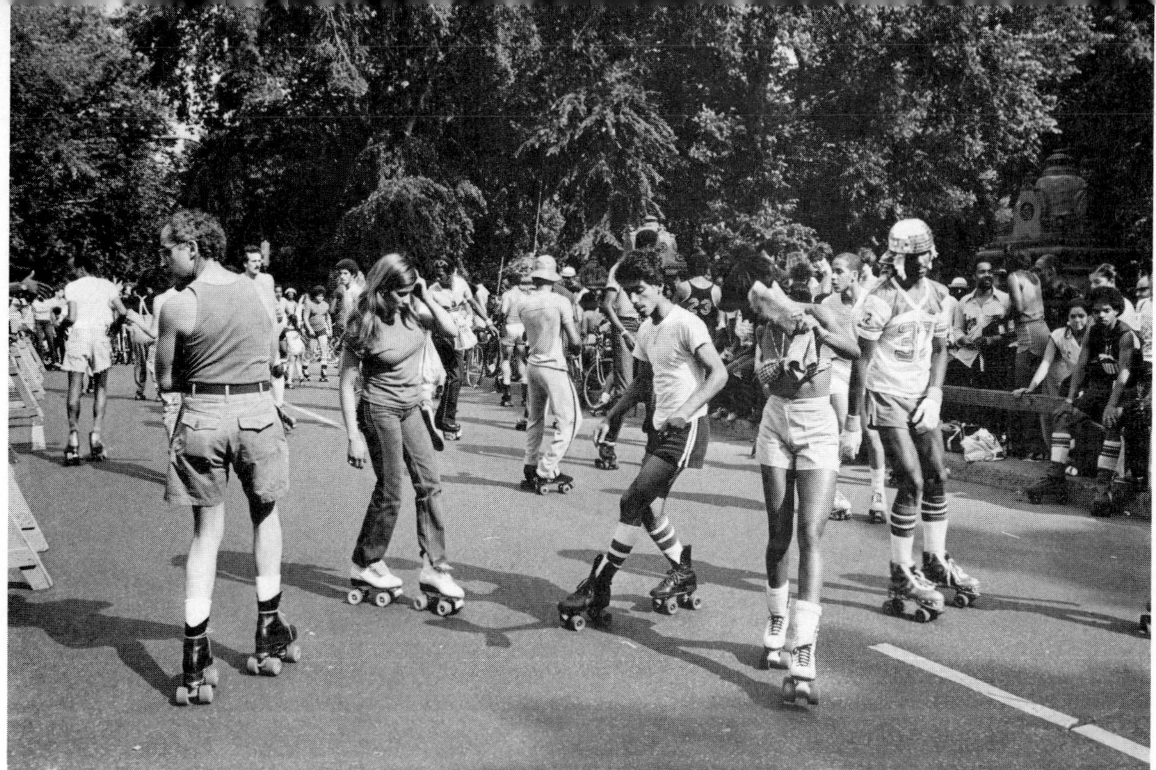

Social well-being is an integral part of wellness. (Photo © Van Bucher 1981/Photo Researchers, Inc.)

These topics will be treated in detail later in this textbook. Note the table of contents to see where each is discussed.

Where Do We Stand?

Americans are, by and large, sympathetic to the idea of **preventive health care.** Polls taken in recent years show that Americans are very much aware of the importance of good health practices. In a poll taken in 1979, 92 percent agreed with the statement, "If we Americans ate more nutritious food, smoked less, maintained our proper weight and exercised regularly, it would do more to improve our health than anything doctors and medicine could do for us." And these attitudes are finding their way into practice. In another survey, 46 percent of American adults said that they had recently changed the life-styles of themselves and their families in order to achieve good health. Statistics show a marked decrease in many types of unfavorable life-style behaviors (although there are important exceptions, such as an increase in smoking in teenage girls and the failure of the public to use safety belts when driving).

Preventive health care Actions taken by the individual to prevent illness.

Individual Responsibility

Health is an individual responsibility. To take responsibility for our health is to recognize that we have the ability to modify the risks inherent in our heredity and social environment. That is, we can modify our risks through changes in our behavior.

Throughout this book, you will be asked to complete Self-Assessment Exercises, which will give you an idea of your attitudes about various health practices, such as smoking and exercise, and life-style factors, such as susceptibility to heart disease. This will give you the opportunity to assess what actions you must take to modify your risk of illness and increase your chances of a longer life of high-level wellness. You can start by completing the Wellness Inventory, in the Appendix.

Gap Between Knowledge and Action

Knowledge about health choices is an important aspect of individual responsibility. Although this knowledge is increasing rapidly, the gap between knowledge and action remains great. For example, approximately 75 percent of lung cancer cases could be prevented if people did not smoke cigarettes. This would mean that more than 80,000 fewer people would die of lung cancer every year. The dangers of smoking are well-known. Every cigarette pack carries a warning that cigarette smoking is dangerous to your health, and public health organizations have launched intensive media campaigns to alert people to the danger. Despite this knowledge, people continue to smoke.

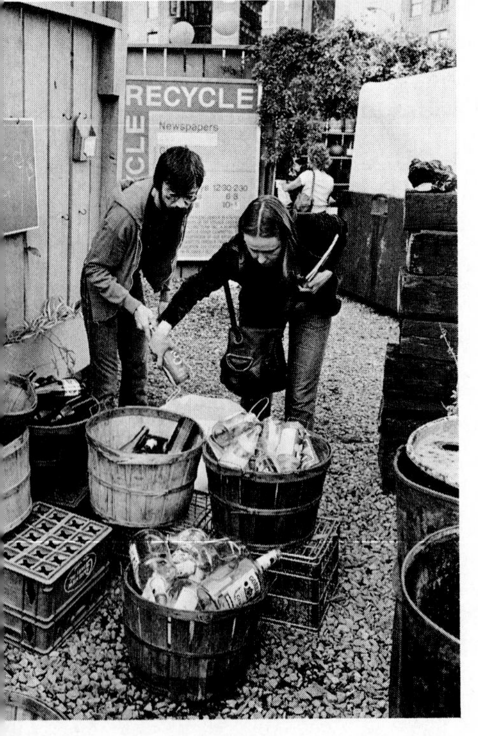

People can interact with their environment to bring about changes for a healthier world. (Photo by Charles Gatewood/The Image Works)

Unfortunately, cigarette smoking is not the only example. Responsibility, the determination to make good health practices a part of one's life, does not come easily, and unless we can see the real problems involved, our desire for a healthy life may become just a hope.

What Is Responsibility?

Responsibility means choosing a healthy alternative over a less healthy one. Many of our health practices are based on habit, not on consciously made decisions. Many of the health practices we learned from our parents or adopted at an early age have become intricately woven into the fabric of our current health behavior. To become aware of them and their potentially harmful effects requires a conscious effort to examine our lives from the perspective of health and then a concerted effort to change habits which die hard.

Sources of Health Problems

Life-Style Choices

Another factor is the quality of modern life-styles, which are often the source of health problems. The fast-paced tempo of contemporary life can lead to a great deal of stress on the mind and body. It has been estimated that stress is a significant factor in 50 to 80 percent of all diseases we now suffer. These disorders are known as the "afflictions of civilization" and are caused by such factors as pollution, poor nutrition, and psychological stress. Most of us cannot isolate ourselves from the world to escape these dangers. Responsibility means obtaining the information to understand the problems and making a conscious effort to cope with them and diminish their effects, even if the problems cannot be totally avoided.

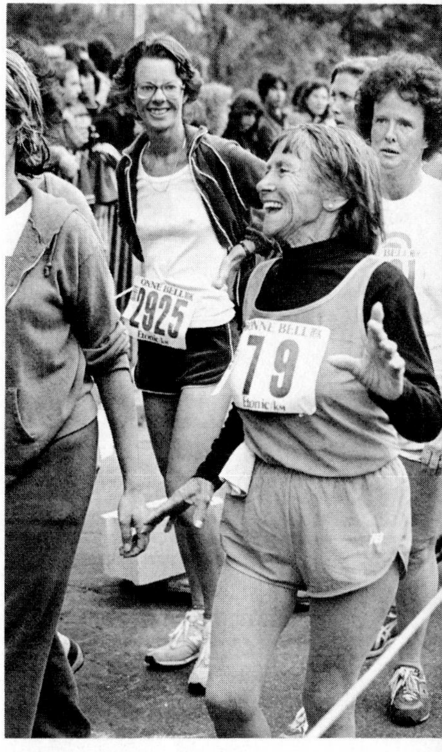

A healthy life is an individual responsibility throughout the life span. (Photo © Susan Lapides 1980/Design Conceptions)

Madison Avenue Marketing

We must also recognize that a great deal of time, energy, and money have been expended to market bad health practices. Advertising in the mass media bombards the public on a daily basis with messages affecting health: weight reduction, vitamin pills, exercise aids, health clubs, personal hygiene products, sugared cereals, dangerous toys, alcoholic beverages, stop-smoking programs, and so on. These messages often contain seductive appeals, based on a promise of easy results. All you have to do is enroll in program X, and the magic formula will solve the problem. All you have to do is eat a bowl of Brand Y a day, and all your nutritional problems will be solved. And if we skip meals, all we have to do is take our daily vitamin pill. Unfortunately, health is not a purchasable commodity. Responsibility requires making a conscious effort to evaluate the various claims made for products and health services and then acting on that knowledge. This is not to say that all claims made for health products and services are false; it is just a reminder of the old saying, "Let the buyer beware."

Lack of Information

Another problem in making good health decisions is incompleteness of our information. For example, everyone knows that smoking is harmful, but very few—particularly smokers—know *how* bad it is or in what precise ways it is damaging to the human body. Obtaining adequate information is essential for understanding the full consequences of your actions. (See Chapter 10 for a thorough discussion of tobacco and health.) Very often, incomplete information leads to mistaken ideas, and many aspects of health, both physical and mental, are distorted in traditional misconceptions.

Well-Being Throughout the Life Span

The goal of well-being throughout the life span demands that we adopt, at least occasionally, a broader perspective on our lives and view our health practices as part of a lifelong process. The human mind and body are extremely flexible, and poor health habits—unless they cause immediate death—can be overcome by our enormous adaptability. It is only too easy to decide to change one's life-style tomorrow or the next day — but not now. Too often people do not value health until they lose it. Under the pressures of day-to-day living, it is difficult to take time out and examine our practices from this perspective, but this is an important part of assuming responsibility for our well-being.

Of course, these are not the only obstacles to making good health decisions, but they do suggest the kinds of problems that must be overcome. In a complex area like health, decisions are not always easy. But if we develop the attitude of responsibility, we will find it easier and easier to take control of our lives.

There is danger in pointing out the problems involved in taking responsibility for health decisions. Too often, good health practices are associated with self-denial, with the idea that good health means giving up good things. An important element in achieving good health is realizing that it is a *positive undertaking.* A healthy person looks better, feels better, and copes with reality more effectively.

Another incentive to make changes is to realize how simple some (although far from all) positive decisions are. Walk three blocks to the grocery store instead of taking the car. Walk up the stairs instead of riding the escalator. Buy yourself your favorite nutritious food as a treat. There are countless ways to do little, everyday things in a more healthy way. Once you begin making sound health decisions, even in small things, the rewards will not be long in coming. But the only way to learn that is to do it.

Review and Discussion

1. How is the concept of well-being different from the concept of health as the absence of sickness?
2. At this stage in your life, what are your goals and how is positive health related to them?
3. How would you define health?
4. Name six life-style risk factors.
5. Why is health an individual responsibility?
6. Describe three specific interactions between the physical, mental, and social dimensions in daily life.
7. Describe some of the obstacles that make good health practices difficult.
8. What simple good health practices could you start today?
9. What long-term health practices do you think you should adopt?

Further Reading

Braverman, Jordan. *Crisis in Health Care* (rev. ed.). Washington, D.C.: Acropolis Books, 1980.
Braverman discusses the economic, social and political problems that affect personal health care for Americans. (Paperback)

Brun, John, and Stewart Wolf. *The Roseto Story*. University of Oklahoma Press, 1979.
A study of traditional family relationships as the cause of the remarkably low incidence of coronary heart disease among citizens of Roseto, Pa.

Dubos, René. *So Human an Animal.* New York: Charles Scribner's Sons, 1968.
Dubos asserts that we are as much the product of our total environment as of our genetic endowment and that interaction with the environment can enhance or severely limit the development of human potential. (Paperback)

Dunn, Halbert L. *High Level Wellness.* Arlington, Va.: R. W. Beatty, L.T.D., 1961.
Dunn discusses the components of high-level wellness and what a person should do to achieve that status.

Pelletier, Kenneth. *Holistic Medicine.* New York: Dell Books, 1980.
The majority of the diseases we fear most are related to life style. Pelletier emphasizes preventive health care based on both psychological and physiological factors.

Rees, Alan, and Blanche Young. *The Consumer Health Information Source Book.* New York: R. R. Bowker Co., 1981.
A description and analysis of sources of health information for the lay person is offered, including an annotated bibliography of current literature and a guide to organizations providing health information.

Remen, Naomi. *The Human Patient.* New York: Anchor Press/Doubleday, 1980.
The premise of this text is that health care professionals must recognize and administer to the total individual if they are to be successful.

The Surgeon General of the United States. *Healthy People: The Surgeon General's Report on Health Promotion and Disease Prevention.* Washington, D.C.: U.S. Government Printing Office (PHS) Publication No. 79-55071, 1979.
A landmark report to the American Public about the health status of the nation's population. The basic health goals that will, in large measure, shape the nation's health care policy for the next decade are included.

Vickery, D. M., and J. F. Fries. *Take Care of Yourself: A Consumer's Guide to Medical Care.* Reading, Mass.: Addison-Wesley Publishing Co., 1976.
A programmed textbook, written by two physicians, that tells the consumer what to do in case of various medical situations—stay in bed and take aspirin, see your physician at once, and so forth.

Part I
Knowing Yourself

Thomas Jefferson wrote in his journal, "A strong body makes the mind strong." There are many who would say that he should have turned the statement around. Certainly, good mental health and knowing how best to cope with the stresses of everyday living are important factors that help ensure general wellness. To know yourself can be a key that unlocks the door to a fuller life. To be aware of what to expect in the development of your personality is as important as to know how best to meet your body's physical needs.

Chapter 2, "Mental Health," and Chapter 3, "Stress," introduce you to positive concepts that will enrich your emotional well-being and contribute to the harmony of your mind and body.

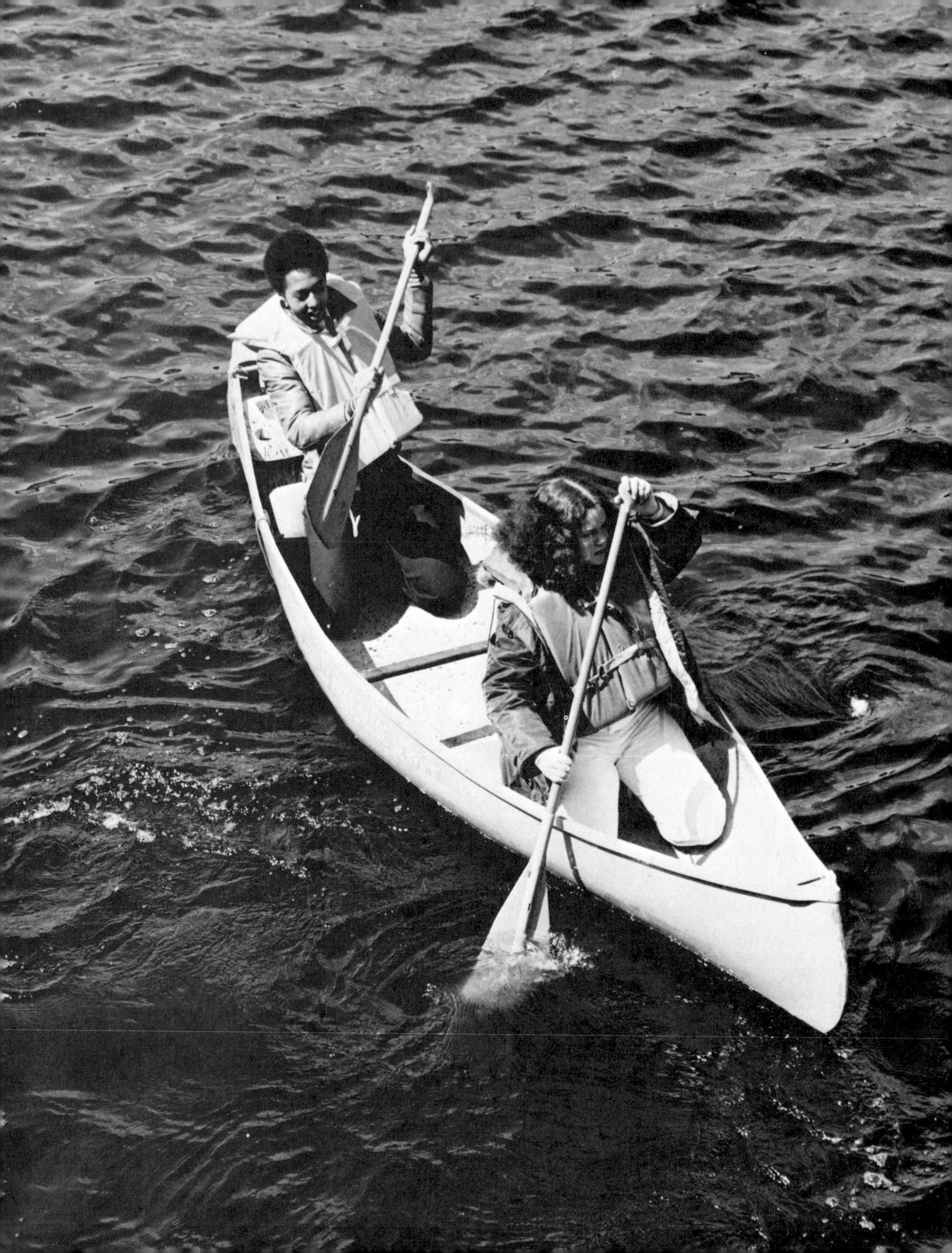

Chapter 2
Mental Health

KEY POINTS

- ☐ Mental health is not simply the absence of mental illness; it is the ability to find happiness and fulfillment, to change and to grow throughout one's life.
- ☐ There is a continuum of mental problems, ranging from mild disturbances to severe problems that may require professional help or hospitalization.
- ☐ Psychological theories, such as those proposed by Sigmund Freud and Abraham Maslow, can be an important help in gaining the self-understanding needed to find fulfillment.
- ☐ Among psychological mechanisms that can interfere with a person's ability to cope with the actual world are defense mechanisms—unconscious mental processes that the mind makes use of in an effort to protect itself against emotional conflicts.
- ☐ All people experience basic emotions, for example, love, elation, anger, fear, and sorrow.
- ☐ Many people experience mild emotional disturbances; these include loneliness, alienation and emptiness, mild depression, and mild anxiety.
- ☐ When psychological problems persist, help should be sought in various forms of counseling.

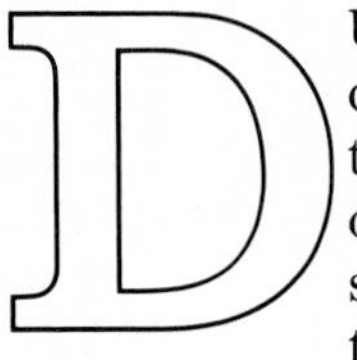

URING the twentieth century, approaches to mental health have changed radically. Traditionally, individuals were considered mentally healthy if they did not suffer from a severe psychological disorder. A fixed line was drawn between the mentally healthy (the sane) and the mentally sick (the insane). Gradually we have come to the understanding that there is a complex variety of mental problems that can affect people's ability to cope with the world and that these problems can range from mild disturbances that everyone suffers from occasionally to severe problems that require professional help, prolonged therapy, or even hospitalization.

What Is Mental Health?

Mental health A state of well-being in which the individual is comfortable in his/her dealings with others and with the challenges of everyday life.

Mental illness A state of being in which the individual is uncomfortable meeting everyday challenges and relating to others.

As we have indicated, **mental health** is much more than the absence of mental illness. According to the National Association for Mental Health, "it has to do with the way each person harmonizes his desires, ambitions, abilities, ideals, feelings, and conscience in order to meet the demands of life as he has to face them. . . . There are many degrees of mental health. No one characteristic by itself can be taken as evidence of good mental health, nor the lack of any one as evidence of mental illness. And nobody has all the traits of good mental health all the time."[1]

Just as we have gained better insight into ***mental illness*** and psychological disturbances, so too we have arrived at a better understanding of the positive goals of mental health. These goals include being comfortable with oneself, being comfortable in interactions with others, and being able to meet the ordinary demands of life without undergoing undue or prolonged stress.

Feeling Comfortable About Oneself

Feeling comfortable about oneself means having a solid sense of self-esteem, based on a reasonable degree of success in achieving one's desires and ambitions. It means knowing your abilities and being aware of your limitations.

Feeling Comfortable in Interactions with Others

Mentally healthy individuals interact positively with those around them. Naturally, there will be times when differences arise, but these conflicts or differences are discussed and resolved through compromise. Mentally healthy people respect the rights of others and try to promote positive interactions.

Meeting Daily Challenges Effectively

Mentally healthy individuals are able to gauge their actions to meet changing situations. They have learned to adapt to their society and

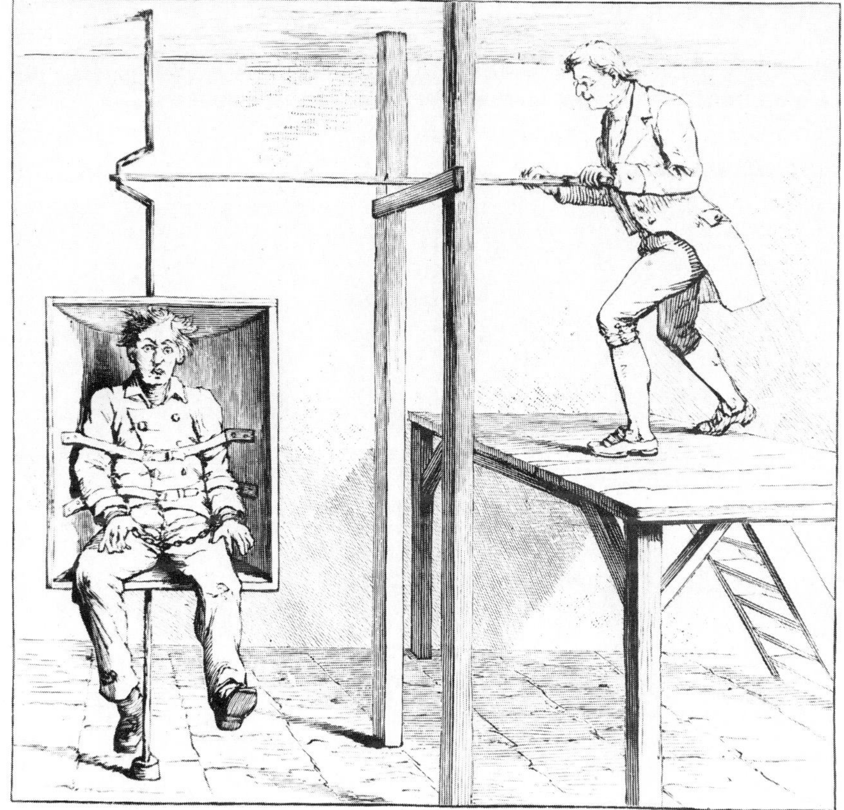

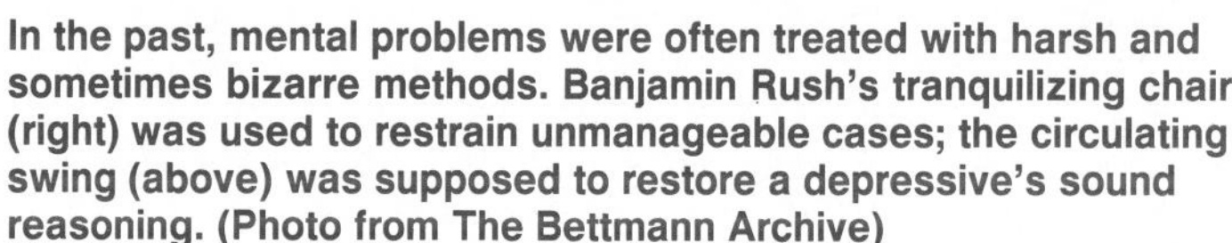

In the past, mental problems were often treated with harsh and sometimes bizarre methods. Banjamin Rush's tranquilizing chair (right) was used to restrain unmanageable cases; the circulating swing (above) was supposed to restore a depressive's sound reasoning. (Photo from The Bettmann Archive)

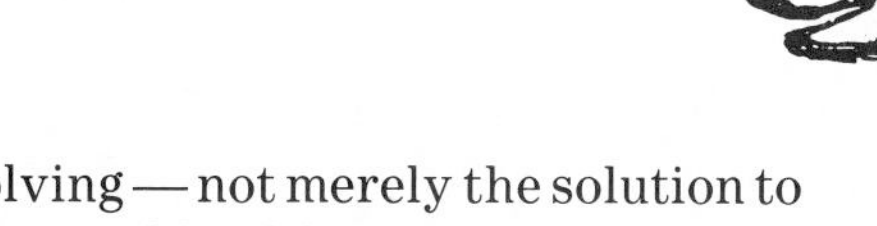

know that the process of problem solving — not merely the solution to the problem — contributes to good mental health.

Understanding Self and Others

Throughout a person's life, change and growth are major aspects of mental health. People are presented with challenges and choices, with opportunities to grow and find happiness and fulfillment. At the same time, this growth is not always easy and can in fact be quite painful. Modern life-styles can create many dilemmas that complicate the already-complex process of choosing between conflicting desires, hopes, and ambitions.

Foundations of Mental Health

One's mental health is shaped by many factors, including hereditary, physiological, and sociocultural factors.

Hereditary Factors

Heredity is what imparts the true limits on our potential, and the environment in which we live and interact sets varying limits on this potential. We bring to our lives generations of hereditary traits, both positive and negative, that are the complex chemical legacy given us by our parents and all our ancestors. What we do with this potential can, in large measure, be determined by each of us through the varying choices we make throughout our lifetime.

Physiological Factors

Our physical health, as evidenced in our actions, is often what is judged as representative of our mental health. Recall that we stated that behavior is our thoughts and feelings put into action. Our physiological health, in great measure, governs those actions. Persons who have good posture, smile, look well-rested, and walk with their head held high seem to exhibit an aura of confidence. They seem to say, "Look at me. I'm alive and I enjoy life."

Sociocultural Factors

Social interaction is a major aspect of total well-being. The sociocultural setting is where personality emerges. Personality is influenced by numerous factors, including one's home, peers, school, and social setting.

A feeling of trust and love are important to the development of positive mental health and a good self-image. (Photo by Franklin Wise/The News Messenger)

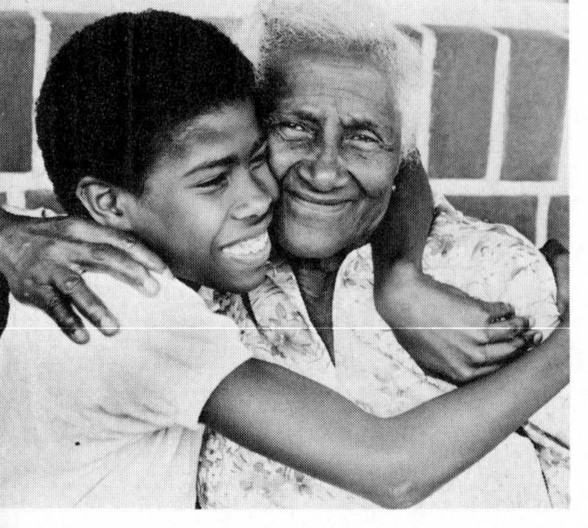

Home. The home is where the socialization process begins. Here you first interacted with a number of persons—your parents, your brothers and sisters, other relatives, and friends and neighbors. In general, most people first imitate the behaviors they observe at home. Our parents and siblings provided our basic concepts of right and wrong and what constitutes socially acceptable or unacceptable behavior.

Peers. Nearly everyone wants to be accepted by society in general, but especially by persons of their own age. Peers are an extremely powerful influence in reinforcing behaviors that contribute to one's health. As a person ages, the individuals and groups that exert influence may change, but the basic need of feeling accepted persists.

Schools. Schools are in a good position to provide a measure of stability in a rapidly changing world. Throughout our years of schooling, including college, we are subjected to varying degrees of authority. In the academic setting we learn to deal with authority and develop both unique skills and generalized ones basic to the total socialization process.

YOUR HEALTH TODAY

Children Learn What They Live

If a child lives with criticism, he learns to condemn.
If a child lives with hostility, he learns to fight.
If a child lives with ridicule, he learns to be shy.
If a child lives with shame, he learns to feel guilty.
If a child lives with tolerance, he learns to be patient.
If a child lives with encouragement, he learns confidence.
If a child lives with praise, he learns to appreciate.
If a child lives with fairness, he learns justice.
If a child lives with security, he learns to have faith.
If a child lives with approval, he learns to like himself.
If a child lives with acceptance and friendship, he learns
to find love in the world.

Dorothy Law Nolte

Community. All persons belong to a community. In its broadest sense, community means a group of people who share common needs, problems, and interests. Community can be looked at on a variety of scales: for example, statewide, regional, national, and in its broadest sense, worldwide. Within all of these contexts we deal with both positive and negative influences, influences that affect our mental health as much as do hereditary and physiological factors. We are constantly interacting with others and our environment, and these interactions help shape the personality that makes each of us unique.

Naturally, not all people will contribute in the same way to community life, nor will the community affect its members the same way. If constant conflict is present in the community, everyone is adversely affected. If adequate employment, health care, fire and police protection, and opportunities for recreational pursuits are present, then everyone benefits.

Theories of Personality and Social Development

In order to alter or build upon our individual foundations of mental health and to meet the challenges of modern life, we must understand ourselves and others. Despite the uniqueness of each individual, there are certain general patterns of human behavior. Psychologists have studied many aspects of human experience and have tried to present a systematic explanation for human behavior that will help people understand themselves better.

Although no single theory of personality development is accepted by all professionals, each theory provides some help in understanding behavior patterns. The various theories can serve as guides in understanding yourself and interpreting the behavior of others.

In this section some basic ideas of Sigmund Freud and Abraham Maslow will be presented. Each of their theories has proven fruitful in providing insight into human nature.

Freud

No one has had a greater impact on studies of personality, the mind, and mental problems than Sigmund Freud (1856–1939). Trained as a neurologist, he became convinced that there were powerful hidden mental processes controlling human behavior. Since people were often not conscious of their feelings and motivations, conflicts arose whose causes remained hidden to them. To explain these unconscious processes, Freud introduced a concept of personality structure based on three subsystems: the id, the ego, and the superego.

Id The primitive part of the psyche that is dominated by the pleasure principle and survival needs.

The **id** is the most primitive part of the personality and consists essentially of basic biological drives geared to survival needs and pleasure, such as hunger, thirst, and sex. These drives are the primary energies of life, although some may be negative in character—such as aggressiveness, selfishness, and self-gratification.

Ego The part of the psyche that consciously directs behavior.

The **ego** begins its development in childhood and is the demand moderator between the id and the outside world. According to Freud, this personality component is not present at birth but develops later in response to parental influence, life experiences, and social norms. A highly developed ego can control the drives and impulses of the id so that a person has more control of self and selfish needs. The ego serves to adapt the individual to the rules and inhibitions imposed by society.

Superego The part of the psyche that incorporates society's moral standards.

The **superego** is the result of learning the moral values of society. It evaluates the demands of the id and advises the ego on what actions are acceptable. It is essentially what we know as our conscience. Until a child's superego develops, the parents are the surrogate superego. This role may be assumed later by teachers and then by society in general. Finally, children develop their own standards for conduct. A person with a weak superego has little or no respect for the laws and customs of society in interactions with other people. On the other hand, a person with an overly developed superego has great feelings of guilt and may even avoid all pleasure-seeking activities.

For Freud the goal of development is the reconciliation of the three components through self-understanding and the development of the ego. By becoming aware of previously unconscious motivations and needs, a person is better able to fulfill real needs without losing sight of the moral bases of human society.

Maslow's Hierarchy of Human Needs

Abraham Maslow developed a five-step pyramid of human needs in which personality development progresses from one step to the next, and the needs of the lower levels must be satisfied before the next level can be reached. Once the needs are met, they must be satisfied throughout life, or else full development can never be achieved.

When needs are met, the individual moves toward well-being. When needs are not met, the person feels frustrated and generally functions ineffectively or in a socially maladaptive fashion.

The primary needs, forming the base of the pyramid, are *physiological*—the satisfaction of hunger, thirst, and sexuality. These are essential biological needs. The second step of the pyramid consists of needs for *safety*—security, order, and stability. The sense of safety is essential in facing potential dangers from the environment as well as from other people. If these needs are satisfied, the individual can progress to the third step in the pyramid, *belongingness and love* needs—the necessity of relating to and being accepted by others, both family and friends. Being accepted in a group and gaining social recognition are important. *Self-esteem* constitutes the fourth step and requires approval, recognition, and acceptance—the elements contributing to self-respect. Finally, at the fifth step, the needs are for **self-actualization**—the utilization of one's creative potential for self-fulfillment. For those who reach this peak position in the pyramid, life is a good experience, meaningful and enjoyable, its problems accepted and surmounted without lapses into despair. Few people reach and then maintain this highest level, the ultimate in personality development, but most people do experience such creative fulfillment from time to time in their lives (see Figure 2–1).

Self-actualization The utilization of one's creative potential for self-fulfillment.

According to Maslow, those persons who are self-actualized act instead of react to their environments. They make independent deci-

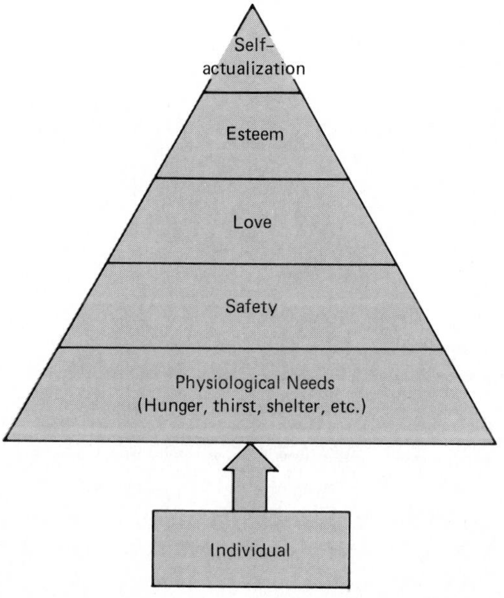

Figure 2–1. The Hierarchy of Needs.

sions as to their life goals, how they perceive themselves, and how they will achieve their goals. According to Maslow, self-actualized individuals—

1. are able to perceive and tolerate reality and are able to accept uncertainty.
2. accept themselves and others.
3. are spontaneous in their thought and behavior.
4. have a problem solving orientation toward life instead of an orientation centered on self.
5. have a keen, unhostile sense of humor.
6. need privacy and detachment sometimes.
7. are relatively independent of their environments; they do not consciously try to be unconventional but follow their own paths.
8. appreciate with continued freshness and pleasure the basics of life.
9. are at times profoundly spiritual.
10. are able to identify with and show concern for humankind.
11. have deep interpersonal relationships with only a few people instead of with many.
12. are highly imaginative and creative in their approach to life.
13. are democratic.
14. are able to view life objectively; they keep the ends distinguished from the means.

Coping with Conflict

In the psychological theories we have discussed, a good deal of attention has been paid to conflicting desires and feelings and the problems that such conflicts can cause. Everyone experiences conflict, and each person develops certain ways of dealing with these conflicts. The ways we cope with conflict become a part of our personality and a part of our everyday life-style.

Defense Mechanisms

Defense mechanisms Unconscious means of protecting oneself from stress.

Certain mental processes or patterns of thought called **defense mechanisms** help to protect us from being overwhelmed by the sheer complexity of living and by situations that are particularly distressing. They provide a sort of security blanket for our psyches. Freud was the first to analyze these; and although defense mechanisms are a normal part of the human psyche, they can hide a person's real motivations and interfere with the perception of reality. While protecting you, the defense mechanisms also enable you to pretend that a situation is other than it is. Since they are unconscious, they are often difficult to recognize—particularly in oneself. The following are brief descriptions of some common defense mechanisms.

Rationalization. Making excuses, often plausible ones, for our behavior, thus deceiving ourselves by refusing to admit our real motivations, is called *rationalization.* For example, you have thought about inviting someone you like—a science major with a very heavy schedule—to go to a jazz concert with you, but you decide not to bother because she or he "is probably too busy." If you looked for the real reason behind the excuse, you might realize that you are not sure how much she or he likes you and you do not want to risk being rejected. Your decision, then, was based on a rationalization.

Projection. When you ascribe your own attitudes or feelings to others, you are engaging in a defense mechanism called *projection.* For example, a person who is afraid of failure may constantly criticize others for his or her fear of failure.

Identification. *Identification* involves attributing to yourself the positive traits of another individual or a group. A person who feels powerless and helpless may gain a sense of strength and independence by identifying with an athlete, a movie star, or a political leader.

Fantasy. In *fantasy* we cease to attend to the demands of the everyday world around us and, for a while, roam around in that delightful, boundless, mysterious world of the imagination. Not only is it relaxing to let the mind wander from time to time; sometimes in such reveries we think of good ideas or suddenly understand something or solve a problem. However, as a defense mechanism, we construct fantasies in which we get want we want, or, as psychologists say, we experience wish fulfillment. The danger is in letting the fantasy become a substitute for reality.

Compensation. *Compensation* (also called substitution) is an attempt to make up for what you perceive as flaws in your personality or behavior by developing different behavior or characteristics. For example, a person who has little athletic ability but would like to be a very good athlete might become a top sports reporter.

Regression. *Regression* is defined as the reversion of behavior or feelings to a more childlike pattern. For example, at college you are responsible for taking care of your own room, and by and large you manage to keep it relatively neat. When you go home, though, you stop making your bed and picking up your belongings (which your mother or father used to do for you). Your behavior at home is regression.

Displacement. An example of *displacement* is the following: when a student fails a course, he goes home and vents the frustration on a spouse, child, pet, or neighbor. The anger felt toward the course or professor is directed toward someone or something considered less "dangerous" to the individual than the professor.

Using Defense Mechanisms

Naturally, these are but a few of the defense mechanisms people use. It should be pointed out that use of these mechanisms is not totally negative behavior. Two individuals may use the same defense mechanism for entirely different situations or in very different ways, one in a healthy manner and the other in an attempt to hide his or her true motivations. When the use of defense mechanisms either becomes all-pervasive or no longer helps in the problem-solving process, one should be concerned. When emotions are so strong that use of a defense mechanism is insufficient protection, it is best to stop what you are doing and concentrate on dealing in a more realistic fashion with the situation in which you find yourself.

Coping with Emotions and Feelings

Emotion Any response of the individual to positive or negative stressors.

Anytime a person feels stress, excitement, or frustration, the person is experiencing **emotions.** An emotion is not merely a mental process, it has a physiological basis as well. The physiological responses to emotional situations will be discussed more fully in Chapter 3.

It is well established that in some respects, all persons are alike. One

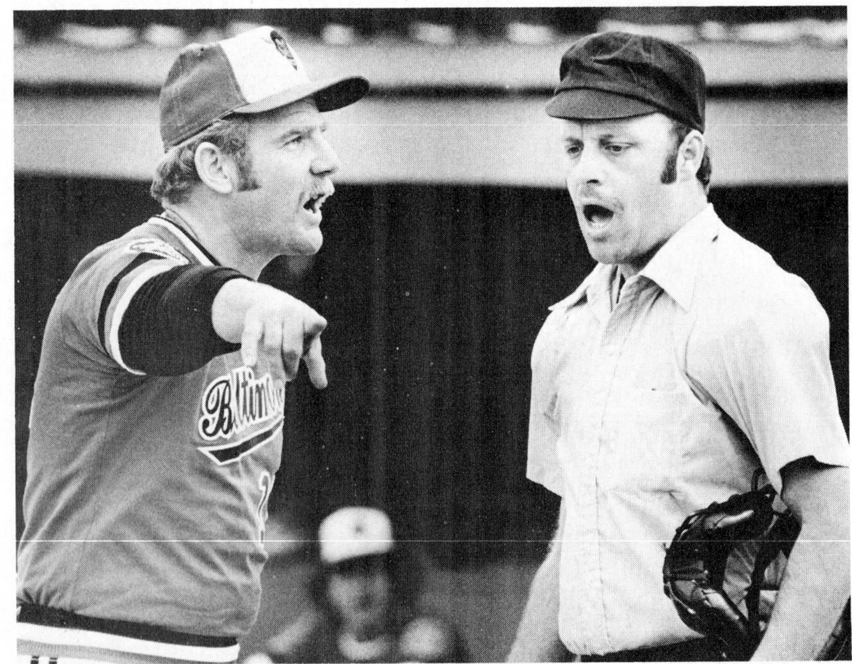

Anger is one of the basic emotions, and individuals should learn socially acceptable ways to express it. (Photo © 1977 Will McIntyre/Photo Researchers, Inc.)

Table 2-1 Sequence of an Emotional Expression

Perception → Appraisal → Emotion → Physiological Changes → Action → Reappraisal

similarity is in the area of emotions. All persons have five basic emotions, which can be characterized by the acronym "LEAFS": Love, Elation, Anger, Fear, and Sorrow. Any of these emotions may surface at any time, depending upon the way we perceive a situation.

There is a generalized sequence of events in an emotional expression. This sequence generally consists of six steps (see Table 2-1).

Our perception of a situation and the way we appraise that situation as either helpful or harmful are what trigger one of the five basic emotions (see box below). The emotion that is elicited causes us to have a physiological response (such as "goose bumps") and we subsequently take an action. Once the action has occurred, the emotionally healthy individual reappraises the situation in light of the response and the degree of satisfaction that has been attained as a result of the action taken.

In the quest for happiness and fulfillment, people often experience emotional letdowns. Most often, these states of mind are temporary responses to an immediate problem. Understanding the nature of these feelings is the first step toward taking effective action to eliminate their causes. In this section we will focus on feelings of **loneliness, alienation** and **emptiness,** mild **depression,** and mild **anxiety** and discuss what we can do about them.

YOUR HEALTH TODAY

Guidelines for Controlling Emotions

1. Try to understand your fears, anxieties, and worries.
2. Remember, your emotions are triggered by the emotional responses of others.
3. Keep your emotions isolated or in context with a situation and don't allow them to affect your general behavioral responses.
4. Learn from mistakes, don't worry over them.
5. Control emotions through direct, positive action.
6. Become reassured after dealing positively with emotionally disturbing situations.
7. Learn from friends who deal with emotional stress calmly.
8. Strive to attain maturity, which involves emotional control.
9. Utilize energy and enthusiasm—positive aspects of emotions—to cope with yourself, others, and your environment.

Source: Adapted from Edward B. Johns, W. C. Sutton and B. A. Cooley, *Health for Effective Living,* 6th ed. (New York: McGraw-Hill Book Company, 1975), 61-62.

Loneliness

Loneliness A feeling that may arise from the absence of a desired relationship.

Individuals differ in their needs for one another; but for an increasing number of people in our fast-paced society, satisfying social needs has become difficult. According to psychiatrist Aaron T. Beck, **loneliness** arises from the perceived absence of a desired relationship. The media have contributed significantly to the problem by establishing images of what life is supposed to be like at various stages. A person who cannot live up to these expectations may feel alienated and lonely.

Moving to a new neighborhood because of school or work breaks up old family and social supports and demands the establishment of new contacts. For many people, television becomes their escape, their window on life. They become spectators rather than participants, and their lack of human contact leads to loneliness.

Occasional loneliness is normal and generally does not last long. A person is soon caught up in activity again. But in chronic loneliness, resulting from unsatisfactory personal and social relationships, the negative feelings are pervasive and prolonged, continuing sometimes for weeks or even months. Lacking are important elements in personality development — for example, in Maslow's hierarchy, the need for belonging and acceptance. Lonely people often lack initiative and wait on the sidelines for something to happen, all the while wishing life were more interesting.

Loneliness should not be confused with aloneness. Everyone needs time to be alone. In periods of solitude, a person sorts out the elements of life and unwinds from the unavoidable pressures of everyday liv-

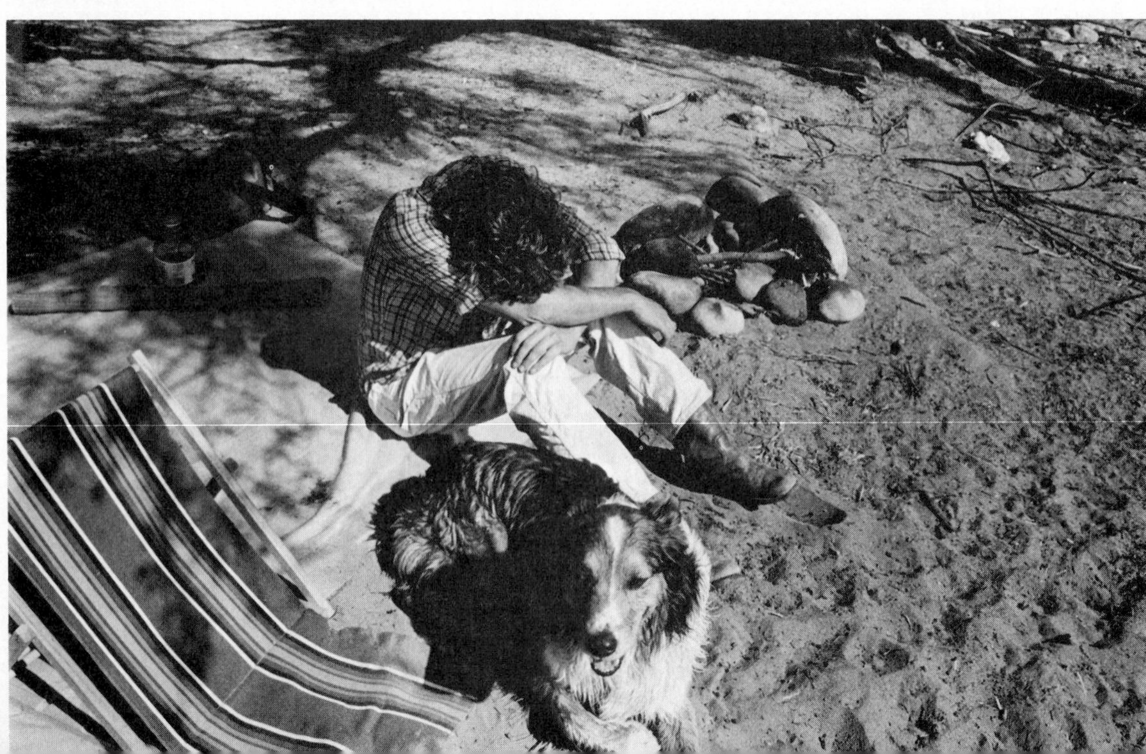

Loneliness is an emotion that most people have felt at one time or another. (Photo by Laurel Eisenberg)

ing. These are times when a person reflects on what has happened and makes plans for the future; such periods are productive interludes of renewal and revitalization, of learning about oneself.

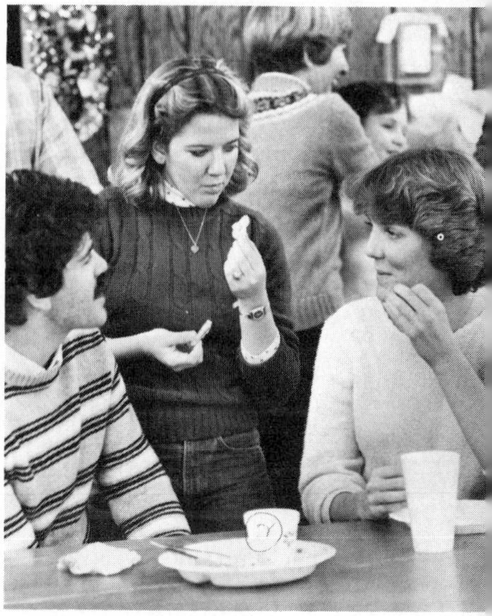

Overcoming Loneliness

To overcome loneliness, one might seek help from a friend, a professor, or a staff member at the student health service. In fact, most colleges and universities have a counseling service within the student health service. However, if one wishes to try and overcome loneliness by oneself, there are some common approaches that can be used: identify the cause, assess the reasons for loneliness, try and learn new skills, and practice the new skills.

Identify the Cause. Try to objectively assess what led to the feeling of loneliness. Was the cause something that had only a temporary effect, or will the effect be more long-lasting? Try and be extremely specific in what you identify as the cause.

Assess the Reasons for Loneliness. Are your thoughts and feelings regarding the cause of your loneliness realistic or idealistic? Could these feelings be of a temporary nature? Are there other things you could do to lessen these feelings?

Try and Learn New Skills. If you rely too much on others for decision making and those others are no longer available, loneliness and depression may result. You must learn how to be more self-reliant and how to apply the decision-making process to various situations. In some cases, you may need to become more assertive. (Complete the assertion questionnaire found at the end of the chapter to gain some insight as to how assertive you are.) There are several basic skills that can be employed to learn how to become more self-reliant and assertive. Some of these skills are discussed in the boxed material that follows.

Practice the New Skills. Merely learning new skills will not overcome feelings of loneliness. As with any endeavor, if you are to improve, you must practice. It is not enough to understand why loneliness occurs; you must actively seek to overcome that feeling.

Social interactions are a help in coping with many mental problems. (Photo by David S. Strickler/The Picture Cube)

Alienation and Emptiness

Alienation and **emptiness** are closely related to loneliness; all are related to a lack of close social ties and friendships. But in alienation there is a feeling that nothing makes sense, a feeling of not knowing exactly what one wants. In this situation, the person is unable to express exactly what he or she feels is lacking. Life seems meaningless, and the person feels powerless to control what happens. These feelings occur partly because the person has been thwarted many times in the past in attempts to achieve goals and desires that may have been unobtainable or unrealistic. Alienation may also be the result of a letdown. When opportunities do not come as quickly as anticipated after a person has spent four years, or more, in college and

Alienation A state of estrangement where the individual feels isolated and confused about his/her interaction with the objective world.

Emptiness A feeling resulting from a lack of close, positive social and personal ties.

YOUR HEALTH TODAY

Assertiveness Skills

Being assertive can contribute to self-esteem. However, there is a fine line between being assertive and being aggressive. Below are seven skills that, if consciously practiced, will help you become a more assertive individual.

1. Speak to others. One must overcome feelings of shyness and begin to initiate conversations. Resolve to begin at least two conversations per day with persons you don't know.
2. Give compliments. Most people don't accept or give compliments well. Try to give a compliment to at least three different people each day. People do care what you think. Tell them.
3. State your beliefs. If you strongly believe in something, don't be reluctant to say, "I think . . ." or "I feel . . ." Let people know your position on issues.
4. Ask for more information. The only "dumb" question is the one that you have but don't ask. If you don't understand what is meant, ask. Be sure you know why something is being done and don't be shy in asking, "Why?" if you don't know.
5. Don't repress your feelings. If you keep your feelings inside, these can build into an explosion. Let your feelings out and express them. Don't be rude, but don't be afraid to run the risk of hurting someone else's feelings; stating your feelings might be better than developing an ulcer or other health problem by not saying anything. Be careful, however, not to be negative.
6. If you know someone is wrong, don't be afraid to disagree. A word of caution must be noted. Be sure you have facts and not conjecture when you confront whoever made the wrong or offensive statement.
7. Look people in the eye. The person who won't maintain eye contact with another person is often perceived as weak. It is quite difficult at first to maintain eye contact; however, you should practice this skill until you can do it without thinking about it.

perhaps has received honors there for superior grades, the rewards in life somehow do not seem to match the effort put forth to attain them. Often these feelings follow rapid changes in living conditions or styles, and the person simply has not had time to catch up to them and absorb them. Negative moods may result because the person has been too dependent on others for decisions and needs to build inner determination and commitment to self.

People who are unable to shake the feelings of alienation and emptiness may need counseling to help them discover personal goals and directions. They may be able to overcome these feelings on their own, however, by making an assessment of their achievements and deciding how to work toward long- and short-range goals. These goals can be listed on a "balance sheet of life," ranked, identified by what must be done to attain each, then mapped through a work plan. (A balance

SELF-ASSESSMENT EXERCISE 2.1

Balance Sheet of Life

GOALS	PRIORITY	METHODS TO ATTAIN GOAL	POTENTIAL PROBLEMS	HOW TO AVOID OR OVERCOME PROBLEMS	WORK PLAN
In next three months					
Play pro baseball	3	Have good season	No contract offer	Free-agent draft	Play to best of ability
Graduate	1	Pass 15 hours	Chemistry	Tutorial help	Balance sport & study
Avoid injury	4	Conditioning	Accidents	Stay alert	Practice hard and stay in shape
Have a positive attitude	2	Stay loose	Poor grades	Study hard	Set priorities for time management
In next year					
In next five years					

sheet of life is presented in Self-Assessment Exercise 2.1. Note that the three-month segment is filled out with sample life problems. You should make up a balance sheet for yourself and fill it out with your own goals and methods of attainment.) The goals must be specific and realistic, of course. If there are career problems, you can probably get counseling on campus. Make certain that the plan includes some goals that can be reached in a relatively short time. Achieving those goals will give you a start on overcoming feelings of powerlessness.

Mild Depression

A major cause of loneliness is **depression.** According to Beck, it is difficult for students to distinguish between a temporary feeling of sadness and full-blown depression. During a mild depression people feel sad, lack energy, lose appetite, and may cry — or at least feel like

Depression A persistent, overwhelming feeling of sadness and lack of motivation.

crying. They have what is commonly referred to as a bad case of the "blahs." These feelings are normal when there is good reason for them, but they must be considered abnormal when the person is overwhelmed by a mood for which there is only a trivial reason or when the depressed mood lasts for a long time.

Sometimes mild depressions come as short-lived moods. They may be related to a temporary situation, such as a forthcoming examination, the loss of a job, or a succession of minor mishaps like a flat tire, a missed ride, and an argument with a member of the family or with a roommate. College students often go through periods of mild depression after the rush of getting back to school and settling into their routines. Or they may become moody after an especially rough semester that demanded a lot of self-discipline and hard work. Rather than having a sense of elation that the pressure is off, they feel let down or depressed for a few days, or sometimes even a week or two, until they adjust to their new routines.

Psychiatrists Aaron T. Beck and David Burns say that people experiencing depression should learn how to recognize negative thoughts and then stop them by redirecting their thoughts to more positive things. The basic premise of this technique is that moods are the result of thoughts, rather than the other way around. Positive thoughts generate positive feelings; negative thoughts bring on negative feelings. Depressed patients who have been given therapy based on this simple, common-sense approach have good recovery rates and do not need long-term drug treatment. Drs. Beck and Burns advise people not to base their opinions of themselves on such things as looks, fame, talent, fortune, or even approval. The basic question is self-esteem: the more you like yourself, the better you will feel. Never put yourself down by focusing on your weaknesses or imperfections.

At the same time, make it a practice to see the funny side of everyday occurrences. Learn to laugh: no other therapy is comparable. Break your depression cycle by doing pleasurable things when you feel a low coming on. This will keep you from getting really down in the dumps. Physical activities, such as riding a bicycle or taking a brisk walk, are often helpful; they keep you from sitting and thinking yourself deeper into the mood of depression. Talking to other people also helps. Try relating to others and their problems rather than thinking of your own difficulties, or do something for someone else.

Mild Anxiety

Anxiety A feeling of fear and apprehension concerning the outcome of an event.

A common reaction to pressures and conflicts is **anxiety**—fear and apprehension concerning the outcome of some event. Most often, anxiety arises because of a definite event—a test, a date, or an interview—and in these cases the nervousness, jitteriness, and uptightness usually pass. Given the pressures of modern life, anxiety is a very common feeling, and it is estimated that one out of three Americans takes anti-anxiety medication at some time.

Free-floating anxiety is anxiety which is not related to any specific fear. There is a general sense of insecurity and apprehension and an inner struggle with conflicting demands. The person suffering from free-floating anxiety is not sure of the causes, and the condition tends to persist.

Free-floating anxiety Generalized apprehension without a specific cause.

Anxiety is a kind of warning that it is time to slow down and take inventory of the reasons for your fears; then you may reappraise the direction you are taking in life. There are a number of techniques that can be used to get rid of, or at least alleviate, anxieties.

One technique—more easily recommended than actually practiced—is to make conscious and regular efforts to relax instead of going full tilt at all times. Many psychiatrists are convinced that anxiety is actually a learned defense mechanism used to counter the pressures of everyday living; consequently, it is also possible to learn how to live with these pressures without permitting them to become internal conflicts. To a large degree, it is a matter of emotional control, of refusing to give in to feelings of anxiety when they occur. When there is a feeling of panic, a person should shift to some other sort of activity. Physical activities of various kinds are good ways to release pent-up feelings. By all means, do not simply sit.

Anxieties can be related also to caffeine, alcohol, or nicotine consumption. If any of these are used, they should be stopped, or at least the amount of intake reduced. Their use may not be the basic reason for existing anxiety, but it can be a contributing factor. Many people turn to tranquilizers in an attempt to deal with their anxieties, but it is best to avoid these drugs. Some tranquilizers can be directly harmful, or they can create other problems.

Getting Help

If any mental or emotional problem continues despite your efforts to reduce it, then you should seek professional help, the sooner the better. After a long period of time, such mental problems can bring on high blood pressure, ulcers, and other physical ills. In addition, the causes of deep-rooted problems are difficult to fathom, and the cure can require months or even years. Getting help early is similar to putting out a fire before it spreads and becomes uncontrollable. Many colleges and communities have hotlines or crisis centers that can be contacted as a first step in identifying other sources of help in dealing with mental and emotional problems. Some clues that a person might need additional help in dealing with mental or emotional problems are as follows:

YOUR HEALTH TODAY

Some Signs That May Indicate a Need for Counseling

1. Intense reaction to problems or disappointments that to most people would appear relatively minor.
2. Inability to get along with or put up with people at home, at school, in recreational activities, or on the job.
3. A fear of having an encounter or confrontation in normal life situations.
4. A mistrust of friends or family.
5. A fear of failure.
6. A lack of interest in or energy toward things that were once stimulating.
7. A preoccupation with anxiety.
8. Beginning to smoke, using alcohol to excess, or using other drugs to solve problems.
9. Insomnia or a disturbance in sleep patterns.
10. A severe increase or decrease in appetite for several weeks or longer.
11. A sense of strain in relationships with peers, spouse, children, parents, or friends.

Short-term personal-problem counseling generally consists of three to ten sessions, with a focus on the kinds of changes that have come into a person's life to cause mental disturbances. A shift in career goals, such as dropping out of pre-med or pre-law training in favor of business or teaching, may demand counseling to smooth inner conflicts. Many young parents need counseling to help them adjust to their new baby, who may suddenly be regarded as an intrusion rather than a blessing. Changes in ways of living necessitated by an accident or a disease can also usually be handled by short-term counseling.

A married couple having problems communicating with each other but wanting to save their marriage may go to a counselor for help. Sometimes both spouses go, but if one refuses, the willing partner can still get counseling assistance.

People having difficulty choosing a career or wanting to make a change in occupations can get counseling service to help determine whether such a change is indeed wise. Career counseling is available free on nearly all college campuses and can also be obtained from government agencies, many industries and businesses, and some professional organizations.

Special Help for Special Problems

Crisis intervention services Counseling services that deal with an immediate problem of an individual.

Crisis Intervention Services. These counseling services are established for handling specific and immediate problems. By telephone, as well as by personal contact, they help rape victims get over feelings of shock, shame, anger, and helplessness for having been victimized.

Crisis intervention services also help people get over the death of a member of the family or a close friend, and they handle such problems as suicide attempts, drug and alcohol abuse, problem pregnancies, family arguments, and beatings or brutality cases. The counseling is available to individuals, families, or small groups. If you or someone you know needs this kind of help, you can often find crisis intervention hotlines listed under "Crisis" in the business section of your local telephone directory.

Self-Help Groups. Some people get needed assistance from self-help groups. Alcoholics Anonymous, for example, has helped many individuals wanting to overcome an alcohol problem. Al-Anon, a related group, was established to aid the alcoholic's family in dealing with the problem. Other self-help groups include such organizations as Emotions Anonymous, Women's Support Group, Men's Support Group, Parents Without Partners, Divorced or Separated Singles, and Make Today Count. People participating in these groups share a common sort of life experience and problems, and they typically rely on their own membership to provide the needed help. Often, however, they turn to professionals for guidance in establishing the framework for their operations. Self-help groups will be listed in the business section or yellow pages of your local telephone directory or in your local newspaper in the classified advertisements.

Self-help groups Support groups that encourage group members to help themselves.

Group Counseling. People with specific problems, such as shyness in relating to other people, may be helped by group counseling. In such counseling the counselor serves as a guide but remains essentially in the background while the members of the group share their feelings and work together in solving difficulties. The technique is especially

Group counseling Therapy method in which a therapist guides a group in discussing their common problems.

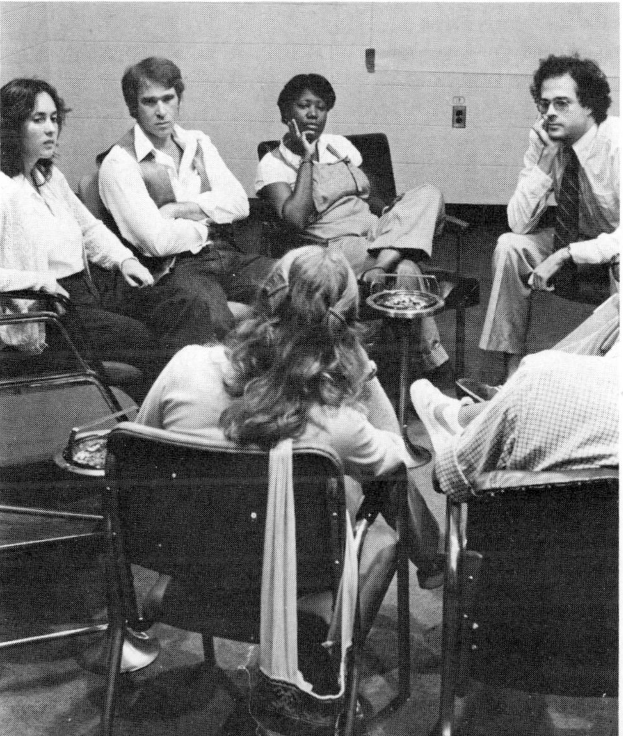

Professional help for mental problems is available to individuals, families, or small groups. College students who need help can usually go to their campus health centers for treatment or reference. (Photo © Bohdan Hrynewych/ Southern Light)

effective for many people because it is helpful to them to learn that others have the same problems and similar emotional reactions to situations. Group counseling may be particularly beneficial to a person who has been unable to relate to others.

Family counseling Therapy method in which a therapist meets with a family to discuss their problems.

Family Counseling. These sessions involve the entire family and aid in resolving such difficulties as drug use, alcoholism, spouse or child abuse, and behavior problems of any member of the family. The counselor has an opportunity during the sessions to observe how the members of the family interact, a help in unraveling sometimes complex and deep-seated problems.

Other Sources of Help

Psychiatrist Medical doctor who specializes in the diagnosis and treatment of mental disorders.

Psychologist Professionally trained individual who helps persons understand and solve their own mental health problems.

Career counselor An individual trained in helping people make career decisions.

Guidance counselor An individual qualified to work with mild mental health disorders.

Pastoral counselor A clergy member specifically trained to work with mental health problems.

Most colleges have counseling centers on their campuses. If they do not, the health center can refer students to local counseling service centers. Often these clinics are in hospitals, community health centers, or health departments. In all metropolitan areas there are therapists in private practice. The local, county, or state medical association can be called for recommendations; or a physician, nurse, social worker, pastoral counselor, or health educator can be asked for suggestions.

In every state there are laws that set up qualifications for the training of people who deal with matters of the mind. **Psychiatrists** are the most highly trained. They are medical doctors who have completed their education for general medical practice and then have continued their education to become specialists. They are qualified not only to put patients through extensive analysis but also to prescribe drugs or other medical treatments if needed. **Psychologists** with Ph.D. or M.S. degrees may work alone or with psychiatrists. They cannot prescribe drugs, but they are well trained and capable of handling most kinds of disturbances. Many psychologists work in health centers where some of the social workers and registered nurses also have advanced degrees and make distress problems their specialty. For less severe problems, **career** or **guidance counselors,** both usually with no less than master's degrees, and **pastoral counselors** can also be turned to for help in solving problems.

What Will It Cost?

Counseling fees typically range from $25 to $75 per session, often more. Some health insurance policies will pay these fees, depending on where the counseling is done and on the qualifications of the counselor. For outpatients in the general community (not on campus) fees may be on a sliding scale based on income. On most campuses counseling is free to enrolled students, or there may be either a minimum fee per visit up to a fixed maximum or fees charged only after a specified number of visits. Sometimes services outside the campus are also free or are a part of the college health-plan coverage, or there may be a standard rate or sliding scale for fees. Patients should discuss fees with the practitioner on the very first visit, so that they know what they are expected to pay and when.

Assessing Your Mental Health

As has been stressed throughout this chapter, everyone experiences periods when they are "down." However, this does not connote mental ill health. What is being emphasized is that most persons can and do practice positive mental health. At a minimum, mental health means that the individual is free of clinical symptoms that may be incapacitating and does not exhibit any signs of mental disorders. At the other end of the spectrum, positive mental health provides a means to enlarge one's capacity for happiness, enjoyment, and life in general. In other words, it allows the person to attain his or her optimal potential.

Characteristics of persons who would be considered mentally healthy can be identified. Among other things, those persons

- experience emotions but are not overwhelmed or ruled by them.
- have a good sense of humor.
- have positive and mature interactions with others.
- are flexible and can adapt to stress.
- know their potential and accept their limitations.
- have a positive self-image.
- see things as they are.
- accept their responsibilities.
- respect the rights of others.
- confront their problems and work to overcome them.
- set and achieve realistic goals.

SELF-ASSESSMENT EXERCISE 2.2

Assertion Questionnaire

INSTRUCTIONS

Go over the list of questions on the next two pages twice.

First, rate each item using the "Frequency Scale." Rate each on how often it has occurred during the past month.

Second, rate how comfortable you were when each situation happened, or how comfortable you would be if it were to happen. For this rating, use the "Comfort Scale."

As Dr. Lewinsohn, the creator of this test, points out, there are no right or wrong answers to the items on this questionnaire.

Frequency Scale

Indicate how often each of these events occurred by marking the Frequency Column, using the following scale:

1 = This has not happened in the past 30 days
2 = This has happened a *few times* (1 to 6 times) in the past 30 days
3 = This has happened *often* (7 times or more) in the past 30 days

Comfort Scale

Indicate how you feel about each of these events by marking the Comfort Column, using the following scale:

1 = I felt very *uncomfortable or upset* when this happened
2 = I felt *somewhat uncomfortable or upset* when this happened
3 = I felt *neutral* when this happened (neither comfortable nor uncomfortable; neither good nor upset)
4 = I felt *fairly comfortable or good* when this happened
5 = I felt *very comfortable or good* when this happened

Important: If an event has not happened during the past month, then rate it according to how you think you would feel *if* it happened. If an event happened more than once in the past month, rate roughly how you felt about it on the average.

Questionnaire

	Frequency	Comfort
1. Turning down a person's request to borrow my car	_______	_______
2. Asking a favor of someone	_______	_______
3. Resisting sales pressure	_______	_______
4. Admitting fear and requesting consideration	_______	_______
5. Telling a person I am intimately involved with that he/she has said or done something that bothers me	_______	_______
6. Admitting ignorance in an area being discussed	_______	_______
7. Turning down a friend's request to borrow money	_______	_______
8. Turning off a talkative friend	_______	_______
9. Asking for constructive criticism	_______	_______
10. Asking for clarification when I am confused about what someone has said	_______	_______
11. Asking whether I have offended someone	_______	_______
12. Telling a person of the opposite sex that I like him/her	_______	_______
13. Telling a person of the same sex that I like him/her	_______	_______
14. Requesting expected service when it hasn't been offered (e.g., in a restaurant)	_______	_______
15. Discussing openly with a person his/her criticism of my behavior	_______	_______
16. Returning defective items (e.g., at a store or restaurant)	_______	_______
17. Expressing an opinion that differs from that of a person I am talking with	_______	_______
18. Resisting sexual overtures when I am not interested	_______	_______
19. Telling someone how I feel if he/she has done something that is unfair to me	_______	_______
20. Turning down a social invitation from someone I don't particularly like	_______	_______
21. Resisting pressure to drink	_______	_______

22. Resisting an unfair demand from a person who is important to me ________ ________
23. Requesting the return of borrowed items ________ ________
24. Telling a friend or co-worker when he/she says or does something that bothers me ________ ________
25. Asking a person who is annoying me in a public situation to stop (e.g., smoking on a bus) ________ ________
26. Criticizing a friend ________ ________
27. Criticizing my spouse ________ ________
28. Asking someone for help or advice ________ ________
29. Expressing my love to someone ________ ________
30. Asking to borrow something ________ ________
31. Giving my opinion when a group is discussing an important matter ________ ________
32. Taking a definite stand on a controversial issue ________ ________
33. When two friends are arguing, supporting the one I agree with ________ ________
34. Expressing my opinion to someone I don't know very well ________ ________
35. Interrupting someone to ask him/her to repeat something I didn't hear clearly ________ ________
36. Contradicting someone when I think I might hurt him/her by doing so ________ ________
37. Telling someone that he/she has disappointed me or let my down ________ ________
38. Asking someone to leave me alone ________ ________
39. Telling a friend or co-worker that he/she has done a good job ________ ________
40. Telling someone he/she has made a good point in a discussion ________ ________
41. Telling someone I have enjoyed talking with him/her ________ ________
42. Complimenting someone on his/her skill or creativity. ________ ________

Total Score ________ ________

INTERPRETING YOUR SCORE

Most people score within the following ranges:

Assertion Frequency: 61–81

Assertion Comfort: 102–137

This means that the typical individual has had most of the listed situations occur at least a few times during the past month. Further, this typical person probably feels at least fairly comfortable with being assertive in several of the situations and neutral to somewhat uncomfortable in some others. If you scored higher than these average scores, you probably know when you're being appropriately assertive (and would very likely write us a letter telling us that we're wrong if we said anything different about you).

If you scored near the bottom of the average ranges, it may just have been an unusually nonassertive month for you. Next month may find you acting (and scoring more assertively, particularly now that you're thinking about it.

If you scored way below the average ranges, however, lack of assertiveness and discomfort with being assertive may be a real problem and major concern for you. See the discussion within the chapter in order to decide what approach to take.

Summary

Two major changes have taken place in approaches to mental health. First, the traditional opposition of mental health versus mental illness has given way to the idea that there is a whole gamut of mental problems, ranging from mild emotional disturbances to severe psychological disorders.

Second, a more positive concept of mental health has arisen, in which mental health is attaining happiness, feeling good about yourself, getting along with other people, coping with the demands of the world without undue stress, and achieving a sense of personal fulfillment.

Understanding psychological theories is an important step in achieving self-understanding. In the theories of Freud, unconscious elements play an important role in human behavior. Three subsystems of the mind—the id, the ego, and the superego—have different natures and present the individual with conflicting demands. Successful personality development depends on reconciling these conflicts.

Maslow's analysis of human nature is based on a five-step pyramid of basic needs: physiological needs, safety needs, belongingness and love needs, self-esteem needs, and self-actualization needs. Individual fulfillment requires the satisfaction of all these needs.

Defense mechanisms are one of the mind's ways of dealing with conflicts and protecting itself through avoidance of real problems. Common defense mechanisms include rationalization, projection, identification, fantasy, compensation, regression, and displacement.

Common emotional problems include loneliness, alienation and emptiness, mild anxiety, and mild depression. Such moods are a normal part of life, but if they persist, psychological counseling may be helpful, or even necessary. In each case there are practical steps that can be taken to solve, or at least alleviate, the problem.

When help is needed, various forms of counseling are available. Short-term personal-problem counseling focuses on coping with changes in people's lives. Other forms of help include crisis intervention, self-help groups, and group counseling.

For persons with more serious emotional problems, long-term psychological help is available from psychiatrists, psychologists, and other mental health workers, both in private practice and in public health facilities.

Much progress has been made in mental health areas, although mental problems continue to be common in our society. Today we have a much better understanding of the positive goals of mental health, and mental problems no longer carry the stigma they did in years past.

Review and Discussion

1. This chapter has described two changes in attitudes toward mental health: the change from a negative to a positive concept and a better understanding of the range of mental problems. In what areas do you see signs of these changes?

2. According to Freud, what are the id, ego, and superego?

3. What are the five types of basic needs according to Maslow?

4. What are defense mechanisms? Name and describe six types.

5. Name four causes of loneliness. What can be done to overcome it?

6. Describe the symptoms of mild depression and mild anxiety. What steps can be taken to alleviate them?

7. Describe four types of counseling that are available to help people with their emotional problems.

8. Discuss the following statement: Some people are too assertive.

9. It is often claimed that modern life-styles are not conducive to achieving positive mental health. Do you agree? (Be prepared to defend your answer.)

Further Reading

Dobson, James. *Emotions: Can You Trust Them?* New York: Regal Books, 1980.
Dobson describes the wide range of human emotions and their universality, despite the fact that they are not always acknowledged or discussed.

Dyer, Wayne. *The Sky's the Limit.* New York: Pocket Books, 1981.
Dyer presents suggestions for living life to its fullest, with a sense of excitement about life. (Paperback.)

Frankl, Viktor E. *Man's Search for Meaning.* New York: Pocket Books, 1975.
A frank discussion of internment in a Nazi prison camp and how the rigor of that life led to the development of the psychological concepts and constructs that, in turn, led to the formation of "logotherapy." (Paperback.)

Harris, Thomas. *I'm OK—You're OK.* New York: Harper and Row, 1969.
Discussion of a sensible approach to the problems that every person, including those who need psychiatric help, face every day. The basic approach is that of Transactional Analysis as a way of accepting responsibility for what happens to the individual.

Kline, Nathan S. *From Sad to Glad.* New York: Ballantine Books, 1975.
The pervasive sadness, hopelessness, and guilt of depressed persons are described, with advice on how to help oneself out of a depression. (Paperback.)

Newman, Mildred, and Bernard Berkowitz. *How To Be Your Own Best Friend.* New York: Ballantine Books, 1974.
The authors develop the idea that our happiness depends on our innate ability and power to be happy and content within ourselves, to accept our flaws but recognize our strengths as well. (Paperback.)

Rogers, Carl. *On Becoming a Person.* Boston: Houghton-Mifflin Company, 1970.
A classic self-revelation by the famous psychologist who describes his own inner feelings and thus helps readers examine their own inner feelings. (Paperback.)

Wassmer, Arthur C. *Making Contact.* New York: Fawcett Books, 1980.
Wassmer helps readers understand the nature of their shyness and gives practical suggestions on how to build meaningful relationships and friendships. (Paperback.)

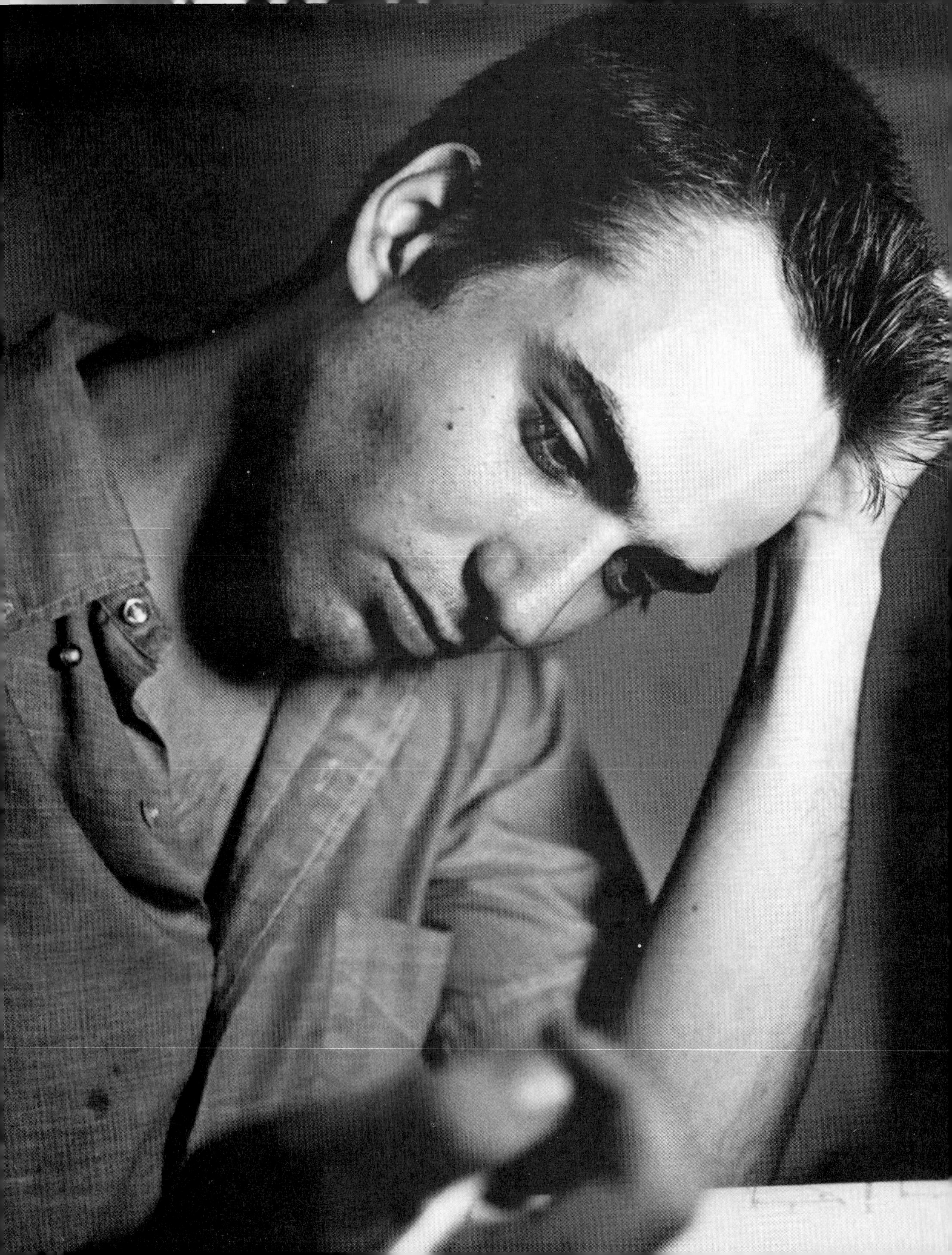

Chapter 3
Stress

KEY POINTS

- ☐ *Stress* is defined as the body's response to any demand—either physical or mental—made upon it; *stressors* are the factors that trigger stress.
- ☐ Response to stressors follows a general pattern called the *general adaptation syndrome,* which includes the *alarm reaction stage,* the *resistance stage,* and the *exhaustion stage.*
- ☐ Bioecological stressors arise from our relationship with the environment and include biological rhythms and noise.
- ☐ Many major stressors are psychosocial in origin; they arise because of the way we perceive and respond to our sociocultural environment.
- ☐ Personality factors, including our self-concept and the way we behave, give rise to stress.
- ☐ Stress is believed to contribute to many different diseases of the body and mind.
- ☐ Setting realistic goals and planning to achieve them are important in reducing stress.
- ☐ Relaxation techniques may begin with either the mind or the body and are effective in reducing the negative effects of stress.

IMAGINE that it is 1900, and you have signed up for a course on health. Can you guess what might have been covered in your classes? You are right if you guessed that you would have spent a lot of time studying anatomy and physiology and learning about such infectious diseases as tuberculosis, cholera, typhus, and influenza. If your professor had been interested in the then-young discipline of health statistics, you might also have learned that the average life expectancy for men was 46 years and for women 49.

Let's return to the present. You are taking a course on health as before, but advances in health care and health maintenance have radically altered the subjects you study. Many of the infectious diseases that plagued our ancestors have been eliminated or controlled. If you were born in 1960, your average life expectancy is about 74 years (this figure is higher for females than for males and also varies with race), and if you make it to that age, you can expect to live as many as 15 more years. Staying well over such a long span of years presents each of us and our health-care providers with a whole new set of challenges. One of the most important of these is not a disease at all but a factor that is believed to contribute to many different diseases of the body and mind. We call this factor *stress.*

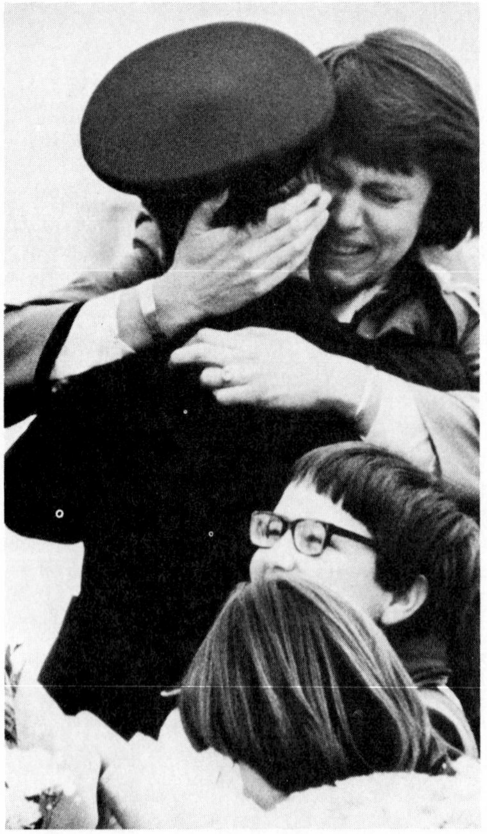

A U.S. Marine returning from overseas. Joyful events, like unpleasant ones, can cause stress. (Photo by Bruce Hoertel)

New Terms for Familiar Feelings

You may be familiar with the use of the term *stress* in physics to mean the action of a system of forces on a body resulting in pressure or strain. Metal for automobiles and airplanes, for example, must be made to withstand such extreme forms of stress as high speeds and sudden starts and stops. The term **stress** has been borrowed from physics to describe the impact of day-to-day events on our minds and bodies.

Stress Mental and bodily responses to day-to-day demands.

Stress and Stressors

Everyone experiences crises throughout life, and each person deals with these crises differently. The great paradox is that even though stress can in some cases be detrimental to health, we cannot live without it. It is our varied reactions to stress that create the will to achieve goals. Stress adds an excitement or flavor to life. It presents challenges to our adaptive resources. Stress is inevitable in today's world; thus, the way we manage stress is what helps determine if we are healthy or unhealthy.

Dr. Hans Selye, a biologist and endocrinologist, was among the first and most influential scientists to borrow the term stress from physics. Selye defined stress as "*the nonspecific response of the body* [which may be elicited by various causes] *to any demand made upon it.*"[1] These demands may be mental or physical, or both, but they always involve the same sorts of psychophysical change. Whether you race to catch a bus or hunt for the answer to a question—or make any one of thousands of similar efforts—your entire body responds. The depth of this response determines the degree of stress.

Stress obviously does not just happen any more than a candle ignites itself. Just as you have to light a match and hold it to the candlewick to get it to burn, so stress is triggered by **stressors.** Stressors may be physical, social, or pyschological (which includes the imaginary expectations about the results of stress).

Stressor A physical, social, or psychological factor triggering a stress response.

Eustress, Stress, and Distress

The growing recognition of stress as a factor contributing to degeneration, disease, and even death has given the word a negative connotation. Most of us, if we think of stress at all, think of it as a bad feeling (or series of feelings) that leaves us confused, anxious, or physically ill. We have only to watch television commercials to learn that too much coffee stresses our bodies and makes us jumpy and irritable. The same medium has taught the world that stress—whether in the form of noisy kids, traffic jams, or bossy in-laws—can cause "tension

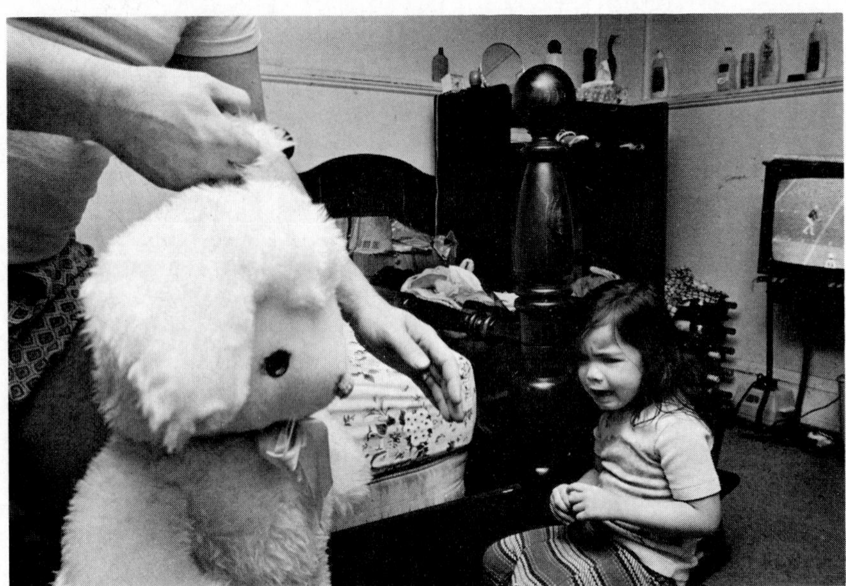

Stressors sometimes lead to destructive responses. (Photo by James Carroll/Archive Pictures, Inc.)

headaches." You can no doubt think of many more examples: we fear that we may be offensive because of acne, bad breath, underarm odor, and even dirty collars.

However, some stress may actually help us perform better. The athlete who "psyches up" for an athletic event, the actor who goes through a self-transformation before representing the character he is to portray, and the student who takes the last examination prior to graduation from college are all experiencing stress. However, unlike the examples in the preceding paragraph, these stressors may well be considered positive. Selye has called our responses to these positive stressors **eustress** (from the Greek word *eu* for "good"). The responses that we have to the negative stressors—**distress**—may gradually erode the strength of our minds and our bodies and lead to disease, disability, and ultimately, to death.

Eustress The body's response to positive stressors.

Distress The body's response to negative stressors.

Change: A Major Stressor

The most prevalent stressor is change. Change and, therefore, stress have been part of your life from the moment you were born, and changes will continue to take place in and around you as long as you live. The biggest visible changes from infancy to adulthood are signaled by growth—in size, intelligence, skills, and relationships. As long as we live, we must confront countless challenges that are associated with major changes: graduating from college, finding a job, succeeding at work, choosing a spouse, parenting, and so on, to the inevitable changes associated with aging.

This description may sound pretty overwhelming and ominous, but is the outlook really all that bad? Are all changes associated with negative stressors? Think about some simple, predictable changes you have experienced during the last 24 hours. At some point you became tired or hungry and you responded in a beneficial way by sleeping or eating. You managed your stress in familiar and effective ways, as we do all the time without even thinking about it. Can you identify more ways in which you almost unthinkingly respond to stress signals?

The General Adaptation Syndrome

In studying numerous laboratory animals and humans exposed to stress, Selye and other researchers were able to show that the response to stressors — be they positive or negative — follows a three-stage pattern. This response pattern has been termed the **general adaptation syndrome (G.A.S.)** (see Figure 3 – 1). It is divided into the alarm reaction, the resistance phase, and exhaustion, as follows:

General Adaptation Syndrome (G.A.S.) The three-stage pattern of response to stressors.

A. *Alarm.* The alarm reaction is like a telephone ringing in the dead of night. The entire body is startled. The pulse rate increases significantly, blood pressure rises, **epinephrine (adrenalin)** and the **adrenocorticotropic hormone (ACTH)** are pumped into the system, and the body is ready to fight or flee.

B. *Resistance.* As the stressor continues, ACTH that was released in the alarm stage begins to drop, and our initial startle response begins to subside. The blood pressure and pulse start to return to normal, and we begin to see what is actually occurring. The reaction to the stressor moves from physical to mental.

C. *Exhaustion.* Despite the fact that we may adapt to a stressor, the organs most frequently aroused may eventually become weakened and wear out if we must continually adapt. In other words, our energy available to adapt can be depleted. If this occurs, the signs of the alarm reaction reappear in increased ACTH levels, but the organ system involved may malfunction or become diseased. Death may follow at once, or the work of the diseased system may be transferred to a healthier system, delaying death for a time. A familiar example of this kind of degeneration is **hypertension** — high blood pressure — in which the elevated pressure makes heavier demands on the heart and kidneys than can be sustained over time. A graphic representation of these three stages is presented in Figure 3 – 1.

Epinephrine Hormone that acts as a stimulant to the circulatory system.

Adrenaline A popular name for epinephrine.

Adrenocorticotropic hormone (ACTH) Hormone that prepares the body for the fight-or-flight response.

Hypertension High blood pressure resulting from buildup along arterial walls.

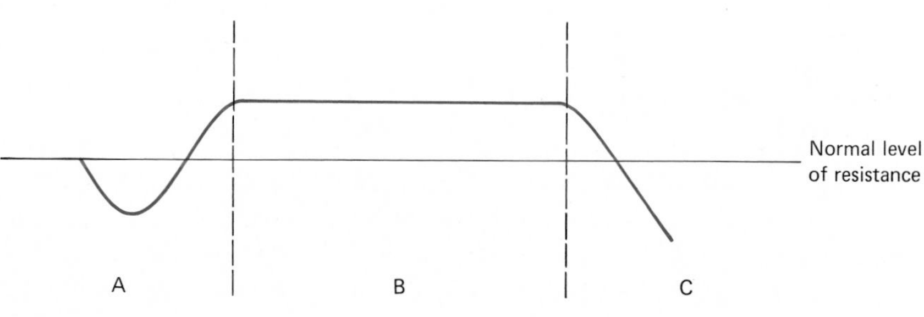

Figure 3 – 1. The General Adaptation Syndrome. **The three phases of the general adaptation syndrome (G.A.S.): *A*, alarm; *B*, resistance; *C*, exhaustion. (Source: Hans Selye, *The Stress of Life* [New York: McGraw-Hill Book Company, 1956], 87.)**

The Body's Response to Stress

Before stress can occur, it must be perceived either consciously or unconsciously. If the individual experiences an event, that event must be interpreted by the body and by the mind. It is this interpretation that will lead to one of three pathways: a constructive (adaptive), a destructive (maladaptive), or a neutral (no) response. The way we interpret an occurrence triggers various physiological mechanisms within the body.

Fight-or-flight The immediate physiological response to stress.

Once the stressor has been perceived and the subsequent emotional response has begun, the nervous system carries the **fight-or-flight** message to the vital organs, increasing the pulse, decreasing the blood supply to parts of the body where it is not needed immediately (like the stomach and intestines), increasing respiration, dilating the pupils of the eyes, and decreasing salivation. These activities contribute to some of the more familiar symptoms of stress: rapid heartbeat, a dry mouth, and stomach pains. They are the body's way of preparing itself to cope with the stressor confronting it.

These symptoms are only part of the story. The body's response under stress includes many drastic changes in body chemistry. Although these reactions are normal and healthy—and in many cases life-saving—they can lead to major health problems if the stress is prolonged. These changes can be seen at work in the endocrine, muscle, gastrointestinal, and cardiovascular systems and in the skin.

The Endocrine System

This system is made up of glands (like the pituitary and adrenals) that secrete hormones into the blood and is closely linked to the nervous system. Stimulation of the hypothalamus during the alarm reaction ultimately results in the release of ACTH into the bloodstream by the pituitary. The ACTH released by the pituitary acts on the outer part of the adrenal glands to produce epinephrine, which helps the body respond to stress. Normally this process has no ill effects on the body. If the stress continues for a long time, however, the protein available for white blood cell and antibody production diminishes, leaving the body more vulnerable to disease. One hormone, **aldosterone,** helps the body prepare for stress by heightening muscle tone and aiding temporary adjustments in temperature and the dispersal of body wastes. If stress remains at a high level, aldosterone acts to keep sodium in the body to retain water, and hypertension (high blood pressure), cardiovascular diseases, and kidney disorders may follow.

Aldosterone A hormone secreted by the adrenal glands, that helps prepare the body for stress.

The Muscle System

The muscle system is capable of responding to precisely two directions from the brain: "contract" and "relax." Hitting a ball with a tennis racket involves a barrage of such messages to different parts of the body, while clenching your fist involves only one command.

This fact is important in understanding stress. As long as the muscles remain contracted, the brain and nervous system stay in a defensive, stress-ready state. In other words, if you allow your muscles to remain tense, your body is going to feel subjected to stress whether or not a stressor exists. The physical results of stress-related muscle tension can range from headaches and backaches to colitis (spasms of the colon) and asthma, and may even include many injuries such as torn muscles and ligaments. Perhaps this is why stress-control and self-help literature concentrate on ways to relax the musculature as a means of preventing stress-related disorders.

The Gastrointestinal System

The gastrointestinal (GI) system, while not directly involved in our impulse to fight or flee, has been found to be a highly accurate mirror of the degree of stress we are under. Hunger and appetite, the triggers that lead us to want to eat, are controlled by the hypothalamus. Each of us knows the signs of hunger and fullness. However, we are likely to overeat or undereat depending upon our emotional state. This can disrupt the GI system, causing spastic contractions of the esophagus, changing the rhythmic movement of the muscles carrying food through the stomach and intestines, and disrupting the elimination of waste products from the intestines.

If stress persists over a long time, physical disorders can result. The most common of the stress-related GI disorders is the stomach, or duodenal, ulcer, probably a result of the stomach's secretion of too much hydrochloric acid and certain enzymes. Diarrhea and constipation also may reflect the impact of stress on the GI system.

The Cardiovascular System

The normal rhythm of the heart can be modified by the nervous system and by epinephrine. Since the heart tends to anticipate, it follows that the blood pressure may be raised even when no true threat exists, as when we go for a physical examination at the physician's office or when we meet new people. As might be expected, blood pressure also tends to go up when strong emotions are aroused.

The blood vessels both anticipate and respond to the hormonal secretions that act as signals of the body being challenged. The cardiovascular system, subjected to chronic stress, may ultimately respond with **hypertension** and **arteriosclerosis** (hardening of the arteries). Loss of elasticity in the arteries usually results in a reduction of the oxygen supply to the heart, and when the coronary arteries are afflicted, the result may be a heart attack.

Arteriosclerosis Hardening of the arteries.

Another disorder that is associated with stress on the vascular system is the *migraine headache.* This syndrome is thought to be caused by a chemical imbalance that acts to constrict the blood vessels leading to and within the brain. To date, the only effective method for preventing vascular headaches is tension and/or stress reduction exercises of the kind that will be presented at the end of this chapter.

The Skin

The *skin*, the largest organ of the body, provides one of the most dramatic views of changes produced during stress. The skin, as you have surely noticed, responds to temperature changes, and its own temperature visibly changes as well. If you are embarrassed, you may blush, as blood rushes to expanding blood vessels near the surface of your face, and your face may actually feel warmer. When you are frightened, the blood drains from the skin to vital organs, leaving you pale and cool to the touch.

Although the skin provides us with a clear view of some of the ways we respond to stress, little research has yet been done on the effects, if any, of stress on the skin. However, it is possible that some familiar skin eruptions, such as hives and acne, may be related to stress.

Types of Stressors

It should be clear from the preceding section that stress manifests itself in a variety of physiological responses. What remains is to examine various types of stressors and, finally, to see how to cope with them. Recognizing the sources of stress should make it easier to determine which ones affect you the most and how you can handle them. The sources of stress may be a result of our biological makeup and how we interact with our environment (bioecological stressors), the way we perceive events in society and how we relate to those events (psychosocial stressors), or the way we perceive ourselves and how we go about living our daily lives (personality stressors).

Bioecological Stressors

Bioecological stressors Environmental conditions that evoke an uncontrollable physiological response.

Bioecological stressors arise from our relationship with our environment, both internal and external. As biological organisms, we are programmed to react in certain fashions when faced with select situations. For example, when it is extremely hot, we tend to perspire in order to maintain temperature balance. Bioecological stressors are the least susceptible to the influence of conscious thought and therefore are least controllable by us.

Time Cycles

The most basic of the bioecological stressors is time. The cycle of the seasons, the light of day and the dark of night, and our division of the day itself into seconds, minutes, and hours tend to dictate what we do, when we do it, and — as you have surely seen in your own experience — how well we do it. In fact, humans are the only creatures on earth that impose a schedule on the natural cycles of dark and light, heat and cold, rather than following the dictates of these natural divisions.

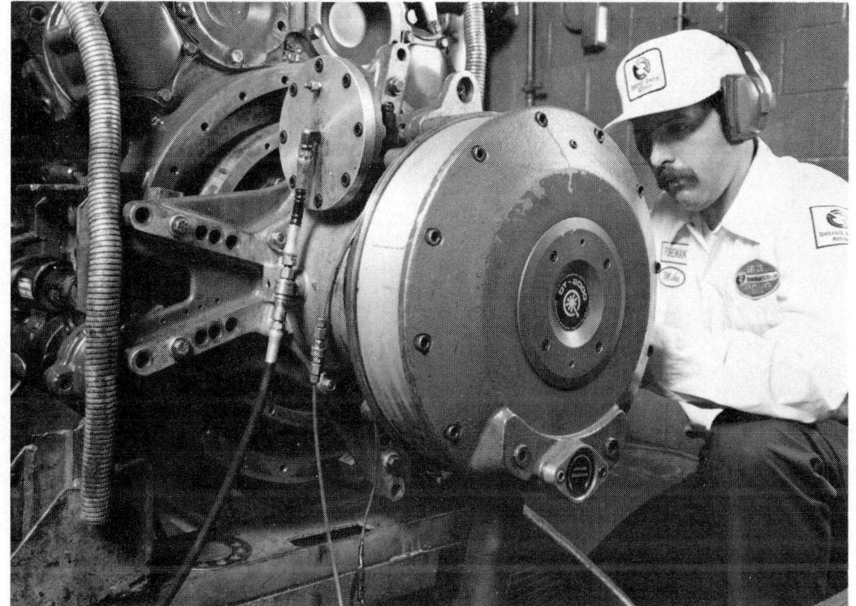

We can protect ourselves from some forms of bioecological stress. Using preventive measures, such as ear protectors in noisy work areas, helps contribute to stress reduction. (Photo by John J. Krieger, Jr./The Picture Cube)

The consequence is that we may sometimes feel "out of sync" with our environment and become moody, irritable, and even ill because we have disregarded natural rhythms. "Jet lag," the problem that often afflicts long-distance air travelers who fly across several time zones, is only one phenomenon in which the natural cycles or biological rhythms to which our bodies are accustomed may be upset. Scientific research is rapidly increasing our understanding of how these cycles affect us within the course of a twenty-four-hour day and even across more limited spans of an hour or so.

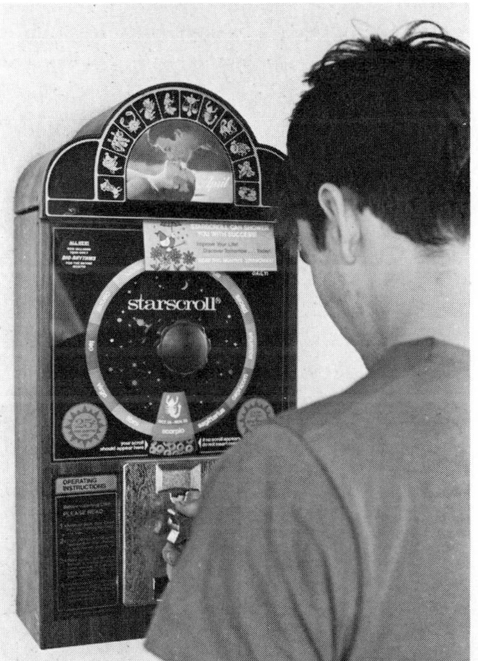

Biorhythms, like horoscopes, are based on the theory that humans live in predictable cycles. In this photograph, a young man pays 25¢ to find out what "the stars" predict for the month ahead and how his biorhythmic time cycles will affect him. (Photo by Paul Waldman)

These naturally occurring cycles which have been termed biological rhythms—not to be confused with bio-rhythms, which are a subcategory within this broad framework—are, for the most part, influenced by the various body hormones, over which we have little control. Three major types of biological rhythms have been identified. These three include **circadian rhythms, ultradian rhythms,** and **infradian rhythms.**

Circadian rhythms Fixed pattern of bodily processes in a 24-hour period.

Ultradian rhythms Cycles that occur in a 90- to 100-minute time span.

Infradian rhythms Relatively long biological cycle, extending over weeks or months.

1. *Circadian Rhythms.* The term *circadian* comes from the Latin for "about one day." Physiological research has shown that basic body processes seem to fluctuate over a 24-hour period according to a fixed pattern. The feeling of hunger most of us experience at noon would be an example of the influence of a circadian rhythm.
2. *Ultradian Rhythms.* Considerably shorter than circadian rhythms, *ultradian rhythms* refer to cycles that occur in 90- to 100-minute time spans. You may have found that as you read a book or listen to your professor for 30 minutes or so, your mind wanders off. You may "come to" with a start, realizing that you do not recall what you read or that you have not heard a word. It is not that the book or professor is dull but rather that the mind can concentrate for only a limited length of time.
3. *Infradian Rhythms.* The longest of the biological rhythms are termed *infradian rhythms.* These cycles may extend over days, weeks, or months. The menstrual cycle and biorhythms (see the box on p. 49) are examples of infradian rhythms.

Sleep and Diet

Although circadian, ultradian, and infradian rhythms may be stressors, they are clearly less controllable by us than are other bioecological stressors to which we can adapt our behaviors in healthy ways. Two such potential stressors, *sleep deprivation* and *poor diet,* have been the subject of a great deal of scientific study that not only teaches us about the stressors but shows clearly how we can reduce their negative effects on health.

Experiments with healthy young adults, for example, have shown that strenuous work schedules combined with little (three–six hours) or no sleep and reduced calorie intake result in changes in performance, mood, and physiology. As a student, you should note particularly that after sleep deprivation, experimental subjects showed marked reductions in reaction time, alertness to signals, motor coordination, and speed of association—all of which are as important to learning as they are to a task like driving a car. There was a clear alteration in mood as well, with many subjects becoming confused, aggressive, obviously despondent, and sometimes even hallucinating. Physical complaints, besides fatigue, included dizziness, thirst, loss of appetite, shivering, tremors, and pains in the back and limbs. It fol-

YOUR HEALTH TODAY

Bio-rhythms: Fact or Myth?

One of the current fads a person may encounter in shopping malls, on home computer software, and even in some wrist watches is the charting of bio-rhythms. A part of the infradian time cycle, the theory of bio-rhythms is based on the idea that beginning at the moment of birth, all humans live in rather predictable cycles (rhythms). These cycles are as follows:

1. *Physical:* A 23-day cycle theorized to govern strength, metabolism or certain hormones, endurance, energy, and resistance to infection.
2. *Emotional:* A 28-day cycle that roughly approximates menstruation, since it is governed by increases or decreases of select hormones. It is thought that men experience hormonal fluctuations similar to menstruation, only no outward signs of the fluctuation exist.
3. *Intellectual:* A 33-day cycle thought to affect, under hormonal control, such things as learning, memory, intelligence, ambition, and other mental functions.

It should be reemphasized that the theory of bio-rhythms is just that—a theory to explain apparent relationships between the physical, emotional, and intellectual states of humans. There is no scientific evidence at this point to prove or disprove the theory.

lows that the combined stressors of sleep deprivation and low caloric intake not only create substantial distress on their own but may, if the pattern persists, reduce one's capacity to deal effectively with other stressors.

Injury and Illness

Other commonly observed biological stressors include pain, injury, and illness. Interestingly, research in this area indicates that the more fully one is prepared for the sensations accompanying illness or injury, the less stressful these sensations are likely to be. Conversely, when information about the sensations is vague and emphasizes the kinds of tension that would be experienced, one's tension tends to increase or acts as a stressor that makes the trauma distressing. Such research suggests that the natural stress associated with physiological change can be reduced by imparting information that concentrates on the process rather than the possibly diffuse psychological reactions it may cause.

Noise

The last of the bioecological stressors we shall examine is noise, to which we may respond as automatically as we do to light and dark. Interestingly, noise may also be a psychosocial stressor, depending upon our personal perception of and response to it.

There are remarkable individual variations in the degree to which noise can act as a stressor. You probably know that if you are under no particular pressure, you can hear all kinds of noises—friends talking, records playing, or a distant television blaring—without being affected. If you are trying to study, however, even one of these noises can distract you and make you irritable and even aggressive. Similarly, if you are waiting for a call that can alter your life in an important way, you may jump every time the phone rings, whereas under normal circumstances the phone bell would be just another sound.

Noise has been found to be a bioecological stressor mainly when it interferes with necessary activities (such as homework) or is a regular part of the work scene, as on construction sites. Prolonged exposure to noise acts as a stressor in creating tissue damage in the ear itself. There are also indications that it may, after long exposure, alter the cardiovascular system, since sustained exposure to high noise levels appears to elevate blood pressure.

Psychosocial Stressors

Psychosocial stress Stress arising from faulty processing of social stimuli.

People who have studied **psychosocial stress** believe that it arises from faulty ways we process the countless and often conflicting messages we get from our social environment. When we have expectations of a situation that are not borne out by experience, psychosocial stress is likely to follow. An analogy to this process is walking into a dark room, touching the switch next to the door, and feeling frustrated when the lights fail to go on. You can surely find examples of the process in your own experience. Have you, for example, expected a high grade on a test and gotten a low one? How did this make you feel? Whatever your explanation for the outcome falling short of your expectation, your view may have been reflected in physiological changes created by your anger and frustration.

Adaptation The body's attempt to maintain balance (homeostasis).

Frustration Inability to do or get what one wants because of uncontrollable circumstances.

Overload Stress resulting from excessive stimulation.

Underload Stress resulting from deprivation of stimuli.

Homeostasis The maintenance of bodily equilibrium.

Four major types of psychosocial stress have been identified: **adaptation, frustration, overload,** and **underload** (deprivation).

Adaptation

We continually try to maintain a state of balance, or **homeostasis,** by *adapting* to the continued influx of information. The way we react to the information we receive can be a source of stress.

Perhaps some of the most significant stressors are those related to changes in our personal lives. Each individual may react differently to any one event. In studying the various social, or life, events that persons experience, Holmes and Rahe found that even those events considered desirable, could influence the onset of disease.[2]

Using Holmes and Rahe's basic research, Girdano and Everly developed a Life-Events Scale for college students. This Life-Events Scale is presented as Self-Assessment Exercise 3.1.

SELF-ASSESSMENT EXERCISE 3.1

Life-Events Scale for College Students

Below are listed events that may occur in the life of a college student. Place a check in the left-hand column for each of those events that have happened to you during the *last 12 months.*

	Life Event	*Point Values*
_____	Death of a close family member	100
_____	Jail term	80
_____	Final year or first year in college	63
_____	Pregnancy (to you or caused by you)	60
_____	Severe personal illness or injury	53
_____	Marriage	50
_____	Any interpersonal problems	45
_____	Financial difficulties	40
_____	Death of a close friend	40
_____	Arguments with your roommate (more than every other day)	40
_____	Major disagreements with your family	40
_____	Major change in personal habits	30
_____	Change in living environment	30
_____	Beginning or ending a job	30
_____	Problems with your boss or professor	25
_____	Outstanding personal achievement	25
_____	Failure in some course	25
_____	Final exams	20
_____	Increased or decreased dating	20
_____	Change in working conditions	20
_____	Change in your major	20
_____	Change in your sleeping habits	18
_____	Several-day vacation	15
_____	Change in eating habits	15
_____	Family reunion	15
_____	Change in recreational activities	15
_____	Minor illness or injury	15
_____	Minor violations of the law	11

Interpretation: Add up your score. If your total score for the year was under 150 points, your level of stress, based upon life change, is low. If your total was between 150 and 300, your stress levels are borderline; you should minimize other changes in your life at this time. If your total was more than 300, your life-change levels of stress are high.

Source: Daniel A. Girdano and George S. Everly, Jr., *Controlling Stress and Tension,* Englewood Cliffs, N.J.: Prentice-Hall, 1979, pp. 56–57. Reprinted by permission of Richard H. Rahe.

It must be emphasized that no single life event, by itself, has ever been identified as being predictive of illness. Rather, it is the accumulation and interaction of these events that could produce a problem. When too many changes occur in one's life in close proximity to one another, logic dictates that an adverse health condition may easily result.

Frustration

At some point, we all have felt frustration. Frustration results when we cannot get or do what we want because of circumstances beyond our control. It is a feeling of being trapped without an avenue of escape. An example of this is the college student studying for an examination who feels that there is no way to prepare sufficiently because of distractions in the dormitory or conflicting demands of college, family, and job.

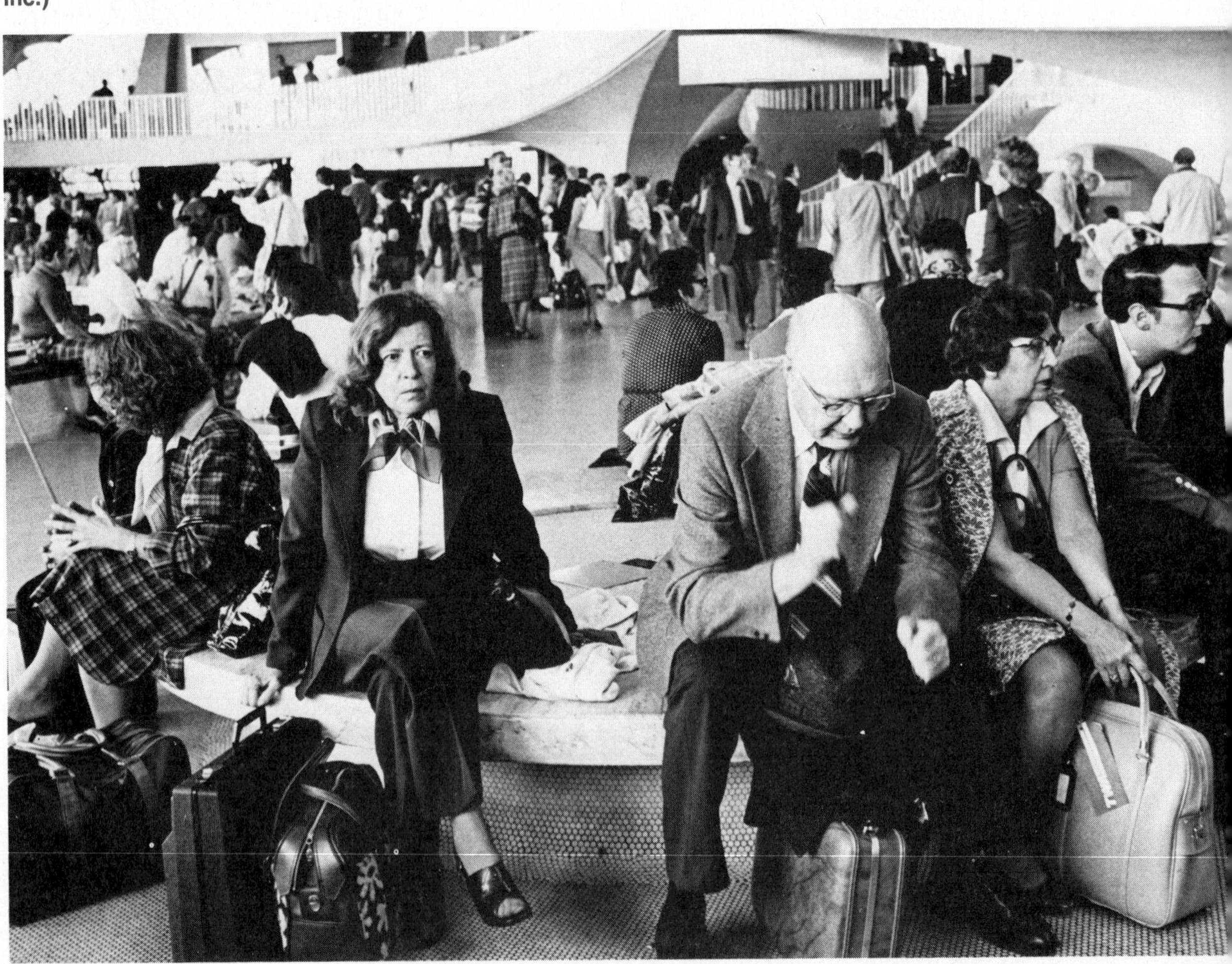

Frustration is a form of psychosocial stress. A delayed flight at an airport is a perfect setting for frustration. (Photo by Ginger Chih/Peter Arnold Inc.)

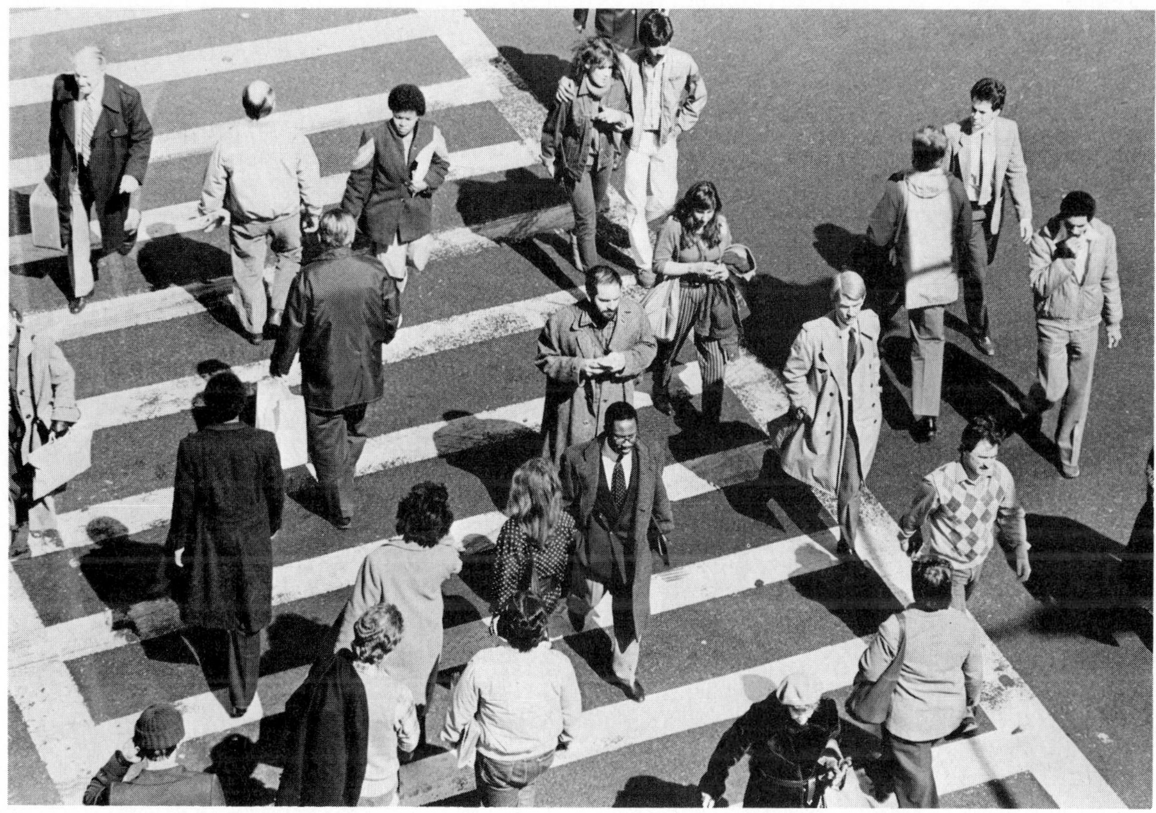

Crowds produce overload, a condition in which there are more stimuli than the mind can process. (Photo by Marc P. Anderson)

Overload

Many of you have probably felt that there just was not enough time in the day to get everything done that must be done. Psychologist Stanley Milgram has termed this condition *overload.* This is a condition in which there are more stimuli than can be processed effectively — whether because of time limitations, the existence of conflicting demands, insufficient help, or unduly high expectations of performance on the part of either the overloaded individual or his or her peers and superiors. People often refer to this condition as **"burnout."**

Burnout Condition of complete overload.

Underload

The opposite of overload, *underload* may result from such things as feeling trapped in a job, having an unstimulating relationship, or experiencing monotony in a highly repetitive job or in one's life-style. An acute sense of isolation, loneliness, and boredom can result. This condition, also called *deprivational stress,* may account for the difficulty uncared-for children have in mastering such seemingly basic skills as speaking. Similarly, the adult who lives alone appears far

SELF-ASSESSMENT EXERCISE 3.2

Susceptibility to Overload

Choose the most appropriate answer for each of the ten statements below and place the letter of your response in the space to the left.

How often do you . . .

_____ 1. Find yourself with insufficient time to complete your work?
(a) Almost always (b) Very often
(c) Seldom (d) Never

_____ 2. Find yourself becoming confused and unable to think clearly because too many things are happening at once?
(a) Almost always (b) Very often
(c) Seldom (d) Never

_____ 3. Wish you had help to get everything done?
(a) Almost always (b) Very often
(c) Seldom (d) Never

_____ 4. Feel that people around you simply expect too much from you?
(a) Almost always (b) Very often
(c) Seldom (d) Never

_____ 5. Feel overwhelmed by the demands placed upon you?
(a) Almost always (b) Very often
(c) Seldom (d) Never

_____ 6. Find your work infringing upon your leisure hours?
(a) Almost always (b) Very often
(c) Seldom (d) Never

_____ 7. Get depressed when you consider all of the tasks that need your attention?
(a) Almost always (b) Very often
(c) Seldom (d) Never

_____ 8. See no end to the excessive demands placed upon you?
(a) Almost always (b) Very often
(c) Seldom (d) Never

_____ 9. Have to skip a meal so that you can get work completed?
(a) Almost always (b) Very often
(c) Seldom (d) Never

_____ 10. Feel that you have too much responsibility?
(a) Almost always (b) Very often
(c) Seldom (d) Never

Scoring: a = 4, b = 3, c = 2, d = 1 **Score:** _______

Interpretation: Total your points and see how stressed you are by overload. A total of 26 to 40 indicates a high stress level; such an excessive level could be psychologically and physiologically debilitating if steps are not taken to reduce it.

Source: Girdano and Everly, *Controlling Stress and Tension,* pp. 67–68, © 1979. Reprinted by permission of Prentice-Hall, Inc.

Table 3-1 Some Psychological and Physiological Disturbances Believed to Be Caused by, Related to, or Aggravated by Psychosocial Stress

Scientists believe that a number of disorders are the end result of our failure to recognize psychosocial stressors and deal with them intelligently. Some of these are as follows:

Emotional: anxiety, insomnia, tension headaches, abnormal aging, sexual impotency, neuroses, phobias, alcoholism, drug abuse, learning problems, general malaise

Psychosomatic: essential hypertension, auricular arrhythmias, ulcers, colitis, asthma, chronic pain, acne, peripheral vascular disease

Organic, triggered by stress: epilepsy, migraine, herpes, angina, coronary thrombosis, rheumatoid arthritis

Psychological adjustment problems: for example, anxiety in classroom learning (moderate interference in satisfying/fulfilling human potential)

Sociological problems: for example, chronic unemployment; delinquency (socially undesirable); socioeconomic impoverishment and instability

Aggravated or prolonged distress in illness of any origin

Source: Adapted from Barbara B. Brown, "Perspectives on Social Stress." In Hans Selye, ed., *Selye's Guide to Stress Research* (New York: Van Nostrand Reinhold Co., 1980), 31.

more likely to develop serious illness than the adult who is married or living with a companion. The American philosopher and psychologist William James summed up the tragedy of deprivational stress when he observed in his *Principles of Psychology:*

> No more fiendish punishment could be devised . . . than that one should be turned loose in society and remain unnoticed by all the members thereof. . . . If every person "cut us dead" and acted as if we were nonexisting things . . . the cruellest bodily tortures would be a relief; for these would make us feel that . . . we had not sunk to such a depth as to be unworthy of attention at all.

Personality Stressors

Often, stress is directly related to the way we perceive ourselves (self-concept) and our behavior. This is called **personality stress.**

Personality stress Stress that arises from one's perception of oneself.

Self-concept

The degree to which any one of us is affected by psychosocial stressors is strongly influenced by how we normally perceive ourselves, and how these perceptions are altered by stress. At Harvard Univer-

YOUR HEALTH TODAY

How Can You Manage Stress?

Listed below are seven basic ways to help you manage stress. A complete discussion of these suggestions is presented in the text.

1. Assess your self-perception.
2. Clarify your goals.
3. Be a participant.
4. Don't be afraid to cry.
5. Avoid self-medication.
6. Organize your time.
7. Get sufficient sleep, diet, and exercise.

sity nearly a century ago, William James's students were shown this basic fact about stress as a formula in which

$$\text{Self-esteem} = \frac{\text{Success}}{\text{Pretensions}}$$

Whether called self-esteem or the currently more popular "self-image," the ideas we have of ourselves are a potent factor in stress. When our pretensions, or goals, meet with success, our self-image is likely to be positive. If we fail to achieve our goals, our self-image becomes more negative.

Whether we succeed or fail, we experience some stress. Moreover, each success and each failure tends to color our self-perception. Not surprisingly, individuals with a positive self-concept are generally more successful in every aspect of their lives than those with a negative self-concept. People with a positive self-concept overcome obstacles that would be catastrophic to others who have a less positive view of themselves.

Behaviors

In the late 1950s and 1960s, Dr. Meyer Friedman and Dr. Ray Roseman developed a model of behavior labeled the Type-A pattern. Type-A persons are aggressive, hard-working, achievement-oriented individuals who tend to be time-conscious, intolerant of interruptions, impatient, and irritable. They are also unable to shift easily into the more relaxed, or Type-B, life-style that would be better for their health. Specifics of Type-A and Type-B behavior are discussed more fully in Chapter 16.

A Basic Approach to Stress Management

Once we realize that stress will occur and that different types of stressors exist, it is important to develop a personal plan to deal with stressors. Ideally, each one of us should learn to set reasonable, achievable goals that take into account those things that tend to act as stressors on us. We should learn to change in positive ways when we can, and accept those things we cannot change.

Assess Your Self-perception

Since it is your perception that makes so many psychosocial stressors hazardous to your health, a first step in coping with stress is to review your self-perceptions. Are they basically positive and healthy? Or do you tend to be overly critical of yourself and fail to appreciate your good qualities? Do you perhaps have an inflated self-image to make up for deep-seated negative feelings? Would you say that you have much interest in the outside world, or are you more absorbed in yourself and your own problems? Do you feel basically sympathetic toward other people, or wary of them? Self-Assessment Exercise 3.3 might be a good starting point for your review.

Clarify Your Goals

In order to set reasonable, attainable goals for yourself, you might find it useful to spend some time considering how you want to lead your life and what your goals should be. Think about what things give you pleasure, what things irritate you, what activities you think would do you good, what things you hope to accomplish in the near and the more distant future, and what aspects of your personality you might like to improve or develop. It may be helpful to actually set your goals down on paper, as well as some means of achieving them. Indicate which goals are most important to you in both the long and short run, which you would like to have done by a certain time, and which are of relatively low priority. Clarifying your goals and identifying which are most important or pressing will help you keep minor stressors in perspective.

Organize Your Time

Having decided what you want to do, try to organize your time so that you can actually accomplish your goals. Schedule your day so that you use the times when you think you work best for the toughest jobs. Again, it may be useful to write out a schedule, as long as it isn't a rigid timetable that does not give you a moment to relax. Even a list of things to do can help you cope with a particularly busy and poten-

SELF-ASSESSMENT EXERCISE 3.3

Self-concept

Choose the alternative that best summarizes how you generally behave, and place your answer in the space provided.

_____ 1. When I face a difficult task, I try my best and will usually succeed.
(a) Almost always true (b) Often true
(c) Seldom true (d) Almost never true

_____ 2. I am at ease when around members of the opposite sex.
(a) Almost always true (b) Often true
(c) Seldom true (d) Almost never true

_____ 3. I feel that I have a lot going for me.
(a) Almost always true (b) Often true
(c) Seldom true (d) Almost never true

_____ 4. I have a very high degree of confidence in my own abilities.
(a) Almost always true (b) Often true
(c) Seldom true (d) Almost never true

_____ 5. I prefer to be in control of my own life as opposed to having someone else make decisions for me.
(a) Almost always true (b) Often true
(c) Seldom true (d) Almost never true

_____ 6. I am comfortable and at ease around my superiors.
(a) Almost always true (b) Often true
(c) Seldom true (d) Almost never true

_____ 7. I am often overly self-conscious or shy when among strangers.
(a) Almost always true (b) Often true
(c) Seldom true (d) Almost never true

_____ 8. Whenever something goes wrong, I tend to blame myself.
(a) Almost always true (b) Often true
(c) Seldom true (d) Almost never true

_____ 9. When I don't succeed, I tend to let it depress me more than I should.
(a) Almost always true (b) Often true
(c) Seldom true (d) Almost never true

_____ 10. I often feel that I am beyond helping.
(a) Almost always true (b) Often true
(c) Seldom true (d) Almost never true

Scoring: 1–6: a = 1, b = 2, c = 3, d = 4
7–10: a = 4, b = 3, c = 2, d = 1

Score: _______

Interpretation: This exercise was designed to provide some insight into your self-concept. If you scored from ten to 19 points, you have a strong self-concept. A score of 20 to 25 indicates a moderate self-concept. If you scored between 26 and 40, your self-concept appears to be in need of bolstering.

Source: Girdano and Everly, *Controlling Stress and Tension,* p. 105, © 1979. Reprinted by permission of Prentice-Hall, Inc.

tially stressful day. (It can be satisfying to check off things done or perhaps award yourself a treat for doing something you'd been putting off.) Be sure to leave time in your schedule for delays and interruptions, which act as stressors. And, a critical thing in scheduling is to make time for fun. Play can be just as important as work. Everyone needs a break from his or her daily routine just to relax, have fun, and enjoy life.

Get Sufficient Sleep, Diet, and Exercise

As we have seen, the lack of sufficient sleep or a nourishing diet acts directly as a stressor, besides reducing our ability to deal with other stressors. Therefore it's important that you meet these physical needs. Regular exercise not only can strengthen your cardiovascular system but also lets you work off negative feelings and relax afterwards. Whether you prefer jogging, bicycling, swimming, walking, or other activities, try to participate in some form of exercise at least three times a week (see Chapter 12).

Learn to React Differently

As you learn more about how you react to stress, physiologically and emotionally, bring these actions under conscious control. Do not always adhere to the old rules. Know when to stand your ground and when to retreat. Need you always be correct? Learn how to compromise; it is not necessary to always have your own way. Do not always push, and you will find others do not push back. Get off the backs of others, and they will get off yours.

Be a Participant

Know what is occurring around you. Do not sit and watch; get involved. Offer to help, but be aware of your time constraints. Overload can creep up quickly.

Don't Be Afraid to Cry

Crying can be a very healthy way to relieve anxiety and tension. There is no need to adhere to the idea that adults do not cry. Laugh when you can, but cry if you have to.

Avoid Self-medication

There are many substances available, both legal and illegal, that are reputed to help a person relax. Reliance on these substances will not make the problems disappear; in fact, they may compound the problem. For women who are pregnant, self-medication can be particularly dangerous.

Relaxation Training

Teaching yourself how to relax is another approach to coping with stress. Naturally, the basic approach which we have just discussed should be followed. However, there are various physical and mental exercise systems that will help you relax. Obviously, not all the suggestions we offer will work for every person, nor should every person try each of the suggestions. As you become more aware of the types and amounts of stress you face, you will probably develop your own ideas or unique combinations to ease the tensions of life.

Psychosomatic relaxation Relaxation technique initiated in the mind and spread to the body.

Somatopsychic relaxation Relaxation technique initiated in the body and spread to the mind.

Relaxation training assumes one of two forms. The first form, **psychosomatic relaxation,** is initiated in the central nervous system, and the second, **somatopsychic relaxation,** is initiated in the periphery of the body.

Psychosomatic Relaxation

Psychosomatic (central) relaxation techniques begin in the mind and move to the body. These techniques work best for persons who react to stress in a random fashion. That is, they may react differently to the same stressor, depending upon the situation in which the stress occurs. Specific psychosomatic relaxation techniques include meditation and biofeedback training.

Meditation. Meditation is probably the oldest systematic method of relaxation known to humankind. It has been shown to effectively alter consciousness through disciplined focus of attention on a single, repetitive or unchanging stimulus. The basic goal of meditation is to reduce mind–body (psychophysiological) arousal or reaction to stimuli.

Numerous methods of meditation exist, and it is not our intent to enumerate all of them. Regardless of the method selected, all forms of meditation share four characteristics: (1) a quiet environment, (2) correct posture, (3) a meditation object, and (4) a passive attitude.

The necessity of having a quiet environment seems fairly obvious. If a person is to focus attention on a single object, the introduction of other variables such as noise will detract from that concentration, especially for the individual who is just learning how to meditate.

Posture plays a major role in meditation, for without good posture, the internal organs become cramped and stressed, exactly what the meditation is supposed to alleviate. It is recommended that you select a comfortable straight-backed chair or sit on the floor with your back against a wall. Do not lie down since that might promote drowsiness. Rest your hands on your thighs at about the knee level with your hands open. As you become more skilled at meditation, you may wish to use some other posture.

The meditation object may be the most important characteristic of the four, for it is upon this object that the individual's attention is focused. The meditation object can be anything that repeats (such as a clock ticking) or does not change (such as a rock). The object may be real or imagined—it does not matter. What does matter is that the object can serve as an element on which to focus your attention.

With practice comes the passive attitude. The passive attitude means that if the mind wanders, the person meditating does not worry about it. It is extremely difficult to keep your attention focused on an unchanging object or stimulus. The mind is used to processing hundreds of bits of information each minute, and you have grown up with that orientation. Even the most accomplished of yogis will experience times when their minds wander.

One form of meditation, **transcendental meditation,** as it is practiced in the United States, has become widely known through the teachings of Maharishi Mahesh Yogi. TM, as it is commonly called, involves two 20-minute periods a day, morning and evening, during which an individual sits quietly and focuses his or her thoughts by repeating a mantra, or Sanskrit word. You can try this on your own, using a word of your own choosing. Wait until two hours after your last meal, since digestion can prevent you from thoroughly relaxing. Meditation is not easy. You must practice it regularly if it is to be effective.

Transcendental meditation (TM) Method of stress reduction involving short periods of concentration on a repeated word.

Relaxation Response. The **relaxation response,** developed by Dr. Herbert Benson, was designed to produce essentially the same basic physiologic responses as the techniques mentioned in the prior paragraphs. The subject is taught to sit comfortably and quietly, eyes closed, muscles completely relaxed, breathing through the nose. With each exhalation the subject says the word "one." No conscious effort is to be directed at achieving the physiological correlates of relaxation.

Relaxation response Relaxation technique used to reduce stress.

Biofeedback. The foregoing techniques may be self-taught, perhaps with the aid of a book, if professional instruction is not available. *Biofeedback,* however, requires sophisticated equipment and is therefore more expensive. What biofeedback machines do is measure physiological changes—such as in blood pressure, muscle tension, skin temperature, and brain waves—and relay the information back to the individual. Through biofeedback, you can become aware of tensions that you previously did not perceive and learn to reduce them. Throughout the training, the individual learns to induce the reactions measured by the machines without their use and eventually the person can do so without relying on the machine.

Somatopsychic Techniques

Somatopsychic (peripheral) relaxation is generally best for those persons who seem to experience the same basic physiologic reaction to a stressor, regardless of the situation or type of stressor. Somatopsychic relaxation techniques include progressive relaxation, breath control, and physical exercise. These types of stress-reduction techniques have been found effective in reducing muscle tension, certain

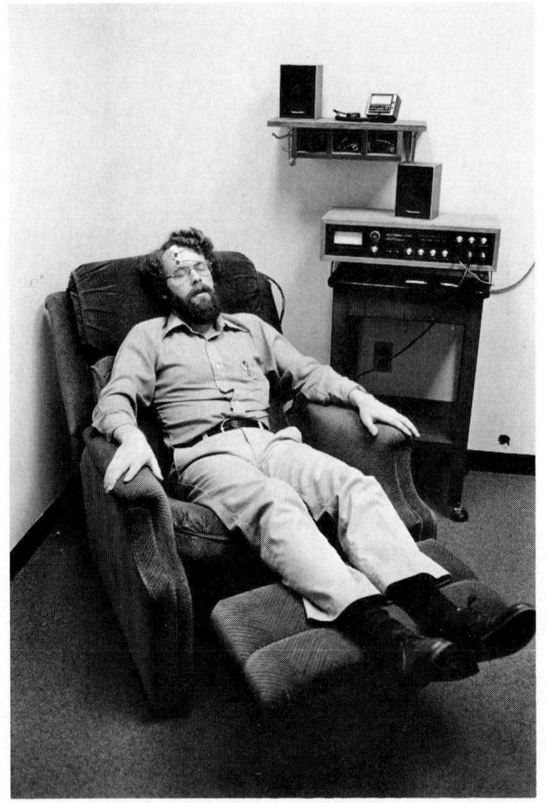

Biofeedback has been shown to be an effective means to reduce stress. (Photo by Ken Robert Buck—University Hospital, Boston/The Picture Cube)

kinds of headaches, and other stress problems by lowering the rate of metabolism, respiration, pulse beats, oxygen use, and blood pressure.

Progressive Relaxation. In this technique, devised by Dr. Edmund Jacobson, the individual is taught to alternately tense and relax the muscles so that tension can be recognized and immediately self-treated. The premise is that if the individual knows when a muscle is tense and how it feels when the muscle is relaxed, the body will learn (as will the mind) to seek the relaxed state.

Jacobson's technique involves tightening a specific muscle group on both sides of the body (such as clenching the fists), holding that particular posture for five to ten seconds and then relaxing the posture for about thirty to forty-five seconds. This process is repeated several times for each major muscle group (thus the term, *progressive relaxation*).

Breathing Control. How many of you have taken a deep breath prior to beginning a particular activity? By inhaling deeply and exhaling slowly, you begin to experience a relaxing feeling. When people are tense, they tend to breathe quite shallowly and rapidly. By consciously inhaling deeply, the diaphragm is forced to expand and tense, and the stomach tends to expand. When you exhale, the diaphragm relaxes and the stomach contracts, thus the term "diaphragmatic breathing." Singers are taught to use this technique, as are those who do a great deal of public speaking.

Physical Exercise. Though not often thought of as relaxation, regular vigorous physical activity promotes both mental and physical health. Recall that we stated earlier that self-esteem has a great deal to do with one's mental health. By engaging in physical exercise, a person accrues numerous psychological benefits while experiencing various physiological changes.

The concept behind regular exercise is that exercise removes various metabolic waste products that can result from experiencing stress. It also strengthens all the body systems and helps the individual attain a positive self-image. This topic is discussed more fully in Chapter 12.

Other Techniques

Numerous other techniques exist that can be utilized to relieve stress. Such things as "Touch for Health," massage therapy, yoga, drug therapy, professional counseling, social engineering, cognitive reappraisal, personality engineering, and nutritional engineering are but a few of the techniques that surpass the scope of this text. Several good texts exist that deal with these topics, and these are listed in the Suggested Readings at the end of this chapter. You might also consult the schedule of classes at your college or university to see if classes on stress reduction are being offered.

What About You?

Developing realistic goals, organizing your time, taking good care of your body, learning a stress-reducing technique—all of these are things you can do to help you cope with stressors. But also important for relieving stress is helping others, and being helped in turn. A talk with a friend not only is a good way to let off steam but also makes you aware that you're not alone with your troubles. In lending a sympathetic ear to someone else, you not only help that person but learn something about another human being and feel good about being useful.

Whatever method you select to reduce the impact of stressors on you now and in the future, there are three axioms that should be followed: (1) do it consistently, (2) do it regularly, and (3) do it right. Remember that by reducing stress you are extending your opportunities to live a long, healthy, productive, and serene life.

Summary

Stress, defined by Dr. Hans Selye as "the nonspecific response of the body to any demand made upon it," is a term borrowed from physics to describe the impact of day-to-day events upon our minds and bodies. Events and conditions that trigger stress, whether physical, social, or psychological, are called stressors. Although the recognition of the contribution of stress to health problems has given the word a negative connotation, stress results not just from negative stressors but from any change in our lives and may sometimes help us perform better. Selye calls the more extreme kinds of stress eustress, when resulting from positive stressors, or distress, when from negative stressors. The term psychosomatic is used to characterize disorders caused or strongly influenced by emotions. It is applied not only to stress-induced imaginary ailments, but also to stress-related disorders with verifiable physical symptoms—real symptoms that are psychogenic, or caused by the mind. The term psychosomatic is also applied to illnesses, called somatogenic, that appear to result from a lowering of immunity due to stress-producing emotions.

Our biological response to stress over time has been shown to follow a three-stage pattern, which Selye calls the general adaptation syndrome. In the first, or alarm stage, the body is mobilized by the secretion of ACTH to fight the stressor or flee from it. When the stressor remains, the second or arousal stage follows, in which the organ systems or processes adapt to cope with or suppress the stressor. In the third, or exhaustion stage—when the stressor persists despite adaptation—energy for adaptation is used up, and death may eventually result.

When the body is under stress, the major organ systems undergo changes in the way they function. If stress is prolonged, major health problems can result.

It is helpful to recognize various types of stressors. Bioecological stressors, including biological rhythms, sleep, diet, pain, illness, injury, and noise, arise from our relationship with the environment. Psychological stressors arise from conflicts between our expectations of a situation and our actual experience. Feeling crowded by many other human beings may also act as a psychosocial stressor. Stress due to being subjected to more stimuli than can be processed effectively is called overload. An opposite condition, underload, or deprivational stress, results from insufficient stimuli and is characterized by a sense of loneliness, isolation, and boredom. Adaptation to multiple stressors is more difficult than to just one.

The degree to which we are affected by personality stressors is determined by our self-concept and behavior. Therefore, an important first step in learning to cope with stress is examining these perceptions. It is also useful to spend some time considering what your goals should be and possible means of achieving them. Then you can organize your time so as to best accomplish your goals. Satisfying your physical needs is essential for coping with stress, and you should avoid unnecessary stressors, such as drugs. You can also reduce stress through such techniques as meditation and biofeedback. Helping others and getting involved with the outside world can help you take care of your own problems.

Review and Discussion

1. In what ways is stress present throughout one's life?
2. What is the difference between eustress and distress?
3. How can stress be a positive factor in a person's life?
4. Describe the three phases of the general adaptation syndrome.
5. Name four types of bioecological stressors. What examples can you find in your everyday life?
6. Name four types of psychosocial stressors. What examples can you find in your everyday life?
7. Define "overload" and "underload." Do you think these are serious problems in our society? Why?
8. What is the most important factor in how people react to psychosocial stress?
9. What are some examples of applied techniques to help people reduce their stress?
10. What practical steps can you take now to reduce stress in your life?

Further Reading

Allen, Roger J. and David H. Hyde. *Investigations in Stress Control,* 2nd edition. Minneapolis, Minn.: Burgess Publishing Company, 1981.
A series of self-assessment exercises that the individual can do to help learn how to manage stress. (Paperback.)

Allen, Roger J. *Human Stress; Its Nature and Control.* Minneapolis, Burgess Publishing Company, 1983.
Contains a basic description of stress and stress-related problems and how they can be overcome through personal control. (Paperback.)

Benson, Herbert, and Miriam Z. Klipper. *The Relaxation Response.* New York: Avon Books, 1976.
An introduction to relaxation techniques, with descriptions of exercises. (Paperback.)

Bolton, Robert. *People Skills.* Englewood Cliffs, N.J.: Prentice-Hall, Inc., 1979.
A basic book that deals with self-assertion, how to listen to others and hear what they are saying, and what to do when conflicts arise. (Paperback.)

Downing, George. *The Massage Book.* New York: Random House, 1972.
A guide to the many techniques of massage. (Paperback.)

Girdano, Daniel A., and George S. Everly, Jr. *Controlling Stress and Tension.* Englewood Cliffs, N.J.: Prentice-Hall, 1979.
A practical description of stress in everyday life, featuring self-assessment exercises. (Paperback.)

Greenberg, Jerrold S. *Comprehensive Stress Management.* Dubuque, Iowa: William C. Brown Company, Publishers, 1983.
A basic book dealing with stress management that is written from the personal perspective. (Paperback.)

Selye, Hans. *Stress Without Distress.* New York: New American Library, 1975.
Description of the author's theory of the general adaptation syndrome and its implications for reducing stress. (Paperback.)

Steinmets, Jenny, Jon Blankenship, Linda Brown, Deborah Hall, and Grace Miller. *Managing Stress: Before It Manages You.* Palo Alto, Calif.: Bull Publishing Co., 1980.
A basic book that gives individuals things to watch for in order to avoid stress and what to do if stresses begin to occur frequently. (Paperback.)

Toffler, Alvin. *Future Shock.* New York: Avon Books, 1976.
A discussion of the impact of rapid changes in today's world and the stress they can cause. (Paperback.)

Tubesing, Donald A. *Kicking Your Stress Habits.* Duluth, Minn.: Whole Person Associates, 1981.
A guide to changing your habits to avoid the minor irritations that can accumulate as major stress. (Paperback.)

Wookfolk, Robert I., and Frank C. Richardson. *Stress, Sanity, and Survival.* New York: New American Library, 1979.
Two clinical psychologists' advice on stress reduction, with guidelines for a low-stress life-style. (Paperback.)

Part II
Life Cycles

"Every cradle asks us 'Whence?' and every coffin 'Whither?' "
R. G. Ingersoll

There are many questions to be answered and decisions to be made between the cradle and the grave. LIFE CYCLES presents information that will help you with some of the answers and decisions along the way. A cycle is a complete course of events recurring in a definite sequence, such as birth, growth, senescence, and death. Chapter 4, "Reproduction," explains the beginning of the cycle—conception and birth. In "Human Sexuality" and "Relationships," Chapters 5 and 6, you will learn of the pleasures, the problems, and the responsibilities that come with maturation. "Aging," Chapter 7, and "Death and Dying," Chapter 8, will add to your understanding of the later cycles of life.

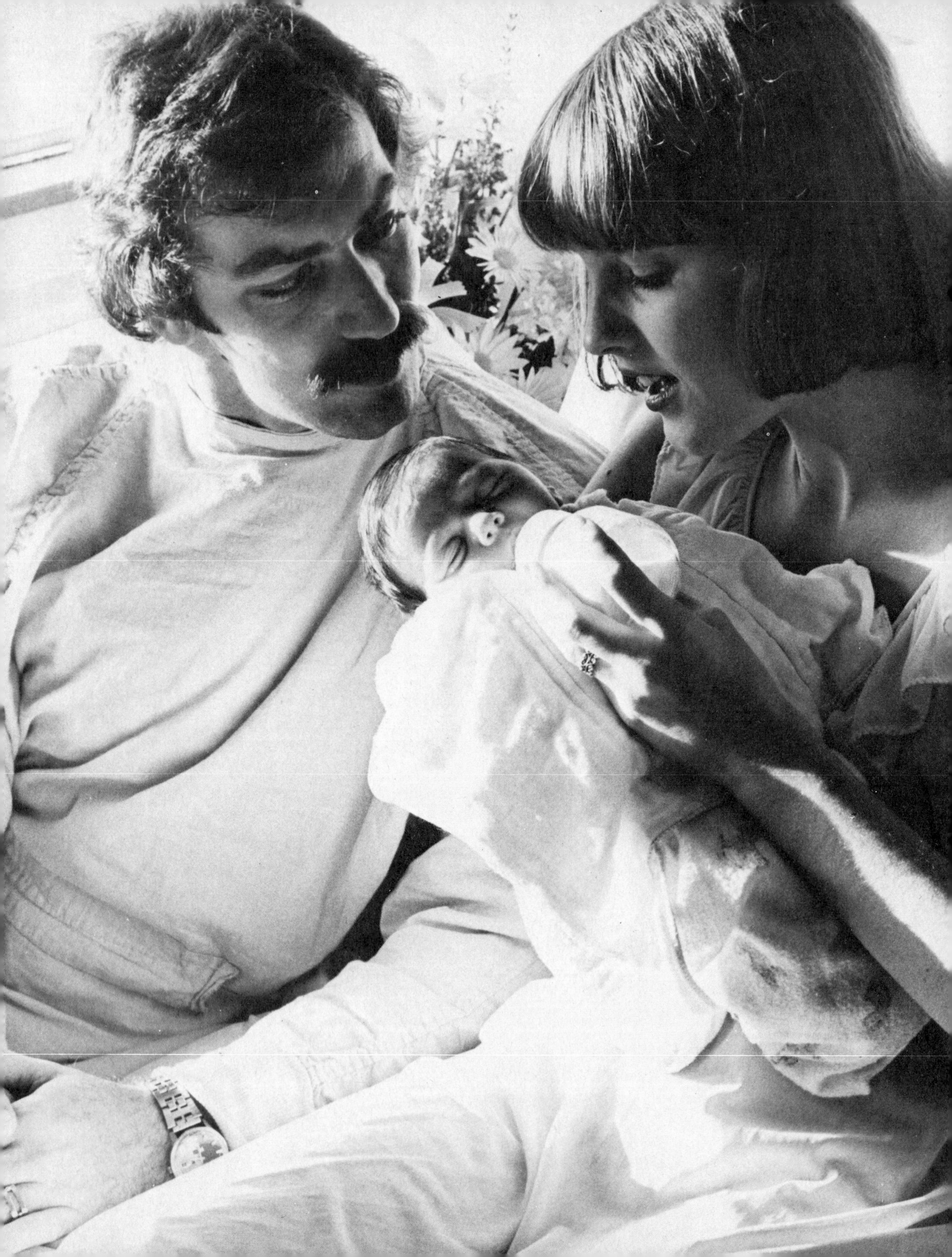

Chapter 4
Reproduction and Birth Control

KEY POINTS

- ☐ Reproduction consists of the production of an ovum, or egg, in the female and sperm in the male; the fertilization of the ovum by the sperm; the implantation of the egg in the uterus; the growth of the fetus during pregnancy; and childbirth.
- ☐ Female sexual organs include the ovaries, fallopian tubes, uterus, vagina, and clitoris.
- ☐ Male sexual organs include the testicles, epididymis, vas deferens, seminal vesicles, prostate, and penis.
- ☐ Menstruation is the final stage of the menstrual cycle, a complex series of events, the purpose of which is the release of a mature egg and the preparation of the female reproductive system for pregnancy.
- ☐ After the egg has been fertilized, it travels down one of the fallopian tubes and implants in the lining of the uterus.
- ☐ Approximately nine months after fertilization, the baby is ready to be born, and the mother begins labor.
- ☐ Various contraceptive methods are available to prevent pregnancy, including the pill, intrauterine device, diaphragm, spermicides, condoms and the rhythm method.
- ☐ Abortion is the termination of pregnancy before the fetus is capable of independent existence outside the mother's uterus.

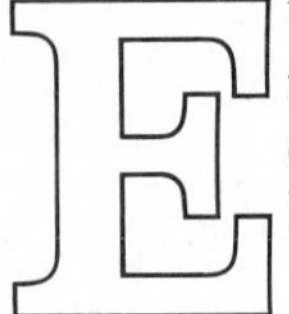

VEN IN these days of unisex fashions, many of the differences between men and women are obvious. Nevertheless, just as the basic design of every human body is the same, there are fundamental similarities in the reproductive systems of both sexes.

In both the male and female reproductive systems the gonads, or reproductive glands, (ovaries in the female; testes in the male) produce the germ cells (ova, or eggs, in females; sperm in males) and manufacture hormones. Pairs of tubes (fallopian tubes in females; epididymides, vasa deferentia, and ejaculatory ducts in males) transport the germ cells. Finally, in both sexes there are organs to receive or deliver sperm (the vagina in females; the penis in males).

The characteristics that distinguish males from females do not become evident in the fetus until approximately twenty weeks after conception, primarily because the reproductive systems of both sexes have the same evolutionary origin. It is thought that every female organ has its male counterpart. The clitoris, for example, is the female equivalent of the penis. Both are highly sensitive to stimulation, but the clitoris has no direct reproductive function.

Genitals The external sex organs.

In both sexes, the reproductive system consists of external organs, or **genitals,** and internal organs, which are located in the bony pelvis.

Female Reproductive Organs

External Organs

Vulva External female anatomy; includes the labia majora, the labia minora and the clitoris.

The external genitalia in the female are collectively called the **vulva** (a Latin word for "covering"). Situated at the entrance to the vagina, the vulva consists of several parts, each of which has its own function.

Mons pubis Rounded pad of fatty tissue over the pubic bone.

The **mons pubis** (or *mons Veneris,* "mount of Venus"), the most visible part of the female genitals, is formed by a pad of fat located over the pubic bone and covered with hair.

Labia majora Major lips of the vagina.

The **labia majora** (major lips of the vagina) are two large folds of skin that contain sweat glands and hair follicles embedded in fatty tissue. Usually close together, giving the female genitals a closed look, the labia majora are less sensitive to touch and pressure than the mons.

Labia minora Inner, hairless lips of the vagina.

Located between the labia majora, the **labia minora** (minor lips) are delicate folds of hairless skin that are rich in blood vessels and oil glands but contain few sweat glands and little fatty tissue. In front, the labia minora split into two folds, one of which passes over the clitoris.

Bartholin's glands Glands that create a genital scent and neutralize the vaginal environment.

Extending toward the back, the labia minora cover the urinary and vaginal openings and the ducts of the **Bartholin's glands.** Until recently it was believed that Bartholin's glands play an important part in vaginal lubrication, but Masters and Johnson's research has shown

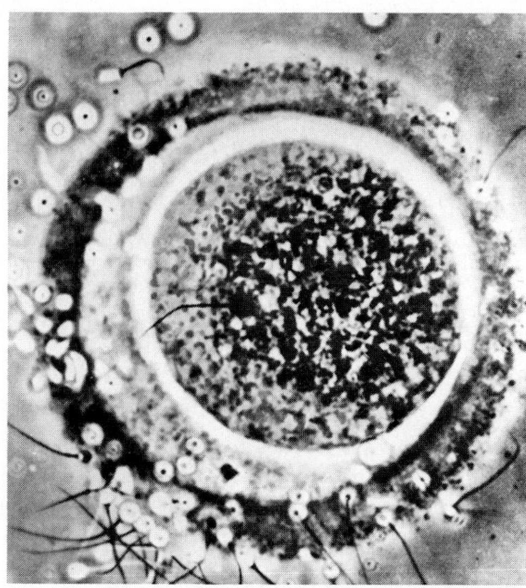

Human egg and sperm cells. (Photo by Landrum B. Shettles, M.D.)

this to be incorrect. It is now believed that these glands play a role in creating a genital scent and neutralizing the vaginal environment so that sperm might be better able to survive.

The **clitoris,** a small organ of spongy erectile tissue located above the opening of the urethra, is the most sensitive of all female genital organs. It is the only known anatomical feature that exists solely to react to erotic stimulation.

Clitoris Small, sensitive organ above the female urethral opening.

The **urethral opening,** the cleft below the clitoris and between the labia minora, is the external opening of the urinary tract. It is located just above the vaginal opening, which is distinguished from the urethral opening by its larger size.

Urethral opening Opening of the urinary tract located just above the vaginal opening in the female.

The **hymen,** or *maidenhead,* a thin fold of membrane that surrounds the vaginal opening, varies in shape and elasticity. Normally, the hymen contains one or more small openings, thus allowing passage of menstrual fluid and other vaginal discharges. In many cases the hymen is ruptured during a woman's first sexual intercourse, resulting in a small amount of bleeding. In some cultures where premarital chastity is of great importance, sheets are inspected for signs of blood soon after a marriage is consummated. Presence of the hymen, however, is an unreliable indicator of virginity because it can be torn accidentally during childhood, or, if it is extremely elastic, it can withstand coitus without tearing. Childbirth results in almost total destruction of the hymen.

Hymen The membrane surrounding the vaginal opening.

Internal Organs

Located in the lower abdominal cavity of either side of the pelvic region, the two **ovaries** are almond-sized, almond-shaped organs, which weigh about three-fourths of an ounce each in the sexually

Ovaries Two small internal female organs that produce ova and sex hormones.

mature woman (see Figure 4–1). The ovaries, which are attached to the pelvic wall, produce the female sex hormones **estrogen** and **progesterone,** as well as small amounts of the male hormone androgen. Although a female child is born with each ovary containing 100,000 to 400,000 germ cells or **ova** (from the Latin word meaning "egg"), during a woman's reproductive years only 400 to 500 eggs reach maturity and are released from the ovaries by a process called **ovulation.** A healthy woman who is not pregnant or using oral contraceptives usually ovulates once per month.

Estrogen Hormone that stimulates female secondary sexual characteristics.

Ova Female reproductive cells.

Progesterone Hormone that prepares the uterus for the fertilized egg.

Ovulation Release of a mature ovum from the ovary.

Fallopian tubes Ducts by which eggs travel from the ovaries to the uterus.

The **fallopian tubes** are about four inches long and, suspended by ligaments, extend from the upper part of the uterus toward each of the ovaries. The cone-shaped outer end of each tube lies close to the ovary but is not attached to it. After ovulation the egg must cross a small gap to enter the fallopian tube, which becomes progressively narrower as it approaches the uterus. The final section of the fallopian tube passes through the thick wall of the uterus and opens into the uterine cavity. Passage of eggs through the tube takes about three or four days, and fertilization usually takes place in the upper portion of the tube. An unfertilized egg eventually disintegrates and is absorbed by the body.

Uterus The womb.

The **uterus,** or *womb,* is a pear-shaped, hollow organ flanked by the bladder in front and the bowel behind. It usually lies bent forward at an angle, resting on the bladder. Thick and muscular, the uterus is suspended by a series of ligaments. The lining of the uterus, called the **endometrium,** contains a wealth of glands and blood vessels and undergoes many changes as a woman ages. It is here that the fertilized ovum embeds and the fetus develops.

Endometrium Uterine lining.

Cervix Uterine mouth projecting into the vagina.

The **cervix** ("neck") is the lower part of the uterus that projects into the vagina. Glands in the cervix secrete mucus in varying amounts to protect the endometrium from infection. During ovulation, the mucus becomes thin and abundant, facilitating the passage of sperm into the uterus.

Vagina The passage from the genital orifice to the uterus.

A thin-walled, muscular tube, the **vagina** ("sheath") is the body cavity adapted to the reception of the semen during sexual intercourse. Unless distended by tampons used during menstruation, by the penis during coitus, or by the passage of a baby during childbirth, the walls of the vagina lie close together. Varying in length from three to four inches, the vagina extends downward and forward from the uterus to the muscular external opening, which is highly sensitive to both pleasurable and painful sensations. The inner vaginal lining, which is similar to the skin covering the inside of the mouth, has few touch and pressure receptors and only a few scattered nerve endings.

The Menstrual Cycle

Puberty Physiological changes resulting in full sexual development.

Puberty refers to the many physiological changes resulting in full sexual development. In a woman this includes breast development,

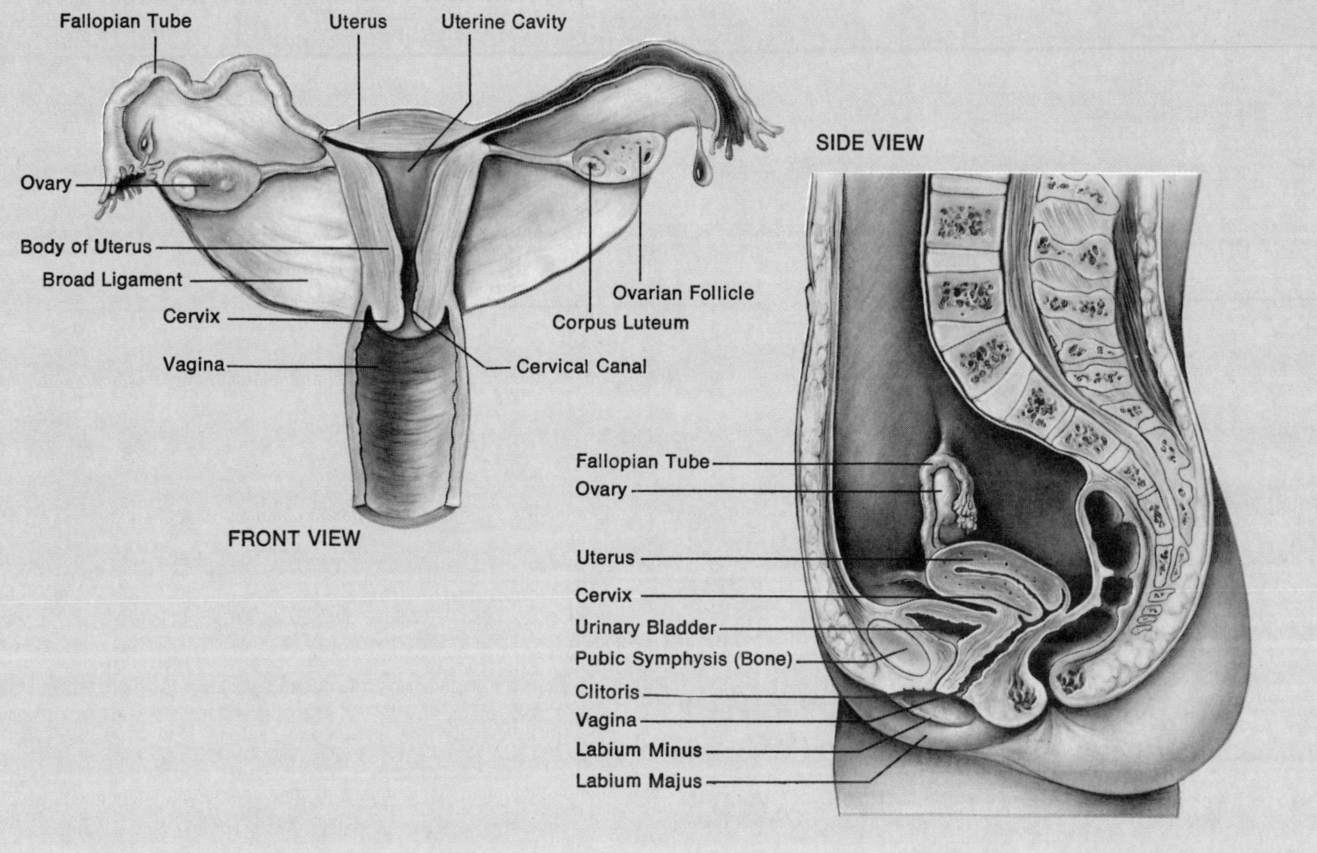

Figure 4–1. Female Reproductive Organs.
Above, **a cross section of the female reproductive organs as seen from the front and *right,* a side-view section.**

growth of pubic and underarm hair, increase in height and weight, widening of the pelvic bones, and the beginning of menstruation. It usually begins when a girl is 10 or 11 years old and culminates 3 to 5 years later when a regular cycle of menstruation is established. The average age for the first menstrual period is about 12½ years, but its occurrence from age 9 to age 17 is considered normal.

Varying in length from 21 to 35 days but averaging 28 days, the menstrual cycle is considered to start on the first day of menstrual bleeding and to end the day before the next menstruation starts. Each month the endometrium is built up in preparation for a possible pregnancy. If pregnancy does not occur, the outer layer of the endometrium is shed as menstrual bleeding. The menstrual flow typically lasts from 3 to 7 days. The amount of fluid lost, which is usually small, varies from person to person but is usually about the same for a given individual.

The menstrual cycle can be divided into three phases: the proliferative phase, the secretory phase, and menstruation (see Figure 4–2). The proliferative, or preovulatory, phase begins when menstrual

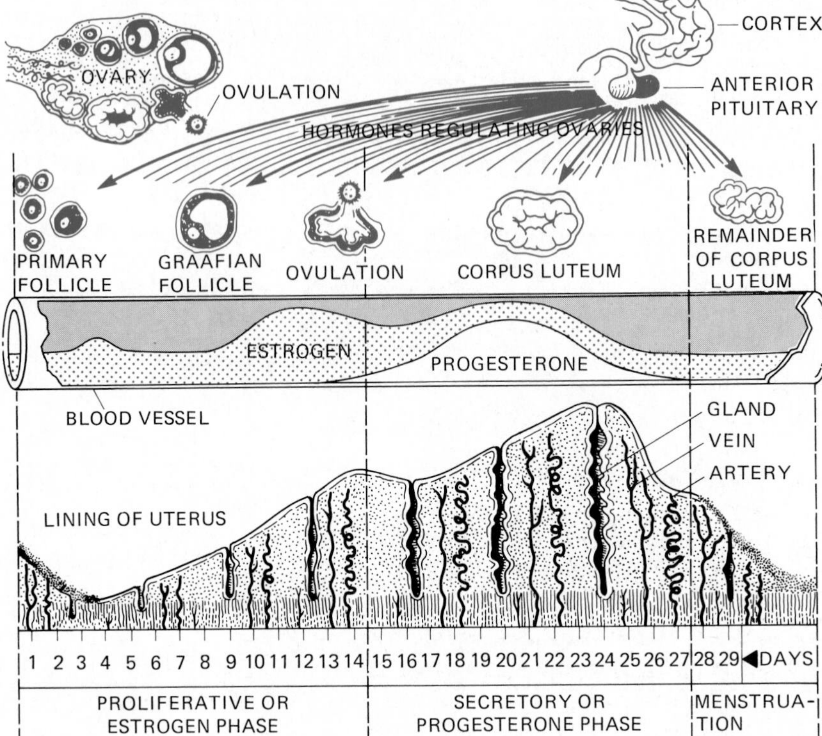

Figure 4-2. The Menstrual Cycle.
This diagram shows the important anatomical and physiological events that constitute the menstrual cycle. (Source: John Burt and Linda Brower Meeks, *Education for Sexuality: Concepts and Programs for Teachers* [© 1975, by W. B. Saunders Company; reprinted by permission of CBS College Publishing]).

bleeding ceases. During menstruation and proliferation the pituitary gland stimulates the maturation of 15 to 20 egg follicles in the ovaries and induces these follicles to produce estrogen. The endometrium, which had become thin during the previous menstrual flow, begins to thicken. As the egg follicles grow, the amount of estrogen continues to rise. About 14 days before menstruation, the most mature egg follicle bursts, releasing the mature egg. The other follicles degenerate and are absorbed by the body. After ovulation, the egg enters the fallopian tube. For approximately 12 to 24 hours, while the egg is in the upper third of the fallopian tube, it is available for fertilization.

Corpus luteum Mass of endocrine cells formed after the release of an ovum.

Ovulation marks the beginning of the secretory, or postovulatory phase. The ruptured follicle becomes the **corpus luteum.** At this point in the cycle the pituitary causes the corpus luteum to produce high levels of estrogen and progesterone, the second major female sex hormone. The progesterone stimulates glands in the endometrium to secrete a fluid suitable for nourishing a fertilized egg.

If pregnancy does not occur, the corpus luteum decomposes. With the destruction of the corpus luteum, estrogen and progesterone levels fall, and the lining of the uterus begins to shrink and decompose, resulting in menstruation, the expulsion of blood, mucus, and fragments of the endometrium through the cervix and vagina.

Menstrual Irregularities

Menorrhagia. Excessive, prolonged menstrual flow, called **menorrhagia,** may require a doctor's attention, since repeated occurrences can drain a woman's body of its iron supply and result in anemia. Heavy bleeding may be related to the loss of pregnancy in its early stages (miscarriage), the use of an intrauterine device (IUD) for contraceptive purposes, or a disorder involving the endometrium.

Menorrhagia Excessive or prolonged menstrual flow.

Amenorrhea. Latin for "without menstrual flow," **amenorrhea** is the natural result of pregnancy, lactation (breast-feeding), and menopause. It is considered normal for girls who are not yet ovulating. However, illness, severe emotional stress, or a drastic change in diet or body weight can also cause menstruation to cease. In cases where no cause can be detected, a doctor may prescribe hormones to artificially trigger the menstrual cycle.

Amenorrhea Absence or abnormal cessation of menstruation.

Irregular periods. After menarche irregular periods are normal for the first year or two, but for some women a predictable menstrual pattern does not develop. The cause is not always detectable, but minor hormone imbalances may play a role, as may physical and emotional stress.

Dysmenorrhea. The most common problem related to the menstrual cycle is **dysmenorrhea,** or painful menstruation. It usually refers to painful cramping in the lower abdomen but may also involve headache, backache, nausea, and diarrhea. Once believed to be mainly psychosomatic, dysmenorrhea is actually often caused by high levels of chemicals in the menstrual fluid called prostaglandins. Drugs that inhibit prostaglandin can greatly reduce dysmenorrhea.

Dysmennorrhea Painful menstruation.

Premenstrual tension. Often experienced as depression, headache, or irritability and involving breast tenderness, weight gain, and a bloated feeling (due to retention of fluids), premenstrual tension, commonly referred to as **premenstrual syndrome** or **PMS** (see box), probably results from an imbalance of estrogen and progesterone just prior to the menstrual period. Although the reaction to PMS by some women is severe enough to warrant medical care, in most women the condition is mild and requires no treatment.

Premenstrual Syndrome (PMS) Distress experienced by some women prior to menstruation.

YOUR HEALTH TODAY

PMS

For some women the four to seven days prior to menstruation can be problematic. The premenstrual distress experienced by these women can be so severe that they can become psychologically and emotionally upset. There have been reported instances in which PMS has allegedly driven some women to violence. Neither researchers nor physicians who have studied PMS are in agreement as to whether or not this condition can lead its sufferers to aberrant behavior. Two points remain uncontested, however: (1) PMS exists and can cause a great deal of distress for some women, and (2) not all women suffer from PMS.

Male Reproductive Organs

External Organs

Penis Male organ for copulation and urination

Glans penis The sensitive, conical head of the penis.

The external sex organs of the male consist of the penis and the scrotum (see Figure 4–3). The **penis** (''tail''), the male organ for copulation and urination, has a conical head, the highly sensitive **glans penis,** which is partially protected by the foreskin, a thin cover that can be pulled back. Circumcision is the removal of the foreskin. The procedure leaves the glans and the neck of the penis exposed, thereby preventing the accumulation of bacteria and smegma, a cheeselike substance secreted by small glands.

The penis of the average man measures three to four inches in length and one inch in diameter when limp. During sexual arousal, blood enters the penis and is trapped in the numerous spongelike cavities, resulting in an erection, which stiffens the organ and causes it to become longer and thicker. Once the penis is erect, the man is ready for intercourse. Contrary to popular belief, the size of the penis is unrelated to a man's race, body build, virility, or ability to give and receive sexual pleasure.

Scrotum Pouch containing the testicles.

The **scrotum,** a multilayered pouch containing the testicles, has many sweat glands and is dotted with pubic hair. The inner layer consists of strong connective tissue and muscle that contracts in response to cold, sexual arousal, fear, anger, and other stimuli, giving the scrotum a compact, wrinkled look. Otherwise, the scrotum is uncontracted and its surface is smooth.

Internal Organs

Testicles Sperm-producing organs.

Sperm Male cells capable of fertilizing the female ovum.

The **testicles** or **testes** (Latin for ''witnesses''—from the early custom of placing the hand over the genitals when taking an oath), are two oval-shaped organs that each weigh about one ounce. the left testicle typically hangs lower than the right. Occasionally, one or both testicles remain undescended after birth (they are contained within the abdominal cavity during fetal development). Unless the condition is corrected, the testicles will not produce **sperm,** since a temperature lower than normal body temperature is essential for sperm development.

Contained within the scrotum, each testicle is enclosed separately in a compact, fibrous sheath of connective tissue that branches on the inside into a series of conical lobes. Each lobe is the site of sperm production, where hundreds of millions of sperm are produced and stored. The formation of sperm in the testes takes approximately 60 days.

Sperm do not mature in the testes. Instead, they continue through several structures that act as maturation and storage sites, produce secretions to increase the sperms' mobility and fertility, and provide

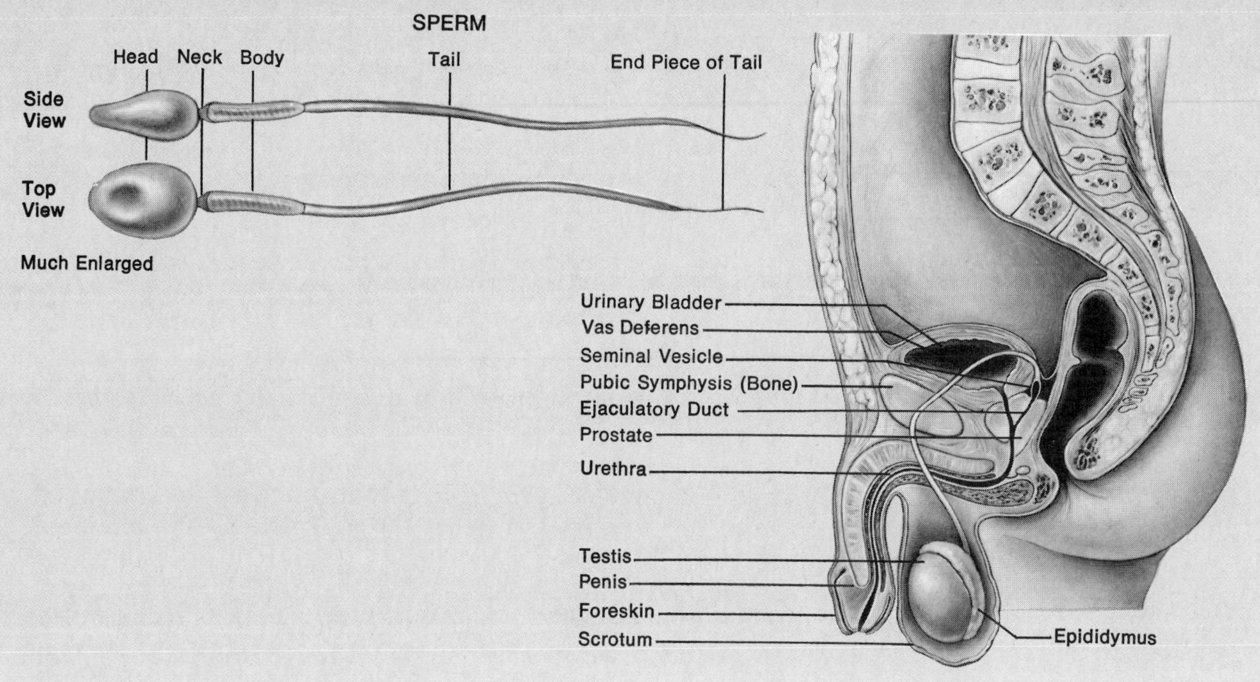

Figure 4-3. Male Reproductive Organs.
Above, **a mature sperm cell, or spermatozoon. The motion of the tail provides locomotion.** ***Right,*** **cross section of male reproductive organs.**

the mechanism whereby the sperm are discharged from the body. The immature sperm move through an intricate system of ducts that combine to form a larger duct, the **epididymis.** A long (about 20 feet) tube, the epididymis is tightly coiled and forms a band on top of and behind the testicle. It leads to the less convoluted **vas deferens,** a cordlike, 18-inch-long structure that travels upward from the testicle into the abdominal cavity. Sperm can be stored in the vas deferens for as long as 42 days without losing their fertility.

Epididymis Coiled duct from the testicle to the vas deferens

Vas deferens Cordlike structure in which the sperm are stored.

The *seminal vesicles,* which lie on the bottom rear surface of the urinary bladder, produce a variety of substances that help nourish the sperm. Each seminal vesicle joins the corresponding vas deferens to form the **ejaculatory duct,** a straight, one-inch-long structure that runs through the **prostate.** During ejaculation, secretions from the prostate and the seminal vesicles and millions of sperm combine to form semen, a sticky fluid propelled through the urethra and out of the body. Unlike egg cells, which are all present in the ovaries by the time a girl is born, sperm are continually being developed in a male's testicles from puberty until old age.

Ejaculatory duct The short structure that runs through the prostate

Prostate Male gland that surrounds the urethral base.

The **bulbourethral (Cowper's) glands,** two pea-sized structures at the base of the penis, secrete a clear bit of fluid that appears on the tip of the penis during sexual arousal. This fluid, called the love drop, is not part of the semen, but it usually contains some sperm. Their presence is responsible for those pregnancies that result from intercourse without ejaculation.

Bulbourethral (Cowper's) glands Fluid-omitting glands at the base of the penis.

Urethra The tube extending from bladder to urethral opening.

The final passage for both urine and semen, the **urethra,** begins at the bottom of the urinary bladder and extends through the center of the shaft of the penis and ends in a small opening at the tip of the glans. A muscle at the neck of the bladder contracts to prevent urine and semen from being released at the same time.

Onset of Puberty in Males

Most boys do not enter puberty until age 10 or 11, and the process may last for as long as 10 years. The first notable changes are growth of pubic hair and enlargement of the penis and testicles at about age 13 or 14. Approximately a year later, hair appears in the armpits, and some fuzz sprouts on the upper lip. During the next few years the beard continues to develop. Under the influence of testosterone, a male hormone, height and weight increase markedly, with the greatest growth in the long bones in the arms and legs and in the shoulder, chest, and thigh muscles. When a boy is about 14 or 15, another hormone triggers the development of mature sperm in the seminiferous tubules of the testes. About this time the boy may begin experiencing *nocturnal emissions,* or wet dreams—erotic dreams that culminate in ejaculation.

Conception

The process of conception, development, and birth of a baby begins with a single sperm and a single egg, tiny cells that contain all the information necessary for the creation of a new life.

Fertilization

Of the approximately 350 million sperm cells deposited in the upper vagina with each ejaculation, relatively few manage to penetrate the mucus-filled cervical canal and begin a 2½-inch upward journey to the fallopian tubes. Sperm reach the egg in the upper third of the fallopian tube, where fertilization occurs, approximately two hours after intercourse and are able to fertilize an egg up to 72 hours after being deposited in the vagina. Conception is unlikely, however, unless the sperm reaches the egg within 24 hours of ovulation. After that time, the egg begins to fragment and disintegrate.

Chromosomes Linear bodies responsible for transmitting heredity.

Only one sperm fertilizes the egg, penetrating its outer membrane and adding its 23 **chromosomes** to the 23 in the egg to form a 46-chromosome human cell. Once the sperm has penetrated the membrane, the egg becomes impenetrable to other sperm. The egg then makes its way down the fallopian tube to the uterine cavity for implantation, a journey that takes from three to five days.

Occasionally, two mature eggs are released from the ovary, resulting in the birth of fraternal twins if both eggs are fertilized. Fraternal

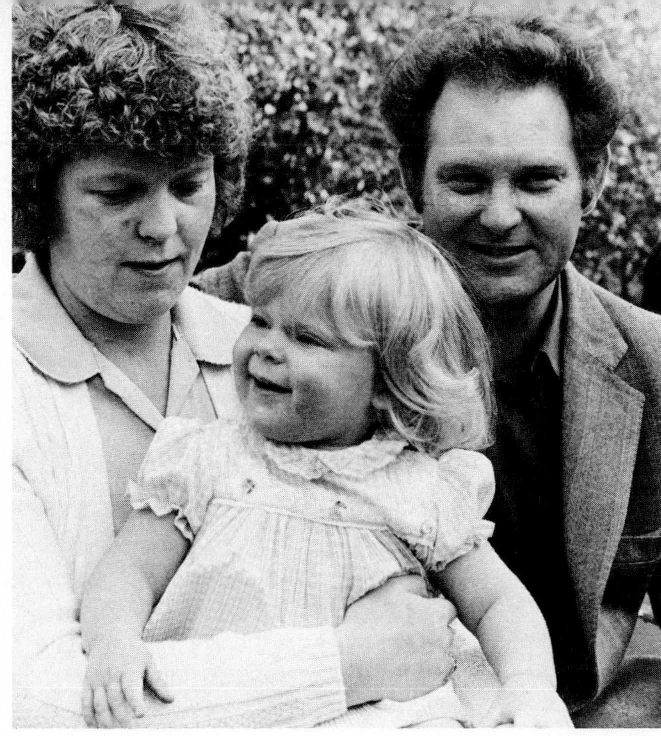

Louise Brown, the world's first test tube baby, with her parents. (Photo from Syndication International/Photo Trends)

twins are not necessarily the same sex, and they may or may not resemble each other. Three fertilized eggs result in triplets, four in quadruplets, and so forth. Identical twins, who originate from a single fertilized egg that splits into identical portions early in its development, are always the same sex and bear a striking resemblance to each other. Some fertility drugs apparently increase the incidence of multiple births by stimulating greater egg production and therefore multiple ovulation.

Infertility

It has been estimated that 10 to 15 percent of married couples in the United States are unable to conceive a child. (This figure does not include those who are voluntarily childless.) About 40 percent of these cases are due to sterility of the male partner. Sterility may result from low sperm production due to hormonal imbalances or genital abnormalities, a blockage in the tiny tubules of the epididymis that prevents sperm from appearing in the semen, or sexual dysfunction (impotence or premature ejaculation). Female infertility can be caused by failure to ovulate, which may be related to menstrual irregularities, hormonal imbalances, or ovarian abnormalities. Malformations, blockages, or infection of the vagina, cervix, uterus, or, most commonly, the fallopian tubes may cause sterility by preventing the journey of either the sperm or egg to the site of fertilization.

Couples are usually advised to try to conceive a child for a year before undergoing diagnostic tests to determine the cause of the infertility. Many treatments are available. Among the most successful are drug therapy to stimulate ovulation and surgery to repair a damaged portion of the reproductive tract.

YOUR HEALTH TODAY

Artificial Processes of Fertilization

If a man is producing no sperm at all or if his sperm count is very low, *artificial insemination* is an alternative. In this procedure a woman is impregnated, usually, with sperm from an unknown donor. The woman comes to a clinician's office daily or every other day around ovulation time, and the donor's semen is placed in her vagina near the cervix. A man with some active sperm, but not enough to father a child, may have his semen mixed with that of the donor so that the child has some chance of having his chromosomes.

The birth of Louise Brown in July 1978 represented a major step in the conquest of human infertility. The British scientists Patrick Steptoe and Robert Edwards removed a mature egg from the ovary of Lesley Brown, who could not conceive naturally because of blocked fallopian tubes. In a process called *in vitro fertilization,* the egg was fertilized by sperm from Mrs. Brown's husband in the laboratory and then placed in the uterus of the mother. There, it implanted itself and grew into a healthy baby, the first so-called test-tube baby in medical history.

While offering hope to many women who have been unable to become pregnant, the Steptoe–Edwards procedure has also raised troubling ethical and legal concerns. For example, what is the legal status of a baby conceived in a laboratory and implanted in the uterus of a woman other than the biological mother? Does the destruction of a fertilized egg in the laboratory constitute murder? Some groups have denounced the process as unnatural and immoral, predicting dire consequences if scientists proceed in their quest to "create life." However, with fewer and fewer babies available for adoption, many couples continue to welcome this means of increasing their chances to become parents.

Pregnancy

By the time a woman consults a doctor about a missed period, she usually has a fairly good idea that she is pregnant. Failure to menstruate (amenorrhea) is usually the first symptom of pregnancy. Many women also experience a pronounced fullness of the breasts as mammary glands enlarge and blood supply to the breasts increases in preparation for lactation (milk production). The breasts become firmer and more tender and the nipples may tingle and feel sore. These sensations usually disappear as the pregnancy progresses, although the breasts continue to increase in size, and the nipples and areolae (areas around the nipples) enlarge and darken.

Some unpleasant symptoms associated with pregnancy in some women are nausea and vomiting. These conditions usually start about two weeks after the first missed period and last for about six to eight weeks. Nausea usually occurs in the morning (hence the popular name, "morning sickness"), but many women feel sick in the evening and throughout the day. In some instances, a suggestible husband may vomit with his pregnant wife.

Pressure on the bladder from the expanding uterus may lead to increased urination as early as the first missed period. This problem lessens somewhat as the uterus rises up into the abdomen, but can become a problem later when the baby's head sinks down and puts pressure on the bladder.

Diagnosis of Pregnancy

By the sixth week of pregnancy (four weeks after a missed period), changes in the breasts, cervix, and uterus are apparent upon pelvic examination. By inserting two fingers of one hand into the vagina and pressing gently on the abdomen just below the navel with the other hand, a clinician can feel the shape of the uterus and tell if it is enlarged, as would be expected during pregnancy. In addition, as a result of increased blood supply, the vagina and cervix take on a purplish color instead of the normal pink.

Laboratory pregnancy tests are based on the presence of HCG (human chorionic gonadotropin), a hormone produced only during pregnancy. A few drops of the woman's urine or blood are put in a test tube or small dish and treated chemically. If HCG is detected, there is a 95 to 98 percent chance that the woman is pregnant. A recent innovation, at-home pregnancy test kits, can, if used correctly, detect HCG in the urine of a pregnant woman as soon as nine days after a missed period. The result of a do-it-yourself test should be confirmed by a clinician.

A woman carries her baby for about 266 days, or approximately nine months. The expected delivery date can be calculated by adding 280 days to the first day of the last menstrual period. For example, a woman who last began menstruating on January 1 can expect to give birth within a few days of October 7, 280 days later. However, two weeks before or after the due date is considered on time.

Most obstetricians divide pregnancy into three-month periods called *trimesters*. The striking changes as the fetus develops during pregnancy are shown in Figure 4–4.

First Trimester

Within 12 hours after fertilization, the egg begins dividing. The solid mass of cells thus formed journeys down the fallopian tube and on about the fourth or fifth day passes into the uterus. By the tenth to twelfth day, the group of cells attaches itself to the endometrium, where it will grow and develop throughout pregnancy. A layer of cells across the center of the group ultimately develops into the fetus; the remaining cells form the **placenta,** the **amniotic sac,** and the membranes that will contain the fetus.

Placenta Organ of interchange between the fetus and the mother.

Amniotic sac Fluid-filled sac that protects the embryo.

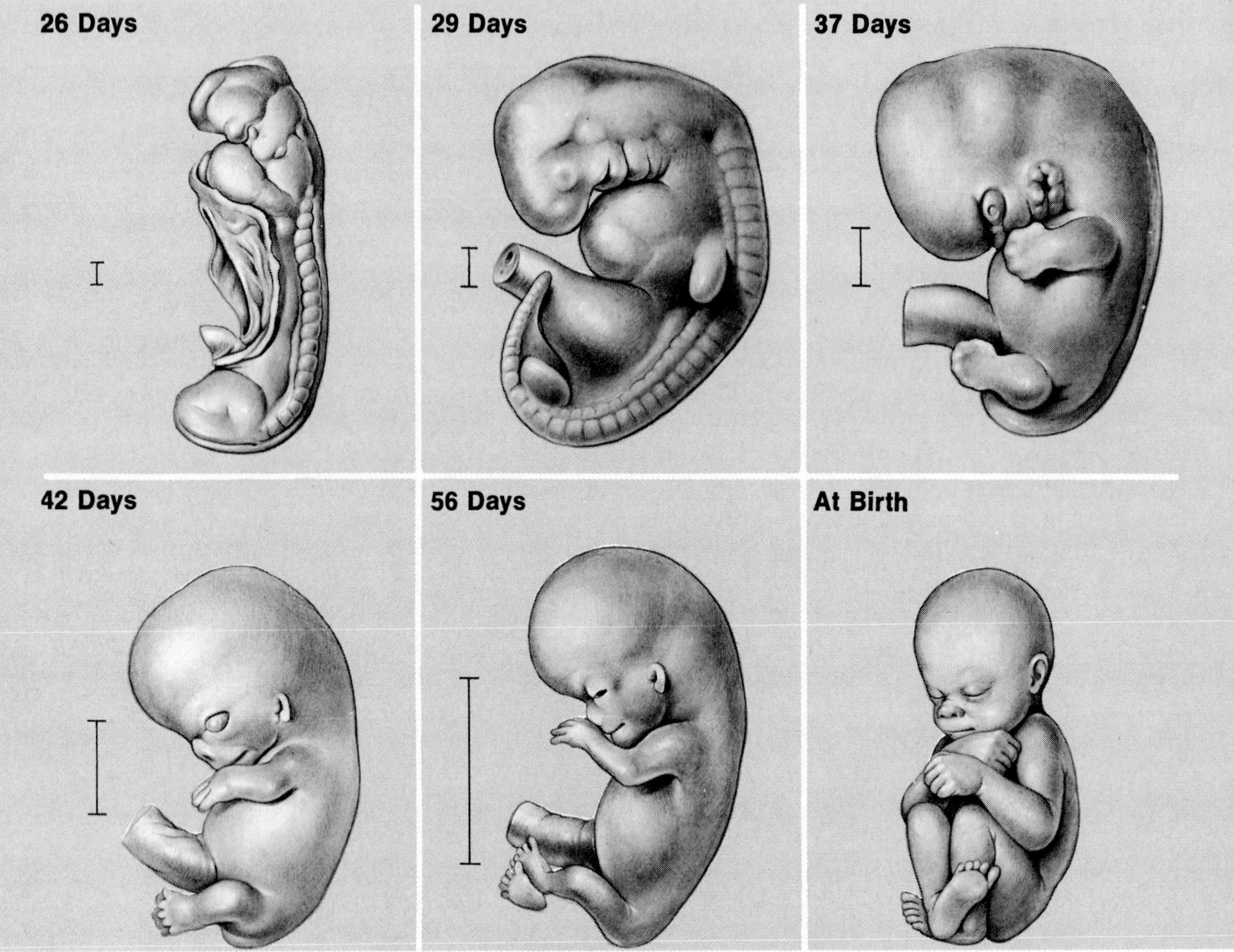

Figure 4-4. Development of the Human Embryo.
The actual length of the human embryo at various stages is indicated by the vertical lines at the left of the figures. At the end of nine months (lower right), it is about 20 inches long.

Connected to the developing fetus by the blood vessels of the umbilical cord, the placenta is the organ through which the fetus receives nourishment from and empties waste matter into the circulatory system of the mother. The amniotic fluid surrounds and shields the fetus, protecting it against cold and heat and acting as a shock absorber should the mother fall or receive a blow to the abdomen. Amniotic fluid is completely replaced about eight times daily.

Embryo Fertilized egg after implantation in the uterus.

Once implanted in the uterine wall, the fertilized egg is called an **embryo.** A 4-week-old embryo is about three sixteenths of an inch long and weighs about one seventh of an ounce. It has a heart that pulsates and pumps blood. The backbone, spinal canal, and digestive system are beginning to form. Small buds that will eventually become arms and legs are present, but no eyes, nose, or ears are visible.

After 8 weeks of pregnancy, the embryo, now called a **fetus,** is about an inch long and weighs about one third of an ounce. Limbs are beginning to show distinct divisions into arms, elbows, forearm, hand, thigh, knee, lower leg, and foot. Facial features are forming, and development of some bones and internal organs are underway. Gonads are present, but the fetus cannot yet be physically distinguished as male or female.

Fetus Embryo from the eighth week until birth.

Second Trimester

The most dramatic occurrence during the middle three months of pregnancy is *quickening:* the first faint, fluttering movements of the fetus are felt by the mother. At first, the motions are so gentle that they may be confused with intestinal gas, but as the pregnancy progresses and the baby becomes bigger and stronger, movements of the fetal arms and legs may feel like powerful thrusts from within. These pokes and jabs are a joyful confirmation that the fetus is alive. As the baby continues to grow, so does the mother's abdomen, and before the second trimester is ended, most women are visibly pregnant.

The second trimester is usually the most relaxing and enjoyable period of pregnancy. The physical discomforts of the first trimester have disappeared, and the growing fetus is not yet a major physical burden.

By the end of the fourth month, the fetus is about 7 inches long, weighs about 4 ounces and has a strong heartbeat and active muscles. Eyes, ears, nose, mouth, and eyebrows are clearly defined.

At 5 months, the fetus's internal organs are maturing rapidly, but the lungs are insufficiently developed to cope with conditions outside the uterus.

By the end of the sixth month, the fetus is about 14 inches long and weighs about two pounds. The skin—quite wrinkled and still somewhat red—is coated with a heavy, creamy protective coating. Eyelids are finally separated and fingernails extend to the end of the fingers. The development of special techniques in the care of premature infants has made it possible for a baby born at the end of the second trimester to survive.

Third Trimester

As the pregnancy progresses, the baby becomes more and more active, occasionally keeping its mother awake nights as it twists and turns within the confines of the uterus. A woman may feel increasingly ungainly as her body swells, and once-easy tasks such as tying her shoes or getting out of bed may require extra effort. Until recently, strict weight control during pregnancy was encouraged to keep the baby small for an easier delivery. Many clinicians now urge women to gain between 24 and 30 pounds, because studies reveal that high-birth-weight babies are usually stronger, healthier, and more intelligent. Excessive weight gain, however, does not benefit the baby, and it places a burden on the mother's heart and lungs.

Smooth-skinned and polished-looking, a full-term baby (one that has remained in its mother's uterus for nine months) is about 20 inches long and weighs about 7 pounds 6 ounces. It is still covered with the creamy coating, but the fine downy hair has largely disappeared (some may remain on the shoulders and arms). Nails protrude beyond the end of fingers and toes, and head hair is approximately one inch long. Lungs are fully mature and able to support life. Ninety-nine percent of the full-term babies born alive in the United States survive.

Amniocentesis

Amniocentesis A process for detecting fetal abnormalities.

Amniocentesis is a procedure used to detect abnormalities in the developing fetus. It is usually performed between the fourteenth and sixteenth weeks of pregnancy and involves inserting a long, hollow needle below the navel into the cavity of the uterus. About 2½ teaspoons of the amniotic fluid that surrounds the baby (and contains cells from the baby) are drawn off and analyzed for chromosomal abnormalities (including Down's syndrome), inherited diseases (such as Tay-Sachs disease and sickle-cell anemia), sex-linked disorders (hemophilia, muscular dystrophy), and structural defects of the spine. The presence of a Y chromosome indicates that the fetus is male.

Amniocentesis is generally preceded by an ultrasound procedure: sound waves are bounced off the amniotic sac to make a picture of the baby and the placenta. The practitioner performing the amniocentesis can then insert the needle into the amniotic sac without harming the baby. There is a very slight risk that the procedure will induce premature labor. Because of this risk, however, it is not recommended that amniocentesis be used solely to discover the sex of the fetus.

At present, amniocentesis cannot detect birth defects that are the result of viruses, X-rays, drugs, or any of the many other environmental factors that could cause fetal damage. It can detect only a small number of the several thousand known defects.

Amniocentesis can be used to determine the presence of chromosomal abnormalities, inherited diseases, sex-linked disorders, and structural defects of the spine. (Photo © William Hubbell 1980/Woodfin Camp & Associates)

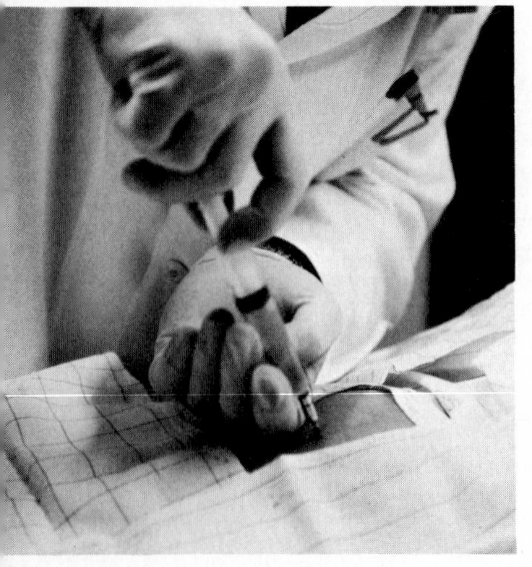

Complications During Pregnancy

Miscarriage and Premature Delivery

Between 10 and 15 percent of all pregnancies end in miscarriage (also known as spontaneous abortion), which is most frequent during the first trimester. Usually preceded by cramps and vaginal bleeding, a miscarriage is said to have occurred if the fetus is expelled from the uterus through the vagina before the fetus has developed sufficiently to survive on its own. At least 50 percent of spontaneous abortions occur because the fetus was not forming properly. One in seven miscarriages is thought to be caused by illness, malnutrition, malformation of the reproductive system, or a serious injury. Women should be warned not to blame themselves for an unsuccessful pregnancy. Miscarriage does not affect fertility, and most women who miscarry eventually produce a live, healthy baby.

Premature labor and delivery, a possible problem during the third trimester of pregnancy, may result from a serious illness of the mother, malfunction of the placenta, or heavy cigarette smoking. At least half the time, however, the cause of premature births is unknown. It has been shown, however, that teenage mothers tend to have more premature births than mothers in their twenties or thirties. Babies born too soon tend to be tiny and frail. They often experience breathing difficulties because oxygen cannot penetrate the membranes of the immature lungs.

Influence of Drugs

It was once believed that the placenta acted like a sieve, filtering out all substances harmful to the fetus; we now know that this is untrue. Some drugs taken by the mother can cause malformations in the fetus, particularly during the first trimester, when fetal development is most rapid. The most widely known drug of this nature is *thalidomide,* a mild sedative that resulted in the birth of several thousand armless and legless children in West Germany and England in the early 1960s. Some drugs used to prevent miscarriage have been linked to fetal abnormalities, particularly *DES (diethylstilbestrol),* a potent estrogen that can cause vaginal cancer and malformations of the reproductive system in late-adolescent girls whose mothers took the drug while pregnant.

Ongoing studies report several areas of concern for sons of mothers who used DES. Such problems as undescended testicles, benign cysts on the epididimus, underdeveloped testes, and sperm and semen abnormalities have been reported.[1]

Drug addiction, excessive alcohol consumption, and smoking are often harmful to the fetus. A heroin- or morphine-addicted mother usually gives birth to a child who will suffer potentially fatal withdrawal symptoms if not treated promptly. A heavy drinker has a greater than average chance of producing a baby with a facial, limb, or heart defect, and infants born to women who smoke are usually smaller and more fragile than babies of nonsmokers. Cigarette smoking also increases the risk of miscarriage and stillbirth (death of the child in the uterus).

Diseases and Infections

Rubella (German measles) can be devastating to a fetus, often causing cataracts, congenital heart disease, deafness, and mental retardation. Women who contract the disease during the first three months of pregnancy are usually urged to consider abortion. Women who have never had the disease should be vaccinated against rubella only if they are not pregnant and are not planning to become pregnant for at least six months (the vaccine contains live rubella virus, which may harm a developing fetus).

Most other viral infections, including influenza, true measles (rubeola), chicken pox, mumps, scarlet fever, and whooping cough, apparently do not cause congenital malformations.

Toxemia

Toxemia, a serious and potentially fatal complication of pregnancy, gets its name from the Latin words meaning "blood" and "poison." The condition is characterized by high blood pressure, protein in the urine, and the retention of fluids by the body. Prompt treatment is necessary to prevent convulsions and possibly death. The causes of toxemia are unknown, but it is believed that poor maternal nutrition is a factor. Treatment consists of bed rest and restricted salt intake (to prevent fluid retention). In more severe cases, hospitalization may be required.

The Rh Factor

Rh incompatibility is a condition that may cause antibodies in the mother's red blood cells to destroy the red blood cells of her baby. The Rh factor (named for the Rhesus monkeys in which it was discovered) is attached to the red blood cells of 85 percent of the population. A woman with Rh-negative blood (one whose blood lacks the Rh factor) may give birth to an Rh-positive baby. As the baby is born, some of its blood cells mix with the mother's blood cells, which, sensing the presence of a foreign invader (the Rh factor), proceed to form antibodies. These antibodies then stand guard, programmed to attack should the same invader ever reappear. If the woman then becomes pregnant with a second Rh-positive baby, the antibodies spring into action, crossing the placental barrier and attacking the blood cells of the fetus, making the baby severely anemic and occasionally causing death.

Modern treatment has succeeded in minimizing the effects of Rh disease. When an Rh-negative woman becomes pregnant, her blood is analyzed for the presence of the antibody. If it is found, and if amniocentesis later reveals that the fetus is severely affected, a blood transfusion can be given to the baby in the uterus. Complete prevention of Rh disease is also possible by injection of a serum into the bloodstream of an Rh-negative woman after any incident during which Rh-positive cells may have entered her bloodstream. These incidents include delivery of an Rh-positive child, abortion, or miscarriage. The serum contains substances that destroy the Rh-positive cells in the woman's body before she develops her own antibodies against them.

Prenatal Care

Surprisingly, there are still women in the United States who walk into a clinic to give birth without having seen a medical practitioner during the entire course of pregnancy.

For healthy women, prenatal care is preventive medicine to verify that the fetus is growing normally and the mother is maintaining good health. For a woman with diabetes or high blood pressure, prenatal care is essential to her own health and the health of the child she is carrying.

Prenatal care begins with the selection of a physician or a certified nurse-midwife to monitor the pregnancy. Midwives are expertly trained to deal with low-risk pregnancy and delivery. They usually work in concert with a physician, or there is a doctor on call should unexpected complications develop.

A woman most often seeks prenatal care to confirm that she is pregnant, and she is seen by a clinician monthly through the seventh month, every two weeks during the eighth month, then every week until the baby is born. Blood pressure and weight are checked at each visit. A rise in blood pressure and an abrupt weight gain warn that toxemia may be developing. Urine is checked for the presence of protein (a sign of toxemia) and sugar (a sign of diabetes). In addition, the clinician palpates the abdomen to determine if the fetus is growing at a normal rate.

Diet during pregnancy should be well balanced and nutritious. A pregnant woman is not really "eating for two," but she does need extra iron and protein, and she should consume increased quantities of vegetables, fruits, meat, fish, eggs, milk, milk products, and grains (bread, cereal, wheat germ, pasta). Vitamin and iron supplements are often helpful but they should be consumed in moderation. A woman should never diet while she is pregnant.

Exercise is as important during pregnancy as it is during any other time of life. Walking, swimming, and many of the exercises taught in natural childbirth classes improve circulation and minimize many ordinary discomforts of pregnancy, including lower back pain and swelling of the legs. Pregnancy is not a good time to take up a new sport, but activities that were standard before pregnancy can be continued. If there is no vaginal bleeding or other complication, sex can be enjoyed throughout pregnancy. Position during intercourse may have to be modified to allow for the woman's expanding abdomen.

Childbirth

Three or four weeks before labor begins, a woman having her first child experiences **lightening:** the fetus drops into the pelvic cavity, relieving pressure on the mother's ribs and making breathing easier.

Lightening The fetus's drop down into the pelvic cavity.

Lightening occurs somewhat later in women who have previously borne children.

As labor nears, the mucus plug that served as a cervical barrier during pregnancy may break loose and pass through the vagina as the "bloody show." In about 10 percent of pregnant women, the amniotic sac bursts, and amniotic fluid spurts through the vagina. Labor, which occurs in three stages, usually begins shortly thereafter.

What triggers and sustains labor in humans? This question has not yet been satisfactorily answered, but it is believed that fetal hormones act upon the placenta and uterus, causing rhythmic contractions to begin. Ultimately, the mother's pituitary gland produces a hormone that causes the powerful contractions needed to expel the fetus. Unlike other pains, labor pains increase and diminish at regular intervals, becoming more lengthy, frequent, and intense as labor progresses. For a baby to be born, it must be forced through the cervix. The first stage of labor is complete when the cervix has dilated to about four inches in diameter—enough to allow the fetus to enter the pelvis and birth canal.

The second stage of labor ends with the birth of the baby. As the uterus continues to contract, the mother begins to "push"—filling her lungs with air, tightening her abdominal muscles, and bearing down. This is indeed "labor," and lasts anywhere from a few minutes to several hours. In some cases, forceps—pincerlike instruments—must be used to assist the baby's head into the birth canal. Such intervention is more likely if the mother has been anesthetized and is unable to bear down sufficiently.

Medical doctor delivering healthy newborn. (Photo by Chester Higgins, Jr./Photo Researchers, Inc.)

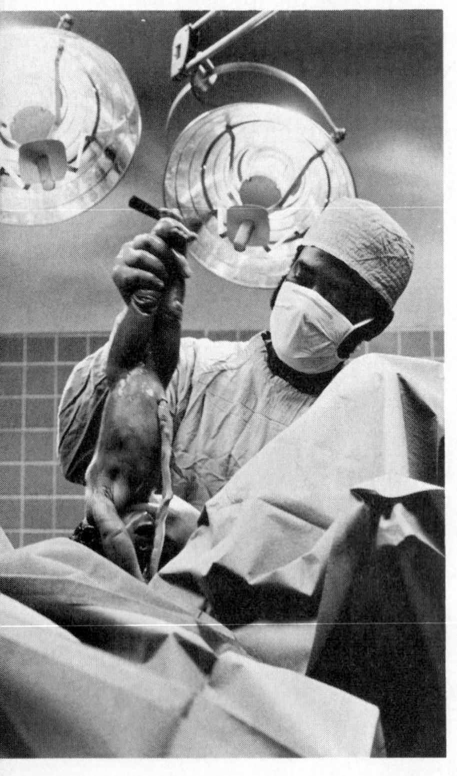

As the mother matches her voluntary pushes with the involuntary contractions provided by nature, the baby's head "crowns" (bulges from the vagina). To prevent tearing the perineum (the tissue lying between the vagina and the rectum), a surgical incision called an *episiotomy* may be made in the perineum. The baby's head is then either pushed or lifted out, spontaneously turning to the side to allow the shoulders to emerge. The rest of the body emerges easily. Using a rubber bulb or tube, the doctor or midwife sucks accumulated mucus and blood from the baby's mouth, and if all is well, the infant responds with a lusty cry, filling its lungs with air for the first time. The mother may have to be distracted from cuddling her new baby and asked to push gently as the placenta separates from the uterine wall and is expelled through the vagina. This third and final stage of labor rarely lasts more than a few minutes.

Methods of Delivery

When anesthesia to ease the pain of childbirth was introduced a number of years ago, many women eagerly welcomed the innovation. However, with the use of pain-relieving drugs, the process of giving birth began to resemble a surgical procedure. The father was banished to a waiting room while the mother was shaved (of pubic hair),

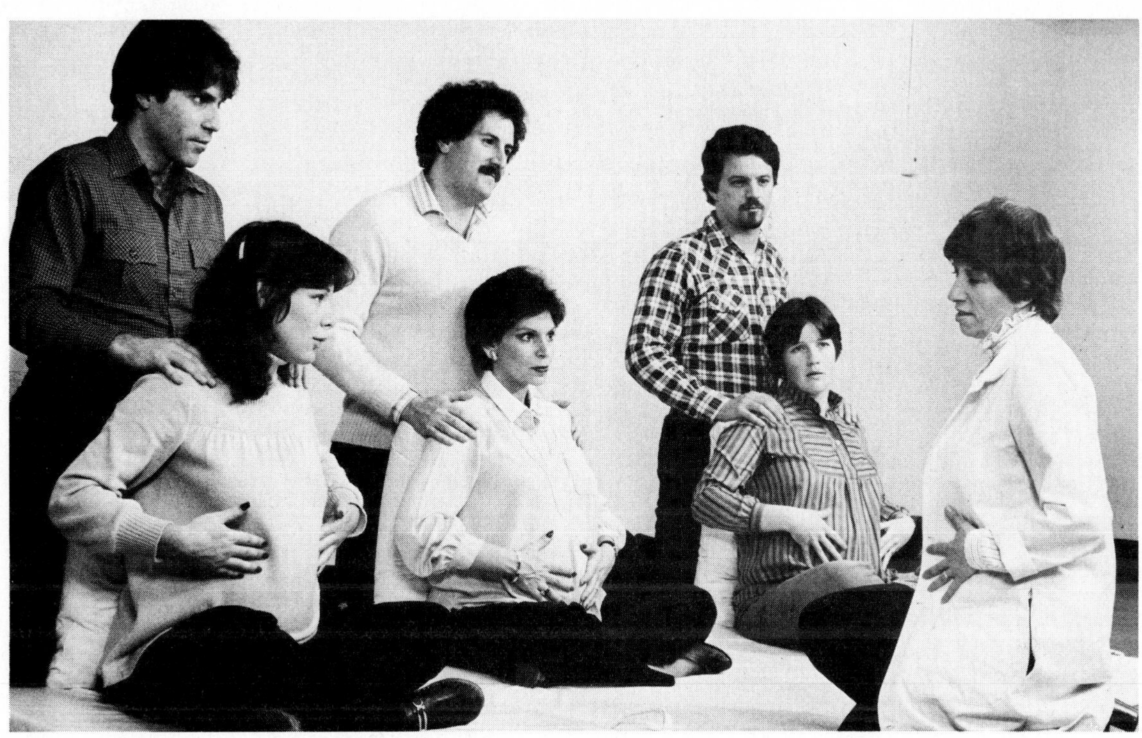

Nurse-instructor teaching the Lamaze method of breathing during labor. (Photo by Robert Goldstein)

bathed in antiseptic, wheeled into a suite resembling an operating room, strapped to a delivery table, and anesthesized. If general anesthesia was used, putting the woman to sleep, she might not even see her new baby until several hours after delivery.

General anesthesia during childbirth is becoming increasingly unpopular, because it entails risks for both mother and baby, prolongs labor, and deprives the mother of the joy of watching her baby emerge. Local anesthetics—novocainelike formulas that are injected into the woman's lower back, inducing a temporary numbness below the waist—are most commonly administered during the second stage of labor. Pain-killers such as Demerol are usually administered in the early phases of labor, enabling the mother to doze off between contractions without actually going to sleep.

Natural Childbirth

Proponents of the **Lamaze method** of natural childbirth (named for the French physician Fernand Lamaze, who developed the technique) have urged women to reject anesthesia, since studies reveal that drugs have a depressant effect on the mother and the fetus (the baby of a woman given general anesthesia may be born asleep). Taught to limit the pain of labor by focusing on a series of breathing exercises, women schooled in the Lamaze method are often able to remain awake and alert throughout labor and delivery. Classes in the mechanics of

Lamaze method Natural childbirth technique involving breathing exercises.

childbirth and exercises designed to facilitate relaxation during labor and strengthen the muscles used in childbirth are also part of the Lamaze method. Husbands who attend Lamaze classes learn how to assist their wives during the various stages of labor, and they are usually allowed to be on hand in the delivery room.

Prepared childbirth Natural childbirth technique designed to reduce tension.

Advocates of **prepared childbirth,** another approach to natural childbirth, believe that fear and tension are the primary sources of pain and difficulty during labor and delivery. As with the Lamaze method, expectant parents attend a series of classes where they learn

YOUR HEALTH TODAY

The Birth Process

Rationale. One of the major causes of uncomfortable pregnancies and also of pain during delivery is fear. Fear is often the result of a lack of information about what is happening or what is about to happen. How much do you know about the birth process?

Objective. To assess one's knowledge of the birth process by completing a crossword puzzle.

Strategy. The following crossword puzzle was designed to give you an opportunity to evaluate your ability to recall the terminology related to the birth process. A glossary of the correct answers with descriptive information follows.

Across

1. When born with weight below five pounds
5. Birth when the buttocks and legs of the baby emerge first
8. Solution injected in amniotic fluid to induce abortion
7. Birth of a dead child
10. Development of fetus within the uterus during the pregnancy
13. Spontaneous premature delivery of a fetus that does not survive
14. The act of impregnation of the ovum by the sperm

Down

1. Interlocking fetal and maternal tissue by which the fetus is nourished
2. Premature expulsion from the uterus of the fertilized ovum
3. The beginning of an organism before it has developed its distinctive form
4. The unborn after the second month of pregnancy
6. Delivery of child by surgery through the abdominal and uterine walls when normal delivery appears impossible
9. The act of giving birth to a baby
11. Fluid surrounding the fetus inside the bag within the uterus
12. The act of bringing forth a child — process of childbirth

Source: Robert Kaplan, Linda Brower Meeks, and Jay Scott Segal, *Group Strategies in Understanding Human Sexuality: Getting in Touch.*

birth procedures and practice relaxation and breathing techniques. The focus is on making childbirth as positive, gratifying, and stress-free an experience as possible for the mother and father.

If for some reason the baby cannot be safely delivered through the birth canal—for example, because the pelvis is too small, the cervix will not dilate, or the fetus is in distress and must be delivered quickly—the baby is removed from the mother's body surgically, through an incision in the lower part of the abdominal wall and through the uterus. The operation is called a **cesarian section.**

Cesarian section Surgical removal of the baby directly through the abdomen.

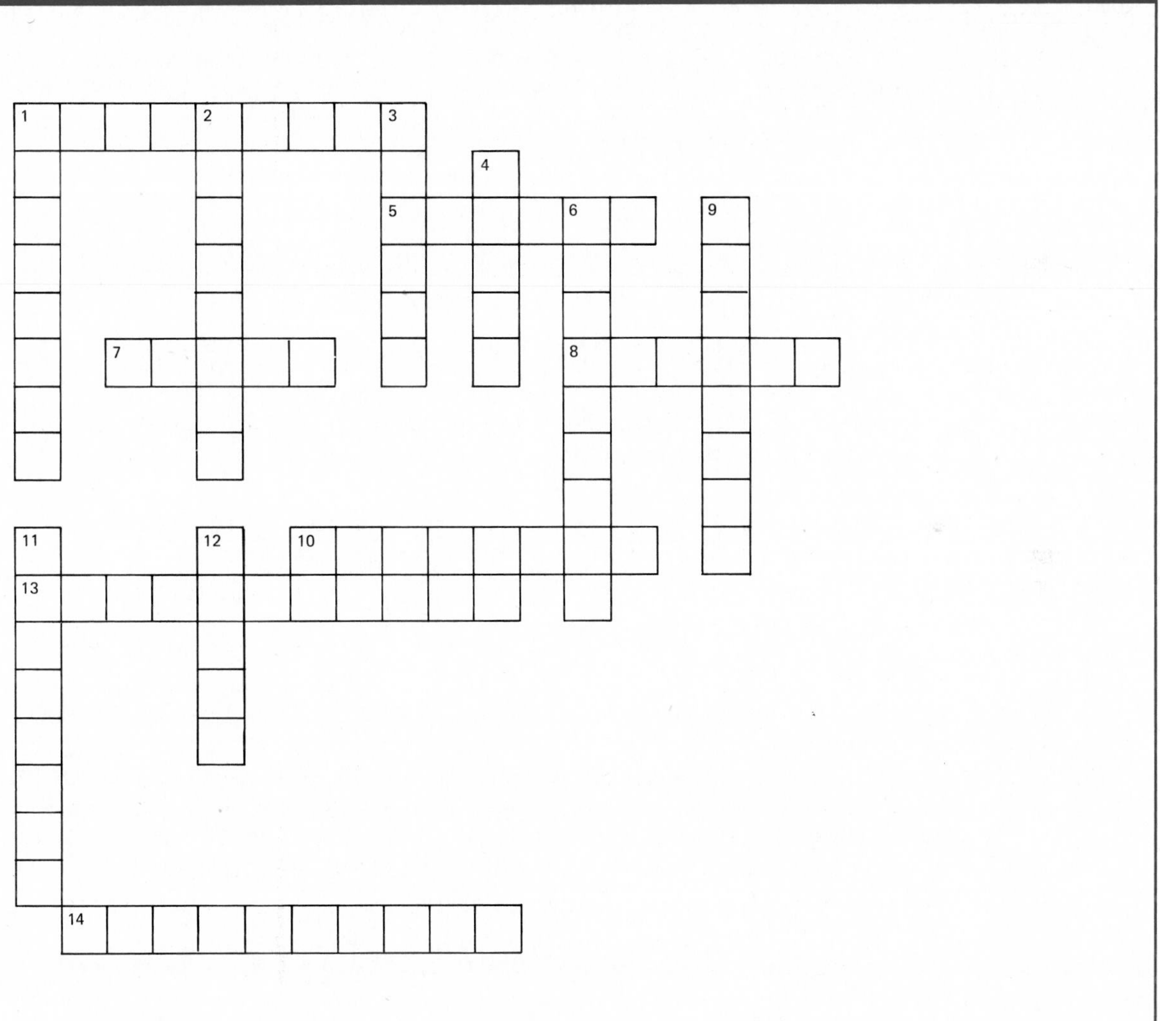

See pages 92 and 93 for answers.

ANSWERS

Across

1. *Premature* refers to infants who weigh less than five pounds, eight ounces at birth; mortality rate among premature infants is directly related to size. About 7 percent of births in the United States are premature. This is a major complication during the third trimester.

5. *Breech* births account for 4 percent of all births. This position is assumed by 50 percent of infants prior to the seventh month of fetal life. A fetus that does not make the turn into the proper position can often be manipulated by the obstetrician during the later stages of birth.

8. *Saline* method for abortion was developed in Sweden and is used after the third month of pregnancy. A needle is inserted through the abdominal and uterine walls and part of the amniotic fluid is removed. This fluid is replaced with an identical amount of strong salt solution and abortion occurs spontaneously within twenty-four to forty-eight hours.

7. *Stillbirths* may be the result of an overdose of hormonal substance called oxytocin that is secreted by the pituitary gland and increased at time of labor to promote uterine contractions.

10. *Prenatal* development is more rapid than growth any other time during one's life span. The most rapid period is from the time of fertilization to the end of the first month.

13. *Miscarriage* occurs in at least 30 percent of all conceptions; it is believed to be nature's way of eliminating an imperfect embryo. Miscarriages may be caused by automobile trips, strenuous physical activity, falls, or emotional shocks. They usually occur in the second or third month of pregnancy.

14. *Conception* is the moment of fertilization; it normally takes part in the upper portion of the fallopian tubes.

Down

1. *Placenta* is a special organ of interchange between embryo and mother. Placental growth is fairly rapid until the fifth month of pregnancy. Shortly after the baby's birth the placenta is detached and expelled through the uterus.

2. *Abortion* is a spontaneous (miscarriage) or induced expulsion of the embryo from the uterus before it has reached a point of development sufficient for its survival.

3. *Embryo* is a stage of the fertilized ovum in early pregnancy; it is unmistakenly human and has a primitive heart beat. After the eighth week it is called a *fetus.*

4. *Fetus* is the term for the unborn child from the third month of pregnancy until birth. At three months it is approximately three inches long.

6. *Caesarian* delivery is the removal of the baby directly from the abdomen. It is a relatively safe procedure; however, physicians usually suggest tying the Fallopian tubes after the third such delivery.

9. *Delivery* is expulsion or extraction of the child at birth.

11. *Amniotic* fluid is the clear, watery fluid in a thin, transparent, tough membrane called the *amnion.* The amniotic fluid serves as a protection for the embryo from jolts and prevents the embryo from forming adhesions to the amnion, which could result in malformations.

12. *Labor* is the first stage of childbirth with any one of three signs: (a) powerful muscle contractions relatively mild at onset and increasing steadily in frequency, intensity, and duration; (b) expulsion of the mucous plug from the base of the uterus; (c) rupture of the amniotic membrane, which causes a flow of clear, waterlike fluid from the vagina.

Postpartum Period

The period following childbirth is called the *postpartum period.* The common, often perplexing phenomenon known as postpartum blues affects many new mothers. Symptomized by sudden crying jags and general feelings of depression, the condition usually disappears gradually as the woman's hormones return to normal and she adjusts to the many changes in her life that motherhood entails.

Lactation

Like natural childbirth, breast-feeding fell out of favor with the advent of modern technology but is now making a comeback. Breast milk is considered the ideal nourishment for a human infant. It is sterile, requires no bottling, contains many vital antibodies, almost never induces an allergic reaction, is always at the right temperature, and is free.

The breast-fed baby's first nourishment is usually **colostrum,** or "early milk," a thin, yellow, nourishing liquid that may drip from the mother's nipples during the last weeks of pregnancy. Within 48 to 72 hours after a woman gives birth, a hormone produced by the pituitary triggers the production of milk in the glands of the breasts. As the infant suckles, the milk is transported through many ducts to the nipples. Assuming that the mother is getting enough to eat and drink, the more the baby sucks, the more plentiful the milk supply. Conversely, if the infant is not breast-fed, the milk dries up.

Colostrum "Early milk" produced in late pregnancy.

Breast-feeding has been called nature's contraceptive, because it tends to delay the return of fertility. However, ovulation can occur at any time, even before menstruation returns. Consequently, this protection is too unpredictable to be depended upon. A nonnursing mother usually menstruates 6 to 8 weeks after giving birth.

Sexual Activity

Normal postpartum bleeding, made up of blood from the site where the placenta was attached and the crumbling lining of the uterus, gradually tapers off and usually stops completely in 3 to 4 weeks. As soon as the flow of postpartum bleeding has ended and the episiotomy or any lacerations have healed, it is safe to resume vaginal intercourse. Sexual activity other than intercourse can resume soon after delivery.

Birth Defects and Genetic Counseling

It is every expectant couple's secret dread that their baby will not be normal. A mother fondling her newborn baby may be simultaneously scanning the tiny body for signs of abnormalities. For most people the odds are excellent that their children will be perfect at birth. Every year, however, more than 250,000 babies in the United States are born with birth defects. Some are the result of environmental influence on the unborn child. Others are genetically caused. Many congenital defects are evident at birth, such as deafness, microcephaly (small head and brain), and spastic cerebral palsy. Other defects appear only later. (See Chapter 18 for a discussion of genetic-related disorders.)

Genetic counseling is available for couples who suspect that they are carriers of a genetic disorder. If a blood test confirms their suspicions, they are advised as to their chances of producing an afflicted child. Should the woman later become pregnant, amniocentesis can detect many genetic diseases prenatally, giving the parents the opportunity to terminate the pregnancy if necessary.

Contraception

It has been said that the only reliable method of birth control is abstinence. This may have been true in the past, when a woman seeking to prevent pregnancy might have resorted to inserting a sponge into her vagina or douching with a variety of exotic concoctions, or, if conception did take place, she might have crudely attempted to abort the unwanted fetus. Today, several effective, medically endorsed methods of contraception are available.

The Pill

Birth-Control Pills. The pill—the popular name for a number of oral contraceptives—was first put on the market in 1960, and by 1977, 54 million women throughout the world were using it. Usually containing synthetic compounds resembling estrogen and progesterone, the pill works by inhibiting secretion of hormones essential to

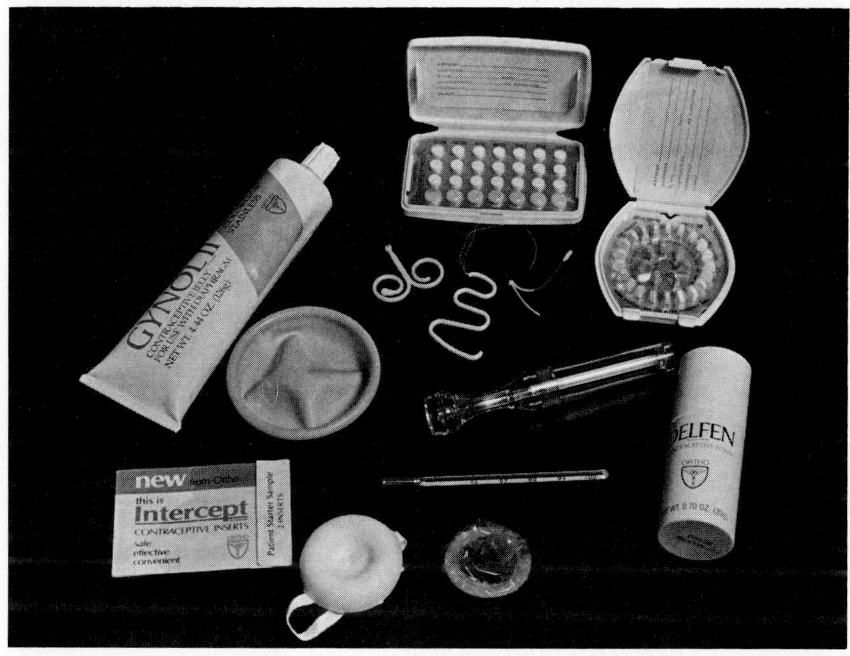

Today various effective contraceptive devices are readily available. (Photo © Alan Carey/The Image Works)

ovulation. True menstruation does not occur when a woman is on the pill, since she has not ovulated; thus, there is a particular advantage for women prone to dysmenorrhea (painful menstrual cramps).

The pill is almost 100 percent effective if used correctly, but in recent years oral contraceptives have been associated with a number of disturbing and potentially lethal side effects, including nausea, weight gain, headache, loss of vision, blood clotting, high blood pressure, and certain types of cancers. If taken during pregnancy, hormonal contraceptives can cause fetal abnormalities. There is an increased risk of heart attack and other circulatory problems, such as strokes, for women who smoke while using oral contraceptives.

The trend has been toward smaller doses of both estrogen and progesterone in an effort to limit side effects.

Mini-Pill. Pill users who experience estrogen-related problems such as high blood pressure and breast tenderness are sometimes advised to switch to the mini-pill, progesterone-only capsules that probably work by interfering with sperm and ovum transport and the development of the uterine lining. Slightly less effective than combined hormonal contraceptives, mini-pills may cause spotting (bleeding between menstrual periods).

The Morning-After Pill. Designed for use after sexual intercourse, the morning-after pill contains DES, a potent estrogen that may cause nausea and vomiting. By law, the morning-after pill can be dispensed only to victims of rape or incest or to a woman whose physical or mental well-being is in jeopardy, as certified by a physician. Because of DES's association with vaginal cancer in the female offspring of women who take the drug while pregnant, women are advised to consider abortion if pregnancy results despite use of the morning-after pill.

Barrier and Mechanical Devices

Intrauterine Devices. An intrauterine device (IUD) is a small plastic object that is inserted into the uterus by a clinician. Precisely how an IUD works is not known. One theory is that the IUD, a foreign body, activates the body's defense mechanisms. Antibodies are produced and create an environment that is hostile to the sperm or the fertilized ovum. A related theory is that the IUD somehow interferes with implantation of the fertilized ovum.

IUDs come in many sizes and shapes. Some can remain in the uterus for years. Others contain copper or progesterone-bearing hormones for additional contraceptive protection and must be replaced periodically. A nylon filament attached to the IUD extends through the cervical opening into the vagina so the user can check to ensure that the device is still in place. IUDs are 95 to 98 percent effective in preventing pregnancy. Undetected complete or partial expulsion from the uterus is the usual reason for failure.

With any IUD there is the risk of serious uterine infection and scarring of the fallopian tubes, which could prevent or hinder later pregnancies. Physicians are commonly advising against use of the IUD for women who plan to have children in the future.

Some women, while using the IUD, experience cramps, longer and heavier menstrual periods, and spotting. Accidental pregnancy with an IUD can result in spontaneous abortion, premature delivery, or stillbirth, and it is now recommended that females who become pregnant with the IUD in place have the fetus aborted.

Diaphragm. A dome-shaped rubber device with a flexible metal rim, the diaphragm fits into the vagina in such a way as to block the entrance to the uterus. For additional protection, the inner surface of the diaphragm — the part that comes into contact with the cervix — is coated with a layer of spermicidal cream or jelly before insertion. A diaphragm must be fitted and prescribed by a clinician.

The diaphragm must be inserted no more than six hours before intercourse for the spermicide to be effective. Afterward, the diaphragm must stay in place for six to eight hours; if intercourse is repeated within that time, a back-up method (foam or condom) is necessary. If used correctly, the diaphragm is 97 percent effective. The failure rate, however, is as high as 17 percent, primarily due to lack of use or improper use. No serious side effects have been associated with use of the diaphragm. Some women, however, complain that the necessity of inserting the device before intercourse inhibits sexual spontaneity.

Cervical Caps. The cervical cap is a small, thimble-shaped cup which fits over the cervix. It is held in place by suction between its

Table 4-1. Birth Control: How Well Does It Work?

Method	Use Effectiveness	Advantages	Disadvantages
Pill (combination estrogen/ progestin)	93-96%	Convenient, extremely effective; does not interrupt sex, and may diminish menstrual cramps.	Medical examination recommended; physician's prescription required. Possible nausea, weight gain, headaches, missed periods, darkened facial skin, depression. Rarely: blood clots in legs, lungs, or brain; heart attacks.
IUD	95-98%	Effective, convenient; both partners usually unaware of it.	Physician must insert after pelvic examination; not all women can use; uterus may "push" it out. May cause cramps, bleeding, spotting, infection—see doctor for pain, bleeding, fever, or severe discharge.
Diaphragm with Spermicide	87-97%	Effective and safe.	Must be fitted by physician, may be difficult to insert; inconvenient, messy, or may cause irritation.
Condoms	90%	Effective, safe; useful precaution against sexually transmitted diseases. Readily available at drugstores.	Interrupts intercourse, may be messy, condom may break; allergic reaction to rubber may occur.
Contraceptive Foams and Jellies	85%	Effective, safe; a good lubricant. Readily available at drugstores.	Must be inserted just prior to intercourse; inconvenient, messy. May cause irritation to one or both partners.
Condoms and Foam (together)	95%	Extremely effective, safe; excellent protection against sexually transmitted diseases. (See also above)	Interrupts intercourse, may be messy or inconvenient. (See also above)
Rhythm	77-98%	Safe, effective if followed carefully; few religious objections.	Difficult to use if menstrual cycle is irregular. Sexual intercourse must be avoided for a significant part of each cycle.

Sources: Based on Planned Parenthood statistics, 1979; and U.S. Public Health Service, *Family Planning Methods of Contraception* (Washington, D.C.: USPHS, 1980).

flexible rim and the cervix. Caps must be fitted just like diaphragms. A snug fit is imperative if the cap is to remain in place. Widely used in Europe, the Food and Drug Administration of the United States has approved the use of the cervical cap only for research purposes.

Spermicides. Available in drugstores without a prescription, contraceptive foams, creams, jellies, and vaginal suppositories contain chemicals that immobilize and kill sperm. A spermicide must be placed high up in the vagina, near the cervix, no longer than 15 minutes prior to intercourse. Failure rate is high—about 23 percent—primarily because spermicides are difficult to use efficiently. They often are not spread evenly over the cervix, leaving gaps where sperm can penetrate. Spermicides are rarely harmful to health, but they are not widely used because many women feel that they are messy and inconvenient.

Sponge. One of the newest over-the-counter contraceptives available is the collagen sponge. This mushroom-shaped device fits into the upper part of the vagina near the cervix. Its effectiveness is similar to that of other vaginal methods. The sponge appears to be a relatively safe device that works by absorbing semen, blocking the cervical opening, and releasing spermicide.

Condoms. Because they are known to prevent the spread of venereal disease, condoms have been making a comeback in recent years. A condom is a rubber or animal-skin sheath that fits over the erect penis, working as a barrier to prevent semen from entering the vagina. After ejaculation but before losing his erection, the man must withdraw while holding the rim of the condom firmly against the base of his penis to make sure that the condom does not slip off and sperm do not spill into the vagina. Condoms do not require a prescription and are 97 percent effective if used properly. Some couples object to interrupting foreplay to put the condom on. Others complain that condoms dull sensation.

Other Methods

Withdrawal. Perhaps the world's oldest birth-control method, withdrawal, or coitus interruptus, requires the man to withdraw his penis from the vagina when ejaculation seems imminent. Obviously, this method requires a great deal of self-control, which is perhaps the primary reason for its high failure rate (20 to 25 percent). Also, small amounts of semen may escape before ejaculation, and even if a man withdraws in time, sperm deposited on the vulva may enter the vagina.

Douching. Douching involves forcing vinegar and water or some other solution into the vagina to wash out sperm after coitus. Not only is this a largely ineffective method of birth control, it may actually aid conception by driving sperm up into the uterus. Also, within one to two minutes after intercourse, some sperm have already penetrated the cervix and are beyond the reach of the douche.

Rhythm Method. The favored method of people whose religious beliefs prohibit artificial methods of birth control, the rhythm method involves abstaining from sexual intercourse during the woman's fertile period—usually the eleventh through the seventeenth days of a 28-day cycle. By keeping track of her menstrual cycle and noting this on a calendar and by taking her basal body temperature (BBT) every day for several months, a woman can determine her pattern of ovulation. When the BBT is elevated for three or four days, ovulation is past and the chance of conception is small. This method is not useful for women with irregular menstrual cycles.

Sterilization. People who have completed their families or who are certain that they wish to remain childless may choose to be sterilized. This is not a decision you are likely to make at this time in your life.

Male sterilization is accomplished by means of a **vasectomy.** Under local anesthesia, a small incision is made in each side of the scrotum, and the vasa deferentia — the tubes through which sperm are carried from the testes to the penis — are tied or otherwise blocked. Sperm are then reabsorbed by the body rather than transmitted in the semen.

Vasectomy Male sterilization by closing the vas deferens.

Female sterilization — called **tubal ligation** — involves cutting, tying, or otherwise closing the fallopian tubes. Once a complex procedure involving major abdominal surgery, tubal ligation can now be effected under local anesthesia. Ovulation continues to occur, but eggs are unable to reach the site of fertilization.

Tubal ligation Female sterilization by closing the Fallopian tubes.

Contrary to myth, sexual performance and response after sterilization remain unimpaired and may even increase because the operation removes fear of unwanted pregnancy. Male and female sterilization must, at this point, be considered permanent. A skilled microsurgeon may be able to reconnect the tubes, but the operation does not always restore fertility.

Abortion

Abortion is one of the most divisive topics in the United States today. Laws will not change the convictions of either the people who believe that every woman has the right to decide to have an abortion or those who believe that every fetus has the right to be born. Self-Assessment Exercise 4.1 will help you discover how you feel about various aspects of the abortion issue. You may want to discuss openly in class your feelings about it after you have all done the exercise.

In 1974 the United States Supreme Court decided that all state laws prohibiting or restricting abortions during the first three months of pregnancy were unconstitutional. It limited the state's intervention in the second trimester to the regulation of the medical practices involved. The Court left decisions concerning abortion in the last trimester, abortion for minors without parental consent, and abortion without the husband's consent to the individual states.

Also, in 1974 the Massachusetts Supreme Court ruled that a husband does not have the right to prevent his wife from having an abortion. Three years later the United States Supreme Court decided that states do not have to pay for an abortion even if matching federal funds are available.

SELF-ASSESSMENT EXERCISE 4.1

Abortion Attitude Scale

DIRECTIONS: This is not a test. The statements ask you to tell how you feel about legal abortion (the voluntary removal of a human fetus from the mother during the first three months of pregnancy by a qualified medical person). Tell how you feel about each statement by circling one of the choices beside each sentence. Here is a practice statement:

SA A S1A S1D D SD Abortion should be legalized.

(SA = Strongly Agree; A = Agree; S1A = Slightly Agree; S1D = Slightly Disagree; D = Disagree; SD = Strongly Disagree)

Respond to each statement by circling only one response.

SA	A	S1A	S1D	D	SD	
5	4	3	2	1	0	**1.** The Supreme Court should strike down legal abortions in the United States.
5	4	3	2	1	0	**2.** Abortion is a good way of solving an unwanted pregnancy.
5	4	3	2	1	0	**3.** A mother should feel obligated to bear a child she has conceived.
5	4	3	2	1	0	**4.** Abortion is wrong no matter what the circumstances are.
5	4	3	2	1	0	**5.** A fetus is not a person until it can live outside its mother's body.
5	4	3	2	1	0	**6.** The decision to have an abortion should be the pregnant mother's.

In order to circumvent the Supreme Court's decision legalizing abortion, Congress and the states now restrict the use of government funds for abortions for poor women. An amendment to the Constitution is being discussed that would prohibit all abortions except when the mother's life is in danger.

Methods

The method used for abortion is determined by the length of the pregnancy.

Vacuum aspiration is the preferred procedure for terminating pregnancies during the first trimester. A suction device is inserted through the cervical canal, and the contents of the uterus are then quickly drawn out.

Dilation and curettage (D & C), an alternative to vacuum aspiration, involves opening the cervix, then scraping the tissues off the inner walls with an instrument called a curette.

SA	A	S1A	S1D	D	SD	
5	4	3	2	1	0	**7.** Every conceived child has the right to be born.
5	4	3	2	1	0	**8.** A pregnant female not wanting to have a child should be encouraged to have an abortion.
5	4	3	2	1	0	**9.** Abortion should be considered killing a person.
5	4	3	2	1	0	**10.** People should not look down on those who choose to have abortions.
5	4	3	2	1	0	**11.** Abortion should be an available alternative for unmarried, pregnant teenagers.
5	4	3	2	1	0	**12.** Persons should not have the power over the life or death of a fetus.
5	4	3	2	1	0	**13.** Unwanted children should not be brought into the world.
5	4	3	2	1	0	**14.** A fetus should be considered a person at the moment of conception.

Source: Adapted from Sloan, Linda A. "Abortion Attitude Scale," *Health Education.* May/June, 1983, pp. 41–42.

Pregnancies of 13 to 20 weeks duration are usually terminated by *dilation and evacuation* (D & E). This method is similar to a D & C, but the fetus is larger and not as easily removed as in the first trimester.

Saline instillation involves injecting a concentrated salt solution into the uterus. Uterine contractions begin within 12 to 24 hours, and after an unspecified period of "labor," the fetus is expelled from the uterus. Rarely performed earlier than the sixteenth week of pregnancy, saline abortions may produce intrauterine infection and hemorrhage. *Prostaglandins,* the fatty acids that function as hormones in the body and can cause strong contractions of the uterus, can also be used to induce second trimester abortions.

Abortion should not be considered a method of birth control. It is both more expensive and risky than conventional means of contraception, and repeated abortions may make a woman more prone to miscarriage if she attempts to carry a pregnancy to term.

Summary

Although reproduction has been the subject of many myths and misconceptions, we now have a basic understanding of the reproductive process, beginning with the ovum in the female and sperm in the male and ending in the birth of a baby.

The external female sexual organs, collectively called the vulva, include the mons pubis, labia majora, labia minora, clitoris, and hymen. The internal sexual organs include the ovaries, which contain the ovarian follicles. The fallopian tubes lead from the ovaries to the uterus, where the fetus grows. The endometrium, the lining of the uterus, is especially adapted to nurture the fertilized egg. The lower part of the uterus, the cervix, projects into the vagina.

The menstrual cycle, which is coordinated by the hormones FSH, LH, and LTH produced by the pituitary gland, consists of three phases: the proliferative phase, the secretory phase, and menstruation. During the proliferative phase, 15 to 20 ovarian follicles mature, and the endometrium thickens in preparation for a possible pregnancy. At ovulation the most mature ovarian follicle bursts, releasing the egg and beginning the secretory phase. The ruptured ovarian follicle becomes the corpus luteum, which then produces hormones, and glands in the endometrium begin secreting. If implantation does not occur, the outer layer of the endometrium is shed during the final phase of the cycle, menstruation.

The external male sexual organs include the penis and the scrotum. Sperm cells are produced in the testicles, or testes, and travel through the epididymides and the vasa deferentia to the prostate, where they join with ducts from the seminal vesicles to form the ejaculatory ducts. The ejaculatory ducts pass through the prostate and empty into the urethra.

During fertilization, the 23 chromosomes in the egg combine with the 23 chromosomes in the sperm to form a new cell with 46 chromosomes, the number necessary to form a complete human cell. The sex of the baby is determined by the sex chromosome contained in the sperm.

After fertilization the egg travels down the fallopian tubes. When it reaches the uterus, it implants itself in the endometrium, where it grows into a fully developed baby. The process takes approximately 266 days, or about nine months, and is divided into three trimesters.

When the baby is ready to be born, the mother enters labor. Strong and painful contractions of the uterus and placenta begin, and the cervix dilates to allow the baby to pass out of the uterus and through the vagina.

Various methods of contraception include the birth-control pills, the mini-pill, the morning-after pill, intrauterine devices, diaphragm, spermicides, douching, condoms, withdrawal, the rhythm method, and sterilization.

Abortion, which should not be considered a birth control method, is a highly controversial issue. The methods used are determined by the length of pregnancy and include vacuum aspiration, D & C, D & E, saline instillation, and prostaglandin induction.

Review and Discussion

1. Name and describe the external female and male sexual organs.
2. Describe the menstrual cycle in terms of its three phases.
3. Describe the path sperm travel from the testicles to the site of fertilization in the fallopian tubes.
4. What symptoms of pregnancy does the mother experience during the three trimesters?
5. What is amniocentesis?
6. Describe the three stages of labor.
7. Discuss the different methods of childbirth.
8. Name four complications that can arise during pregnancy.
9. What are the main methods of contraception? How do they compare in effectiveness?
10. Why is abortion controversial?

Further Reading

Francke, Linda Bird. *The Ambivalence of Abortion.* New York: Dell Publishing Co., 1981.
A study of people's reactions to abortion, based on interviews with couples.

Guttmacher, Alan F. *Pregnancy, Birth, and Family Planning.* New York: New American Library, 1973.
A detailed presentation of practical information on pregnancy, birth, and family planning, based on the author's experience as a doctor.

Kitzinger, Sheila. *The Experience of Childbirth.* 4th edition. Baltimore: Penguin Books, 1978.
A sociologist, childbirth educator, and mother of five discusses pregnancy and childbirth and how to prepare for the experience, with particular attention to the emotional and psychological aspects involved. (Paperback)

Lamaze, Fernand. *Painless Experience, With Particular Attention to the Emotional Childbirth.* New York: Pocket Books, 1972.
A description of the Lamaze method by its founder.

Rugh, Roberts, and L. B. Shuttles. *From Conception to Birth: The Drama of Life's Beginnings.* New York: Harper & Row, 1971.
A detailed description of the development of the human embryo and fetus in the womb, with a number of striking color photographs. (Paperback)

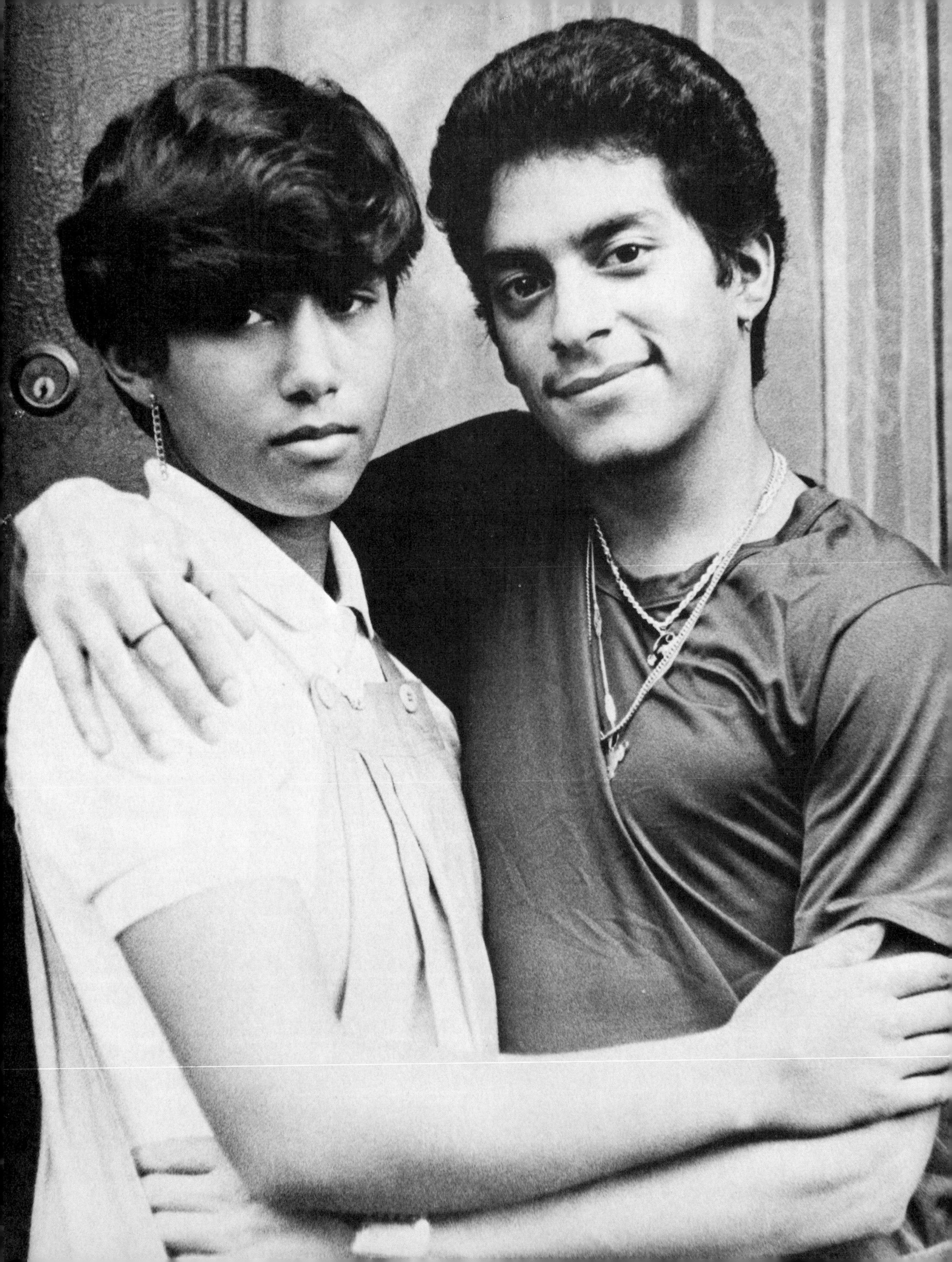

Chapter 5
Human Sexuality

KEY POINTS

- ☐ Human sexuality is the subject of many myths that can prevent it from being a fulfilling expression of the whole person.
- ☐ The male or female biological identity given us at birth is reinforced by learned sex roles.
- ☐ Androgyny is the concept that male and female are not opposites but that people can and should display the best human traits.
- ☐ The human sexual response, which is very similar in both men and women, follows four phases: the excitement phase, the plateau phase, the orgasmic phase, and the resolution phase.
- ☐ People suffering from physical disabilities or mental handicaps do not lose their sexuality but may need special help to overcome their problems.
- ☐ Deviant sexual behavior includes those actions that are discouraged or punished by society.
- ☐ Many aspects of sexual behavior are governed by laws, including private sexual practices, rape, prostitution, and pornography.
- ☐ Sexuality pervades all that we are and much of what we do; it is both a joy and a responsibility.

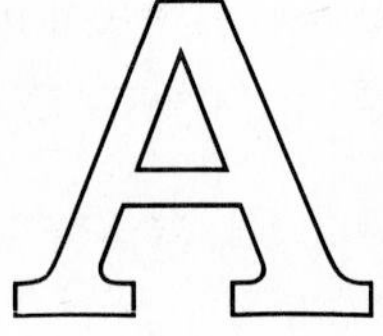

HEALTHY sexuality reflects a concern for our body and emotions and also for those people with whom we share our sexual life. Sex is therefore both a joy and a responsibility. Luckily, the choices we make about our sexual expression can enhance rather than detract from our enjoyment and growth. A satisfying sexual life is more than technical mastery or acrobatics; it is the total consequence of all our sexual decisions and an expression of the whole person. The ways we express our sexuality reveal as much about the many sides of our personality as the ways we work, dress, paint a picture, write a paper, or fix a meal.

No other area of human behavior is as obscured by myth as sexuality. Today little children know that babies are not brought by storks, yet we continue to believe and perpetuate myths about every aspect of sex. These myths confuse us and reinforce our fears of inadequacy and sexual failure. They compound our ignorance of our bodies and can create guilt feelings about normal sexual desires and practices. Because fear and guilt tend to cause much sexual distress, we need to discover the truth about our sexual selves and put the myths to rest.

There are many ways to express our sexuality in public and in private. When society disapproves of sexual acts, it labels them variant or deviant. But deviance is not an absolute, since attitudes vary widely from society to society and from individual to individual. We therefore have to make many decisions about sex roles, sexual practices, partners, and the use of our reproductive potential. Most important, this awareness of our sexual nature forces us to decide not only how to exercise it but with whom and when. These choices can have a profound effect on our entire well-being. To make them we need to examine our values and moral beliefs and seek knowledge about our human sexual development, functions, and behavior.

Sexual Identity

Sexual Development

We are sexual beings from the moment of conception, when our genetic sex is determined. Each month a woman's ovaries usually produce one ovum, or egg. The ovum always contains an X (female) sex chromosome. The testes in a man manufacture millions of sperm cells every day; half of the sperm carry an X chromosome and half carry a Y (male) chromosome. If an X-carrying sperm cell fertilizes the ovum, the embryo is destined to be a genetic female; if a Y-bearing sperm reaches the egg first and penetrates it, the XY combination makes a male embryo. This is the first step toward our sexual identity.

In the first few weeks of embryonic life, the tissue that will become the sex organs (the *genital ridges*) is the same whether the embryo is

YOUR HEALTH TODAY

Some Common Sexual Myths and Fallacies

- All transsexuals are gay.
- The size of the erect penis is related to the size of the penis before erection.
- Sexual desire and ability decrease markedly after the age of forty.
- Women have different sexual needs from men.
- Masturbation will render you sterile and drive you crazy.
- Once a man or woman is sterilized, sex drive diminishes.
- Retarded people are easily sexually aroused.
- Real men do not exhibit tenderness in public.
- There is a difference between vaginal and clitoral orgasms.
- Women who get raped asked for it.

female or male. About six to eight weeks after fertilization, the undifferentiated tissue begins to change. In the female the ridges start to form into the structures they were programmed to become—ovaries, uterus, vagina, clitoris, vulva. Nothing is needed other than the original genetic instructions. In the male things are different. The inner core of the genital ridges becomes testes, which begin to produce two hormones: **testosterone,** which prevents the genital tissue from changing into female organs, and **androgen,** which stimulates the development of both the internal and the external male genitals. If it were not for these two substances, even the genetic male would have female genitalia.

Testosterone A male sex hormone that prevents female development.

Androgen A sex hormone that stimulates development of male characteristics.

Because the growth of the male's sexuality is so dependent on the simultaneous stimulation and repression by male hormones, it seems that there is a greater chance that something will go wrong at this very early stage. The male embryo is fine-tuned at a very vulnerable period in a way that the female is not.

Momentous changes stimulated by hormones occur again about twelve to fifteen years later. At puberty the testes and the ovaries mature and prepare to fulfill their biologic destiny: to create new life. The testes produce testosterone, which is essential for the creation of spermatozoa. By the time the adolescent boy experiences his first ejaculation, he is probably capable of becoming a father. The male hormones radically alter the young boy's body. Muscle mass increases, the voice lowers, hair grows, and the skin toughens.

In the girl the ovaries begin to release, one by one, the ova that have been stored there since before birth. The ovaries produce the female hormones estrogen and progesterone, which regulate the girl's menstrual cycle, round her hips, and cause her breasts to develop.

Male and female hormones are produced in both sexes, but the delicate balance influences our reproductive potential and our total sexual identity. The often-disturbing hormonal and body changes at puberty force us to come to terms with our sexual self.

Gender Roles

Gender Identity Awareness of one's maleness or femaleness.

Gender identity refers to our consistent awareness of our maleness or femaleness. This identity is assigned to us at birth and, according to research, is firmly established by the time we are 12 to 18 months old. No one tells us how to behave in the uterus, but this changes the instant the obstetrician announces, "It's a boy!" or "It's a girl!" From then on we are treated in certain ways according to the sex indicated by our genitals. Mothers have been seen to respond to a boy infant's cry differently than to a girl baby's cry. In one study[1] a mother wheeling her infant in a carriage told half of the people she met that the infant was a boy and the other half that the child was a girl. When people thought the baby was a male, they remarked on his strength and gave him a gentle swipe. The ones who believed they were looking at a girl remarked how pretty she was and softly patted her arm.

We first learn gender or sex roles by imitating our mother and father. During childhood our parents and teachers reward us when our behavior is appropriate ("Such a lady!") and discourage it when it

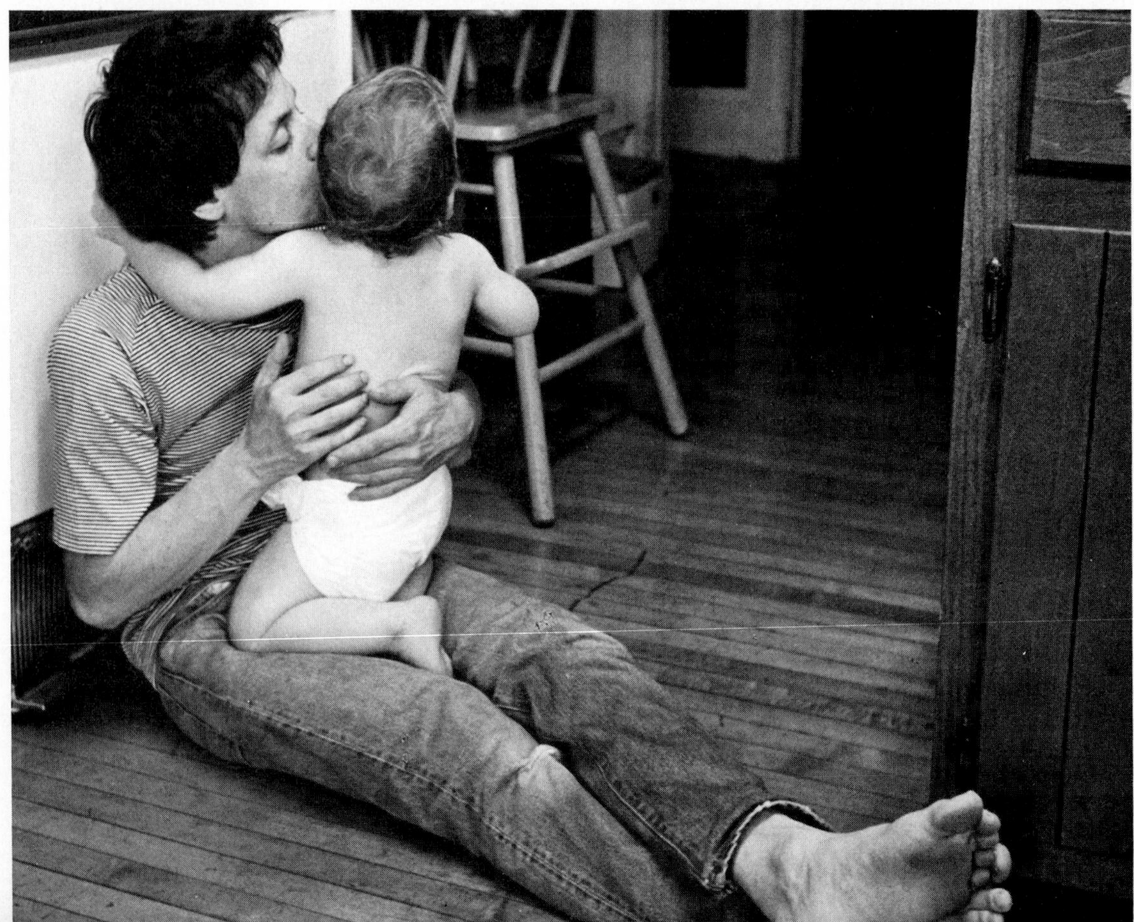

Father and son. Changing attitudes toward male roles encourage father love as well as mother love. (Photo Marjorie Pickens 1982)

is inappropriate ("Don't be a sissy!"). A typical example of how rigid the standards are for male and female behavior is the father who scolds his small son for crying over a scraped knee, telling him, "Big boys don't cry." Over and over, we are given clues as to the kinds of behavior society expects from us. The media, our religious training, and — perhaps most important — our peers continually reinforce the learned roles, and there is intense pressure to conform.

Androgyny Versus Sex-typing

The "he-man" and the "total woman" are mythical creatures. Each sex secretes both male and female hormones, and, as we saw, the sexual organs of both sexes evolve out of exactly the same tissue. The specifics of masculine and feminine behavior are partly a result of hormonal influences, but they are largely culturally imposed. The traits assigned to men (for example, strength and assertiveness) and women (for example, gentleness and tenderness) are subject to change from age to age and from culture to culture. Recently, both feminists and advocates of men's liberation have renewed an interest in the concept of **androgyny** (from the Greek *andro-*, male, and *gyne*, female). Androgyny emphasizes that both men and women can and should display the best human traits, whether the characteristics are considered masculine or feminine.

Androgyny Having both male and female characteristics.

Psychological studies show that rigid sex typing is associated with anxiety, low self-esteem, and neuroticism in adults of both sexes. It also correlates with lower intellectual and creative potentials. Sexual stereotyping may simply set impossibly high standards of behavior.

Strongly sex-typed persons may find that they cannot function according to their talents or respond to the needs of every situation, simply because a whole range of behavioral options is closed. The totally masculine man, for example, cannot react with warmth and compassion; the totally feminine woman is helpless in an emergency.

The androgynous person, free to engage in both feminine and masculine behavior, is not limited to these labels. Androgynous men are not afraid to do "woman's work," and androgynous women can function in a "man's world." In short, they can do what they *can* and *want* to do, not what they have been told they *should* do. Today, more and more women seek partners who are gentle and yielding as well as independent; more and more men find they prefer women who are as decisive as they are compassionate. The modern world requires people to cope with diverse situations in the home and in the world; androgyny frees people to deal more effectively with all kinds of situations without feeling emasculated or unfeminine.

Some adjectives, such as "dominant" or "athletic," are commonly applied to males in our culture today; others, such as "tender" or "submissive" are commonly used to describe feminine behavior. Are there any terms that are completely inappropriate for one sex or the other? Make a list of those traits you see in yourself. Are you masculine, feminine, or androgynous?

Human Sexual Response

Vasocongestion Enlargement of the blood vessels, as occurs during sexual arousal.

Myotonia Muscle tension, as occurs during sexual arousal.

Human sexual response is an intensely personal, whole-body reaction to sexual stimulation. It is not restricted to the pelvic organs, and it is greatly affected by emotions. The two physiologic changes that occur in both men and women during sexual stimulation are **vasocongestion,** the congestion of the pelvic blood vessels that causes tissue swelling, and **myotonia,** or muscle tension. The swelling and tension build until orgasm releases them and returns the body to its relaxed state.

The duration and intensity of sexual responses vary from person to person. Even the same person will experience different degrees of pleasure in different sexual situations. Those parts of the body that are exquisitely sensitive to stimulation on one occasion may be less so at another time. As personal and variable as sexual response is, the general response pattern remains the same regardless of the person or the situation.

The Sexual Response Cycle

Coitus (intercourse) Sexual activity involving insertion of the penis in the vagina.

William H. Masters and Virginia Johnson, the now-famous sex-research and therapy team, measured and analyzed the sexual reactions of hundreds of volunteers in various situations, including manual and mechanical stimulation and natural **coitus** or **intercourse.** They described the anatomic and physiologic changes as a cycle with four phases: the excitement phase, the plateau phase, the orgasmic phase, and the resolution phase (see Figures 5–1 and 5–2). Some might add another phase to precede these, the desire stage.

In *Human Sexual Response*, Masters and Johnson offer an astonishingly detailed description of what, until then, only lovers and writers had tried to capture. Surprisingly, most of the details point up the similarities — not the differences — between the male and female response cycles.

People of both sexes proceed through the phases in the same order. None of the phases is skipped, but each may vary in length and intensity. If the stimulation is inadequate, the cycle will stop. Outside stimuli — a telephone ring or a child's cry — can short-circuit the sexual reactions, as can guilt, anxiety, or boredom.

The phases are not clear-cut events, of course, but are part of a process. They overlap and flow into one another. They are, in short, a simplification that offers an arbitrary but convenient way to look at the many ways men and women respond to sexual stimuli. Human sexual response follows the same pattern regardless of the type of sexual activity or the heterosexual or homosexual orientation of the participants.

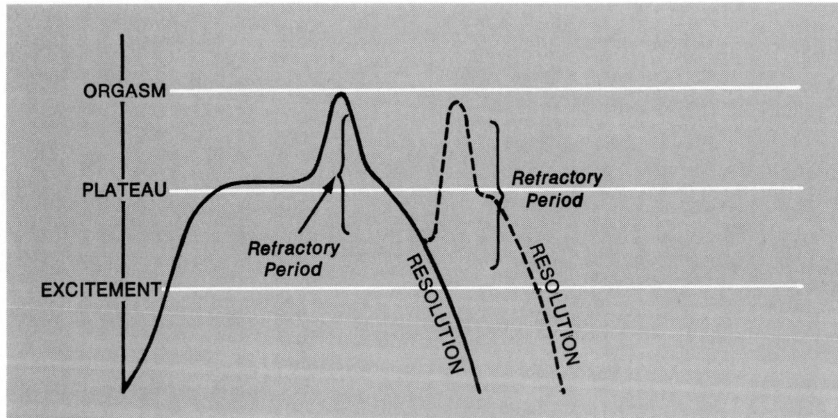

Figure 5-1. The Male Sexual Response Cycle.
Although there are variations in intensity and duration, the male sexual response follows an almost standard pattern. (Source: William H. Masters and Virginia E. Johnson, *Human Sexual Response* [Boston: Little, Brown & Co., © 1966], 5.)

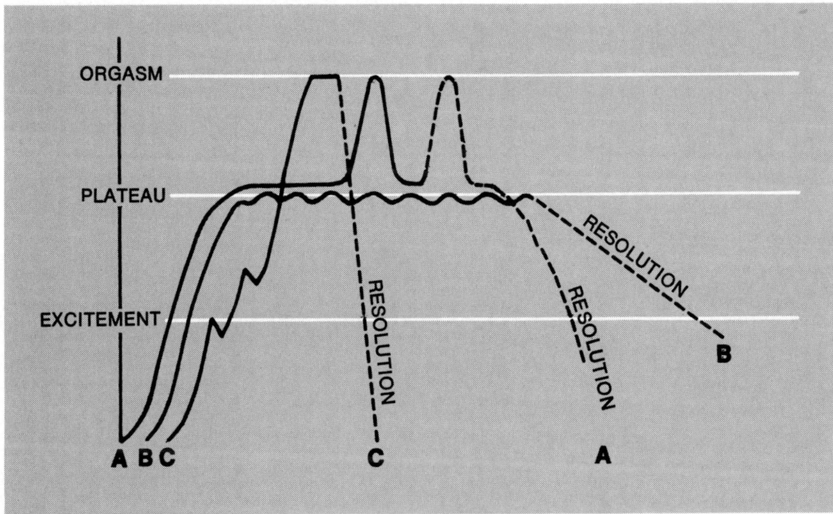

Figure 5-2. The Female Sexual Response Cycle.
There is greater variation in the female sexual response cycle than in the male. Curve *A* represents a cycle with multiple orgasms, curve *B* a cycle without orgasm, and curve *C* a cycle with one orgasm. (Source: William H. Masters and Virginia E. Johnson, *Human Sexual Response* [Boston: Little, Brown & Co., © 1966], 5.)

Excitement Phase

Excitement phase The first phase of sexual response.

The first stage is the **excitement phase.** In both men and women this phase is initiated very quickly, within seconds of the first sexual contact or even the first erotic thought. It can last for minutes or hours.

The woman's sexual involvement is signaled by reactions in both the genitals and other parts of the body. Within 10 to 30 seconds the vagina becomes lubricated with a fluid "sweated" from the vaginal walls. The vaginal barrel expands, lengthens, and changes color. Blood rushes through the pelvic arteries faster than it can be removed by the veins. This is called **tumescence,** and it causes the vulva and clitoris to enlarge. If the woman has not had a baby, the labia majora flatten and separate; in the woman who has delivered children, the labia swell. The labia minora thicken and expand, and the uterus lifts slightly.

Tumescence Genital swelling due to the rush of blood in sexual arousal.

Away from the genital area, the breasts increase in size and the dark areas around the nipples (the **areolae**) swell. Heart rate and blood pressure rise with the growing muscular tension, pumping blood into the congested genital area, which becomes even more sensitive. Late in the phase a rash, the sex flush, may appear on the abdomen and spread to the breasts.

Areolae Dark areas around the nipples.

Within seconds of the start of sexual activity, the man experiences an erection of the penis, caused by tumescence. (The size of the erect penis is in no way related to the size of the penis before erection.) The scrotal sac flattens and the testes lift. The nipples may become erect, and, as in his partner, blood pressure and heart rate increase.

Plateau Phase

Plateau phase The second phase of sexual response, involving lubrication and enlargement of genitals.

The **plateau phase** is more intense and may last 30 seconds to 3 minutes. During this brief interval the woman's vagina develops the orgasmic platform. The lower third of the vagina becomes enlarged by blood and distended. The upper two-thirds further expands and lengthens to accommodate a penis and to prepare a reservoir for semen. Lubrication increases, and the uterus elevates more. The body of the clitoris withdraws from its normally overhanging position and retreats under its swollen hood. The labia become even more enlarged and, if orgasm is imminent, the labia minora undergo a startling color change, going from pink to bright red or from red to deep wine. A pair of glands just inside the labia (Bartholin's glands) secrete a lubricating fluid.

In the man the penis increases in circumference, and the glans may change color. The testes elevate further, and blood congestion may increase their size by 50 percent. Cowper's glands produce fluid, the **preorgasmic ejaculation.** This small, uncontrollable emission may contain millions of active sperm.

Preorgasmic ejaculation Drop of fluid secreted from the penis during sexual arousal.

In both partners muscle tension increases: facial muscles twitch into a grimace, nostrils widen, the back arches. Heart rate and blood pressure continue to race, and late in this phase the woman may hyperventilate.

Orgasmic Phase

The briefest phase of all, the **orgasm,** is the peak of sexual tension. It lasts just a few seconds, sending waves of pleasurable release throughout the body. The orgasmic experience varies from person to person. If orgasm does not occur, there may be several reasons, including inadequate stimulation and emotional conflict interfering with stimulation and release.

Orgasm Climax of sexual tension.

The woman experiences 5 to 12 contractions of the muscles around the orgasmic platform at 0.8-second intervals and may feel the uterus contract as well. Various muscles in the hands, feet, and rectum contract spasmodically.

In the man orgasm and ejaculation occur at the same time. Ejaculation is the most specific difference between the female and the male sexual responses, because the woman has no comparable reaction. Contractions of the male accessory organs give the signal that orgasm is about to happen, and contractions along the urethra propel the semen out of the penis at 0.8-second intervals.

Resolution Phase

The **resolution phase** points up some significant differences between the sexual reponses of men and women. During this relaxing phase, the woman can be restimulated into one or more orgasms, but the man usually enters the refractory stage, during which he is relatively immune to further stimulation. This stage can last from 15 minutes to many hours. The periods usually become longer as the man gets older.

Resolution phase Final relaxation phase of the sexual cycle.

In the woman the pelvic organs return to their normal positions and lose their tumescence. The vaginal walls relax and regain their usual color. The mouth of the uterus, or *cervix,* descends into the pool of semen deposited in the upper vagina. The labial congestion diminishes, and the whole body moves into its relaxed state.

The man loses his erection in two stages. First, the penis regresses to about one and one-half its normal size; then it slowly returns to its usual dimensions. The scrotum relaxes; the testes descend. Breasts, muscles, skin, blood pressure, heart rate, and breathing all return to normal.

Looking at sexual responses as a four-phase cycle merely provides us with a way to analyze it scientifically. Every person's experience will not exactly match the simplified pattern, and not everyone will experience all the biological changes. Masters and Johnson's model shows that despite the obvious differences between male and female anatomy, the physiology, or functioning, of sex in men and women is remarkably similar. This awareness should help lead to easier communication between partners about their sexual needs and preferences. Our understanding of each other's individual sexual needs should not be obscured by our imagined differences.

Normal Patterns of Sexual Behavior

Intercourse (coitus) Sexual activity involving insertion of the penis in the vagina.

Aside from **intercourse,** various other patterns of sexual behavior are considered common.

Sexual Fantasies

It is often said that the most important sex organ is the one between the ears. A troubled mind can disrupt or even prevent sexual sensations. It can completely destroy a man or woman's sexual responsiveness and prevent orgasm.

Both men and women fantasize during sex, but their fantasies are different. Men tend to fantasize more than women, and, some say, may fantasize more about events they would not attempt in real life. Fantasies are not necessarily the expression of real wishes; they do, however, allow people to experience situations and sensations they would not normally have—to try out some new, forbidden pleasure while retaining complete control over the situation.

Fantasies may be bizarre or coherent, conventional and romantic, or aggressive and violent. They are always personal. Many people claim that their enjoyment of sex is greatly increased when they allow themselves to imaginatively change, embellish, and exaggerate details of the actual experience.

Masturbation

Masturbation Manipulation of one's own genitals.

The **masturbation** *will drive you crazy* myth is a particularly deadly one. If any of the warnings were true, we would certainly see a much greater prevalence of insanity, warts, hairy palms, or any of the other distressing consequences attributed to masturbation. Millions of normal children have suffered needless guilt, and millions of parents have given their children an unhealthy introduction to sexuality. From the first "No!" and handslap, the young child learns that his or her body is bad. Most boys and girls nonetheless do masturbate. Particularly during adolescence, when sexual urges run high, masturbation offers young people a way to release tensions in a nondestructive way. It also allows them to learn about their bodies and personal sexual feelings.

Sex therapists have found that masturbation offers an important way to treat failure to achieve orgasm. Masters and Johnson reported that all female orgasms are caused by direct or indirect clitoral, not vaginal, stimulation. (There is no truth to the notion that vaginal orgasms are mature ones, whereas clitoral orgasms are the sign of immature sexuality.) *The Hite Report* notes that even women who did not reach orgasm with intercourse easily attained it with masturbation.[2]

Masturbation, like other sexual actions, is a private activity. Children can engage in it privately without being told that what they are doing is bad. It is known that adults continue to masturbate. But myths die hard. Many adults report that they feel "lonely, guilty, selfish, silly, and generally bad" when they masturbate.[3]

Oral-Genital Stimulation

For many people, oral-genital stimulation is an important form of sexual expression. These individuals find **cunnilingus** (oral stimulation of the female's genitals) and **fellatio** (oral stimulation of the male's genitals) acceptable, pleasurable, and arousing.

Cunnilingus Oral stimulation of the female's genitals.

Fellatio Oral stimulation of the male's genitals.

Oral-genital stimulation is not an acceptable practice for some, however. Meeks and Heit offer the following reasons for this nonacceptance:

1. Because of religious beliefs, some individuals feel that any sex that does not result in the possibility of reproduction is immoral.
2. Some people feel that oral-genital contact is dirty. This may be because the urinary openings are closely connected to the genitals.
3. Some people feel that oral-genital contacts are acts practiced only by homosexuals.[4]

Petting and Foreplay

Petting and **foreplay** are noncoital forms of sexual expression. Petting, which is any act of touching or kissing and excludes intercourse, can be extremely pleasurable and arousing. Petting is a term that is often used to describe adolescent behavior. Foreplay, on the other hand, generally refers to those acts of touching and kissing which precede intercourse. Some foreplay techniques are kissing, gentle carressing, manual stimulation of the genitalia, oral stimulation of the genitalia, and anal stimulation.

Petting Any act of touching or kissing that excludes intercourse.

Foreplay Any act of touching or kissing that precedes intercourse.

Variant Sexual Behavior

Societies have always distinguished between normal sexual behavior and behavior that varies from the norm. Today this labeling is controversial, and various words are used to describe those sexual actions

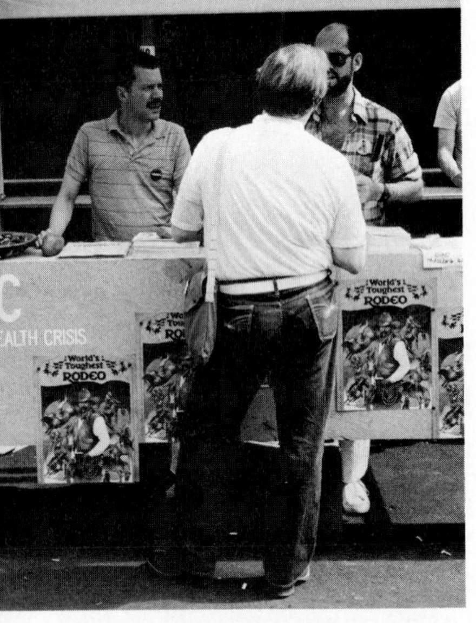

Homosexuals remain one of our most discriminated against and misunderstood groups (Photo by Marc P. Anderson © 1983)

not sanctioned by the culture—variant, deviant, atypical, alternative, diverse.

Variant behavior, as we shall call it, does not imply biological or psychological abnormality. It merely denotes actions discouraged or punished by the society in which they occur. In primitive societies, where continuation of the species is essential for the group's survival, sexual acts that do not result in reproduction—homosexual acts, for example—are usually strongly forbidden. Behavior that threatens the family or may result in defective offspring (such as incest) has been almost universally condemned.

Today many people maintain that any kind of sexual activity between consenting adults is *normal.* They reason that any behavior seen among mammals is normal for humans also and that any activity observed in human societies is acceptable for all humans in any society.

These arguments do not hold up completely. Many of the sexual patterns of mammals are irrelevant to human behavior. Many mammals mate only during the female's fertile period or require a certain amount of pain to stimulate ovulation. Human sexual desire does not depend on the woman's state of fertility.

Is it really true that "anything goes"? We must make decisions about our sexual behavior. To do this we have to distinguish between actions that, besides satisfying sexual needs, harm us or erode our social groups and those that contribute to our personal and interpersonal growth.

There are many laws governing sexual behavior, and we must evaluate whether these rules actually harm or benefit us. Like everything else in life, sex brings responsibilities. We must ask, "What are the consequences of our actions to ourselves, to others, and to society?"

What cannot be denied is that humans engage in a wide variety of sexual activities. The following are examples of some of the sexual behaviors that vary from the norm in our society.

Homosexuality

Homosexuality Sexual desire for a member of the same sex.

Few areas of human sexuality are as consistently controversial and provocative as **homosexuality.** Homosexuality refers to emotional or erotic attraction to and behavior with a member of the same sex.

The terms heterosexual and homosexual tend to mislead people into thinking that, at least with regard to human sexual behavior, people can be grouped in an all-or-none fashion. On the contrary, Kinsey's research has shown that the range of possible sexual behavior goes from completely homosexual to completely heterosexual (see Table 5-1). Many writers and researchers have attempted to make Kinsey's findings in this area general knowledge. Yet, despite their efforts, homosexuals remain one of our most discriminated-against and misunderstood groups.

Table 5-1 Heterosexual-Homosexual rating scale

0	1	2	3	4	5	6
entirely heterosexual	largely heterosexual with incidental homosexual activity	largely heterosexual but with distinct homosexual activity	equally heterosexual and homosexual	largely homosexual but with distinct heterosexual history	largely homosexual but with incidental heterosexual history	entirely homosexual

Source: A. C. Kinsey, W. B. Pomeroy, E. E. Martin, and P. H. Gebhard, *Sexual Behavior in the Human Female* (Philadelphia: W. B. Saunders Co., 1953). Reprinted by permission of The Kinsey Institute for Research in Sex, Gender, and Reproduction, Inc.

Bisexuality

Bisexuality is the engagement in both homosexual and heterosexual behavior. Public reactions to bisexuals are mixed. Many people feel that bisexuals are suffering from an identity conflict, while others believe that bisexuals have the best of both worlds. Regardless, it appears that more and more people today are professing to be bisexual.

Transsexualism

Twenty years ago Christine Jorgensen shocked the world with a sex-change operation. Several years ago a male-to-female transsexual, Rene Richards, successfully won the right to play women's tennis.

Transsexuality is the belief by a person that his or her true gender identity is that of the other sex. Such individuals feel trapped in the wrong body with the wrong genitals. The majority of transsexuals are anatomical males with female gender identities. They may seek to change their sex with hormones and surgery.

Before an operation is done to remove the original genitals and

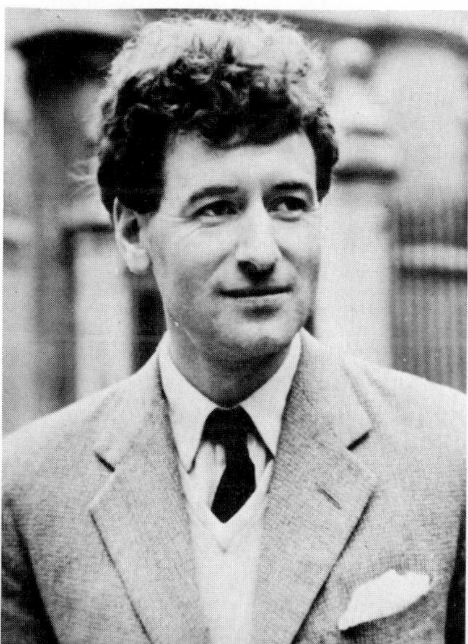

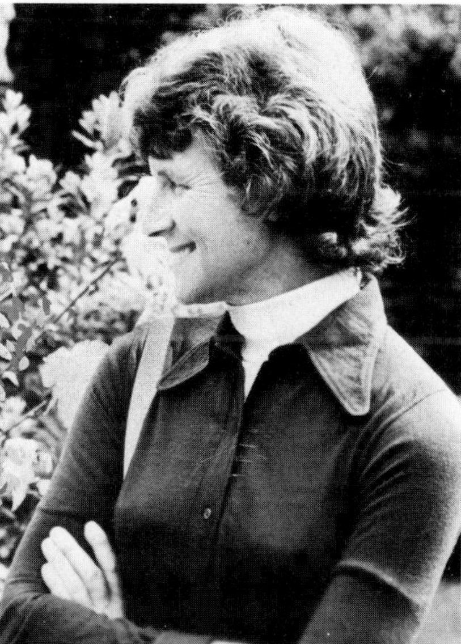

James Morris, a noted British journalist, underwent a sex change and is now Jan Morris. (Photo left by Jerry Bauer; photo right by Bruno de Hamel)

SELF-ASSESSMENT EXERCISE 5.1

Attitudes Toward Homosexuality and Bisexuality

A LOOK AT YOUR LIFESTYLE

You have decided to live in a dormitory for the coming school year. Two different persons have approached you to share a room. One, however, is your favorite. You feel especially close to him/her. It seems you can be very honest, and you are completely accepted. This person approaches you and says, "Before you decide to room with me, I want you to know that I am bisexual."

What is Your Reaction to This Statement?

Identity the key issue or problem. ______________________

Identify three possible solutions or alternatives. ______________________

____

____

GATHERING INFORMATION

What are three things you would like to know about your friend?

____

____

____

EVALUATING THE INFORMATION

Identify at least one reason for and one reason against each alternative you identified. ______________________

____

____

MAKING RESPONSIBLE DECISIONS

What alternative would you select? ______________________

Give the most important reason for your choice. ______________________

____

create new ones, physicians first determine why the person wants to change sex and whether or not all the practical aspects of assuming the new sexual identity are clearly understood. A trial period with cross-dressing, living the new role, and taking hormones comes first. Many transsexuals have other, even more serious psychological problems than their confused gender identity, which prevent them from successfully changing sex.

Other Forms of Sexual Variance

Transvestism and Fetishism

The transvestite is neither a homosexual nor a transsexual but a person who gets pleasure from dressing in the clothes usually worn by the other sex. Transvestites are heterosexuals who are able to engage in successful sexual relationships with the opposite sex. The person who loves to cross-dress is typically a male, often one who has children. Psychologists propose that transvestism is a way for a man to escape the rigors of the masculine role. Children may experiment with cross-dressing, but this does not necessarily signal a life-long future of transvestism.

Like the transvestite, the fetishist is sexually stimulated by inanimate objects. Fetishists find sexual pleasure in a multitude of things, such as shaving soap, handkerchiefs with purple stripes, and roses.

Exhibitionism and Voyeurism

The exhibitionist, or flasher, exposes his genitals in public. Jokes and comedy routines commonly identify him by a trench coat and bare legs. The obscene phone caller gets sexual pleasure from making sexually explicit calls to unsuspecting listeners. The caller, like the flasher, rarely resorts to violent behavior. The voyeur, or "peeping Tom," obtains sexual stimulation from watching the sexual acts or naked bodies of others. Voyeurism usually refers to the observation of people who do not know they are being watched. The profusion of sexually explicit films, books, and magazines signals that there is a little bit of voyeur in many of us.

Sadomasochism (S/M)

The underground, or counterculture, newspapers are full of advertisements for sadomasochistic services. Sadists enjoy inflicting pain on their sexual partners. Real sadomasochism involves one person giving pain, often through burning or whipping, and one person receiving it. It can lead to serious injury and even death. Sadomasochism should not be confused with normal, playful biting and scratching that many lovers employ and that are not meant to be malevolent.

Nymphomania and Satyriasis

When the desire for sex becomes the most important part of life, overshadowing all others, it is called nymphomania in women and satyriasis in men. It is perhaps a comment on the pervasiveness of sexual myths that nymphomania is a commonly known phenomenon, whereas satyriasis is rarely mentioned. Presumably, excessive sexual desire in men is considered a normal condition, but in women it is thought to be deviant.

Nontraditional Partners

Bestiality

Sexual activity with animals is known as bestiality. Societies have generally scorned the person who enjoys sex with animals, although the topic is becoming a familiar one in movies, plays, and cartoons. Pornographic productions commonly use the theme, usually portraying a woman with an animal. There is no reason, however, to think that the real incidence of human-animal contact is increasing.

Pedophilia and Incest

Pedophilia refers to the sexual contact between a child and an adult. Some societies have freely allowed pedophilia, and many others tolerate it. Most modern cultures condemn it, but an increasing number of prostitutes in the large cities of the United States are children, many of them boys.

Incest is sexual activity — not necessarily intercourse — between people who are too closely related to be legally married. It is the universal taboo; nonetheless, it has always existed and continues to exist. Historical studies indicate that incest was once rare in the United States and was generally restricted to noncoital activity between siblings and to cousin marriages.

Today incest is called the most unreported form of child abuse. Given the relationships involved and the tactics used, forcible rape is rarely the case but, incest can lead to seriously troubled lives for the typically young female children who are involved. Families may protect the abuser out of shame and fear. Many child abuse experts now believe that family counseling is the best way to help both the victim and the other members of the family.

Sexual Problems

Discussion of human sexual response would not be complete without mentioning potential difficulties, or problems. Most people experience some unfulfilling sexual responses at some time in their lives. Many times the problem is simply a temporary reaction to stress, fatigue, or illness. It is frequently a symptom of an interpersonal conflict. But it can also be a serious and distressing result of a significant emotional or physical disability. Masters and Johnson observed that 90 percent of sexual problems are caused not by disease but by "hostility, poor communication, maintenance of the double standard, unrealistic expectations, deceptions, differences in reproductive goals" and fears of sexual failure.[5]

People differ in their sexual needs and responses. We need not experience or even desire orgasm with each sexual encounter in order to be normal. The solution to sexual problems usually requires us to look at the whole person or at the couple, not just at the malfunctioning organ. Treating the emotional conflicts is probably more important than improving the techniques.

Problems of Women

Orgasmic dysfunction, sometimes referred to as *frigidity,* describes an inability to reach the orgasmic phase of the sexual cycle. It may be *primary,* if the woman has never experienced orgasm. If it is *secondary,* or *situational,* she has had orgasm in some situations—such as masturbation—but not in others, or she has stopped having orgasms.

Orgasmic dysfunction Inability to reach orgasm.

Vaginismus is the powerful, often painful contraction of the outer third of the vagina, which can impede and even prevent intercourse. It is often associated with **dyspareunia,** or painful intercourse. Dyspareunia can be due to vaginal infection or chemical irritation from douches, hygiene sprays, or contraceptives. Emotional problems that interfere with adequate lubrication are also likely causes. In postmenopausal women or women who have had their ovaries removed, hormonal changes cause thinning of the vaginal mucous membranes, leading to soreness during intercourse.

Vaginismus Strong, painful contraction of the vagina.

Dyspareunia Painful intercourse.

Problems of Men

Erectile dysfunction, commonly called *impotence,* is the inability to attain or maintain an erection. A man who has never had an erection of sufficient strength for intercourse has *primary* dysfunction. If he has intermittent problems or has ceased having erections, he has a *secondary* problem.

Erectile dysfunction Inability to attain or maintain an erection.

Many cases of erectile dysfunction are caused by psychological problems and are cured by counseling, but recent studies show that disease (usually endocrine, cardiovascular and central nervous system disease, diabetes mellitus, and prostatitis) appears to play a greater role than had been previously thought.

Premature ejaculation is defined as the inability to postpone ejaculation. Just how long it should be controlled during lovemaking is, of course, variable and a personal preference. The absence of all voluntary control identifies a true dysfunction.

Premature ejaculation Inability to postpone ejaculation.

Retarded ejaculation, or *ejaculatory incompetence,* occurs when a

Retarded ejaculation Inability to ejaculate despite erection.

man is unable to ejaculate even though he has achieved an erection. Frequently the man simply cannot ejaculate in the vagina.

The causes of *dyspareunia* in men are usually physical. Poor hygiene, leading to infection, and allergic reactions to vaginal contraceptives or douches can cause discomfort during intercourse.

Sexual problems can be helped with education, counseling, improved communication between partners, and, of course, treatment of any physical causes. Masters and Johnson and many other sex therapists have developed specific techniques to help individuals and couples with their sexual problems.

Sexuality and the Law

Laws are meant to control behavior, and cultures have always found it necessary or desirable to control both the private and the public expressions of sexuality—but without much success. It has been estimated that 95 percent of Americans have committed a sexual offense, if all the laws on the books are taken into consideration.

States differ in their sex laws, but most of them consider any sexual activity other than penile-vaginal intercourse a felony. Obviously most infractions of such laws are not punished because they are difficult to detect and prove and because there are so many offenders. Yet the potential for conviction and punishment exists. As long as the laws remain, the question remains: should society tell individuals what they can do in the privacy of their own homes, as long as their actions do not harm anyone? The Model Penal Code developed by the American Law Institute recommends that all private acts between consenting adults be decriminalized.

Fornication Sexual intercourse between unmarried consenting adults.

Cohabitation A man and a woman living together without being married.

Adultery Sex between a married person and someone other than the spouse.

Some of the private activities punishable by law include fornication, cohabitation, and adultery. **Fornication** is sexual intercourse between unmarried consenting adults. **Cohabitation** is a man and woman living together without being legally married. After a couple have cohabited for seven years, most states consider that they have a common-law marriage, which confers on them certain legal property rights. **Adultery** is sex between a married person and someone other than the spouse. Adultery does not include sex with a prostitute, however.

In most states today, homosexuality itself is not a crime. However, the sexual acts performed by homosexuals and many heterosexuals—oral-genital contact, anal intercourse (sodomy), mutual masturbation—are crimes. In some cities and counties, homosexuals are not allowed to teach in public schools or live in their chosen communities.

Rape

Other crimes punished by society, however unsuccessfully, include those that involve sexual attack. **Rape** is legally defined as "carnal knowledge of a person by force, against the person's will." Many states, however, determine that only a woman can be raped and that only a man can be a rapist. Although laws are changing, in many places a wife cannot charge her husband with rape. Traditionally and legally, a wife was required to render sexual services as part of her marriage agreement, even when she chose not to do so.

Rape Sexual intercourse forced against the victim's will.

The rapist is not simply an oversexed man. The major motivation for rape is not considered to be sex but anger and the desire for power over a woman. Rape is a violent crime that uses sex as the weapon. There are seldom any witnesses, and rape trials often become a credibility battle between the victim and the rapist. Faced with a threatening attacker, each women copes in a different way, some by struggling and others by giving in to avoid injury or death. The lack of a struggle does not, however, imply consent.

Rape is probably the only crime in which the victim has to defend herself. She may have to prove that she resisted, and her sexual history may be open to scrutiny. Until recently, hospitals and police were not known to be supportive of the rape victim. Today more emergency room physicians and police officers are specially trained in treating the rape victim and in trying to ensure that the rapist is caught and punished. Still, conviction is difficult and 50 to 90 percent

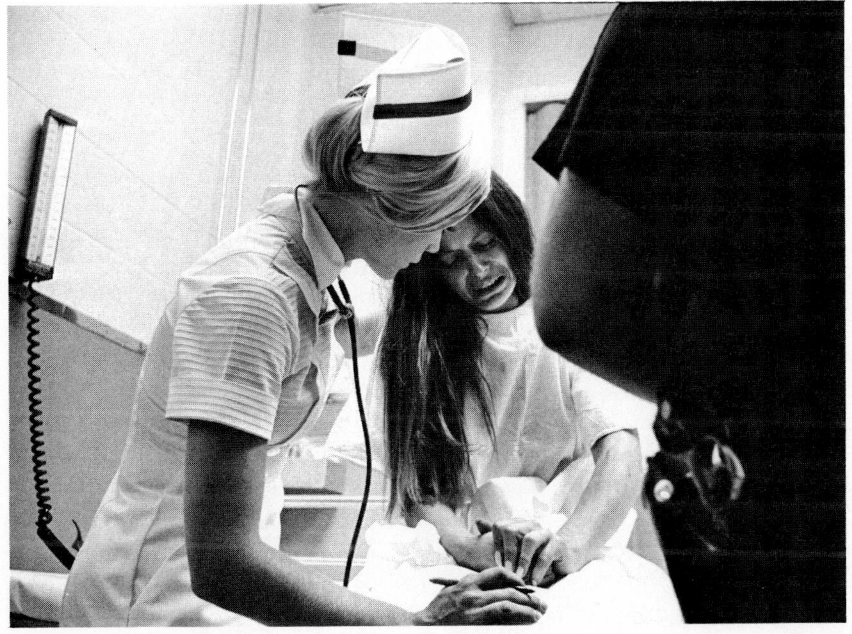

The psychological effects of rape can be severe. Today, more emergency-room personnel and police officers are specially trained in working with the rape victim. (Photo © Robert Goldstein 1983/Photo Researchers, Inc.)

YOUR HEALTH TODAY

Rape Prevention

The prevention of rape is laid on the potential victim's shoulders. She should take precautions not to put herself in dangerous situations. *But* excessive fear and anxiety only interfere with freedom of movement and cause unnecessary worry. They do not eradicate the crime.

There are at least six common-sense ways to protect against rape:

1. Be aware that most rapists are known to their victims.
2. List only your initials on your mailbox and in the phone book. Do not let it be known that you live alone.
3. Try to stay in well-lighted areas. Before getting into your car, check the back seat.
4. Never hitchhike.
5. If you think you are being followed, do not go directly home.
6. Do not open your door to strangers.

If rape occurs, the victim should call the police or rape-crisis center immediately. She must not change clothes or bathe, which would destroy any evidence. She will be asked to go to a hospital for examination and for treatment of any injuries and prevention of venereal disease and pregnancy, if necessary. Rape-crisis centers have been established in many cities. A counselor will assist and support the victim throughout the procedures and will offer psychological counseling to help the victim recover as fast as possible.

of rapes are never reported. (For information on rape prevention see the Box entitled "Rape Prevention.")

Prostitution

The so-called world's oldest profession is sexual activity in return for payment or some other form of material reward. It is outlawed in every state except Nevada. Prostitution causes the most alarm when prostitutes are prevalent on the streets and harass passers-by, especially if it occurs in residential areas.

Some people consider prostitution a victimless crime. Others point to the fact that the procurer, or pimp, often abuses his prostitutes and that the industry is associated with drug traffic, robbery, organized crime, and child prostitution.

Prostitution is a billion-dollar industry, and male prostitution, especially homosexual, is increasing. Because the many cases would clog the courts, prostitution is rarely punished. Police use decoys to arrest prostitutes, and sometimes their clients, but release most of them after payment of a small fine. The arrests are merely attempts to discourage open prostitution.

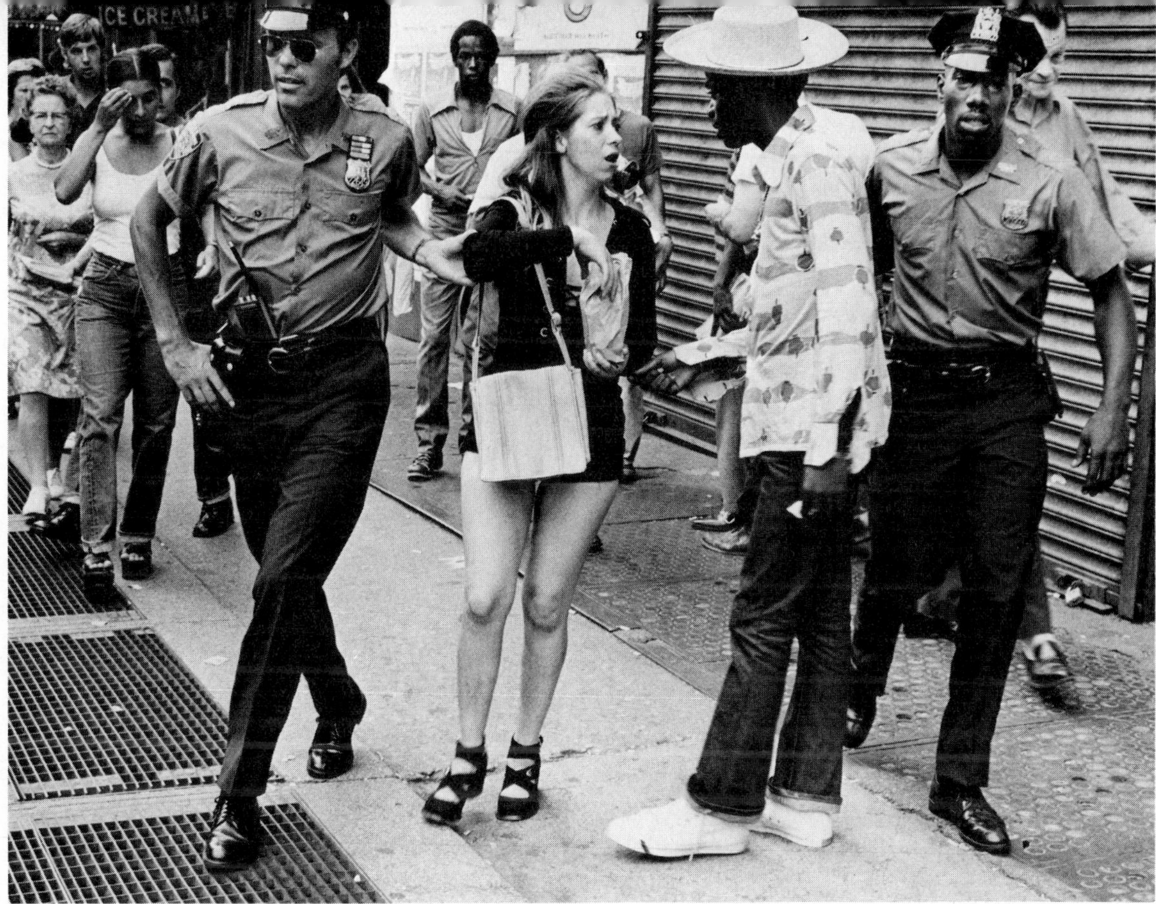

Prostitution, "the world's oldest profession," although illegal in nearly every state, is difficult to control because of its continued prevalence. (Photo © Michael Hanulak/Photo Researchers, Inc.)

Pornography

Pornography is the use of written or visual materials for sexual arousal. Many people believe that pornographic materials lead to bizarre sexual behavior, particularly assault. In 1971 a presidential commission, however, reported that pornography appears to have no harmful effects on adults. The commission found that male sex offenders had had less exposure to pornography than other men. It recommended that pornography be legally available to consenting adults. Congress and the President rejected the findings.

Denmark legalized all pornography in the 1960s, with surprising results. After legalization, there was a decrease in the number of all types of sexual offenses reported in Copenhagen, except rape. The largest decrease was in voyeurism and in child molestations. This suggests that the materials may provide a sexual outlet—a safety valve—for potential offenders of children.

Recent studies on violent pornography report dramatically different results. The portrayal of rape in which the victim became sexually aroused by or sympathetic with her attacker tended to reinforce men's belief in rape myths *(all women want to be raped).* A film depicting rape increased male aggression toward women, whereas a nonviolent film did not. It appears that *violence,* not *eroticism,* is the factor that can lead to serious antisocial behavior.

Summary

Despite the increased openness in discussing human sexuality, we still believe myths about every aspect of sexuality. These myths can reinforce our fears of inadequacy and sexual failure. We need to put these myths to rest so that we can see sexuality as an expression of the whole person.

We should distinguish between *public sexuality*—learned, stereotyped patterns—and our *private sexuality*—our personal genital responses to sexual stimulation. In both areas we have many decisions to make about the ways in which we express our sexuality.

Genetic sex is determined at conception. An ovum contains an X, or female, chromosome; sperm can have either an X or a Y (male) chromosome. If the ovum is fertilized by an X-bearing sperm, the embryo will be female; if fertilized by a Y-bearing sperm, a male results. At first the development of sex organs in the embryo is the same in both sexes, but at about six to eight weeks hormones in the male stimulate the development of male organs.

The masculine or feminine identity given to us at birth is reinforced throughout life by learned behavior, or sex roles. Certain ways of acting are considered appropriate for a given sex: according to sex-role stereotypes, males, for example, are supposed to be strong and independent, females weak and dependent. Recently, however, there has been interest in the concept of androgyny, the belief that people can and should feel free to express the best human qualities, regardless of whether they are considered masculine or feminine.

The human sexual response follows a four-phase cycle: the exitement phase, the plateau phase, the orgasmic phase, and the resolution phase. This cycle is essentially the same in men and women, and an awareness of the similarities can help lead to easier communication between partners about sexual needs and preferences.

Most people experience some unfulfilling sexual responses at some time in their lives. Many times the problem is a temporary reaction to stress, fatigue, or illness; in many other cases it is a symptom of psychological conflicts between partners. Occasionally more severe problems arise, such as orgasmic dysfunction in women and erectile dysfunction in men.

Variant, or deviant behavior, consists of those sexual actions that are not sanctioned by society. Some forms that are, or have been, considered variant are transsexualism, trasvestism, fetishism, exhibitionism and voyeurism, pedophilia, incest, and sadomasochism.

There is much controversy today concerning the regulation of sexual behavior by the law. Many private sexual practices are illegal, although the laws are rarely enforced. Prostitution and pornography are both areas where laws and their enforcement vary widely. Rape is clearly illegal, but it remains difficult to get convictions; often the victim ends up being put on the defensive.

In conclusion, it is essential to understand the facts about human sexuality. Sex is both a joy and a responsibility, and an understanding of medical and psychological truths and honest communication can enhance our enjoyment and personal growth.

Review and Discussion

1. Describe the differences between the fetal development of males and females.

2. What psychological characteristics are assigned to masculine and feminine roles in our society?

3. Define androgyny. Can you give examples of cases where sex roles may interfere with a person's fulfillment?

4. Describe the four phases of the sexual response. What are the major differences between the male and female responses?

5. Describe four common male and female sexual dysfunctions.

6. Describe six forms of deviant sexual behavior.

7. What types of sexual behavior are governed by law? In what areas do you think the laws should be changed?

8. What myths about sexuality are involved in the difficulties in getting convictions in rape cases?

9. In your opinion, what responsibilities are part of a full expression of sexuality?

10. List and explain some common sexual myths.

Further Reading

Carrera, Michael. *Sex: The Act, The Facts and You.* New York: Crown Pbl. 1981.
A frank and open discussion of the facts of human sexuality.

Farrell, Warren. *The Liberated Man.* New York: Bantam Books, 1975.
Explores the idea of male liberation and freeing men in their most intimate relationships. (Paperback.)

Filene, Peter Gabriel. *Him-Her Self: Sex Roles in Modern America.* New York: New American Library, 1976.
A historical look at the effect of sex roles on life in America. (Paperback.)

Friday, Nancy. *Men In Love.* New York: Dell Publishing Co., 1981.
Offers an intimate look at the sexual fantasies of men while exploring the role fantasy plays with regard to sexuality. (Paperback.)

Hite, Shere, *The Hite Report.* New York: Dell Publishing Co., 1981.
A nationwide study of female sexuality. Includes the candid responses of 3,000 women, ages 14 to 78. (Paperback.)

Lehrman, Nat. *Masters and Johnson Explained* (revised edition). New York: Playboy Press Paperbacks, 1981.
Highlights and analysis of Masters and Johnson's Human Sexual Response *and* Human Sexual Inadequacy, *endorsed by the authors. (Paperback.)*

Talese, Gay. *Thy Neighbor's Wife.* New York: Doubleday and Company, 1980.
A novel that deals with morality and sexuality. (Paperback.)

Tschirhart, Linda S. and Ann Getter. *In Defense of Ourselves: A Rape Prevention Handbook for Women.* New York: Doubleday and Company, 1979.
A frank discussion of rape and how women can prevent rape.

Woodbury, John and Elroy Schwartz. *Silent Sin.* New York: New American Library, 1971.
A case history of a young girl's incestuous relationship with her father and the ultimate effect it had on her life. (Paperback.)

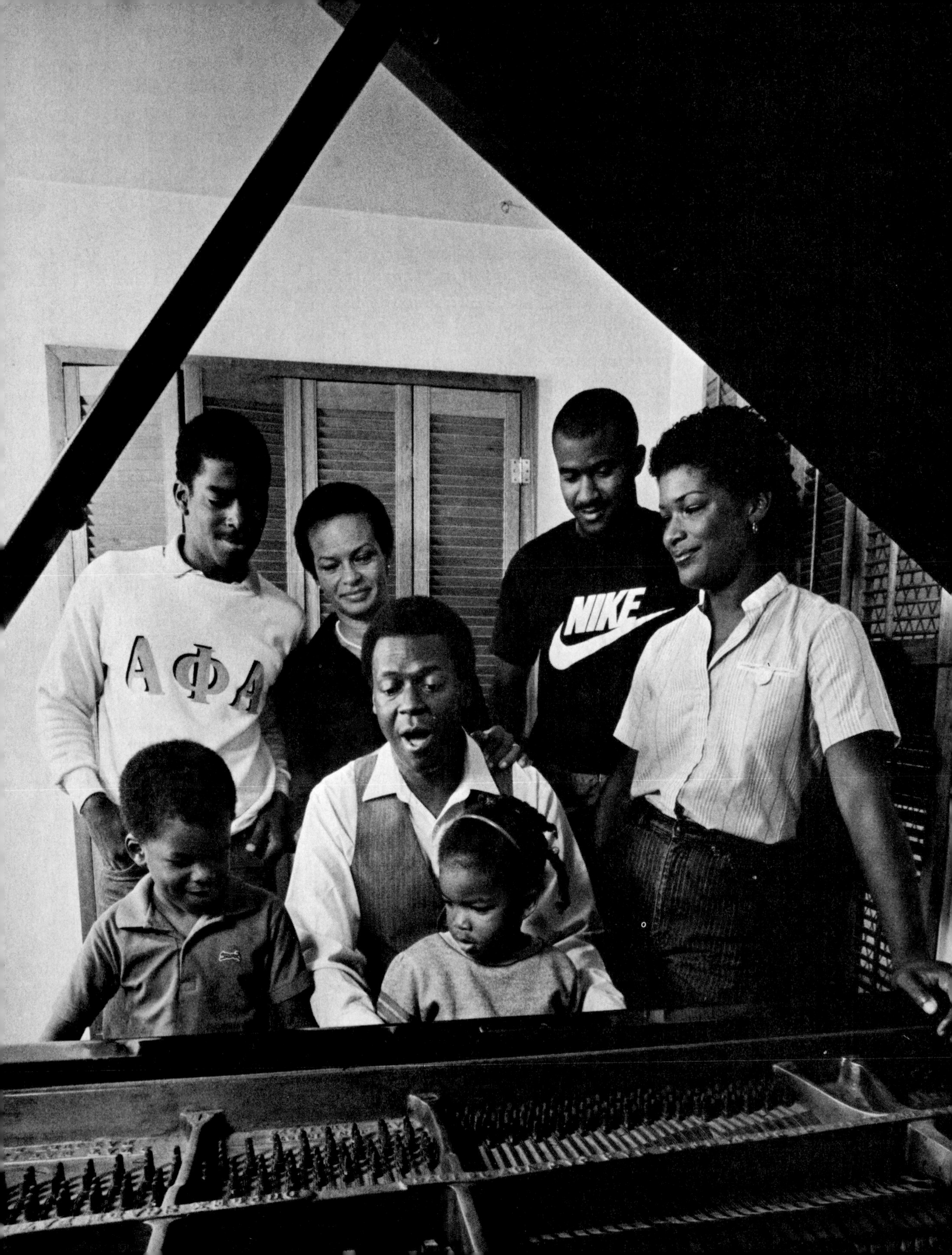
ΑΦΑ
NIKE

Chapter 6 Relationships

KEY POINTS

- ☐ The sexual revolution was not a sudden change but rather one stage in the gradual evolution of personal relationships and the family.
- ☐ Sexual freedom brings with it the need to use an effective means of birth control and to be aware of the dangers of sexually related diseases and psychological problems.
- ☐ Although its bases have changed somewhat, marriage retains its predominant position in our society as a means of propagating offspring and expressing affection.
- ☐ Having children can be very satisfying and can strengthen a good marriage but will not solve marital problems.
- ☐ The number of couples getting divorced has reached record levels, and there has been an even greater rise in the proportion of single-parent families.
- ☐ Alternatives to conventional family life include open marriage, group marriage, part-time marriage, bisexual or homosexual marriage, celibacy, and cohabitation.
- ☐ Although the choices in relationships have become broader and freer in recent years, they should be made seriously, on the basis of careful thought and self-understanding.

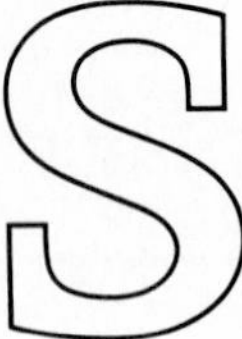

URELY you know by now that there is more to health than keeping your body's systems in good working order. Your mind and emotions are involved, too. For example, you have to make choices among different options, which can be difficult and even stressful, with important consequences for your total well-being for the rest of your life. And of these choices, none is more important than what sorts of lifetime commitments you make to others — whether you will marry, have children, or live with others in alternative arrangements.

What choices you make may ultimately be determined by when, where, and to whom you were born; the code of beliefs you have learned; and such significant outside influences as school, friends, and the media. Nevertheless, the decisions are yours, and they require careful thinking about who you are and how you want to live your life. Because of recent changes in attitudes toward relationships, more possibilities are open to you than would have been in the past, and making life-style choices now may be harder than in previous eras.

The Sexual "Revolution"

At first glance, it may appear that you are living in a completely different world from that in which your parents grew up and that the choices you face have a very recent history — dating back, specifically, to the 1960s. Since that decade there has been much talk about the sexual revolution that supposedly took place then. With that decade came the opportunity to choose from numerous life-styles — ranging from the traditional American-as-apple-pie marriage to homosexual parenthood. The central actors in this revolution were young people. Breaking sharply with the past, they were said to be engaging in sexual intercourse at ever earlier ages, with the consequences of unwanted pregnancies, high divorce rates. This added to concern about the disintegration of the family — with all that such an event would imply for society.

Increasingly, though, social scientists are coming to the conclusion that the rumors of revolution were greatly exaggerated. Most historians who specialize in the study of social change agree that the sexual revolution of the 1960s was mainly a new awareness of events that have been underway for decades. The most important of these events are the following:

1. As the science of medicine has progressed over the last century, the mortality rates have declined steadily, providing a major reason to limit family size.
2. Nearly perfected methods of birth control have transformed sex from an act primarily for procreation to one primarily for pleasure.

3. A century of technological innovation has led to the gradual reduction of the number of household chores women have to perform, thus freeing them for activities outside the home.

As these few sentences suggest, substantial changes in the family and the perception of appropriate roles for men, women, and children have evolved to their present state slowly. Just as slowly, the old taboos against talking about or depicting sex have disappeared. The sexual revolution of the 1960s is more accurately seen as one step in the evolution of the family, a time when certain gradual changes in sexual roles and behavior were openly acknowledged.

Choosing a pattern for living with others at this point in the evolution of our sexual attitudes, however, is perhaps more difficult than ever before because there are so many options. The family, which not too long ago was declared all but dead, is still with us—although it has changed considerably in recent years and apparently is continuing to change. According to the best available statistics, marriage is taking place at later ages than was the case until recently, both partners usually work at jobs outside the home, and the number of children produced by each couple is declining. The challenge for the future, in the view of one authority, is "the problem that has no name: . . . how to juggle work, love, home, and children"[1]—in other words, how to mesh our traditional values with new life-styles.

Dating

Whether called "dating," "going out," or just "getting together," this is the first step most young people take toward developing the social skills involved in building satisfactory relationships. At whatever age you start dating and for however long you continue to build your social life around dating, it plays an important role in shaping your image of yourself.

It may seem self-evident that there is a considerable difference in the dating "script" for high school freshmen, college freshmen, and single or recently divorced people in their twenties, thirties, forties, or later years—but often all are described as going through the same experience.

Young Teens: Dating as a Rehearsal for Adulthood

As practiced by younger teens, dating has been aptly described as a rehearsal for more serious courtship. Early dating is a part of the larger preparation for maturity that goes along with the gradual establishing of independence from family, learning to drive, getting work experience, and developing other social skills. Naturally, young

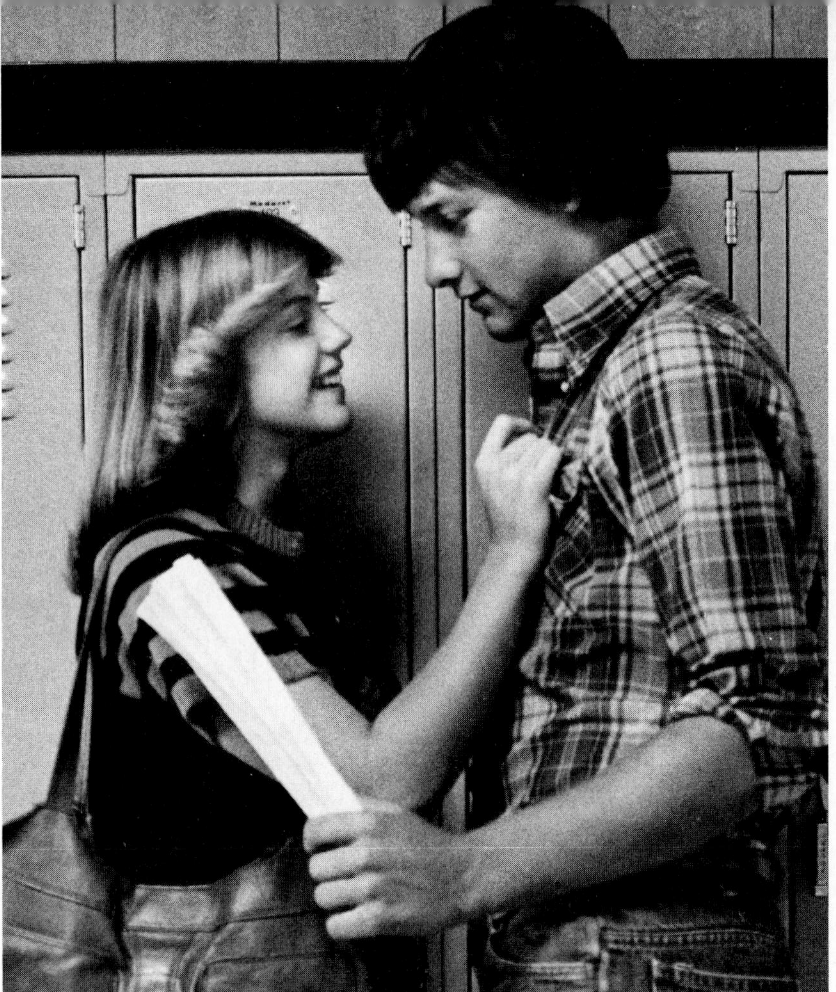

Dating among young teenagers is a rehearsal for adulthood. (Photo by Nancy J. Pierce/Photo Researchers, Inc.)

teens bring preconceptions to each of these experiences. The expectations and vocabulary they bring to dating are derived from what they have seen and heard in their own environments, including such sources as movies, television, and popular music.

Within this framework, young teens tend to perceive dating as a way of discovering the promise of romantic love. In this initial experimentation with adulthood, physiological signs—butterflies in the stomach, blushing, perspiring, rapid heartbeat—are accepted as virtually certain indications of love, although these are the same physiological signals of fear, anger, excitement, and joy. Learning to recognize these signs for what they truly represent is a part of what we call growing up.

Whether the signals are interpreted correctly or not, the attachments formed in dating sometimes grow into what the partners perceive as love, which in turn may lead to sexual experimentation.

Pairing Off: The Sexual Experiment Begins

An important shift in attitudes toward sexual experimentation as a part of dating usually begins to emerge in the later years of high school. Progress from a simple kiss to prolonged sessions of necking and petting now seems increasingly to culminate in sexual intercourse. More recent studies show that the percentage of women aged 15 to 19 who have had sexual intercourse has risen steadily, from about 30 percent in 1970 to 50 percent in 1979. The mean age at first intercourse in 1979 for these women was 16.2 years.[2]

From 1970 to 1980, at the same time that the national birthrate was dropping, the percentage of pregnancies that were out-of-wedlock rose from 9 to 16. Only about one-half of those teens who were pregnant married the father of their child—a fact that has been attributed partly to the increased availability of abortions.[3]

The Case for Contraception

Not surprisingly, figures like these have created a great deal of concern about moral, social, and medical issues. From a medical point of view, neither pregnancy nor abortion is desirable for women under 18. The risks of going through pregnancy before one's own body is completely developed can have serious health consequences for both the mother and her child. The young pregnant woman is likely to deny her condition longer, so instead of the simple surgical procedure appropriate for early pregnancy, a complex and hazardous abortion method may be necessary. And whether abortion occurs promptly or not, it can generate serious psychological problems.

Physicians and social scientists are also perplexed by the rise in teenage pregnancies, perhaps less because it reflects on the moral

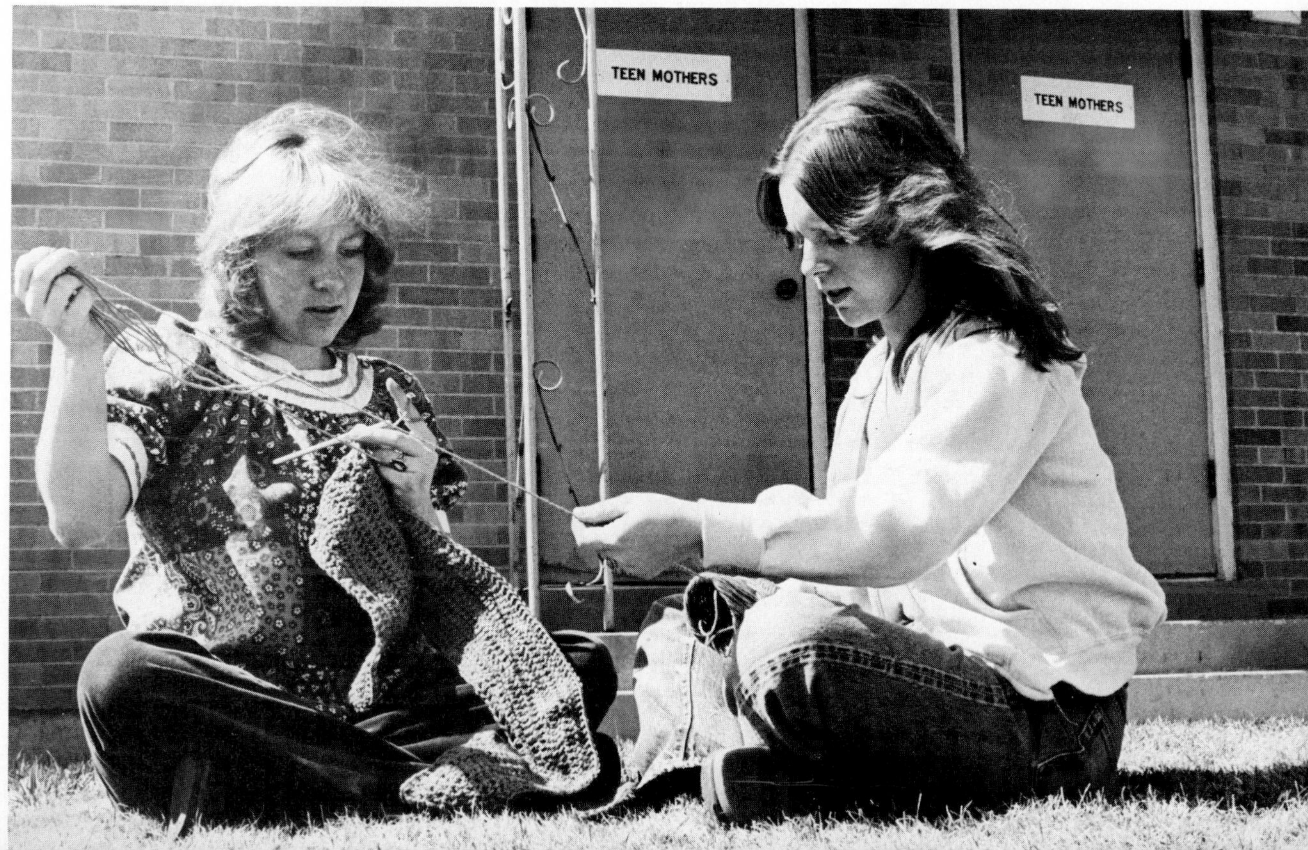

Two unwed 17-year-old girls, one a mother (right), the other pregnant, at a special school for teen mothers. Recent statistics show a dramatic increase in teenage pregnancies. (Photo from Associated Press)

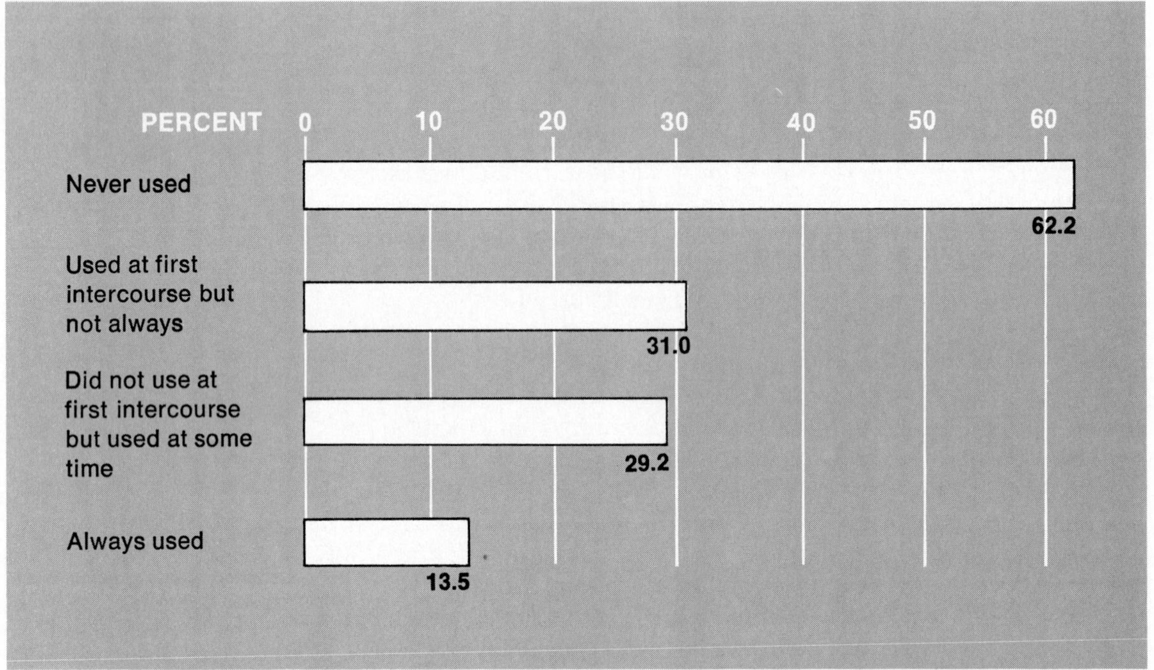

Figure 6–1. Contraceptive Use and Pregnancy Among Teenagers. Percentage of sexually active unmarried women aged 15 to 19 who became pregnant before marriage, by contraceptive-use status. Note that 13.5 percent of those who reported always using contraceptives still became pregnant. (Source: Adapted from M. Zelnik and John F. Kantner, "Sexual Activity, Contraceptive Use, and Pregnancy Among Metropolitan Area Teenagers, 1971–1979." Adapted with permission from *Family Planning Perspectives* 12 [Sept.–Oct. 1980]: 236.)

climate of the nation than because it suggests a remarkable ignorance of the kinds of contraceptive techniques that are available and effective. Interviews with pregnant teens tend to support the view that there is still a profound reluctance (despite the abundance of sources —see Chapter 4) to consult with anyone about how to prevent pregnancy.

Data such as those shown in Figure 6–1 may cause justifiable concern. When considered along with the rising trend toward marrying at a later age, they suggest that early intercourse often occurs without the goal of serious partner selection in mind. However, there is a growing body of research showing that the more goal-directed teens —those who plan to attend college or have fairly well-delineated life schemes—not only are more likely to defer first intercourse but also are more likely to use contraceptives.[4] The weaker her self-image and the greater her need for love and companionship, the more likely a girl is to engage in unprotected intercourse and, if pregnant, to go to term in hopes of acquiring a longtime companion and source of love. Unfortunately, the expectation and reality rarely mesh.

College Dating: A Changing Picture

The traditional image of a date that many people have — an attractive, well-dressed young couple at a prom — was a collegiate creation of the 1920s, the first time in our history when young men and women found themselves together in large numbers away from home. This image persisted during the three decades that followed, in part because it was portrayed as typical behavior in movies and television and, perhaps, because it was reported as typical by social scientists who studied it.

Sexual Freedom

Although good looks and charm have not disappeared as criteria for date and mate selection in college, the rules of the game appear to have changed substantially. According to the old rules, a well-brought-up young man could have sex before marriage (often with prostitutes), while an equally well-brought-up young woman was expected to remain a virgin at least until she was engaged and, properly, until she was married. As we have seen already, the rules were not always kept; but the open acknowledgment and acceptance of the transition away from the double standard did not come until the 1960s, along with the atmosphere of naturalness, openness, and sexual permissiveness. The apparent consequence has been to make premarital sex the norm rather than the exception among college students.[5]

Health Problems of Sexual Freedom. Before turning to the customary sequel to dating — marriage and child rearing — it is important to stop and think about some of the health problems that accompany the new sexual freedom. Besides the need for using an effective form of birth control, one should be aware that sexual experimentation may lead to problems ranging from bladder infections to disorders such as herpes, gonorrhea, and other sexually transmitted diseases (see Chapter 15).

Sexual permissiveness may also present psychological problems. It has been reported, for example, that though it was once the norm for psychiatrists to see patients suffering from sexual malfunctions, it is now common for them to treat patients who are overwhelmed by the sexual options that are open to them.

Making choices that may affect the course of one's entire life is never easy. Indeed, the most ordinary kind of decision making can be stressful. When these decisions involve choosing between old and hallowed customs and those that are new and not as widely accepted, the task becomes even more difficult.

Making Your Own Decision

If you feel uncomfortable about engaging in sexual activities outside of marriage, you have the right and obligation to yourself to say, "No." You may feel a little bit out of it, but there is no reason why you

YOUR HEALTH TODAY

Making Your Own Decision

If you believe that living together before marriage—for whatever reason—is desirable, you should prepare yourself for some problems that could arise. The following questions are offered for your consideration:

- How will my family and friends react to my decision to live with someone?
- How will I feel about their reaction?
- What do I want from my partner's and my relationship? Is living together the best way to fulfill this need?
- What rules will govern sexual behavior both in and out of this relationship? Are these rules fair to both of us?
- If my partner is sexually active outside this relationship, how will I react?
- Will my partner and I be supportive of each other if our families are resistant?

cannot make and live with this decision—perhaps becoming happier with yourself as a result, since your solution is consistent with your feelings.

Marriage: Myth and Reality

All kinds of statistics are cited to support the contention that marriage is no longer a popular institution. According to the U.S. Census Bureau, for example:

- The proportion of the population age 18 and over that is married is down from 76.4 percent of males and 71.6 of females in 1960 to 67.8 of males and 62.4 of females in 1981.
- The rising median age at marriage for females is up from 20.3 in 1950 to 22.3 in 1981; for males, from 22.8 in 1950 to 24.8 in 1981.
- The number of divorces is up from 385,000 in 1950 to 1,182,000 in 1980.

Although often cited, such data are scarcely enough evidence that we should mourn the passage of a custom that has had a central place in Western culture for hundreds of years. In fact, over 90 percent of all individuals in the United States will marry at some point in their lives. There is widespread agreement among most students of marriage—physicians, psychologists, sociologists, family counselors, ministers, and others—that many of the problems that bedevil marriages could be avoided if people simply brought more realistic expectations to marriage.

Love and Kinship

It may surprise you to learn that even today social scientists are not in agreement about the value of **romantic love** in building a lasting marriage. Some regard it as a feeling so impossible to define properly that it cannot accurately be factored into research.

Love (romantic) Intense affection, concern, and attachment to another individual.

Nevertheless, in a youth-oriented culture like our own, love becomes a primary motivation for marriage, as the reduction of family ties leaves a young person free to fall in love and through love and marriage to form an alternative to the traditional extended network of kinfolk. The partners in such a love marriage are potentially better able to concentrate on building an effective relationship, because of the minimal number of kin.[6]

While it is obviously true that the kinship ties of today are less important than they were in the past, they have not disappeared completely. In fact, the chances of marrying someone who is totally repugnant to the most important of kin – parents – are limited because parents continue to have and exercise a substantial degree of social and economic control (which may, of course, be extended as long as financial dependency remains).

We may conclude that although the bases for marriage have changed somewhat, the institution itself remains the primary way sanctioned by custom, faith, and law for the expression of affection and the propagation of offspring.

The institution of marriage has changed somewhat over the years. However, it still remains the accepted means for propagating offspring and expressing affection in our society. (Photo © Peter G. Aitken/Photo Researchers, Inc.)

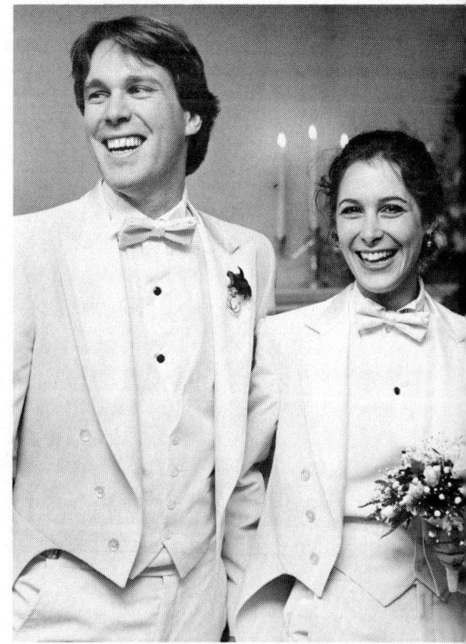

Readiness for Marriage

Just as there is no universally accepted definition of love, so there is no sure technique for predicting readiness for marriage. However, most authorities agree that such factors as age, emotional and social maturity, and financial resources should be carefully considered.

Age

Age heads the list because it has been found again and again that early marriages (made between the ages of 16 and 22) are statistically the least likely to last. Social and economic factors may be involved, since younger persons are less likely to have the education and financial security that help make a marriage succeed.

Early adulthood is also commonly a time in which each of us changes some tastes, standards, and goals. If these directional changes take place within marriage, they are likely to create friction, particularly if one's taste in people is undergoing revision too. The boy or girl who was appealing in high school may no longer seem even mildly interesting just a few years later. If one has married during that first stage, the danger is obvious.

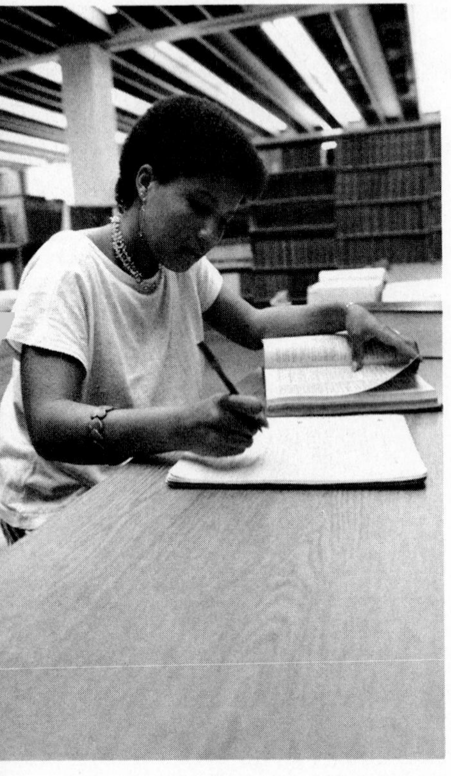

Woman graduate student in a university library. The changing aspirations of women have led to new patterns of marriage. (Photo © Frank Siteman 1983/Stock, Boston)

Emotional and Social Maturity

Still another reason advanced against early marriage is that it can be emotionally and intellectually stultifying. Since fewer and fewer people are getting married when they are young, the young marrieds are likely to be cut off from the activities of the peer group, literally growing old before their time, and possibly bitter about all the missed fun.

Age and emotional maturity contribute to social maturity by adding experience in all kinds of social interactions. Most authorities agree that social maturity requires not only the standard social experiences of high school and college but also a significant length of time in which each partner had demonstrated the ability to live independently of emotional and financial support from his or her family. It is also important to be independent before marriage simply to have a more objective understanding of whether marriage is truly the desired alternative to freedom to do what one likes when one wants to do it. If the answer is "yes," the marriage is more likely to succeed than if no basis for comparison existed.

Financial Readiness

If one is ready for marriage in terms of age and emotional and social maturity, one other basic criterion that remains to be met is the thorny one of financial readiness. This may seem like a small concern when both partners are working, but it is important to consider not only one's present financial situation but also possible future changes. What if one or the other partner wants to return to school for an advanced degree? Or loses a job? What if the wife becomes pregnant? What if a parent or sibling has to move in? The list of possibilities is potentially longer and more disturbing than even these examples suggest, but they should serve as a reminder of the fundamental importance of not only earning enough but also having reserve funds for emergencies.

Selecting a Partner

A good deal of time, study, and effort have been expanded by family researchers on trying to identify the factors that lead to successful marriages. The findings of one group of researchers can be stated as follows:

> The chances of a happy marriage are determined by one's own personal traits, those of one's chosen partner, and how those traits act upon each other. Consider, then, some of the traits to look for in a potential mate. Right away let us dispel the notion of the "one and only" or the "marriage made in heaven." For every person there are thousands of potentially good mates. If the person you might be considering for marriage seems to have some serious deficiency in some respect, just keep looking. On the other hand, if no one

SELF-ASSESSMENT EXERCISE 6.1

LoveMeter: A Technique for the Measurement of Love

Below is a list of items concerning love. Please read all statements very carefully and respond to all of them on the basis of your own actual feelings without consulting any other person.

Do this by reading each item and then writing, in the space provided at the left, only one of the following numbers: 0, 1, 2. The meaning of these figures is:

0 absent
1 weak
2 strong

In other words, each of the following statements refers *only* to *your own actual feelings, attitudes, desires, wishes,* and the like regarding *only a specific person.* So always keep that person in mind and answer every item with 0, 1, or 2, depending on how you feel about that person only. For instance, if *your* willingness to accept responsibility for the other person's actions is absent, write 0; if it is weak, say 1; and if it is strong, reply 2.

Please check here who that person is: spouse_____, fiancé(e)_____, dating partner_____, other (indicate relationship)_____.

Remember: Each statement refers only to your own feelings about that person only!

_____ **1.** Willingness to accept responsibility for the other person's actions.

_____ **2.** Feeling as if we were one person.

_____ **3.** A sense of loyalty.

_____ **4.** A desire to be together forever.

_____ **5.** Loneliness when separated.

_____ **6.** A desire to make the other person a source of my security.

_____ **7.** Putting the partner's welfare before mine.

_____ **8.** Helping the partner financially when possible.

_____ **9.** A feeling of intellectual closeness to the other person.

_____ **10.** A desire to share religious convictions.

_____ **11.** Longing to experience things together.

_____ **12.** Making the other person secure.

_____ **13.** Making financial decisions together.

_____ **14.** A general feeling of dependence on the partner.

_____ **15.** Sacrificing for the partner.

_____ **16.** Longing to do things together.

_____ **17.** Realizing financial limits and expecting what is possible.

_____ **18.** Helping the partner improve.

_____ **19.** Sharing the partner's unhappiness.

_____ **20.** Acceptance of the partner's ideas about family size.

_____ **21.** Sharing the partner's opinions.

_____ **22.** Acceptance of the other person's ideas about child rearing.

(Continued)

_________ **23.** Efforts to make our relationship grow.

_________ **24.** Unselfish giving.

_________ **25.** Sharing the partner's interests.

_________ **26.** Sharing a philosophy about dividing labor between male's and female's.

_________ **27.** Finding joy in the partner's happiness.

_________ **28.** Helping in sickness.

_________ **29.** Enjoying just being together.

_________ **30.** Pride in the partner.

_________ **31.** Giving moral support.

_________ **32.** Avoiding things that hurt our relationship.

_________ **33.** Doing things for the other person's friends and relatives.

_________ **34.** Helping solve the partner's problems.

_________ **35.** Enjoying just talking with the partner.

_________ **36.** Patience when problems arise.

_________ **37.** Forgiving faults and weaknesses.

_________ **38.** Speaking about my daily experiences.

_________ **39.** Acceptance of the other person's goals.

_________ **40.** Lifting the other person's ego.

_________ **41.** Willingness to settle differences constructively.

_________ **42.** Willingness to share responsibilities.

_________ **43.** Willingness to plan together.

_________ **44.** Sharing a philosophy of family life.

_________ **45.** A sense of trust.

_________ **46.** Expressing my feelings openly.

_________ **47.** Enjoying listening to the other person.

_________ **48.** Respect for the partner's actions.

_________ **49.** A need to be wanted by the partner.

_________ **50.** Making the other person feel important.

(Score equals the sum total of fifty numerical responses. Range: 0, no love, to 100, strongest love.)

Source: Adapted from Panos D. Bardos, "Erotometer," *International Review of Sociology* 1 (1971): 71–77.

---

seems to fit your ideal for marriage, you might well be overcritical, or just not ready for marriage.[7]

Traits to Look For

It is generally agreed that it is advantageous for the partners to be fairly well matched in age, background, level of education, and aspirations. When the match is good in these aspects, there is considerably less likelihood of disappointment and disagreement on such touchy issues as what faith to follow, how to rear children, and with whom to socialize than there is in marriages in which the partners have less in common. This is not to suggest that the marriages of people from widely different backgrounds are doomed from the start, but that it takes above-average adaptability to make them work.

There is also a consensus that the partners should be open with each other about their health and their hereditary disorders, if any, simply because these issues may be singularly important in the decision of whether or not to have children.

Engagement

Historically, the announcement of the pledge by a man and a woman to marry was described by the now somewhat archaic word *betrothal.* Betrothal, like the marriage that followed, was binding on both parties—except in extraordinary circumstances. The contemporary equivalent of betrothal is, of course, **engagement**—a custom that is far less constraining or burdened with rules than the formal betrothal. Nowadays, couples can become engaged with a minimum of fuss or as much as they want, including public announcements, an exchange of tokens (customarily a ring for the bride-to-be), and parties to celebrate the event.

Engagement Pledging oneself to marry a certain individual.

Purpose of the Engagement. Delightful as all this may be, the engagement period has a serious purpose. Mainly, it gives the couple

YOUR HEALTH TODAY

Traits to Look for in a Partner

1. Ability to adapt to new situations and demands.
2. A usually optimistic view of life and the future.
3. Ability to laugh.
4. A concern for the well-being of others.
5. Maturity.
6. Ability to express and experience love and intimacy.
7. Compassion, warmth, and understanding.
8. Ability to set realistic goals.
9. Honesty.

Traits to Avoid in a Partner

1. Jealousy.
2. Anxiousness.
3. Inability to set realistic goals.
4. A generally negative outlook on life and the future.
5. Depression and withdrawal.
6. Inability to express and experience love.
7. Unrealistic expectations of the relationship.
8. Total dependency.
9. Dishonesty.

the opportunity to see each other more nearly as they may be in marriage because they are paired off, not dating other men or women, and probably spending more time together than previously. In other words, the couple are on their own, much as they will be, if their marriage endures, for years to come.

Length of the Engagement Period. Society imposes no fixed length on the engagement period, and in practice it may vary from as little as a month to several years, usually depending on whether both partners have completed their schooling and are established in their careers. Because marriages between mature adults have been shown to be more durable and happier than those between young people, it is probably a good idea for a young couple to test their commitment for a somewhat longer time than an older, more experienced couple might feel is necessary.

Reasons to Break the Engagement. Neither partner should hesitate to break the engagement if the relationship seems to be in trouble — for example, if it should become clear that the woman is a "clinging vine" in search of a surrogate father or the man becomes jealous of his fiancée if she does more than say a cool hello to the men she meets. Other danger signals to watch out for are mood swings, irrational outbursts of anger, a reluctance to talk things through, and undue involvement by parents and relatives. Remember, it is far less complicated and painful to end an engagement than to go through a divorce.

Developing a Healthy Relationship

It might seem that if each partner in a marriage has carefully chosen a life companion — subjecting him or her to all the "tests" that have been mentioned so far — there would be no more to worry about and the newlyweds would, in fact, live happily ever after. Unfortunately, this is seldom true because marriage is different from engagement, and even from living together. In principle, at any rate, there is no easy exit from marriage as there is from the other two relationships.

Adjusting to One Another's Habits

Given this sense of indissolubility, a couple may find as early as their honeymoon that it is necessary to adjust to each other's small but sometimes irritating habits, such as regularly leaving clothing on the floor, not refolding the newspaper, or squeezing the toothpaste from the middle rather than tidily rolling it up from the bottom of the tube. Trivial, yes — until one thinks of a possible lifetime of such petty aggravations. As one newlywed observed:

> Marriage is like taking an airplane to Florida for a relaxing vacation in January, and when you get off the plane you find you're in the Swiss Alps. There is cold and snow instead of swimming and sunshine. Well, after you buy winter clothes and learn how to ski and learn how to talk a new foreign

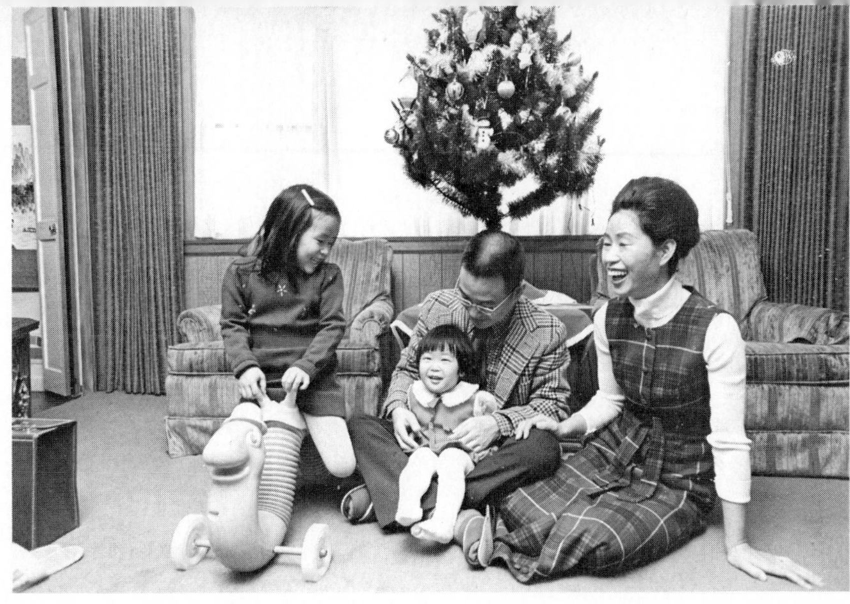

Developing a healthy family requires the efforts of all family members. (Photo © 1981 Peter Menzel)

language, you can have just as good a vacation in the Swiss Alps as you can in Florida. But I can tell you it's . . . a surprise when you get off that marital airplane and find that everything is far different from what one had assumed.[8]

Recognizing Partner's Worthwhile Characteristics

When differences and problems are less than acute, a couple may come to recognize that no one can live in ecstasy forever, and realize that although each may have chosen the spouse for all the wrong reasons (looks, wealth, sexiness) he or she has other complementary qualities that are at least as worthwhile as and more lasting than the superficial characteristics responsible for the original attraction. As William Lederer and Don Jackson have pointed out,

In a workable marriage both parties may be better off together than they would have been on their own. They may not be ecstatically happy because of their union, and they may not be "in love," but they are not lonely and they have areas of shared contentment. They feel reasonably satisfied with their levels of personal and interpersonal functioning. They can count their blessings and, like a sage, philosophically realize that nothing is perfect.[9]

Moving Beyond Romantic Expectations

Sex. If one wisely accepts that nothing is perfect, it follows that even the romantic expectations of an ideal sex life created by popular magazines and how-to books are also exaggerations. Good sexual relations are, of course, vital to marriage, but this does not mean that fireworks are going to go off every time or that you have to practice gymnastic contortions to hear the proverbial bells ringing. Moreover, there is no rule specifying how little or how much sex is necessary for a marriage to be successful. The only two people who are involved in making the how-when-where decisions are the couple themselves, and if their pattern of sexual relations suits them it is totally irrelevant what the ads say, the movies portray, or the sex advisers write.

Fantasies. Another romantic fallacy that dies hard in marriage is embodied in the words of the old song, "I Only Have Eyes for You," which suggests that after marriage a kind of blindness to others of the opposite sex not only can but must set in. This fallacy not only runs counter to all we know of human nature but encourages a virtually unattainable degree of fidelity of mind and heart. There is needless guilt when such fidelity is violated. Ask any honest long-married couple you know if they have ever fantasized about another man or woman and the answer will be "Yes." This does not mean they acted on their fantasies but simply that they had them without violating a lifelong commitment to the spouse. Indeed, there are some authorities who feel that these fantasies can be healthy since they serve as a substitute for the far more dangerous extramarital affair.

Roles. Until relatively recently, a predominant myth of the ideal marriage held that the woman should be content to keep house, rear the children, and wait on her husband, who, in turn, would be the sole financial supporter of the family. However, a new myth has evolved —that both partners should take perfectly equal roles in a marriage. Just how any individual marriage should work is best determined by the wants, needs, and values of the individuals involved.

Anticipate and Avoid Causes of Conflict

Talk About Potential Problems. To avoid conflict over differing views about how your marriage should be structured, you and your prospective spouse should consider all the practical aspects of your impending marriage. It is probably impossible to talk too much or

YOUR HEALTH TODAY

Healthy Families

The following are generally held to be some of the characteristics of healthy families:

- They spend time together.
- There is appreciation and concern for the welfare of each family member.
- They are able to make decisions efficiently.
- They are expressive and supportive of each other.
- They have good communication.
- They are committed to maintaining the integrity of the family.
- They handle adversity well.
- There is a well-defined power structure.

Sources: Adapted from C. A. Gantman, "A Closer Look at Families That Work Well," *International Journal of Family Therapy* 2 (1980): 106–119; and from N. Stinnett, "In Search of Strong Families." In *Building Family Strengths,* edited by N. Stinnett, B. Chesser, and J. DeFrain. (Lincoln: University of Nebraska Press, 1979).

think too hard about a step in your life as important as this one. (Think about how much time can be spent making out a guest list or choosing flowers for a wedding. Certainly, how often each partner will do the dishes or balance the checkbook or spend an evening alone is worthy of at least as much consideration.)

Write Down Expectations. Putting your thoughts in writing can help you clarify some of your ideas and expectations about marriage. Although a marriage contract is not legally binding, some couples find that making out such an agreement can help them learn what is most important to each other and prevent conflict by anticipating and avoiding its causes. In marriage it is important not only to know yourself but to know your partner.

Realize You Are Different from Your Parents. Keep in mind, too, that probably the only models of marriage that each of you is really familiar with are your parents'. Those may or may not be good models. However, your marriage will be different from theirs because of the two different personalities that are joining.

Five Types of Marriage

In a fascinating study of "enduring marital relationships," John Cuber and Peggy Harroff found five different styles of marriage that they saw again and again in their research.[10] They labeled these "the conflict-habituated," "the devitalized," "the passive-congenial," "the vital," and "the total." A brief review of these types is included here not because these are the only kinds of marriages but rather to show how a host of different patterns can be encompassed by the word marriage.

The *conflict-habituated marriage* is distinguished by its tension and verbal battles, which interestingly act more effectively than cement to keep the couple together. It may be that the absolute freedom to express resentments, with no pretense at politeness but with no threat of physical abuse, is a form of openness that can support true comradeship effectively. The husband in one such marriage, a physician, said that he had never even considered divorce seriously. Perhaps more important, he added, "A number of times there has been a crisis, like the time I was in the automobile accident, and the time she almost died in childbirth, and then I guess we really showed that we do care about each other. But, as soon as the crisis is over, it's business as usual."[11]

The *devitalized marriage,* as its name implies, is a polar opposite of the conflict-habituated and tends to take on its dominant characteristic only after the marriage is well-established—or after the first flower of romance has faded—when a kind of tolerant acceptance of the mate sets in. The fact that there is no more excitement in the relationship is taken for granted as a part of the aging process. Cuber and Harroff describe such partners as caught in "a habit cage" from which escape is not sought because it runs counter to expectations and the belief in the binding nature of the marriage contract.

The *passive-congenial* couple differ from the devitalized in that they start out by accepting the premise that married life is going to be undramatic. Passive-congenials commonly assert that the glue that holds their marriage together is a common interest or shared tastes. These people appear to emphasize peace and orderliness above such elements as sexual attraction, since this frees them to do other things that may seem more significant to them personally than any individual aspect of the marriage itself.

Partners in a *vital marriage* usually are dedicated to their work and children, but the excitement in their lives comes from shared experiences. They prefer to do things together rather than to tell each other about what each did independently. When disagreements arise, they usually are about fairly substantive issues and are settled quickly, never to be warmed over in future arguments as would be the case with the conflict-habituated.

The *total marriage* is just what its name implies, a complete meshing of personalities and interests in which husband and wife are friends, lovers, and partners. As in the vital relationship, shared experiences outnumber separate ones, conflicts are settled once and for all as they arise, and mutual supportiveness is carried to a high degree.

Cuber and Harroff found that these types of marriage are neither mutually exclusive nor divorce-proof. However, the greater the bond and expectations — as in the total marriage — the more damaging the consequences of change or infidelity are likely to be. Couples with more modest expectations of the institution of marriage are seemingly somewhat less despairing about the impact of their fights and failures to achieve some rare state of bliss.

Children: To Have or Have Not?

Couples who decide not to have children are among the first generation for whom such a choice is not only possible but actively supported by some segments of society. Many people now advocate zero population growth on the grounds that uncontrolled expansion will lead to depletion of natural resources, overcrowding, famine, and disease. Adherents of the traditional view that marriage is ordained for the purpose of child raising offer equally compelling arguments and have developed data to show that technological innovations will offset the predicted shortages in resources, space, health care, and food.

How many children should a couple have?
Three? Two? One? None?
It depends on how many children they really want.
How many they feel they're ready for—emotionally, not just financially.
And when they feel they're ready. (It could also depend on their concern about population growth!)
The important thing is that the question is asked.
Because asking leads to thinking.
And thinking leads to planning.
And planning leads to us.
Planned Parenthood
Children by choice. Not chance.

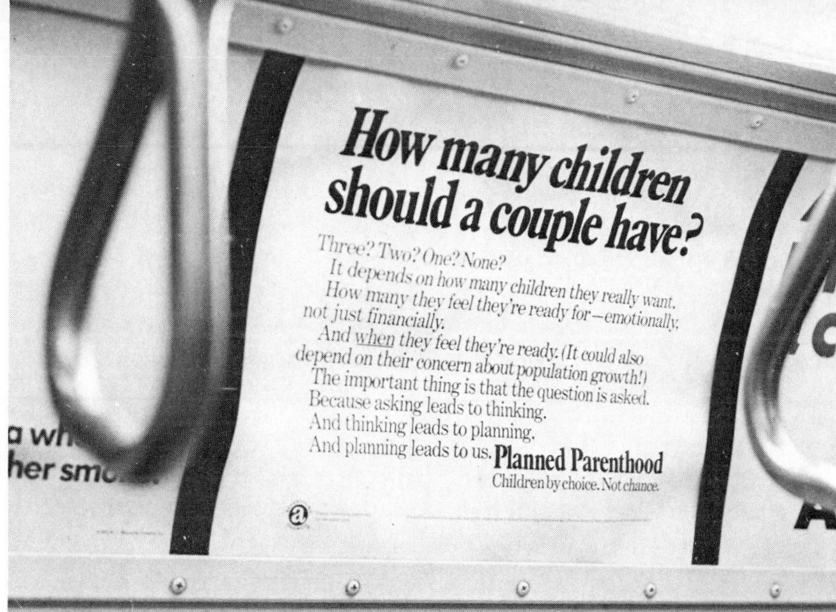

Planned Parenthood poster in subway. Organizations like Planned Parenthood provide information that allows couples to have a child by conscious decision rather than by unwanted accident. (Photo © Yvonne Freund/ Photo Researchers, Inc.)

Reasons for Not Having Children

For many couples, however, the decisions about whether to have children, when, and how many result primarily from personal rather than global considerations. In any case, it is important to remember that having children is never a solution for marital problems and may, on the contrary, serve to increase them. An equally poor reason for having children is to prove that one is masculine or feminine.

Some people choose not to have children simply because they do not like them. Others are opposed to the idea of giving up 18 or more years of their lives to the nurturance of another being. Some view children as a burden that will interfere with their careers. Still others have hereditary conditions that may make childbearing dangerous. In all cases the decision is the couple's and should be honored by parents, friends, and acquaintances for the simple reason that it is a private decision and should not be subjected to outside standards.

Economic Considerations

Another and increasingly widespread reason for having no children or only a few is purely economic. It has been estimated that in 1980 having a child and caring for it at home for 18 years plus four years at a public college costs an average middle-class family $85,000. (It is worth noting that these costs grew by about 33 percent between 1977 and 1980 alone and include only childbirth, food, clothing, medical care, and education at a public university — gifts, private education, and frills were excluded.)

Benefits of Having Children

Having heard so much about the drawbacks of having children, you may wonder whether there are any benefits. Of course there are. Having children acts as a bond between parents and makes a good marriage even better. Besides, if one is mature, having children can be a constant source of pleasure. By sharing one's life with children, one has a day-to-day source of new ideas and new outlooks, which is stimulating and refreshing. And having children gives people a sense of their own immortality by providing a link with the future.

Delays in Having Children

While deciding to have children is not simple, it is the course followed by most married couples. Current statistics show, however, that most couples will have children at a somewhat later age than was the norm in past generations. The reasons for the delay seem often to be tied to career goals and to the obvious need to have a fair degree of financial security.

How Many to Have

A debate has raged in social science circles for years about what number of children is ideal for the development of children themselves and about the impact on each child of its place in the birth order. Two tentative conclusions are suggested by this research. One is that the more children there are in a single family, the greater the likelihood that one or more will show signs of intellectual and emotional deprivation. The second is a convincing reversal of the dictum of psychologist G. Stanley Hall (1844–1924) that "being an only child is a disease." In fact, only children, being the sole focus of parental attention, seem to show such desirable traits as above-average intelligence, high achievement, and good relationships with adults.

Straining and Breaking the Bonds

Living in wedded bliss is the dream of every bride and groom. Unfortunately, the reality often falls far short of expectations.

Marital Abuses

Some of the worst abuses of the married partnership—violence and infidelity, which were once only whispered about—are now the subject of intensive study. And a variety of support groups have been mobilized to help individuals with such problems.

Violence

Marital rape Forcing one's wife to have sexual relations.

Of all kinds of marital violence, the one that is still least reported is **marital rape,** which may be defined as "nonconsenting sexual encounters" in which the typical pattern is for the male to trick, pressure, intimidate, or physically force his wife to have sexual relations.

It is estimated that the incidence of marital rape may be as high as two million offenses a year. Both husband and wife require psychotherapy—the wife to alleviate fear, distrust, anxiety, and possible sexual dysfunction; the husband to gain insight into and control over his behavior. If treatment is refused by the husband, the wife is probably well advised to seek sanctuary and legal aid.

The battered wife, battered child, and even battered husband syndromes are other patterns of familial abuse that have recently received considerable attention. These are clearly threatening to marital stability but, even more seriously, may carry with them the seeds of future destructive behaviors. A child who has grown up witnessing physical abuse or being victimized by it is considered likely to carry the pattern forward in his or her adult life.

Infidelity

Perhaps the most common of all the strains on a marriage is **infidelity.** Experts on marriage and the family agree that sexual infidelity is usually seen as a way out of the ordinary problems of marriage by individuals who are immature, are frightened of close and permanent relationships, and, in fact, are apt to derive some pleasure merely from the clandestine nature of their affairs. There are also data to suggest that in some instances the spouse contributes to the flight from the realities of marriage by failing to communicate, not meeting sexual needs, or engaging in any one of a wide range of covertly or overtly hostile behaviors.

Infidelity Unfaithfulness in a relationship.

The most difficult marital decisions sometimes hinge on whether to confess an affair and possibly end the marriage or to look for professional help to eliminate the problems that led to the affair. There is no simple answer to a problem that is so individual. Most authorities agree, however, that it is preferable to be open about one's infidelity if one wants to preserve a marriage, since this communication—plus possible therapy—may be the most effective way to eliminate the problem and begin rebuilding the relationship.

Breaking the Bonds: Divorce

Current estimates show that 40 to 50 percent of marriages made now will be dissolved—often with serious consequences for the couple and their children. Four possible causes for these statistics are often mentioned. One is that society as a whole has become more tolerant of **divorce.** The second is that changes in the law have made divorces easier to obtain. A third reason, which is more debatable, is that couples are now more stressed than ever before in history. (Some point out, however, that in the old days couples were so overwhelmed by the work they did—on farms, for example—that there was little time left over for the consideration of whether one was feeling fulfilled and satisfied by marriage.) A fourth cause given is that the

Divorce Legal dissolution of a marriage.

expectations of marriage regarding emotional fulfillment have risen markedly.

Psychic Costs of Divorce

Whatever the causes, the number of people getting divorced has reached record levels. The U.S. Census Bureau in 1981 reported that there were approximately 2 million marriages and 1 million divorces. These figures represent a doubling of the divorce rate since 1976. The immediate and long-term psychic costs are difficult to calculate. The process of divorce, no matter how civilized, is almost always stressful. It usually involves pain, anxiety, and depression. Hardly any couple can go through a divorce without feeling self-doubt and probably exaggerating real or imagined shortcomings. Such feelings may, in turn, make them more fearful about ever committing themselves to another person, in the future.

Clearly divorce can be traumatic and a trauma of this magnitude is going to take its toll on one's performance at work as well as many other areas of life. Most significantly, the children of the divorced couple must face tremendous adjustments. It has been found that some children, particularly young ones, even feel a sense of guilt that they have somehow contributed to the divorce through some shortcoming of their own. Most will be puzzled by their place in the settlement, whether it is joint or sole custody.

Single Parents

One consequence of the rise in the divorce rate has been an increase in the number of single parents. In 1981, according to the U.S. Census Bureau, approximately 10.4 percent of all households in this country had only one parent, up from 6.2 percent in 1970. (For both years, nearly 90 percent of these single parents were women.) Actually, single-parent families are increasing somewhat faster than the divorce rate, partly because of a decline in the rate of remarriage. Some of those divorced persons who in the past might have been driven to remarry as soon as possible by what was considered a stigma attached to their condition are now choosing to stay single.

Ordinarily, rearing children should be easier for two adults together than for either separately, since being responsible for even one child is a large task. However, a divorced person who has left an especially burdensome marriage may feel that it is far easier to care for the children alone, without having also to respond to the demands of the former spouse. Small but increasing numbers do make this choice. Some parents in this situation develop close friendships with other single-parent families, which may provide some of the emotional and practiced support ordinarily given by a spouse in a conventional family.

Alternatives to Traditional Marriage

We have concentrated in this chapter on the life-style that is followed by the majority of Americans—dating, marriage, and parenthood. There are a number of other patterns that are accepted and some that are more distinctly experimental and chosen by a much smaller number of people, but which should not be overlooked since they provide some people with satisfaction.

Alternative Types of Marriage

Open Marriage. One such alternative is the **open marriage,** which is founded on the premise that traditional marriage based on the exclusive fulfillment of human needs by one partner does not permit continued intellectual and emotional growth. In open marriage, time is permitted for privacy and psychological regeneration. Role flexibility and exchange (as opposed to the traditional homemaker/breadwinner division) is stressed to promote understanding. Open communication is taught and its use encouraged. Finally, freedom to have sex outside the primary unit is considered permissible as a way of fostering individual growth. Clearly, entering into such an agreement requires a rare degree of mutual trust, tolerance, and ego-strength.

Open marriage Marriage in which both partners permit sexual freedom beyond the primary unit.

Group Marriage. Other heterosexual alternatives include triads (three adults as a primary unit) and the larger aggregations variously called group marriages, communes, cooperatives, and collectives. These involve significantly more sexual freedom than monogamous marriage; they have been found even less likely to succeed because of the extraordinary level of ego-strength, shared goals, and trust that must exist for such groups to survive—and most do not.

Part-Time Marriage. Still another heterosexual alternative that may prove more durable is the part-time marriage, which simply reflects the accommodation to dual-career marriages, where partners work in widely separated locales and meet on weekends and holidays. There are obvious built-in strains on such an arrangement, as well as financial costs, which may argue against this alternative for most people. Part-time marriage usually is considered inappropriate if children are to be included in the family. Sometimes, however, such an arrangement may, at least temporarily, seem preferable to uprooting the entire family when a significant career opportunity for one partner requires a transfer.

Bisexual and Homosexual Alternatives

Another variation in life-style is the bisexual marriage or relationship in which one or both partners are attracted to both men and women. Marriage offers one solution since it presents a commonplace facade to the world while preserving sexual freedom for the man and the woman.

Among the more recently evolved alternatives is the open union of homosexuals in a long-term relationship similar to marriage, often with well-defined "husband-wife" roles, and in some still-rare instances the adoption and rearing of children.

Cohabitation

Cohabitation, which is sometimes described as an alternative life-style but which may also be a trial marriage, is the increasingly widespread custom of living together as if married but without the legal or religious ties. According to the U.S. Bureau of the Census, the approximately 1.8 million U.S. couples who were living together in 1981 represent a tripling in the number of cohabitants since 1970. These data support current research which suggests that in the U.S., attitudes toward the primacy of marriage have been progressively changing. Two reasons have been offered for these attitudinal changes:

1. Increased opportunities for singles to achieve financial independence from their families.
2. Changes in the work environment that enable women to achieve financial independence, thus making the economic offerings of marriage less attractive.

These alternatives serve to underscore the point made at the beginning of this chapter — that the sexual evolution that began decades ago has reached a point where many life-style options are now openly practiced and discussed, although not all are widely accepted.

The Single Life

The single life has always been an acceptable alternative to marriage, although not always a very popular one. Today it is becoming increasingly popular as more and more people make a conscious decision not to marry. In the past, people remained single because they had not found anyone they wished to marry or they had not been asked. Increasingly, however, large numbers of people are single as a result of a commitment to a career that is so demanding that their potential for marrying has been reduced. Many other people enter singlehood as a result of divorce or marital separation. Many singles find the single life to be rewarding, enjoyable, and demanding. Some singles, however, have found it difficult to establish a sense of identity. One way many singles have attempted to establish a sense of identity has been through the "singles scene."

Singles scene The mingling of unmarried people with emphasis on sexuality and youthful life-styles.

Singles Scene

The **singles scene** is a very popular way for singles to express themselves heterosocially. The "scene" is very complex in part be-

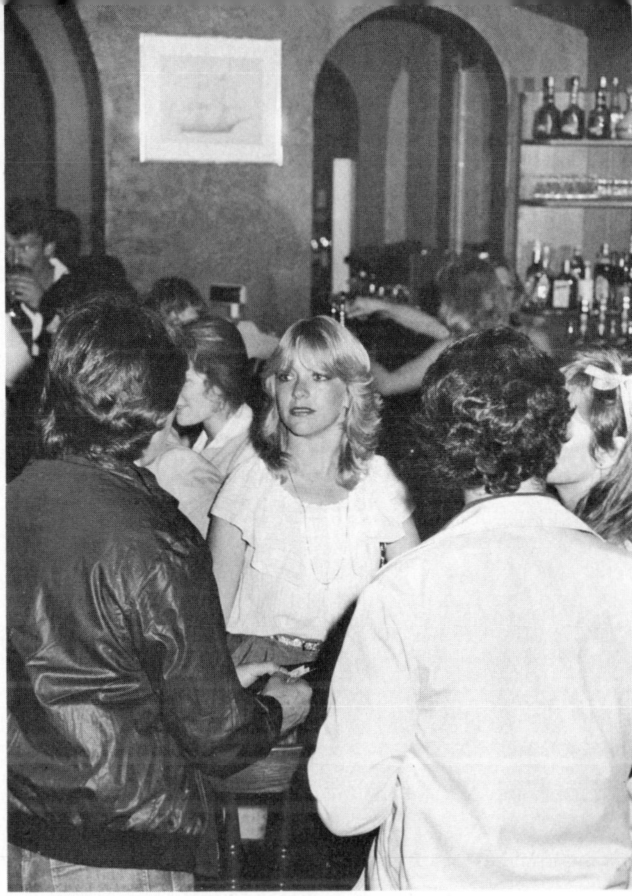

The singles scene can produce feelings of anxiety and tension, or it can be an enjoyable and rewarding experience. (Photo © Bill Bachman 1982/Photo Researchers, Inc.)

cause the goals and expectations of its members vary. To help people through the complexities of the singles scene, a number of magazine articles have been written emphasizing sex, physical attractiveness, and youthful styles. While promising to help people "make it" in the singles world, many of these articles only create anxiety among their readers. The emphasis on sexuality, physical attractiveness, and youth has no doubt contributed to the fact that membership in the singles scene tends to be brief and of limited importance to most singles.

Whatever the reason a person has for becoming or remaining single, it is a style that many people are embracing and finding as rewarding as marriage, if not more so.

Celibacy

Another style worthy of mention is one that has been accepted for centuries, though practiced only by limited numbers and not likely to increase much in popularity—that is, **celibacy.** In some religions, including the Roman Catholic, in order to join the priesthood or serve in certain other capacities, the individual is required to put aside sexual fulfillment. However, some persons remain celibate simply because they have no desire for sexual relations. Although most of us do have sexual needs which are best met by others, sex is by no means necessary for intimate and nourishing friendships. For some people, then, a celibate life may be a satisfying one.

Celibacy Abstinence from sexual involvement.

Summary

The variety of options open today may make choosing a pattern of lifetime commitment to others more difficult than in the past. Contrary to the image of sudden upheaval that the term sexual revolution suggests, recent changes in sexual behavior and roles are just one stage in the evolution of the family that has been going on since the Renaissance.

Dating—the first step most of us take toward building satisfactory relationships—plays an important role in the development of self-image. Sexual experimentation during dating has tended increasingly to culminate in sexual intercourse, which has resulted in an increase in pregnancies and abortions among teenagers.

Although the bases of marriage have changed somewhat, the institution remains the primary accepted means for expressing affection and propagating offspring. Readiness for marriage includes such factors as age, emotional and social maturity, and sufficient financial resources. Important traits to look for in a spouse include adaptability, optimism, a sense of humor, and an interest in promoting the well-being of others; similarity of the partners in background, age, education, and aspirations increases the chances for success in marriage. The engagement period, which may precede marriage, gives a couple a chance to see each other more nearly as they may be in marriage.

No marriage is perfect. Although good sexual relations are important in a marriage, only each married couple can best judge what kind of sex life suits them. Until relatively recently a common myth about marriage maintained the woman should be content to keep house and wait happily for her husband to get home from work. The opposing myth, that both partners must take perfectly equal roles in marriage, is not true for everyone either. It is important to consider what both you and your partner want out of marriage.

Marriages come in many different patterns, including the conflict-habituated, the devitalized, the passive-congenial, the vital, and the total marriage.

Today, the decision not to have children receives support from some segments of society. One should not have children to try to solve marital problems, which may be worsened by the presence of children. Other reasons people may choose not to have children include not liking them, not wanting to devote so many years to their nurturance, seeking to focus on one's career, having hereditary disorders that may make childbearing dangerous, and not feeling financially able to support children. However, children can strengthen a good marriage, provide pleasure to the parents, and give the parents the sense of having a link with the future.

The most extreme strains on marriage are violence and infidelity. According to current estimates, from 40 to 50 percent of marriages entered into now will dissolve. The process of getting divorced involves pain, anxiety, and depression and takes a toll on children as well.

The rise in the proportion of single-parent families has been even greater than the rise in the divorce rate, partly because of a decline in the rate of remarriage after divorce. Some single persons choose to have children without marrying or living with a partner.

Unconventional alternatives to marriage include open marriage, group or communal marriage, part-time marriage, homosexual or bisexual marriage, and celibacy.

Review and Discussion

1. In what ways is the sexual revolution the culmination of long-term social changes?

2. Explain the statement "Dating is a rehearsal for adulthood."

3. What reasons have been suggested for the increase in teenage pregnancy in recent years?

4. What are the advantages and disadvantages of living together before (or instead of) marriage?

5. What are the criteria that tend to lead to a lasting marriage? What should be taken into account in selecting a mate?

6. Describe several myths about love and marriage. What problems can these myths create?

7. What are the five types of marriage described by Cuber and Harroff?

8. What are some of the benefits and drawbacks of having children?

9. What are the most serious strains on a marriage, and what can be done about them?

10. Describe three types of alternative life-styles. What psychological and social problems may be faced by individuals who choose them?

Further Reading

Bach, George R., and Ronald M. Deutsch, *Pairing.* New York: Avon Books, 1971.
A sensitive discussion of relationships and their role in a fulfilling life. (Paperback.)

Fromm, Erich. *The Art of Loving.* New York: Harper and Row, 1974.
A well-known psychologist's discussion of love and its central place in human experience. (Paperback.)

Greenwald, Jerry. *Creative Intimacy.* New York: Jove Publications, 1977.
An analysis of intimacy and the myths surrounding it. (Paperback.)

Kephart, William M. *The Family, Society, and the Individual.* 5th ed. Boston: Houghton Mifflin Company, 1981.
A collection of articles providing more detailed analyses of family structure, sex roles, and alternative relationships. (Paperback.)

Krantzler, Mel. *Creative Divorce.* New York: New American Library, 1975.
An autobiographical account of the author's experience of divorce. (Paperback.)

Oettinger, Katherine B. *Not My Daughter.* Englewood Cliffs, N.J.: Prentice-Hall, 1981.
A description of the growing problem of teenage pregnancy, with practical recommendations. (Paperback.)

Pietropinto, Anthony, and Jacqueline Simmenauer. *Husbands and Wives.* New York: Berkley Publishing Corporation, 1981.
A study of contemporary marriage, based on extensive interviews with husbands and wives. (Paperback.)

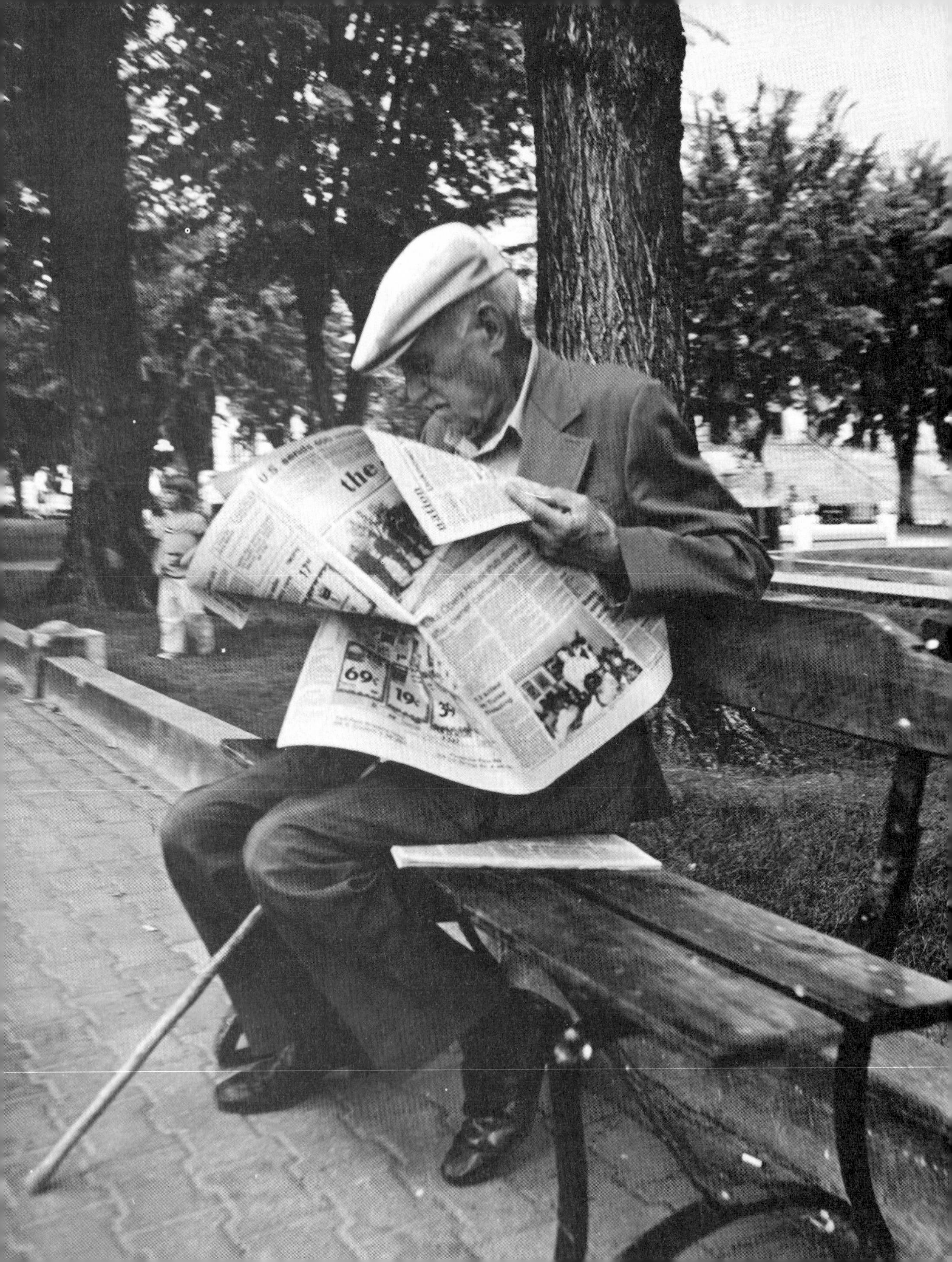
the
nation
69¢
19¢

Chapter 7
Aging

KEY POINTS

- ☐ Aging begins at conception and continues until we die, and the ability to grow old gracefully is an essential part of a person's well-being.
- ☐ Aging, senescence, ageism and gerontology are defined and discussed.
- ☐ The three major social theories of aging are the activity theory, the disengagement theory, and the continuity theory.
- ☐ Our society believes many myths about elderly people that are in sharp contrast to the realities.
- ☐ Factors contributing to a longer life include proper nutrition, regular exercise, avoidance of negative stress, and life satisfaction.
- ☐ The elderly have much to contribute to society, and society can do much to help them.
- ☐ Organizations representing the elderly are doing much to change negative stereotypes of aging.
- ☐ Aging is, most of all, an opportunity to live more: to work more, play more, learn more, and experience more.

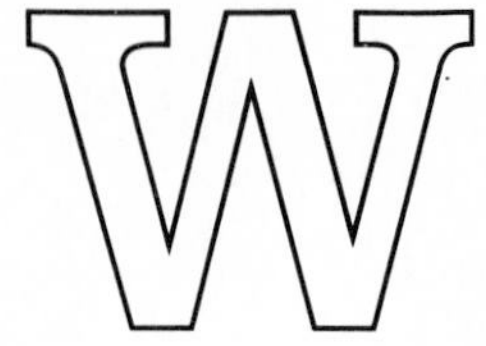

WE BEGIN aging at the moment of conception and continue to age until we die. But old age, the time of life that nineteenth-century British prime minister Benjamin Disraeli labeled "a regret," is as often feared as it is misunderstood. Children who eagerly count the days from one birthday to the next may grow into adults who dread the passage of the years. Yet the visible presence of many politicians, judges, artists, writers, businesspeople, homemakers, and other healthy, active, and creative individuals in their seventies, eighties, and even nineties proves that old age need not be synonymous with senility and idleness.

Indeed, far from being a burden to themselves and society, the aged may often be better citizens than their younger counterparts. They are more likely to observe laws, participate in the political process, and volunteer their services to charitable and religious organizations. Older workers perform as well as or better than younger workers in most jobs and have less turnover, fewer on-the-job accidents, and less absenteeism. Contrary to stereotype, older drivers have safer driving records than those under 65. Although not all of the elderly are financially secure, most have their economic needs met through Social Security, other pensions, and Medicare and are eligible for many programs and services at reduced rates. The aged are usually free from the day-to-day responsibilities of child care and full-time jobs, and thus, health permitting, are able to enjoy leisure time, travel, and the company of friends.

This chapter focuses on what we know, how we feel, and what we can do about aging. It deals not only with the physical aspects of getting older but with the psychological and social aspects as well. We consider both the individual's experience of aging and how society deals with the aging individual. Naturally our perspective of aging changes as we grow older, but whatever age we may be, it is important that we examine our attitudes toward our own aging and that of others. If we become conscious of the fears and stereotypes that stand in the way of our appreciating older people, we can learn to experience our own aging positively — as an opportunity for growth and satisfaction.

What Do You Know About Aging?

Aging The process of physical, mental, emotional, and social change experienced throughout life.

Senescence Biological deterioration associated with age.

For many of us the term **aging** brings to mind an image of a wrinkled, white-haired person. Actually, the word refers to the many physical, mental, emotional, and social changes that we experience throughout the life cycle. The deterioration that we associate with old age is the result of **senescence.** After we reach maturity, our bodies begin to degenerate: we can no longer run as fast, hear as keenly, or react as quickly. These changes occur at varying rates in different people, but they are inevitable, and they culminate in death.

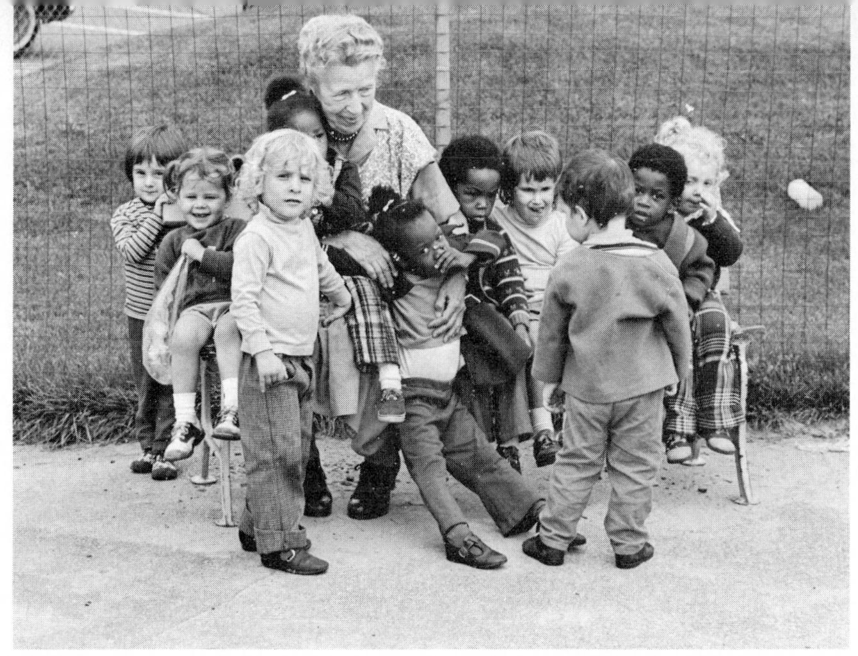

Old age can be a time of continued fulfillment and interest in life. Unhurried by daily responsibilities, the aged are freer to enjoy personal growth and satisfaction. (Photo © Paul Sequeira/Photo Researchers, Inc.)

The exact age at which a person is considered old varies from culture to culture and, to a certain extent, from individual to individual. Bernard Baruch, the vigorous "adviser to Presidents" who lived to be 95, declared, "To me, old age is 15 years older than I am." However, in American society a person is usually considered *aged* or *elderly* after reaching the age of 65. **Ageism** is the deliberate stereotyping of and discrimination against people because they are old. In our youth-oriented culture, the elderly are viewed by many as forgetful, nonproductive, and old-fashioned; as a result they are often forced out of the job market, ridiculed, or ignored. Like its counterparts, racism and sexism, ageism cheats not only its victims but its practitioners, depriving them of the talents, company, and wisdom of a large portion of humanity.

Ageism Discrimination against and stereotyping of the elderly.

Gerontology, the study of aging, is a relatively new area of learning. Gerontologists draw their knowledge from the aged themselves, from professionals engaged in working with the aged, and from the growing body of research studies having to do with the processes of aging and their consequences. Gerontology is an interesting field of study, in which much remains to be learned. (To find out how much you really know about aging, do Self-Assessment Exercise 7.1, "Facts on Aging.")

Gerontology The study of aging.

Biological Theories of Aging

Despite mankind's eternal search for a fountain of youth, the key to halting or reversing the aging process remains elusive. Senescence, the biological decline that accompanies aging, remains unstoppable by any means known to science.

Senescence is a gradual, irreversible process. It is not something that happens overnight, nor does it occur accidentally. The changes that characterize senescence come from within the individual. Envi-

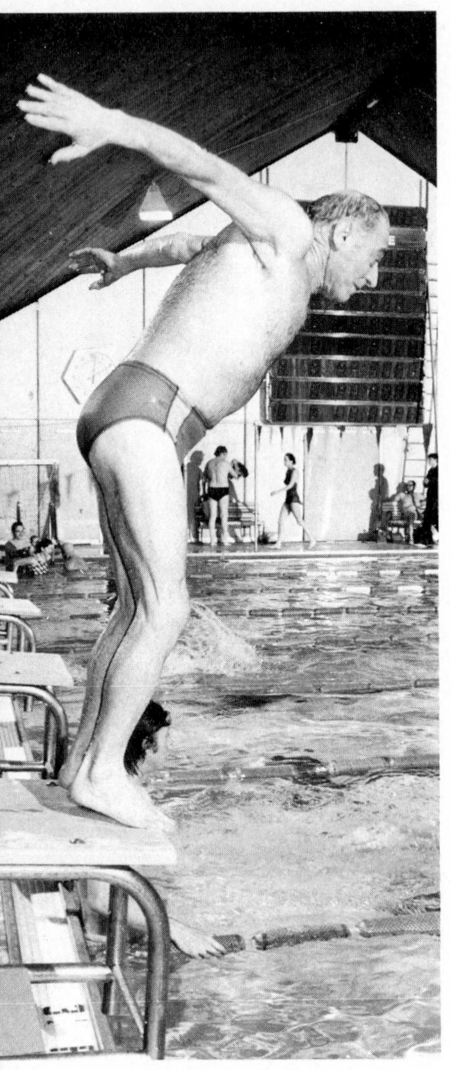

Many elderly people continue to lead active and vigorous lives. (Photo by Ira Wyman/Sygma)

ronmental factors hasten aging (sunlight, for example, ages the skin), but they do not cause it. The causes of senescence continue to baffle scientists, though numerous theories have been offered to explain the many processes that appear to be involved.

Wear and Tear Theory. Proponents of the *wear and tear theory* argue that the body is a complex piece of machinery that wears out and ultimately breaks down. The wear and tear theory, however, does not apply in all cases. It has not yet been proved that any one organ or system wears out in *all* people. Also, unlike most pieces of machinery, the human body can often repair itself.

Rate of Living Theory. The *rate of living theory* holds that we are each programmed to live a specific length of time, but we can speed up our biological clocks — and thus accelerate aging — by expending our energy too quickly. Those who subscribe to this theory recommend avoiding excitement, resting frequently, and avoiding strenuous physical activity. Studies have shown, however, that exercise usually prolongs life, a fact that would seem to discredit the theory in part.

Waste Product Theory. Chemical wastes that accumulate in some parts of the body are the basis for the *waste product theory* of senescence — which, however, has been generally discounted because these wastes do not appreciably hinder cell functioning.

The preceding three theories can be classified as general theories of aging and have been popular and influential. The theories that follow are attempts to explain the causes of senescence on the basis of biochemical changes.

Collagen Theory. A factor more likely to be significant in aging is central to the *collagen theory.* The basic component of cartilage and connective tissue, collagen, is an elastic, rubbery substance that stiffens over the years. As a result, tissues containing collagen lose elasticity and become more brittle as we grow older. However, although there is agreement that this change in collagen contributes to aging, it is not believed to be the basic cause of senescence.

Mutation Theory. The *mutation theory* attributes aging to changes (mutations) in DNA, the basic genetic material in human cells. Mutated cells continue to divide, eventually becoming so numerous that they damage the organs that contain them. Scientific research has provided considerable support for the theory. However, there are still many unanswered questions blocking its full acceptance.

Error Theory. The *error theory* focuses on "mistakes" in such vital bodily functions as enzymatic reactions and the synthesis of proteins and RNA (a substance similar to DNA). As yet, however, there is a lack of research to support this theory.

Genetic Theory. The *genetic theory* relies on the assumption that the human cell is like a miniature computer programmed to mature, age, and die in a specific way. Some proponents of this theory believe that our genetic makeup dictates from the beginning how long we will be able to live; others believe that random gene mutations can alter an individual's genetic equation and thus affect aging.

Autoimmune Theory. The *autoimmune theory* holds that the body reacts to changes within itself. When we are vaccinated against a disease such as polio, our body develops defenses against the deadly virus. In other words, we acquire immunity. Occasionally the body develops excessive immune reactions: it treats its own tissues as if they were foreign invaders and acts to destroy them. Some theorists believe that the cellular changes caused by aging trigger such a reaction, because the body's defenses do not recognize the aged cells as part of the "self."

Free Radical Theory. Another theory holds that *free radicals*—substances released by polyunsaturated fats—produce chemical reactions that alter and damage body cells. Proponents of this theory believe that the consumption of vitamin E, vitamin C, and the food additive butylated hydroxytoluene (BHT) retard the aging process by interfering with the activity of free radicals.

RNA Tumor Virus Theory. The *RNA tumor virus*, which can be transmitted both horizontally (person to person) and vertically (genetically from parent to child), may play a role in aging. In these viruses the genetic material consists of RNA and can cause changes in the cell's metabolism and form new proteins, the effects of which are not yet completely known. Environmental stress, various hormones, and other viruses can serve to activate RNA tumor viruses, resulting in the production of either cancerous or age-inducing proteins.

The biological key to aging remains elusive, primarily because there is so much variation in how people age. These differences have thus far defied categorization, and no one has been able to fit them into a single, all-encompassing theory. We all come into contact with different environmental influences, eat different foods, have different lifestyles, react to stress differently and, perhaps more significantly, differ in genetic makeup. We also differ in attitude toward life—which may well prove to be highly important in how we age.

Social Theories of Aging

Scientific knowledge, data, and statistics are of little use if they cannot be applied to real-life situations. Social gerontologists have developed theories that are designed to tie together what is known about aging, especially about the changes in emotional and social life that elderly people go through, thereby providing guidance for those who work with and plan programs for senior citizens. The three theories that are currently receiving the most attention in social gerontology research are the activity theory, the disengagement theory, and the continuity theory.

Activity Theory. A variation on the theme "You're only as old as you feel," the *activity theory* holds that the happiest, best-adjusted older people are those who look, act, and feel younger than their years. Keeping busy, maintaining social contacts, developing new interests, and finding ways to channel productivity and creativity—even after retirement—are seen as the keys to successful aging.

Disengagement Theory. A very different view, the *disengagement theory,* hold that as people age—and approach death—they focus inward, on themselves and those close to them, rather than on less personal matters. Proponents of the theory believe that this gradual withdrawal is a natural step in the order of things, permitting the individual to make the most of whatever time remains. Supposedly, disengagement also benefits society by allowing younger—and presumably more able-bodied and efficient—people to take over the work that is necessary to maintain the social, economic, and political systems.

Continuity Theory. According to the *continuity theory,* people in maturing develop personality patterns (habits, preferences, associations, commitments, etc.) and seek to continue them as they grow older. How well one adjusts to events associated with aging, therefore, depends upon one's accumulated experience, established lifestyle, and one's physical, mental, and emotional predisposition to cope with changes. Since adjustment is an adaptive process, one who has always adapted well and has developed a flexible personality is most likely to adjust well to old age. The fact that problems are new or different does not change the nature of the person who is dealing with them.

Dispelling Myths: The Realities of Aging

The stereotypical old person—embittered, inflexible, bored, lonely, short-tempered—is an invention of dramatists and comedians and is no more representative of the entire elderly population than a leather-jacketed, unkempt hoodlum is representative of all teenagers. If we are to benefit fully from living and working with older people, and if we are to dispel our own fears about aging, we must first separate truth from fiction. Begin by taking the Self-Assessment Exercise 7.1, which deals with common attitudes about aging, then compare your notions with the following realities.

Myth: *Old people are basically alike and are aging in the same ways.*

Reality: *There are great individual variations in the ways that physical changes occur as one ages. Remember, growth and development follow a predictable but unique process for each individual.*

SELF-ASSESSMENT EXERCISE 7.1

Facts on Aging

Mark each statement true or false.

1. The majority of old people are senile.
2. All five senses tend to decline in old age.
3. Most old people have no interest in, or capacity for, sexual relations.
4. Lung vital capacity tends to decline in old age.
5. The majority of old people feel miserable most of the time.
6. Physical strength tends to decline in old age.
7. At least one-fifth of the aged are living in long-stay institutions (nursing homes, mental hospitals, homes for the aged, etc.).
8. Aged drivers have fewer accidents per driver than drivers under age 65.
9. Most older workers cannot work as effectively as younger workers.
10. About 80 percent of the aged are healthy enough to carry out their normal activities.
11. Most old people are set in their ways and unable to change.
12. Old people usually take longer to learn something new.
13. It is almost impossible for most old people to learn something new.
14. The reaction time of most old people tends to be slower than the reaction time of younger people.
15. In general, most old people are pretty much alike.
16. The majority of old people report that they are seldom bored.
17. The majority of old people are socially isolated and lonely.
18. Older workers have fewer accidents than younger workers.
19. Over 15 percent of the U.S. population are now age 65 or over.
20. Medical practitioners often tend to give low priority to the aged.
21. The majority of older people have incomes below the poverty level (as defined by the federal government).
22. The majority of old people are working or would like to have some kind of work to do (including housework and volunteer work).
23. Older people tend to become more religious as they age.
24. The majority of old people report that they are seldom irritated or angry.
25. The health and socioeconomic status of older people in the year 2000 will probably be about the same as that of today's older people.

Answers: *All odd-numbered statements are false. All even-numbered statements are true.*

Source: Erdman Palmore, "The Facts of Aging Quiz: A Review of Findings," *The Gerontologist,* vol. 20 (1980), no. 6, p. 671.

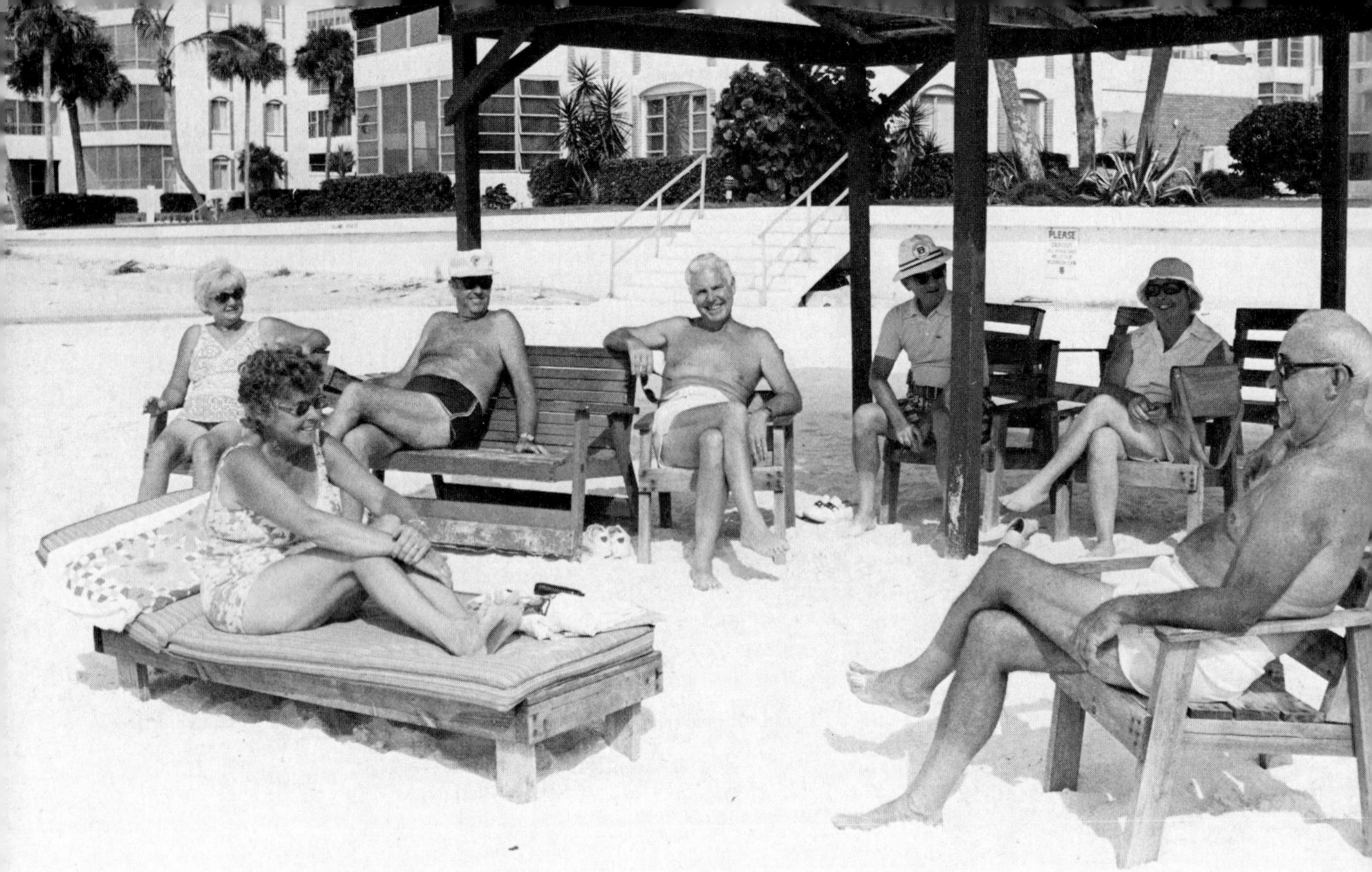

Contrary to the stereotype, many of the elderly have sufficient income to live comfortably. (Photo by Eric Kroll/Taurus Photos)

We all age differently, and within each person various organs and tissues age at different rates. Person A needs a cane to walk but reads without glasses, while person B wears a hearing aid but plays an hour of tennis each day. And while physical changes invariably accompany old age, they are rarely as debilitating, as massive, or as rapid as is commonly believed. The changes are gradual, almost always occurring slowly enough to allow individuals to make necessary adjustments and continue functioning capably and autonomously.

Myth: *Old people are frail and feeble and must greatly limit their activities.*
Reality: *The majority of older people are in good health and able to engage in their normal activities throughout life, a little more slowly, perhaps, but with enjoyment and commitment.*

Debilitating physical or mental conditions afflict fewer than one-fifth of all older adults. The remaining 80 percent perform tasks and pursue interests in accordance with life-style and personal preference.

Myth: *Most old people become senile.*
Reality: *Senility is not synonymous with old age.*

Two-thirds of those who live past age 80 exhibit no signs of the memory loss, intellectual decline, or psychotic symptoms that characterize senility. The idea that senility is inevitable for all is a myth.

Myth: *Most old people are lonely and miserable.*
Reality: *An older person's personality and mental health are related to many factors and do not necessarily deteriorate with time.*

When we age, we do not leave our younger selves behind. Much of what we were remains with us, subtly altering not in response to age but in response to the physical, environmental, and social changes that affect us throughout life. Stereotypical old people do exist, but far more noteworthy is the fact that the majority of senior citizens are well adjusted. Young people do not have a monopoly on happiness.

Myth: *Old people are set in their ways and unable to learn or change.*
Reality: *Although older people may require more time to learn new things, learning can occur at any age.*

The keys to learning are motivation, interest, and energy. In the absence of brain damage, debilitating illness, and depression, a mind that has been exercised and developed throughout youth and middle age remains active throughout the rest of life as well. In fact, many retired people seize the opportunity to return to school, learning new skills, studying a wide variety of subjects, and even earning college and graduate degrees. Older people may have to study harder or review material more frequently than do younger students, but they are just as able to absorb and apply new information. Indeed, their life experiences and knowledge of the history of their times may give them a richer perspective of what they learn than younger people have.

Myth: *The high proportion of old people in our population is due to medical advances that can keep people alive much longer than in the past.*
Reality: *The increasing proportion of the population that is 65 years of age or older is primarily a result of increased fertility and decreased infant mortality rather than increases in longevity.*

In 1981 there were 25 million senior citizens; it is expected that by the year 2000 this figure will have increased to 31.8 million. However, advances in medical technology have not made it possible for the human body to survive substantially longer, as is commonly believed.

Until recent decades, the elderly population was small because many people died before reaching adulthood. Improved sanitary conditions and the conquest of many diseases have resulted in a dramatic increase in the number of people who survive past infancy and young adulthood into old age. While *average* life expectancy has indeed increased greatly, *possible* life expectancy has not.

Myth: *A large proportion of the elderly are in nursing homes or other institutions.*
Reality: *Less than 10 percent of the aged reside in long-stay institutions.*

The notion that nursing homes and hospitals house a substantial proportion of senior citizens is erroneous. Most older people value their independence and successfully maintain their own households.

Myth: *Most old people are living at or below the poverty level.*
Reality: *A majority of the aged have a sufficient income and are not living at the poverty level.*

Surprisingly, aging parents are more likely to assist their adult children financially than vice versa. However, while there are those who retire in luxury and comfort, a quarter of the elderly population have incomes at or below the poverty line, and many others must sacrifice and plan their budgets very carefully in order to make ends meet.

Myth: *Few old people are able to work.*
Reality: *Many older people are doing some type of work or would like to work.*

Approximately one-third of persons 65 or older are able and willing to work, but only 12 percent are actually employed. The reluctance of employers to hire senior citizens persists, despite evidence that in most jobs older workers perform as effectively as younger workers.

Myth: *Most old people have little interest in sex.*
Reality: *Most healthy people over age 65 maintain their interest in and capacity for sexual relations.*

While it is true that sexual capacity peaks in the late teens and early twenties and wanes thereafter, many couples continue to engage in intercourse to orgasm throughout their lives. Factors that may inhibit sexual response in older people include changes in hormonal levels, which may make intercourse painful for women; changes in the central nervous system and other physical infirmities; fear of failure; lack of privacy (for couples in nursing homes); the absence of an interested — and interesting — partner; and societal attitudes regarding sexual behavior of the elderly.

Senescence

Senescence Biological deterioration associated with old age.

Senescence, the inevitable biological deterioration that accompanies old age, begins at different ages and progresses at different rates for all people. In general, it results in a person having a lowered resistance to disease and a diminished ability to withstand stress.

The senses, our links to the outside world, commonly become less acute with age. Senses of taste and smell may dull, and thickening nerve endings interfere with the sense of touch. Some elderly people thought to be paranoid (afflicted with "distorted thinking" or delusions of persecution) are actually suffering from undiagnosed hearing loss, a condition that usually begins with the inability to hear high-frequency sounds (whistles, the ringing of a telephone or doorbell, children's voices). A hearing aid, if properly fitted and maintained, is usually of some help, and instruction in lip reading may also be useful. Those attempting to communicate with a hearing-impaired individual should face the person and speak slowly and clearly. Shouting is usually counterproductive, since it causes the voice to become high pitched and distorted.

Changes in vision that accompany aging are caused by decreased effectiveness of the pupil, the lens, and the retina. Usually both eyesight and color perception are damaged (pastel shades are lost on people with eye problems). Some visual disorders, such as cataracts, are surgically correctable, but other eye diseases, such as glaucoma (which is controllable if treated in time) may result in partial or total blindness. Several organizations specialize in helping visually handicapped people to maintain their independence by teaching them to substitute their remaining senses for sight. Those afflicted with multiple handicaps, such as loss of both sight and hearing, can keep in touch with the world through rehabilitative techniques, their own ingenuity, and the support, care, and patience of those around them.

Respiratory, digestive, reproductive, and temperature control systems also decline with age, but these changes are rarely disabling.

Alzheimer's Disease

Alzheimer's disease Condition characterized by memory lapses and periodic confusion.

Some elderly people suffer from **Alzheimer's disease,** which is a condition characterized by memory lapses or periodic confusion, or both. This disorder can lead to — among other things — behavioral and personality changes, forgetfulness, confusion, and motor activity problems. The individuals at greatest risk of suffering from Alzheimer's disease are those with relatives afflicted by it. The cause of Alzheimer's is unknown, and currently there is no cure for it. It can, however, be successfully managed through a regimen of daily exercise, proper diet, prescription medications, and social contact.

How Do You Feel About Aging?

Defining all people over 65 as "the elderly" implies a uniformity that does not exist. If anything, as people age they become more diverse. Usually older people are less under pressure to conform than are the young, less likely to wear clothes just because they are in style, and more eclectic in their tastes in music, literature, television shows, and movies. Still, ageism persists. Even those in the helping professions —doctors, nurses, social workers, physical therapists, psychiatrists —resist specializing in geriatrics. Moreover, social services for the elderly are often insufficient and inappropriate, and there is evidence that the elderly receive inferior medical care and treatment. Some nursing homes are notoriously understaffed "dumping grounds" for homeless and infirm senior citizens. Occasional nursing home scandals have popularized the image of the impoverished, feeble, dependent elderly person.

For many, retirement is an opportunity to pursue creative interests. Here a woman is engaged in fine art bookbinding. (Photo © Joel Gordon 1981/Joel Gordon Photography)

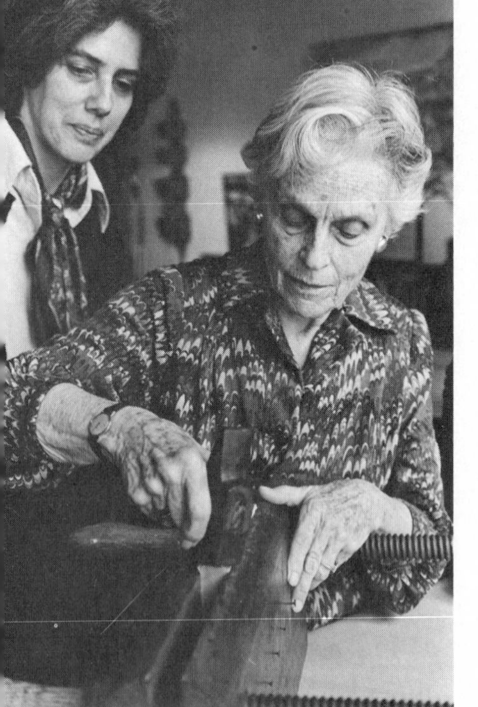

Sources of Our Fears and Misconceptions About Aging

Older people have not always been neglected. In preindustrial societies, the wisdom and experience of age were valued. In such societies, where most people died at a much younger age than they do now, reaching an advanced age was considered an achievement. In those societies most work was centered in the home, so that most people could continue to work until death, surrounded by several generations of their families.

However, along with industrialization came a tendency to value the maximization of production above all else. Although some of the elderly might have been only slightly less capable of doing physically demanding work than those much younger, on the assembly line this was not good enough. At the same time, as more and more of society's goods were produced or processed in factories, the kinds of money-earning work an elderly person could do at home were greatly reduced.

The accompanying breakup of the extended family, especially during the last few decades, has meant that fewer and fewer young people have frequent contact with the aged. No longer are elderly people as much a part of our daily lives as they once were—people with whom we grow up and who give us a sense of all the wonder and experience we have to look forward to in a long, full life. Although we may see them daily walking down the street, many of us ignore them. If we knew older people well, they would remind us of life—of the long lives they are leading and the lives we have ahead of us. But because we do not know them, they seem strange and forbidding, and remind us of death—of our own mortality, which we would rather not think about.

Personal Concerns About Aging

Simone de Beauvoir has written, "It is this very awareness that one is no longer an attractive object that makes life so unbearable for so many elderly people."

Self-Assessment Exercise 7.2 is designed to counter the notion that to be old is to be unattractive. Begin by picturing your body as it is now, inside and out, and answer the questions in the exercise. Then, as if you were looking into a crystal ball, picture as much as you can about your "older" self—your skin, eyes, hair, legs, arms, torso. How do you feel? Anxious? Resigned? Sad? Pleased? Do you feel or look much different than you did a week ago, a month ago, a year ago, 5

SELF-ASSESSMENT EXERCISE 7.2

Body Images

1. What is the strongest part of your body?
2. What is the weakest part?
3. What is the oldest part?
4. What is the youngest part?
5. What do you consider the most attractive part of your body?
6. What is the least attractive?
7. Where does your body have the most warmth?
8. Where is your body coldest?
9. What is the most vulnerable part of your body—the place most quickly or easily hurt?
10. What is the smoothest part of your body?
11. What is the roughest part?
12. What is the hardest part?
13. Where do you carry tensions in your body?
14. What part of your body do you most want to change?
15. What do you least want to change?
16. What part of your body are you ashamed of?
17. What part of your body do you feel most proud of?

Source: Lillian R. Dangott and Richard A. Kalish, *A Time to Enjoy*, Englewood Cliffs, N.J.: Prentice-Hall, 1979, p. 2.

years ago? Observe and record as many details as you can. Our tendency to equate aging with deterioration may cause us to lose sight of those aspects of our lives that are enhanced or remain unchanged over the years.

Many of what we consider the drawbacks of aging have positive aspects as well. For example, needing more time to learn or do things may also mean *taking* more time: being more attentive to whatever you're doing, often enjoying it more than a younger person who rushes through things. Feeling that your physical attractiveness is no longer your most important asset can relieve you of worrying about how you look and let you pay more attention to other people. And having lived through the events of many decades may give you a fuller sense of the issues, problems, and possibilities of the present than you had at, say, age 21.

Exploring Expectations About the Future

Now that you have a mental picture of your older self, can you imagine what life will be like when you are old? Self-Assessment Exercise 7.3 should help you explore your attitudes toward your own old age.

Fate and chance enter all lives. By and large, however, our feelings, perceptions, fears, expectations, and prejudices profoundly influence what we will become. Many people act and feel old not because their bodies have failed them, but because they are functioning in accordance with prejudices and misconceptions about old age. By adopting a narrow, negative view of what it is like to be old, we may inevitably move toward fulfilling our own prophecy. For example, a person who believes that loneliness is an inescapable part of old age may make little effort to preserve or develop friendships, thereby guaranteeing solitude. On the other hand, a healthy, optimistic outlook contributes to continued growth throughout life.

What You Can Do About Aging

Women live longer than men. "Thin" people outlive "fat" people. Other predictors of longevity include not smoking, drinking moderately, maintaining a balanced diet, being healthy, getting enough rest, being financially comfortable, having social and recreational outlets, exercising regularly, feeling useful and needed, and having satisfying work.

For reasons that are not yet clear, longevity tends to run in families. Scientists believe that the genetic makeup of some people may retard the aging process or provide greater resistance to disease.

Self-Assessment Exercise 7.4 at the end of this chapter, the Life-

SELF-ASSESSMENT EXERCISE 7.3

Your Old Age

1. What personality qualities do you most like to see in old people?
2. What do you most fear about growing older? What is the worst thing that can happen to you in old age?
3. Would you like to retire? At what age? Will you have a choice? How do you feel about retirement? What do you picture your economic situation to be?
4. What kind of housing would you like? What kind of neighborhood do you want? What kind of community?
5. How will you like to spend your leisure time? What kinds of activities do you expect to find pleasurable?
6. What changes do you expect in your sexuality?
7. What will be the quality of your friendships? Will you make new friends easily? (Who would you like for your friends?)
8. What do you imagine your health will be like when you are old? What health problems do you anticipate?
9. What advantages do you see in being old? What kinds of pleasures are more possible in your later years than in your youth?

Source: Lillian R. Dangott and Richard A. Kalish, *A Time to Enjoy*, Englewood Cliffs, N.J.: Prentice-Hall, 1979, p. 5.

Score test, will give you an idea of how long you might expect to live. The exercise may also help you to pinpoint—and correct—those habits that may shorten your life span.

Nutrition

At any age proper nutrition is essential to good health. The quality of your diet, even in infancy, affects how long you will live, and it will continue to do so throughout life. Therefore, it is important to establish good eating habits early in life and to maintain them.

In old age, however, some physical changes can make it harder than in youth to get a balanced diet. Although fortification of bread, cereal, milk, and other food staples has made malnutrition a less common occurrence among the aged, for some the use of certain drugs, a sluggish digestive system, poor kidney function, or dental problems interfere with the body's absorption and utilization of nutrients. Spicy foods, which once produced only minimal discomfort or no trouble at all, may cause digestive disturbances and aggravate intestinal disorders in older people.

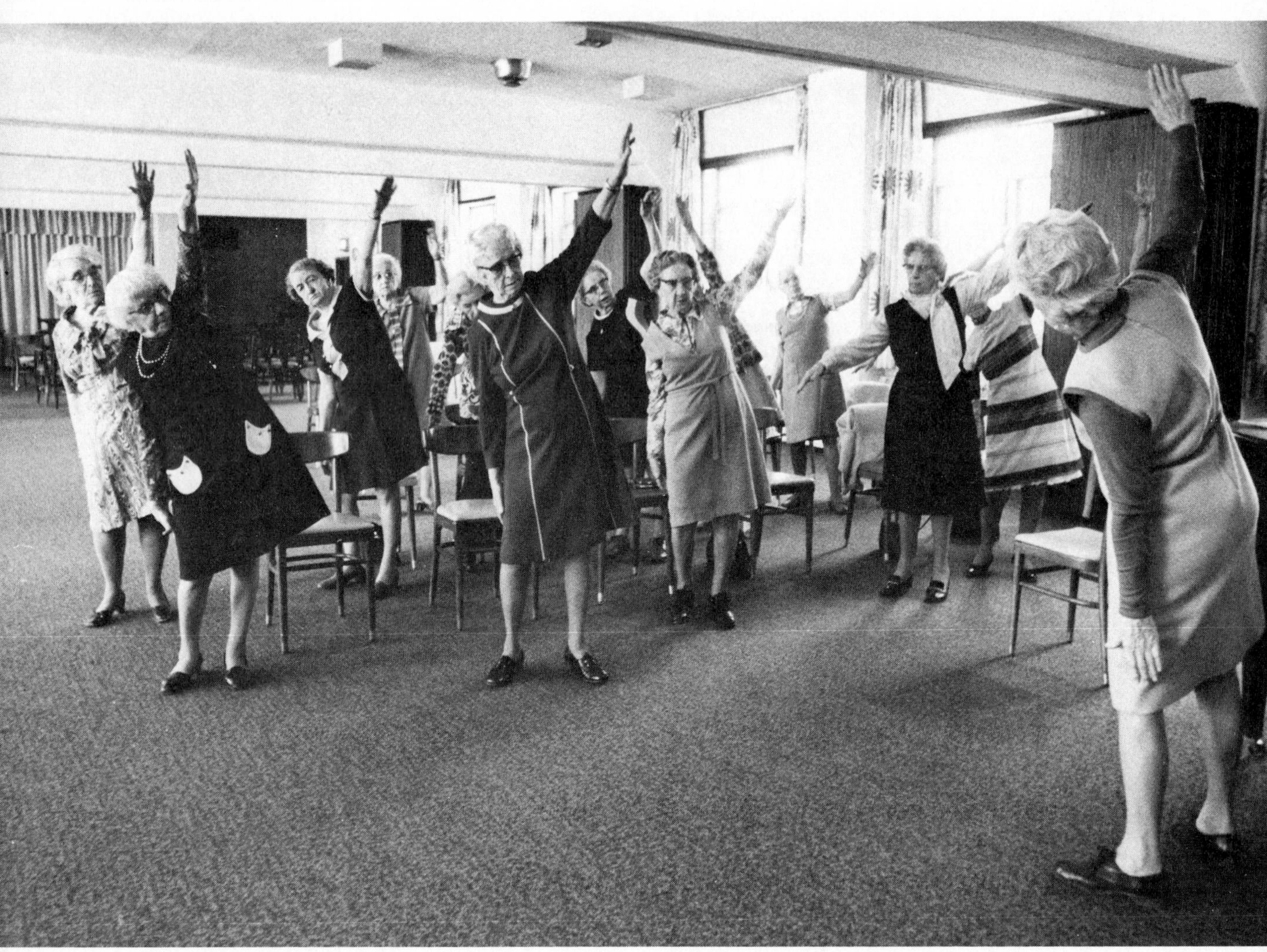

Exercise is as important in later years as it is earlier. (Photo by Ben Ross/Photo Trends)

Deterioration in the senses of taste and smell may result in loss of appetite or a tendency to overuse salt, sugar, and spices to make food more palatable. Decreased mobility and impaired vision may make the selection and preparation of food more difficult. Finally, a healthy variety of foods costs money. A financially strapped older person, who once thrived on meat, potatoes, vegetables, and cheese, may have trouble maintaining an adequate diet on a reduced income.

Recommended dietary allowances (RDA), which have been fairly well established for children and adolescents, offer no clear nutritional guidelines for older people. It is believed, however, that the dietary needs of healthy senior citizens are similar to the food requirements of younger adults of the same sex. Regardless of age, calorie requirements vary in accordance with physical activity, although, given the same level of activity, you can expect to require somewhat fewer calories in your forties than in your twenties and fewer still in your sixties.

In our society choosing a nutritious diet is not something that comes naturally: it must be learned, and it requires time and thought. If you have any doubts about whether you're eating the right foods, now is the time to think about your diet and make changes that will stand you in good stead in your later years.

Exercise

Prolonged inactivity results in a number of physical changes—all of them bad. On the other hand, regular exercise throughout the life span significantly increases the likelihood of good health and long life. It increases energy, retards deterioration of vital organs, sharpens appetite, controls weight, promotes restful sleep, and may improve the condition and appearance of the skin. Recent research indicates that exercise may help slow or stop bone loss, or **osteoporosis,** a condition that causes bones to break easily and heal slowly. (The addition of calcium to the diet is also thought to aid in counteracting this condition.)

Osteoporosis Bone-weakening disease.

Like good eating habits, a regular exercise program (at least three times weekly) is best established during the early years. Exercise is beneficial, however, even if it is delayed to late adulthood, provided that one begins gradually and slowly works up to a more vigorous regimen, under the guidance of a physician.

Stress

A 70-year-old woman who enjoys community activities and socializing with friends is compelled, because of financial hardship, to sell her home and move to a small apartment in an unfamiliar neighborhood. A 72-year-old man who takes price in his carpentry and gardening skills is stricken with a painful arthritic condition. A 65-year-old woman who has devoted herself to her job is forced to retire. An 80-year-old man who has never lived alone is widowed. A 35-year-old quarterback, who has slowed down too much to continue to play football professionally, must turn to coaching or another career.

Negative stress, which may stem from physical ailments or being forced to relinquish the roles that have shaped one's life, threatens an individual's health and sense of well-being. Acceleration of the aging process, serious illness, and even death can result. A bereaved person, for example, may seem to "age overnight," and you may have noticed how U.S. presidents seem to age considerably in office.

Counseling is often useful in helping people give vent to their emotions and reorder their lives. Stress is less likely to affect permanently those with a certain degree of adaptability, a willingness to let go of the past and live in the present, and the ability to relax.

Walking, swimming, and stationary bicycling are relaxing exercises that can be done by most individuals at any age. But healthy individuals who have exercised regularly over the years may continue to participate in more vigorous sports, like jogging, into their nineties—and even beyond. Kenneth H. Cooper in *The New Aerobics* (Evans, 1970) cites the example of a 102-year-old man who ran six miles and walked five or ten miles nearly every day.

Life Satisfaction

In addition to proper exercise and adequate nutrition, people of all ages have emotional needs that must be met in order for them to lead satisfying lives. Among these are needs for self-esteem, sufficient privacy, contact with other people, spiritual comfort, the feeling of being cared about, a sense of independence and of being able to control one's life, and the ability to communicate thoughts, feelings, and convictions. Economic security, intellectual stimulation, and participation in a variety of recreational activities also contribute to health and longevity.

Think about what you know of your own needs—whether they are being met and how you are meeting them. As you work now and in the future to have a full and satisfying life, you can develop emotional strength and intellectual curiosity that will keep life interesting and rewarding for you in your later years.

What Society Can Do for the Elderly

Society as a whole benefits when senior citizens find outlets for their skills, talents, and energies. Some older people have come to view lifelong employment as their right and resist pressure to step aside in favor of younger workers. Suggested changes in the Social Security laws, which will reward people who retire later, reflect the trend toward encouraging older workers to remain in the labor force. Other options include part-time employment and volunteer work as tutors, consultants, teacher's aides, and so forth. Innovative programs such as part-time job sharing may enable more older people to continue working as long as they are willing and able to do so.

In recent years, day-care centers for children have been set up in nursing homes, benefiting young and old alike. The youngsters profit from their exposure to many eager teachers and storytellers, and the elderly gain by feeling useful and involved. Foster grandparent programs offer children in hospitals, day-care centers, and institutions the support, companionship, and assistance of an older person for about 20 hours each week. Participants, who are paid a small salary,

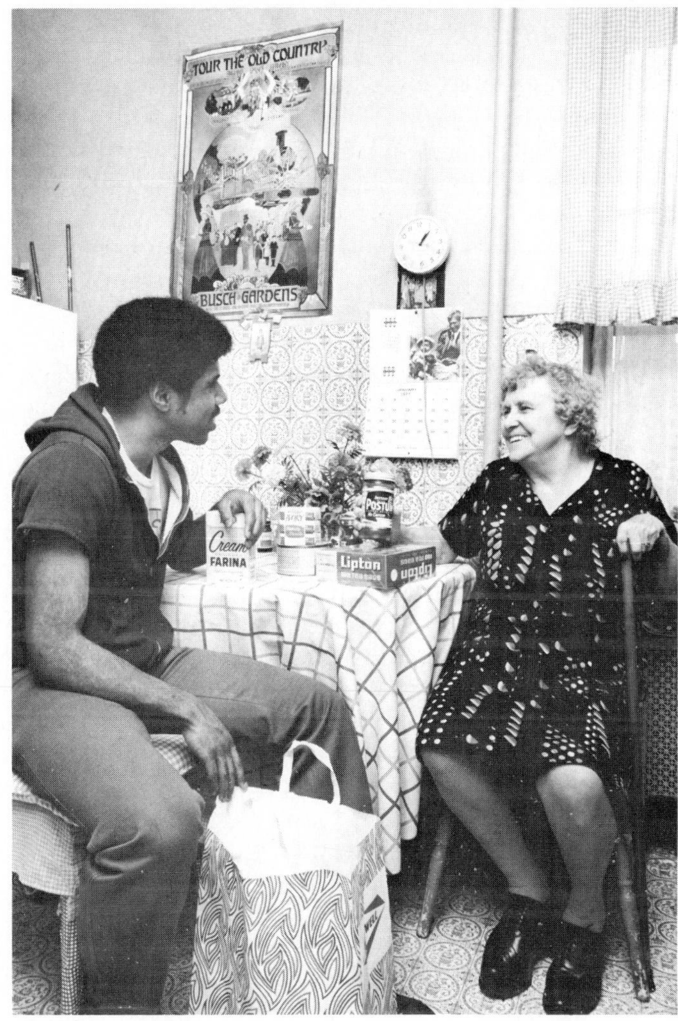

One of the ways society can help the elderly is by providing home day care services. (Photo © Guy Gillette/Photo Researchers, Inc.)

have worked effectively with severely handicapped and emotionally disturbed children. Such programs can be of special benefit for older people who particularly enjoy being around children.

Community Services for the Aged

Until the second half of this century, it was not unusual for several generations of one family to live under the same roof. This arrangement is now uncommon, and young people who are able to support themselves usually establish their own homes. Most older people, too, strive to assert and to maintain their independence—and the majority succeed. However, the trend toward separate households for senior citizens has introduced a new social problem: what happens when aging persons are no longer able to care for themselves? Do they move in with a son, daughter, or other relative? Can they remain in their own home with the help of a housekeeper or home attendant? Is a nursing home or a senior citizen's hotel a feasible alternative?

Most older people fear dependence and isolation more than they fear death. Supportive family relationships—which are needed throughout life—become increasingly important as a person ages. Although children are not legally responsible for their parents, sons and daughters usually acknowledge a moral responsibility based on love and obligation, and they often provide financial assistance, help with chores, run errands, and intervene in the event of an emergency.

Community services designed to help ailing and infirm older people remain in their own homes include the following:

- Meals on Wheels. Nutritious breakfasts, lunches, and dinners are delivered to the homes of elderly shut-ins at mealtimes. Some community centers also serve balanced meals at moderate costs.
- Domestic help such as housekeepers and homemakers who provide companionship and assist with marketing, cooking, laundry, and housework.
- Inexpensive and accessible transportation. Some organizations provide vans to take infirm older people to senior centers, special events, classes, and the theater.
- Home-centered health services such as mobile medical offices (doc-mobiles), doctors who make house calls, visiting nurses, and home attendants who assist with bathing, dressing, feeding, household maintenance, and other essential services.
- Day-care centers for the elderly, modeled after centers for children of working parents. Staffed by professionals paraprofessionals, social workers, and volunteers, such facilities provide a haven for physically and psychologically disabled persons who live alone or whose families are not at home during the day.
- Volunteers who call the homes of the elderly on a daily basis.

Education

Today, as never before, many educational institutions provide information about aging. Young students, few of whom have any contact with senior citizens on a day-to-day basis, can—by studying about the lives and needs of the elderly—rid themselves of preconceived notions, glimpse their own futures, and discover the keys to successful aging.

And just as courses in aging have been incorporated into many college and postgraduate curricula, adult education programs have been expanded to help meet the needs of older Americans. "Life span education," which deals with specific aspects of aging, includes vocational rehabilitation, exercise, self-assertion, leadership training, and crafts courses, as well as classes that deal with the legal rights, personal concerns, sexual problems, biological changes, and health needs of older adults. Many colleges offer free or half-cost tuition in their traditional curricula to students over 65. For the elderly, as for the rest of us, continuous education is not only possible but essential for growth, development, and adaptation to a changing world.

Looking Toward the Future

We should hope that the elderly of the twenty-first century will fare better than the elderly of the twentieth century because of advances in health care, improved educational and occupational opportunities, increased retirement benefits, and a decreasing tendency to stereotype and segregate older people. Organizations like the Gray Panthers — a political action group run and staffed by militant, energetic, vocal senior citizens — have already done much to dispel the myth that the aged are a homogeneous mass of people who have outlived their usefulness. Advocates for the elderly, including the National Council on Aging, the National Council of Senior Citizens, and the American Association of Retired Persons, have attempted to promote a more positive image of the elderly and have campaigned actively to secure legislation that is favorable to senior citizens. Nevertheless, a great deal more remains to be done if the image of the elderly in America is to be substantially improved.

Choosing What We Will Become

Aging has been called "one of the most difficult chapters in the great art of living." We pattern our lives according to a vaguely outlined plan, choosing one option over another based upon our hopes, fears, and opportunities. The more positive our expectations, the greater the likelihood that our senior years — indeed, all of our years — will be fulfilling, challenging, and productive.

Think of aging, most of all, as an opportunity to live more — to work more, play more, love more, learn more, and experience more, without some of the constraints and responsibilities of earlier years. Although eventually age brings some deterioration of the body, you need never stop growing intellectually and emotionally.

Imagine the sheer quantity of experience and memory that someone 70 or 80 years old is able to draw upon, and that you, too, will be able to enjoy, if you reach such an age. But at the same time, you will be experiencing just as many fresh and exciting things as when you were 20.

SELF-ASSESSMENT EXERCISE 7.4

Life Score

I. Habits

1. Exercise

To qualify as a minute of conditioning, it must be a minute with the heart rate at 120 beats per minute, or more. Beware of overestimating activities in which there may be a lot of standing about, e.g., tennis. As a rule, golf, bowling, baseball, and volleyball do not result in conditioning. If you have:

		Your Score
Less than 15 minutes of conditioning per week, score	0	____
15–29 minutes	+ 2	____
30–44	+ 6	____
45–74	+12	____
75–119	+16	____
120–179	+20	____
180 or more	+24	____

2. Weight

Look at the weight table to determine how many pounds overweight you are. If you are:

		Your Score
0–5 pounds overweight, score	0	____
6–15 pounds	− 2	____
16–25 pounds	− 6	____
26–35 pounds	−10	____
36–45 pounds	−12	____
46 or more	−15	____

3. Diet

		Your Score
If you eat a well-balanced diet, score	+ 4	____
If you avoid saturated fats and cholesterol, score	+ 2	____

4. Smoking

One cigar is considered to be the equivalent of one cigarette. If you smoke only a pipe, enter −4. If you smoke:

		Your Score
0 cigarettes per day, score	0	____
1–9	−10	____
10–19	−13	____
20–29	−15	____
30–39	−17	____
40–49	−20	____
50 or more	−24	____

5. Drinking

Cocktails are assumed to contain 1½ ounces of hard liquor. If you are pouring doubles, multiply accordingly. One pint equals 16 ounces or about 10 cocktails. One 8-ounce beer is the equivalent of one cocktail. Six ounces of wine also is the equivalent of one cocktail. If you drink:

		Your Score
0–1 cocktails per day, score	0	____
2–3	− 4	____
4–5	−12	____
6–8	−20	____
9 or more	−30	____

6. Seat Belts

The actual time you wear a seat belt while driving is probably one-half your first guess (unless that guess was zero). Take a minute to come up with a more accurate estimate. If you wear a seat belt:

		Your Score
Less than 25 percent of time, score	0	____
About 25 percent	+ 2	____
About 50 percent	+ 4	____
About 75 percent	+ 6	____
About 100 percent	+ 8	____

7. For Women Only

Contraception—If you have had a hysterectomy, tubal ligation, or have reached menopause, skip this section. If you use:

		Your Score
Nothing and would not have an abortion, score	−10	______
Mechanical method and would not have an abortion, score	0	______
Birth control pills and would not have an abortion, score	+ 4	______
Nothing, but would have an abortion, score	+ 4	______
Birth control pills and would have an abortion, score	+ 5	______
Mechanical method and would have an abortion, score	+10	______
Bad Bonus: If you smoke and use birth control pills, score	−10	______
Habits Total		______

II. Stress

Fill out the Holmes Scale at the end of this test, then record your score in the appropriate space. If your Holmes score is:

		Your Score
Less than 150, score	0	______
150–250	− 4	______
250–300	− 7	______
More than 300	−10	______
Stress Total		______

III. Immunity (Age 13 and up)

If you are not sufficiently current on:

		Your Score
Tetanus (booster every 10 years), score	− 4	______
Diphtheria (booster every 10 years for those with high risk of exposure only), score	− 2	______
Immunity Total		______

IV. Personal History

		Your Score
Tuberculosis—If you have been in close contact for a year or more with someone with tuberculosis, score	− 4	______
Radiation—If you have had radiation (x-ray) treatment of tonsils, adenoids, acne, or ringworm of the scalp, score	− 6	______
Asbestos—If you work with asbestos regularly and do not smoke, score	− 2	______
If you work with asbestos regularly and do smoke, score	−10	______
Vinyl Chloride—If you work regularly with vinyl chloride, score	− 4	______
Urban Environment—If you live in a city, score	− 6	______
For Men and Women (risk of venereal disease)—		
If sexual activity has been frequent and with many different partners, score	− 1	______
For Women Only (risk of uterine cancer)—		
If you began regular sexual activity before age 18, score	− 1	______
If sexual activity has been frequent and with many different partners, score	− 1	______
If you are Jewish, score	− 1	______
Personal History Total		______

Source: Donald M. Vickery, *Life Plan for Your Health,* © 1978, Addison-Wesley, Reading, MA., pp. 57–63. Reprinted with permission.

V. Family History

		Your Score
Heart Attacks (myocardial infarction)		
For each parent, brother or sister who had a heart attack before age 40, score	− 4	______
For each grandparent, uncle or aunt who had a heart attack before age 40, score	− 1	______
High Blood Pressure (hypertension)		
For each parent, brother or sister with high blood pressure requiring treatment, score	− 2	______
For each grandparent, uncle or aunt with high blood pressure requiring treatment, score	− 1	______
Diabetes		
For each parent, brother or sister with juvenile-onset diabetes, score	− 6	______
For each grandparent, uncle or aunt with juvenile-onset diabetes, score	− 2	______
For each parent, brother or sister with adult-onset diabetes and required treatment with insulin, score	− 2	______
For each grandparent, uncle or aunt with adult-onset diabetes and required treatment with insulin, score	− 1	______
Cancer of the Breast (women only)		
If your mother or a sister has had cancer of the breast, score	− 4	______
Glaucoma		
If you have a parent, grandparent, brother, sister, uncle or aunt with glaucoma, score	− 2	______
Gout		
If you have a parent, grandparent, brother, sister, uncle or aunt with gout, score	− 1	______
Ankylosing Spondylitis (a type of arthritis)		
If you have a parent, grandparent, brother, sister, uncle or aunt with ankylosing spondylitis, score	− 1	______
Family History Total		______

Adding Up Your Lifescore

I. Habits	______
II. Stress	______
III. Immunity	______
IV. Personal History	______
V. Family History	______
TOTAL	______
Now Add	**200**
To Obtain Your Lifescore	______

Be sure to get the plus and minus signs right so that you add or subtract correctly.

A LifeScore of 200 is about average. A LifeScore about 210 indicates a positive life style, which gives you an excellent chance of enjoying health beyond the average life expectancy of 69 years for men and 77 years for women. A LifeScore below 185 means your chance of a healthy future is clearly decreased. If your LifeScore is below 170, consider your life to be in danger. Below 150, make out a will and get your affairs in order.

To determine how long you might expect to live on the basis of this test, make these simple calculations.

For men, the formula is:

$$\underset{\text{LifeScore}}{\underline{\hspace{2cm}}} \div 200 \times 70 \text{ years} = \underset{\text{Life Expectancy}}{\underline{\hspace{3cm}}}$$

For women:

$$\underset{\text{LifeScore}}{\underline{\hspace{2cm}}} \div 200 \times 75 \text{ years} = \underset{\text{Life Expectancy}}{\underline{\hspace{3cm}}}$$

Summary

Aging is a process that many of us fear and misunderstand, but the examples of many active and creative older individuals show that graceful aging is possible. The term *aging* refers to the various transitions we experience throughout the life cycle; and the term *senescence,* to the deterioration associated with old age, which affects all of us, although at different rates. *Ageism* is stereotyping of and discrimination against the elderly on the grounds of age. *Gerontology,* a relatively new field, is the study of aging.

Although various theories have been developed to explain aging and senescence, none has yet been shown by research to account for all the individual variations in the aging process. Other theories, offered by social gerontologists, seek to explain how people adjust to aging and what constitutes successful aging.

In order to benefit from living and working with elderly people and to overcome our fears of aging, we must learn to distinguish false ideas about aging from the facts. Contrary to stereotype, the physical changes of aging occur much more gradually and are much less debilitating than is commonly believed; most elderly people remain healthy and able to engage in their normal activities throughout life; a large majority of those over 80 show no symptoms of senility; elderly people can remain in good spirits and continue to learn as long as they live; fewer than 10 percent of the aged reside in nursing homes and institutions; a majority have sufficient income for their needs; many remain able and willing to work; and most maintain their interest in and capacity for sexual relations. Misconceptions about aging have arisen partly because the decline of the extended family in our society has resulted in fewer young people having frequent contact with the elderly.

To a large extent, people choose how they age. It is important that we examine our prejudices about aging so that we can replace them with positive attitudes that will affect how we age. A helpful exercise is to imagine your older self: how your body will look and feel and what your life will be like.

Although heredity seems to affect longevity, other important factors that contribute to long life are maintaining good nutrition and regular exercise, successfully coping with stress, and leading a satisfying life.

It is important for society to help the elderly find ways of continuing to use their abilities and energies in paid or volunteer work, including programs designed especially for them. The decline of the extended family has meant an increase in the number of elderly persons living alone; such community services as Meals on Wheels and day-care centers for the elderly can help them remain in their own homes when ill or infirm, as most would prefer. Besides offering information about aging to the young, colleges now offer courses designed to meet the needs of the aged.

Organizations such as the Gray Panthers have helped to combat negative stereotypes of the aged and lobby in favor of their interests. More positive expectations about aging will help the young, in their turn, lead fulfilling lives in the later years.

Review and Discussion

1. Define aging, senescence, ageism, and gerontology.
2. What examples of ageism do you see in daily life? What signs of changing attitudes can you think of?
3. Describe ten physical changes that occur with aging.
4. Describe the main social theories of aging. Which one do you think leads to the most successful old age?
5. Name six examples of community programs to help the elderly. Are there other needs that community programs could help meet?
6. American society has often been criticized for being too youth-oriented and not placing enough value on old age. Do you think this criticism is justified?
7. Discuss the main factors leading to a long and healthy life. What can you do now to improve your Life-Score?
8. How do you think the wisdom and experience of older people can be put to better use?

Further Reading

Anderson, Barbara. *The Aging Game.* New York: McGraw-Hill Book Company, 1979.
A frank discussion of how to take control of one's life and age successfully. (Paperback.)

Biegal, Leonard. *The Best Years Catalogue.* New York: G. P. Putnam's Sons, 1978.
A wealth of information on aging, food, shelter, health, safety, creative leisure, transportation and travel, money, joing and sharing, communicating, rights and legacies. (Paperback.)

Bumagin, Victoria E., and Kathryn F. Hirn. *Aging is a Family Affair.* New York: Thomas Y. Crowell Company, 1979.
Interesting and useful information for individuals of all ages on health, dependence, communication, money, sex, marriage, senility, and grief.

Comfort, Alex. *A Good Age.* New York: Simon & Schuster, Inc., 1978.
A discussion by an internationally known gerontologist of attitudes towards aging. (Paperback.)

Dangott, Lillian R., and Richard A. Kalish. *A Time to Enjoy.* Englewood Cliffs, N.J.: Prentice-Hall, Inc., 1979.
Includes questionnaires and other activities for readers to gain deeper insight into their own aging as well as the aging of others. (Paperback.)

Louis Harris and Associates, Inc. *Aging in the Eighties: America in Transition.* Washington, D.C.: National Council on Aging, 1981.
An extensive investigation of public opinion about aging, commissioned by the National Council on Aging.

Montague, Ashley. *Growing Young.* New York: McGraw-Hill Book Company, 1983.
Discussion of the development of childhood traits as applied to aging, such as the ability to learn, love, and explore, and not just forgetting these traits as aging occurs. (Paperback.)

Schwartz, Arthur. *Survival Handbook for Children of Aging Parents.* Chicago: Follett Publishing Company, 1977.
A nontechnical and readable book aimed at helping adult sons and daughters understand and deal with aging parents. (Paperback.)

Zarit, Steven H. (ed.). *Readings in Aging and Death: Contemporary Perspectives.* New York: Harper & Row, Publishers, 1977.
A collection of articles from books, journals, and other periodicals for students interested in exploring major issues in gerontology. (Paperback.)

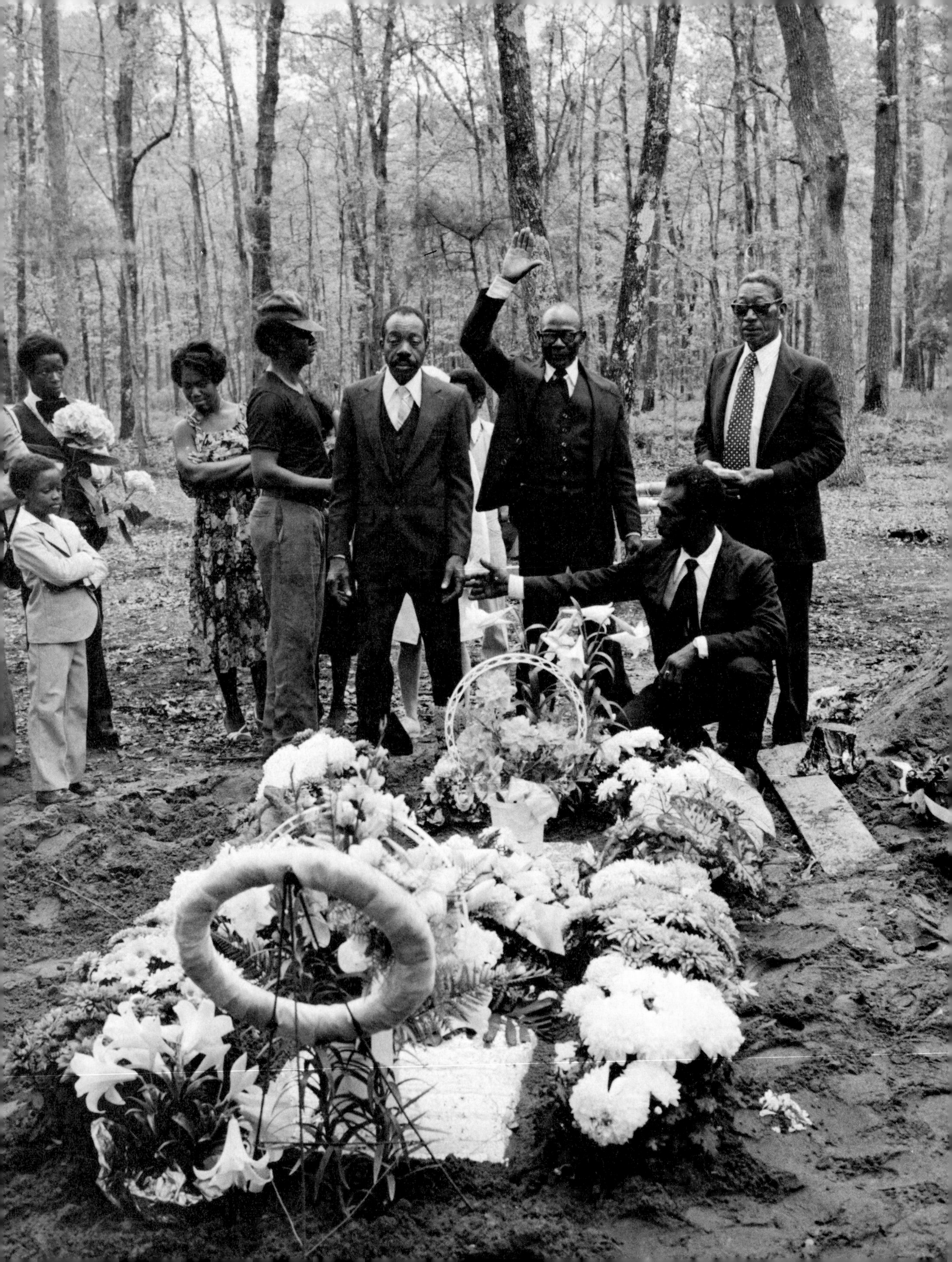

Chapter 8
Dying and Death

KEY POINTS

- ☐ The study of death can lead to a fuller life through understanding the relationship between death and life.
- ☐ Dying persons, given time, pass through five stages: denial and isolation, anger, bargaining, depression, and acceptance.
- ☐ Active and passive euthanasia are defined and discussed.
- ☐ Children need special help in understanding dying and death.
- ☐ For the terminally ill, hospices, whose aim is to provide a warm, caring environment for dying individuals, are an alternative to hospitals.
- ☐ Suicide is usually an expression of helplessness, hopelessness, and loneliness; it remains a major problem in today's society.
- ☐ When a person dies, the family members—despite their grief—must make many practical arrangements and decisions.
- ☐ Grieving plays an important role in helping survivors return to their normal lives.
- ☐ Memorial services often help in coping with the loss of a loved one.

Fear no more the heat o' the sun,
Nor the furious winter's rages;
Thou thy worldly task hast done,
Home art gone, and ta'en thy wages.
Golden lads and girls all must,
As chimney-sweepers, come to dust.

WILLIAM SHAKESPEARE

DEATH has always fascinated poets. John Dryden likened it to "landing on some distant shore," George Henry Boker, a nineteenth-century American writer, called it "that blessing which men fly from," and the English poet and dramatist John Heywood declared, "Death makes equal the high and low." Woody Allen summed up the modern attitude toward death when he observed, "I'm not afraid to die. I just don't want to be there when it happens."

Death in Contemporary American Society

Terminal illness An incurable illness.

Until the last century, death was a highly visible phenomenon in American society. Wars, famine, epidemics, and infant mortality were commonplace. Most people died at home, and until the development of the funeral industry in the 1860s, the dead were usually carried from the house and buried in private by members of their own families. Death was unwelcome, but it was expected and accepted. Today we can save many people who previously would have died, so we segregate the aged and the sick and place them in hospitals to be cared for by strangers in a sterile, white-walled world. Even those whose illnesses are **terminal** often remain hospitalized, usually in intensive care wards. Family and friends attempting to communicate with the dying person must compete with physicians, nurses, respirators, pain-relieving drugs, plasma bottles, heart monitors, and other medical equipment. As death nears, the patient is isolated even more, presumably to shield others from the actual death scene. Family and friends often remain at a distance and do not share the reality of death.

Surprisingly, while death is hidden from us in the real world, it is common in the books we read, the television shows and movies we watch, and the songs we hear. Children's literature—such as *The Three Little Pigs*, *Bambi*, and *Little Red Riding Hood*—often deals with violent death. Playwrights—from Euripides to Shakespeare to Ibsen to Arthur Miller—have used death to dramatize their themes. Often, popular movies contain numerous gruesome death scenes. In many of these films, however, and in other forms of popular enter-

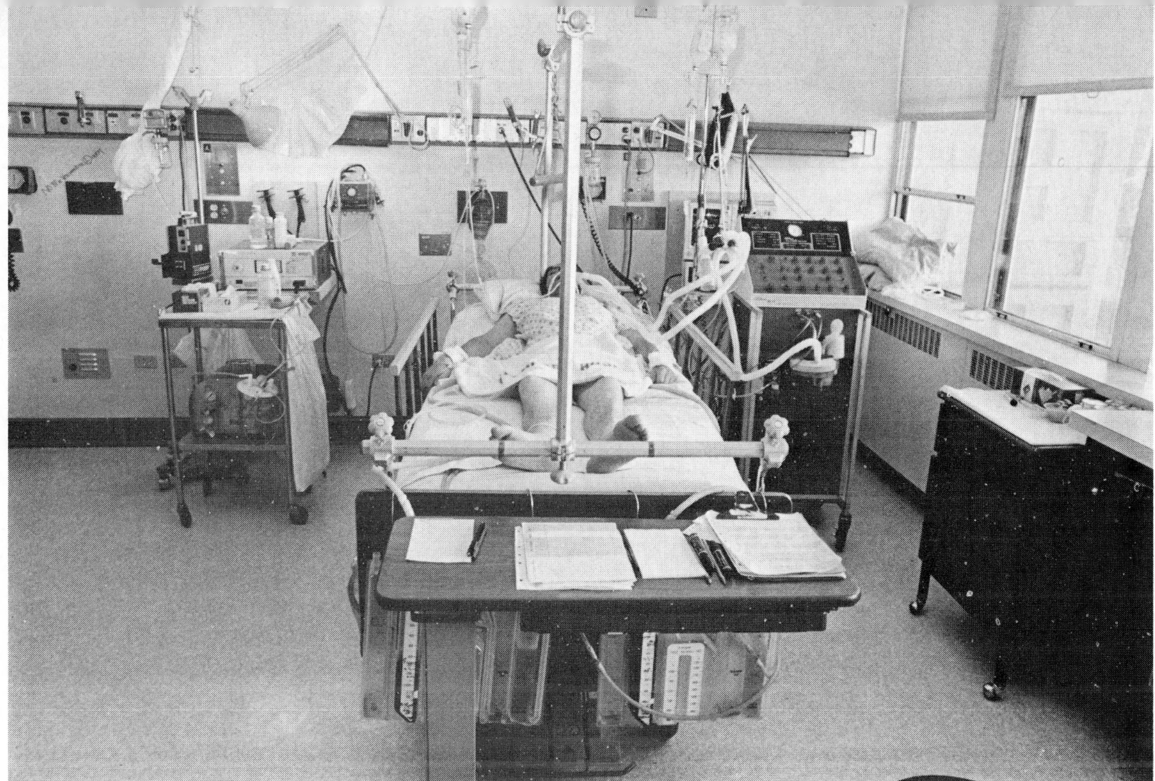

It is becoming more and more common to sustain dying persons' lives in hospital rooms, such as this intensive care unit. (Photo by William Thompson/The Picture Cube)

tainment, the actual treatment of death is too far removed from reality to stimulate reflection about the meaning of death and the experience of dying. Murders in television programs and crime dramas usually exist either as casual, bloodless acts or violent, gory ones that take place so that the hero or heroine can pursue the murderer. Indeed, deaths on stage are usually plot devices that may shock us or make us cry, but they tell us as much about death as watching an airplane fly tells us about being a pilot. Actors playing death scenes in movies or on television usually speak clearly and look attractive, even when they have supposedly been mortally wounded or are in the final stages of a long and painful illness.

Television news, with its graphic coverage of wars, airplane crashes, floods, and political assassinations, brings images of death into our living rooms, but these reports rarely give us any insight into what a dying person needs, feels, or experiences.

The Fear of Death

Are Americans obsessed with death? Studies reveal that some people think about death frequently — sometimes as often as every day — and these thoughts focus on what psychologists call "death anxiety." Specific anxiety, or fear, is a response to a concrete threat (one fears a tornado or a mugger), whereas free-flowing anxiety is generated by a more vague menace, like the dark. Death may be a genuine threat, but it is so vaguely understood that it gives rise to both specific anxiety (fear) and free-flowing anxiety.

Fears associated with death include:

- *Fear of death,* or, primarily, fear of nonbeing. This involves the perception that death is the loss of everything—all human contact, our possessions, our identity, our selves.
- *Fear of dying.* Perhaps greater than the fear of death itself is the fear of the many negative experiences associated with the process of dying: pain, loneliness, physical deterioration, loss of self-control, surgical mutilation, dependency, humiliation, and loss of self-respect as the ability to care for oneself diminishes.
- *Fear of the results or consequences of death.* One might worry about divine judgment, an afterlife, reincarnation, the possibility of going to hell, or what will happen to people, possessions, and unfinished business left behind.
- *Fear of the death or dying of others.* This includes the fear of losing a loved one, of being abandoned, or of seeing someone we care about suffer and die.

Self-Assessment Exercise 8.1 is designed to help you gain insight about how you view dying and death.

The Dying Person

It has become increasingly difficult to tell when a life has ended. There appear to be differences among the legal, medical, and theological professions as to when death has occurred. The classic, or legal, definition of death is when heartbeat and breathing cease. Medical scientists agree that death occurs when the brain ceases to function (a flat **electroencephlogram**). From the standpoint of religion, death does not occur until the soul has exited the body.

Electroencephlogram
Graphic tracing of the electrical impulses of brain cells.

The Five Stages of Dying

For many years it was widely believed that a dying person should be shielded from the news of impending death. This philosophy is no longer generally accepted, primarily because most dying people sense their plight and need help in coming to terms with it. Just as we can learn how to live, we can learn how to die, but it is a difficult, gradual process often made harder because there is so little time. Elisabeth Kübler-Ross, author of *On Death and Dying,* observed that terminally ill people go through five stages: denial and isolation, anger, bargaining, depression, and acceptance, although some may not go through these stages in order.

Denial and Isolation. Informed that one is dying, the initial response is usually, "There must be some mistake," or, "No, not me, it

SELF-ASSESSMENT EXERCISE 8.1

How Do You Feel about Death and Dying?

The statements listed below are indicative of how some people feel about dying and death. Read each statement and check how you feel about the item. Give yourself 5 points for each time you respond "Very Acceptable," 4 points for "Acceptable," 3 points for "Unsure," 2 points for "Unacceptable," and 1 point for "Very Unacceptable."

	Very Acceptable	Acceptable	Unsure	Unacceptable	Very Unacceptable
1. Attending a funeral					
2. Living forever					
3. Seeing a dead person					
4. Writing a living will					
5. Telling someone they are dying					
6. Visiting a hospital for the terminally ill					
7. Dying quickly					
8. Dying rather than being unable to walk again					
9. Visiting a cemetery					
10. Being able to choose when you will die					
11. Dying before your spouse					
12. Talking with a dying person					
13. Dying after your spouse					
14. Planning for your own funeral					
15. Being unhooked from a life-support system					
17. Dying in your sleep					
18. Being told that you have a terminal illness					
19. Dying with the hope there's an afterlife					
20. Refusing to try a "miracle" drug that might work					

Scoring: If your total score for all 20 items is 80 or above, you have a positive attitude toward dying and death. That is, you do not appear to fear dying and death. If you score between 40 and 79 points, you appear to accept some things about death, but are not comfortable about other things dealing with death. If you scored 39 or fewer points, you may wish to do additional reading or a follow-up analysis of your feelings about dying and death.

Source: Donald A. Read, *Looking In: Exploring One's Personal Health Values,* Prentice-Hall, Englewood Cliffs: 1977, & Walter Sorochan: *Promoting Your Health,* NY: Wiley, 1981, p. 447. Used by permission.

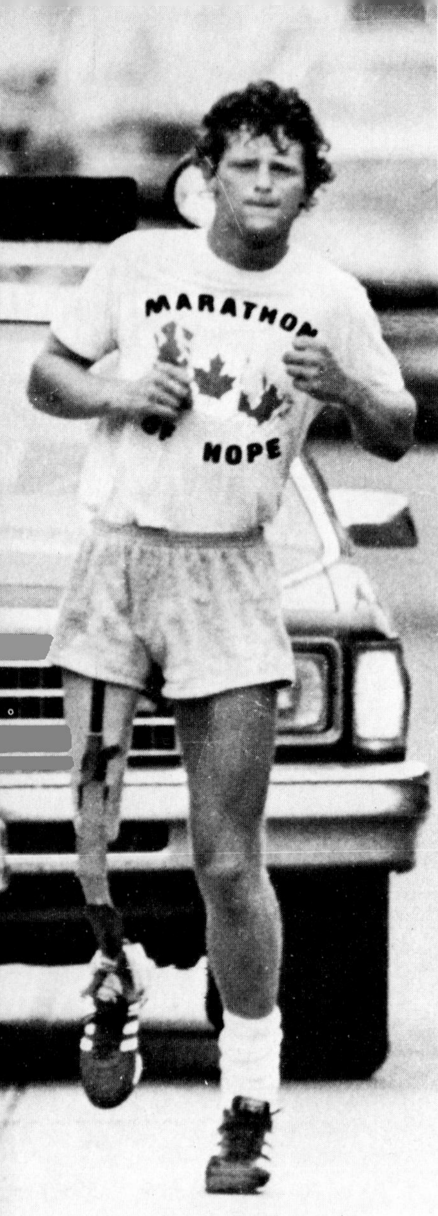

Terry Fox, who lost one of his legs to cancer, ran halfway across Canada to raise money for cancer research before his death on June 28, 1981. Many of the dying make contributions to humanity during their last days. (Photo from United Press International)

cannot be true." As people attempt to shield themselves from the truth, isolation occurs. Denial and isolation are defense mechanisms that afford temporary protection until other, less extreme methods of defense can take over.

Anger. Denial usually gives way to anger, rage, envy, and resentment. Now, instead of saying, "It cannot be me," the patient asks, "Why me?" and looks for someone to blame for the situation. This stage is characterized by hostile outbursts directed at hospital personnel, family, friends, or God.

Bargaining. This is an attempt to postpone the inevitable — a way of buying time. Most bargains are made with God in the hope of earning an extension of life or freedom from pain.

Depression. As the patient's physical condition deteriorates and as his worsening illness continues to take its toll on his family, the dying person experiences remorse, anguish, and guilt. This overwhelming sadness is also a form of mourning for oneself, a deep sorrow in anticipation of losing everything and everybody.

Acceptance. For many people — but not all — denial, anger, and depression fade into a peaceful acceptance of the inevitable if they are given enough time and support. As death nears, the dying person is likely to prefer nonverbal communication. A gentle touch or the quiet presence of a loved one can offer great comfort at this time.

Talking to the Dying Patient

Because most of us do not fully understand death, we are uncomfortable when visiting a dying person. We worry about finding the right words, about reacting to the patient's expressions of grief, anger, and despair, and about controlling our own emotions. Like the rest of us, dying people appreciate kindness, understanding, thoughtfulness, someone to talk with, and a gentle touch. Listen carefully, respond honestly, and avoid expressions of pity. Gifts of books, magazines, or a favorite food may be appreciated more than flowers, and loving notes or carefully chosen cards can brighten the day. When an adult family member is hospitalized and the spouse must spend many hours at the hospital, friends can be of invaluable assistance by doing household chores, caring for young children, preparing meals, and making themselves available to help whenever possible.

Organ Transplants

With the increased success in transplanting body organs, the dying individual can attain a special type of immortality. In the same way that a person leaves belongings to others, the individual can now bequeath body parts. Eyes and kidneys, for example, can live for many years in another body if removed and transplanted quickly

YOUR HEALTH TODAY

The Dying Person's Bill of Rights

This bill of rights was created at a workshop on "The Terminally Ill Patient and the Helping Person," sponsored by the Southwestern Michigan Insurance Education Council and conducted by Amelia J. Barbus.

- I have the right to be treated as a living human being until I die.
- I have the right to maintain a sense of hopefulness, however changing its focus may be.
- I have the right to be cared for by those who can maintain a sense of hopefulness, however changing this might be.
- I have the right to express my feelings and emotions about my approaching death in my own way.
- I have the right to participate in decisions concerning my care.
- I have the right to expect continuing medical and nursing attention even though "cure" goals must be changed to "comfort" goals.
- I hve the right not to die alone.
- I have the right to be free from pain.
- I have the right to have my questions answered honestly.
- I have the right not to be deceived.
- I have the right to have help from and for my family in accepting my death.
- I have the right to die in peace and dignity.
- I have the right to retain my individuality and not be judged for my decisions which may be contrary to beliefs of others.
- I have the right to discuss and enlarge my religious and/or spiritual experiences, whatever these may mean to others.
- I have the right to expect that the sanctity of the human body will be respected after death.
- I have the right to be cared for by caring, sensitive, knowledgeable people who will attempt to understand my needs and will be able to gain some satisfaction in helping me face my death.

Source: Copyright © 1975 by American Journal of Nursing Company; reproduced with permission from *American Journal of Nursing,* January 1975, vol. 75, no. 1.

enough. Some states provide people the opportunity to specify, on their drivers' licenses, that they want to be organ donors. State laws vary with respect to being an organ donor, so the individual should check with the local medical authority or medical school to determine what the law is in the state in which he or she resides. In those cases where state law does not afford the opportunity to specify on one's driver's license the wish to be an organ donor, individuals desiring to bestow usable tissues are advised to carry a Uniform Donor Card,

UNIFORM DONOR CARD

OF ______________________________

Print or type name of donor

In the hope that I may help others, I hereby make this anatomical gift, if medically acceptable, to take effect upon my death. The words and marks below indicate my desires.

I give: (a) _____ any needed organs or parts

(b) _____ only the following organs or parts

____

Specify the organ(s) or part(s)

for the purposes of transplantation, therapy, medical research or education;

(c) _____ my body for anatomical study if needed.

Limitations or special wishes, if any: ______________________________

08-21-81 100M/81

Signed by the donor and the following two witnesses in the presence of each other:

Signature of Donor	Date of Birth of Donor
Date Signed	City & State
Witness	Witness

This is a legal document under the Uniform Anatomical Gift Act or similar laws.

For further information consult your physician or

National Kidney Foundation, Inc.
2 Park Avenue, New York, N.Y. 10016

Figure 8–1. A Sample of a Uniform Donor Card. Copies are made available from the National Kidney Foundation.

such as the one provided by the National Kidney Foundation (see Figure 8–1).

Euthanasia

Euthanasia Withdrawing life-support systems from an ill patient.

An unconscious person who cannot be revived and who is unable to function in any meaningful way can often be kept alive indefinitely by means of artificial life-support systems, placing an intolerable emotional and financial burden on the patient's family. In such cases, proponents of **euthanasia** (or "easy death," from the Greek word *thanatos,* meaning "death," and the prefix *eu,* meaning "easy" or "good") advocate withdrawing the life-support systems—or "pulling the plug"—thus allowing the patient to die naturally and with dignity.

In reality, euthanasia can be active or passive. Active euthanasia—which is illegal—is a deliberate merciful act undertaken when a person's mind or body has deteriorated beyond repair. Purposely administering a drug overdose is an example of active euthanasia.

Living will A document indicating the signer's desire to die as quickly and painlessly as possible once he or she is diagnosed as terminally ill.

The decision to "pull the plug" or to withhold heroic medical treatment—passive euthanasia—has been common practice for years but has only recently been endorsed by courts of law. Passive euthanasia is usually performed by a physician, often at the request of the patient or the patient's family. If—as is usually the case—the patient if unconscious, the decision is sometimes aided by the existence of a **living will,** a document that indicates the signer's desire to die as quickly and painlessly as possible once it has been specified that he or she is terminally ill.

To My Family, My Physician, My Lawyer and All Others Whom It May Concern

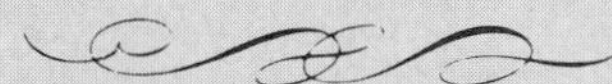

Death is as much a reality as birth, growth, maturity and old age—it is the one certainty of life. If the time comes when I can no longer take part in decisions for my own future, let this statement stand as an expression of my wishes and directions, while I am still of sound mind.

If at such a time the situation should arise in which there is no reasonable expectation of my recovery from extreme physical or mental disability, I direct that I be allowed to die and not be kept alive by medications, artificial means or "heroic measures". I do, however, ask that medication be mercifully administered to me to alleviate suffering even though this may shorten my remaining life.

This statement is made after careful consideration and is in accordance with my strong convictions and beliefs. I want the wishes and directions here expressed carried out to the extent permitted by law. Insofar as they are not legally enforceable, I hope that those to whom this Will is addressed will regard themselves as morally bound by these provisions.

Signed______________________________

Date ______________________________

Witness______________________________

Witness______________________________

Copies of this request have been given to ______________________________

____

____

____

Figure 8–2. A Sample of a Living Will.
Copies are available from Concern for Dying, 250 West 57th Street, New York, N.Y. 10107

Care of the Dying Patient: The Hospice

Hospice Institution that provides medical care for the terminally ill.

Given a choice, most people would prefer to die at home or in a warm, caring, homelike environment. **Hospices,** which originated in England and have recently taken root in the United States, were developed to meet the special needs of the terminally ill. Staffed by doctors, nurses, clergy, physical therapists, dieticians, legal counselors, pharmacists, and volunteers, a hospice can function as an in-patient facility, providing 24-hour care; as a home care program; or as a day-care facility for patients who can return home at night, where relatives and friends supply necessary assistance. In a hospital the focus is on avoiding death at all costs. The aim of the hospice is to provide a supportive, life-enhancing environment for dying individuals and their families. Medication is prescribed to control pain while affording maximum mental alertness. As much as possible, patients' personal needs are given priority, and patients make decisions regarding their own care. However, the specific structure of hospices varies from location to location, and their price structure, particularly with respect to Medicare reimbursement, also varies. An individual needs to contact the hospice in which he or she is interested and discuss these factors prior to making a decision about which facility to utilize.

Freed from costly, strength-sapping treatments and frustrating, desperate searches for a cure, hospice patients are given the opportunity to make constructive use of the time that they have left. Hospice care does not end with the death of the patient. Bereavement follow-up, which benefits the family, friends, and members of the hospice staff who worked with the deceased, continues for at least a year.

Children and Death

As difficult as it is for adults to envision their own death, children are at an even greater disadvantage. Children feel immortal and may have to be restrained from attempting to skate on thin ice or fly like Superman. With the conquest of most childhood illnesses, it is the rare child who must face the prospect of dying, but such situations do occur, creating a unique ordeal and challenge for all concerned.

Whether or not they are told that they are dying, critically ill children usually perceive their situation by first realizing that they are very sick, then gradually observing that—contrary to their expectations—they are not getting better, and eventually reaching the conclusion that they will never get better and will die. How

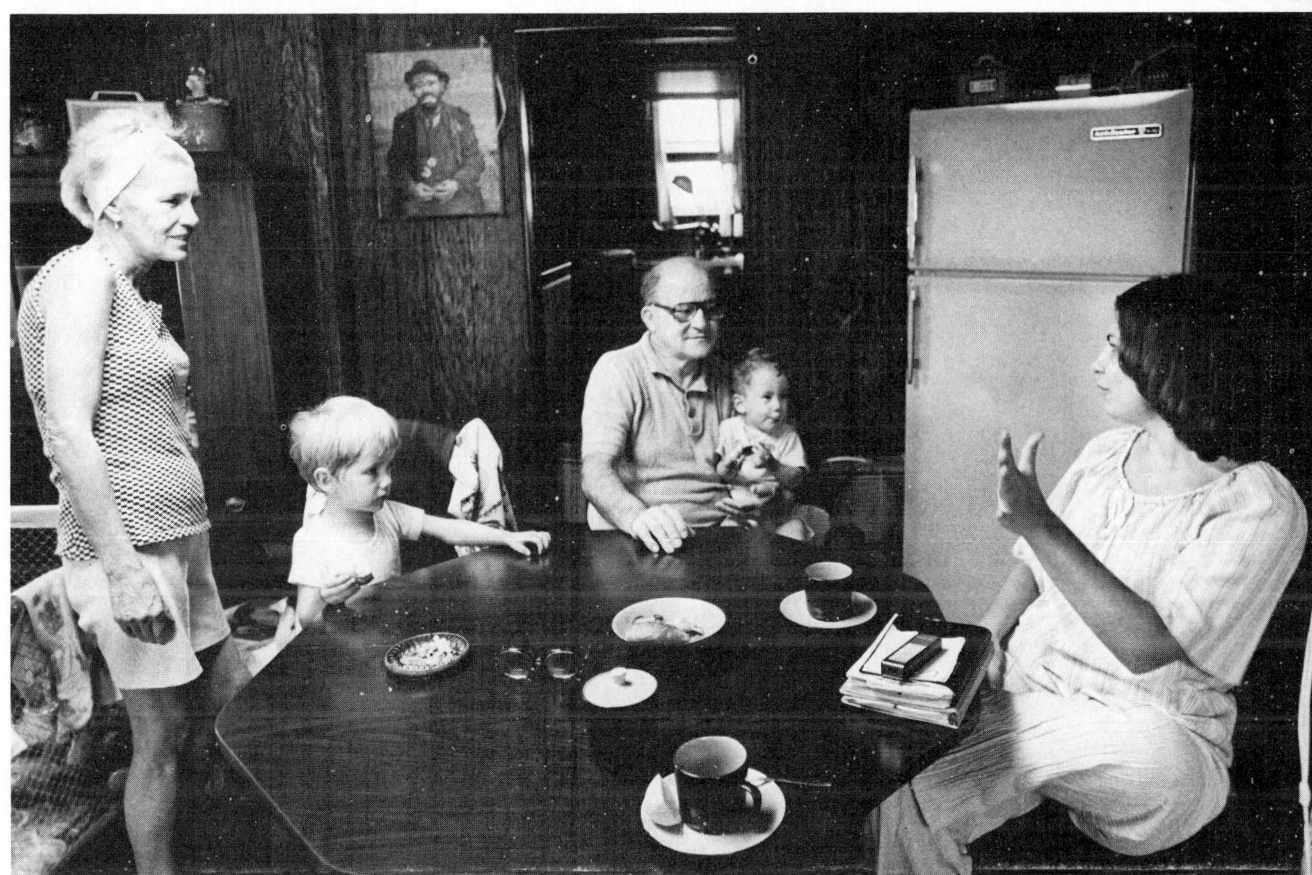

Hospice patient (left) with her husband and two grandchildren talking to hospice nurse in the home. Many hospices offer home-care programs as well as inpatient services. (Photo by Linda Bartlett/Woodfin Camp & Associates)

quickly this information is sorted out and absorbed depends on the child's stage of development, the child's understanding of death, and the readiness of adults to listen and respond honestly to questions. Like healthy youngsters, dying children are curious, impatient with dishonesty, and in need of loving comfort and support. Parents should not try to hide the fact that the child is dying. It should be discussed with the child, however, that many children and young people have survived an apparently terminal illness or injury. In such cases the child or young person often needs help in dealing with the emotional trauma of surviving a seemingly terminal situation.

A child who has lost a loved one needs help in expressing a confusing tangle of emotions that may include bodily distress (inability to sleep, lack of appetite), hostility toward the deceased ("If Daddy really loved me, he wouldn't have left me."), guilt ("I wished my brother would go away and now he's dead. I killed him."), replacement (attempts to get others to take the place of the deceased), ideal-

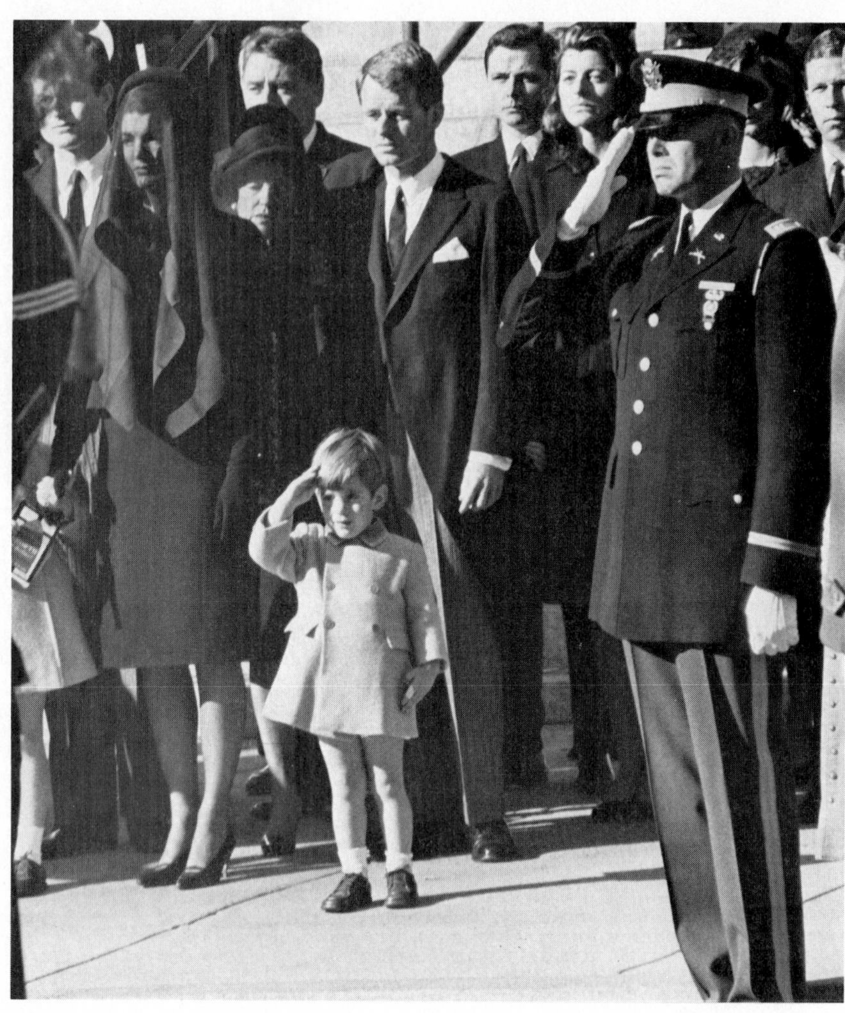

Children must be allowed to face death in their own way. (Photo from United Press International/Bettmann Newsphotos)

ization (attributing almost saintlike characteristics to the deceased), and panic ("Who will take care of me now?").

Children need to be allowed to mourn in their own way and at their own pace, but like bereaved adults, they benefit most from being gently encouraged to focus on life, not death. Keeping a grief-stricken child out of school and away from friends is probably counterproductive.

An adult attempting to explain death to a child should lovingly and directly convey the message that death is final, universal, and inevitable. Careless, evasive answers can create fears and misconceptions that may haunt a child for years. A child who is told that a dead person is "on a long journey" or "asleep" may refuse to travel or become terrified of going to sleep.

Suicide

In most cultures the taking of a life, even one's own, is considered a crime against society. For centuries, a person who committed suicide was refused burial in church or local cemeteries, the family was ostracized, and all property was confiscated. Today, suicide is still illegal in many states. Although families of suicide victims are no longer faced with legal action, they suffer a heavy burden of guilt and shame.

Many people contemplate suicide, but the instinct for self-preservation is so powerful that most hold back long enough for the feelings of despair to lessen. It is almost impossible to determine how many people attempt suicide each year, but some 30,000 succeed in the United States alone. Particularly alarming is the increase in suicide among the college population. One study revealed that one-third of the college students who die during their university years take their own lives. Second only to accidents as the major cause of death among persons 10 to 25 years old, suicide is usually a desperate response to helplessness, hopelessness, depression, and loneliness. Many teenagers who end their own lives do so under the influence of drugs or alcohol, which may intensify feelings of depression, panic, and anxiety.

Other groups that have a high suicide rate are divorced persons, American Indians, Hispanics, the elderly, the sick, and, surprisingly, highly successful professional people, particularly physicians and dentists. Health care practitioners often devote themselves to their careers to the exclusion of all else, leaving huge gaps in their lives that result in feelings of despondency.

A person who has absolutely resolved to die usually chooses a highly lethal method, such as a gun or jumping from a tall building. When such people accidentally survive, they will almost certainly try suicide again. In other cases, the determination to die is not as strong. People who flirt with death, such as those who play Russian roulette or drive recklessly, are thought to have strong suicidal tendencies and may well succeed in killing themselves. Other suicidal gestures are actually cries for help or attention, though they still may end in death.

Help for the Suicidal Person

Anyone who threatens suicide should be taken seriously and, if possible, referred to psychological counseling. Many self-destructive individuals have been helped by suicide prevention and crisis intervention centers, community-based organizations that have 24-hour telephone hotlines. These can be found in the front of your telephone book, or call Information in the nearest major city. If you are in need of help to prevent suicide, a long-distance phone call is worth the price. A caller can talk, listen to calm reassurance, and find out where to go for additional help. Some crisis intervention workers respond to an acute emergency by visiting the suicidal person, planning "something to live for," and arranging follow-up care.

A suicidal person faces a critical choice: life or death. Those who choose to live may emerge from their experience with a heightened appreciation of life's complexity and promise.

The American Way of Death

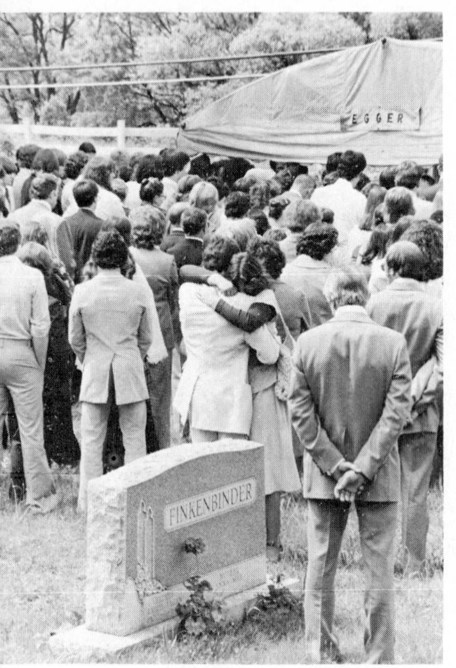

Memorial services are one way of helping us cope with the death of a loved one. (Photo by David S. Strickler/The Picture Cube)

Ceremonies and rites such as wakes and funerals and viewing the body in the casket are thought by many to be useful in helping survivors grieve and accept the reality and finality of death. We have come a long way, however, from the time when a person was buried in a simple pine box following a brief service. Today's funeral usually involves using a funeral director's facilities, equipment, and services, which may include removal of the deceased to the funeral home, preparation of the death certificate, coordination of all details of the funeral service, and help in filing death benefit claims. Other expenses include the clergyman's honorarium; a casket, cemetery plot, and monument or grave marker; a hearse for the deceased and limousine service for some of the mourners; gravediggers to open and close the grave; and perpetual care of the gravesite, monument, or marker.

In an attempt to limit the high cost of dying, some individuals donate their bodies to science. Others have joined memorial societies, nonprofit organizations made up of people who have preplanned their own simple, economical funerals. Membership in a memorial society is not required for one to prearrange one's death ceremony and body disposal with most funeral homes.

Cremation, which is usually less costly than burial, involves burning the body and either storing the ashes that remain or scattering them over land or water. Customarily, the ashes are deposited in an urn that is placed in a niche, a sealed or hollow in the wall of a funeral vault. Costs vary depending on the size, location, and design of the niche. The urn can also be buried in an earth grave or kept by the family of the deceased. An ancient practice, cremation is currently popular in densely populated areas such as England and Japan. Only five percent of the people who die in the United States are cremated, but this number is reportedly increasing.

Executor Person appointed to ensure the carrying out of an individual's will.

It is important to know that most persons should have a will—a legal document stating what is to be done with their property or estate—and should name someone to be **executor,** or person who sees that the stated wishes are carried out. Making a will can save the survivors a great deal of emotional trauma and thereby help the grieving process.

Grief

Grief is our reaction to the loss of a loved one. We grieve not only for the person who is gone but also for ourselves. We feel personally diminished, as though a part of us has died too. Grief releases a flood of emotions that must be understood, freely expressed, and ultimately mastered through the process of mourning.

Those close to a person who is terminally ill often begin mourning before the actual loss occurs. This phenomenon — known as anticipatory grief — results from fear of the impending loss, disruption of life patterns, and uncertainty about the future. A person experiencing anticipatory grief has an urgent need to be with the dying person, to know that the dying person is being helped in every way possible, to be informed about the dying person's condition, and to be able to talk about and express feelings.

As painful difficult, and emotionally draining as mourning can be, it is a normal, healthy, and necessary adjustment process that is made easier if we keep as busy and active as possible. In time, our emotional ties to the deceased person weaken, and social outlets, family, hobbies, work, and everyday chores resume their normal places in our lives.

Grief Patterns

Grief patterns may include shock, emotion, depression and isolation, physical symptoms, guilt, hostility and resentment, and hope and affirmation of reality.

Shock. In the same way that dying people initially refuse to believe they are terminally ill, a person who has lost a loved one may respond, "I don't believe it," or "It can't be true."

Emotion. Initial shock generally yields to a flood of emotion. Crying during this stage is both necessary and desirable. Those who struggle to "be brave" or to deny feelings may only prolong the mourning process.

Depression and Isolation. Still struggling to come to terms with our loss, we experience overwhelming sadness. Places and activities that were once pleasant and familiar seem foreign and uninviting, adding to feelings of loneliness and alienation.

Physical Symptoms. Overwhelming fatigue, dizziness, headaches, and nausea may overcome a grieving person.

Guilt. Most of us would agree with William Faulkner that "Between grief and nothing, I will take grief." Mingled with our sadness at having lost a loved one is our happiness — and guilt — that we are still alive.

Hostility and Resentment. The pain of loss often leads to anger

YOUR HEALTH TODAY

Planning for Death

When an individual dies, there are numerous details that must be considered. Many of these details can be taken care of by friends, and others require the attention of the family. Some persons put these provisions into their will so that some of the burden is taken off of the family. The items in the following checklist indicate details that most often should be taken care of.

- Decide on time and place of funeral or memorial service(s).
- Make list of immediate family, close friends, and employer or business colleagues. Notify each by phone.
- If flowers are to be omitted, decide on appropriate memorial to which gifts may be made (such as a church, library, school, or charity).
- Write obituary. Include age, place of birth, cause of death, occupation, college degrees, memberships held, military service, outstanding work, list of survivors in immediate family. Give time and place of services. Report these details in person or by telephone to newspapers.
- Notify insurance companies.
- Arrange for members of family or close friends to take turns answering door or phone, keeping careful records of calls.
- Arrange appropriate child care.
- Coordinate the supply of food for the next several days.
- Consider special needs of the household, as for cleaning, etc., which might be done by friends.
- Arrange hospitality for visiting relatives.
- Select pallbearers and notify. (Avoid men with heart or back difficulties or make them honorary pallbearers.)
- Notify lawyer and executor.
- Arrange for disposition of flowers after funeral (as to a hospital or rest home).
- Prepare list of distant persons to be notified by letter and/or printed notice and decide which to send each.
- Prepare copy for printed notice if one is wanted.
- Prepare list of persons to receive acknowledgments of flowers, call, etc. Send appropriate acknowledgments. (Can be written notes, printed acknowledgments, or some of each.)
- Check carefully all life and casualty insurance and death benefits, including Social Security, credit union, trade union, fraternal, and military benefits. Check also on income available to survivors from these sources.

Source: Adapted from Ernest Morgan, *A Manual of Death Education and Simple Burial* (Burnsville, N.C.: The Celo Press, 1973), 30.

toward those who made us suffer: the dead person for leaving us, the physician for not saving the person, and God for not answering our prayers.

Hope and Affirmation of Reality. We can emerge from the experience of grief with a new vision of oursevses and our world. We might still feel diminished—after all, someone who was once a major part of our lives is no longer there—but we are whole again and able to continue with the business of living.

How To Comfort a Grieving Person

For many of us, comforting a grieving person is much like talking to a dying person: words fail us; we fear that what we say may be inadequate or may add to the person's pain. A simple "I'm sorry"—coupled with an arm around the shoulder or a firm grip of the hand—is usually appreciated. Encouraging the grieving person to deny reality ("He's not dead, he's just away") and insincere expressions of empathy ("I know how you feel") are rarely useful. Being available to listen, talk, reminisce, and assist with chores can be helpful, but well-meaning friends and relatives should avoid doing too much for the grieving person, since some maintenance of one's normal routine usually facilitates the grieving process. In some cases a wake is held, and this assists in the grieving process, for it brings family and friends together to remember the attributes of and good times with the person who has died.

Life and Death

Life and death are not two distinct states of being. Each is an integral part of the other, and to understand one we must understand both. Death education, therefore, is a process whereby we explore our relationship with life. We emerge from a study of death with a heightened awareness of our own mortality and, hopefully, with a new resolve to use our time on Earth creatively and wisely. The greatest loss is not that we will die but that so many of us go through life mechanically, unable to appreciate life's joys, sadness, and mysteries.

For all of its physical, emotional, and spiritual pain, dying presents a singular opportunity for growth and discovery. Like soldiers on the eve of battle, terminally ill people often experience a heightened sensory awareness, relishing sights, sounds, tastes, and smells that they had never before noticed. Freed from everyday chores, some dying people use their last months to put their affairs in order, enjoy the company of family and friends, heal shaky relationships, or visit places that they have always wanted to see. Indeed, all of us, by conquering our fear of death, become more able to take risks, try new experiences, and savor each moment of our lives.

Summary

Life and death are inseparable, and understanding death is necessary if we are to understand life. But death is a taboo subject, one that most people try to avoid talking about. Death education can play an important role in helping us understand our own fear of death and achieve a heightened awareness of the possibilities of life.

Despite the attempt to isolate death or present it in a superficial way, many people still have fears. They may fear death itself as the loss of everything—contact with others, identity, self—or the process of dying, with its pain and loneliness. They may also fear the results or consequences, either divine judgment or the unfinished business they are leaving behind. These fears can also be for others as well as for oneself.

With advances in medicine, it has become increasingly difficult to determine exactly when a person has died. The old criteria—the stopping of the heart and breathing—are not always applicable, and a new criterion—brain death, or irreversible coma—is now gaining acceptance in the medical community. However, there still exists conflict between some theological and biological definitions of death.

Terminally ill patients often go through five stages of coping with dying: denial and isolation, the refusal to believe that they are dying and to discuss it with others; anger, when the patient looks to someone to blame; bargaining, the attempt to postpone the inevitable; depression, when the dying person experiences remorse, anguish, and guilt; and acceptance, when the person accepts the inevitability of death and feels at peace. Most of us find it difficult to talk to dying persons, but they appreciate kindness and attention.

An alternative to the traditional care for the terminally ill is the hospice. The aim of the hospice is to provide a supportive, life-enhancing environment for dying individuals and their families.

Children have even greater problems than adults in facing death and need loving comfort and support. A child who has lost a loved one needs help in coming to terms with a confusing tangle of emotions.

Suicide remains a major problem. It is usually a response to helplessness, hopelessness, and loneliness. Researchers have discovered that some suicide attempts are really calls for help (although the person may actually succeed). The person threatening suicide should be referred to psychological counseling.

Funeral ceremonies are thought to be useful in helping survivors accept the reality and finality of death. Among the alternatives to burials are cremations. When death arrives, there are many things that have to be done, and a checklist is provided as a guide.

Death affects not only the person dying but those close to the person. Grief is the normal, healthy, and necessary process of adjustment to the loss of a loved one. Finally, the acceptance of death is an important factor in living a full life. It can make us see and appreciate the joys, sadness, and possibilities of life.

Review and Discussion

1. Name and describe the five stages of coping with dying according to Kübler-Ross.

2. What is the difference between active and passive euthanasia? How far do you think doctors should go in the attempt to keep people alive?

3. Name five types of fear associated with death. What can be done to overcome them?

4. Name six common grief patterns. Describe how you think people experiencing grief can be helped.

5. How can children be helped to face death?

6. What is a hospice? How is it different from a hospital?

7. What are the psychological symptoms of potential suicides?

8. Describe some images of death you have seen on television. Do you think that death is presented realistically?

9. How does acceptance of death as an inevitable part of life lead to a fuller life?

10. Do you think dying adults should be told of their impending death? Should children be told about their own impending death?

Further Reading

Aries, Philippe. *Western Attitudes Toward Death.* Baltimore: Johns Hopkins University Press, 1974.
A discussion of the changing attitudes toward death in Western culture from the Middle Ages to the present. (Paperback.)

Becker, Ernest. *The Denial of Death.* New York: The Free Press, 1973.
An analysis of human attempts to deny the reality of death. (Paperback.)

Bluebond-Langner, Myra. *The Private Worlds of Dying Children.* Princeton: Princeton University Press, 1980.
A study of children with leukemia, describing the stages children pass through as they learn they are dying. (Paperback.)

Gunther, John. *Death Be Not Proud: A Memoir.* New York: Harper & Row, 1965.
A writer's moving account of the death of his seventeen-year-old son. (Paperback.)

Kübler-Ross, Elisabeth (ed.). *Death: The Final Stage of Growth.* Englewood Cliffs, N.J.: Prentice-Hall, Inc., 1975.
How to live more fully with the knowledge that everyone must die. (Paperback.)

Schneidman, Edwin. *Death: Current Perspectives.* 2nd ed. Palo Alto, Calif.: Mayfield Publishing Co., 1983.
A comprehensive treatment of dying and death from contemporary personal, psychological, anthropological, and sociological perspectives. (Paperback.)

Stoddard, Sandol. *The Hospice Movement.* Briarcliff Manor, N.Y.: Stein & Day, 1977.
A sympathetic account of hospices based on the author's own experience working in a London hospice.

Tolstoy, Leo. *The Death of Ivan Ilyich.* New York: Bantam Books, 1981.
A short novel about a dying man who finally learns to accept his death. (Paperback.)

Part III

Drugs: Use and Abuse

Almost everyone, directly or indirectly, comes in contact every day with drug use or abuse. The three chapters that follow, "Alcohol," "Tobacco," and "Drugs," build a foundation that should help you better understand the types of drugs you may encounter, how they act in the body, and their impact on society. The drug scene is a varied one that includes licit and illicit drugs, street drugs, prescription drugs, over-the-counter drugs, drugs for pleasure, and drugs to ease pain. We are part of a drug culture in which public control and personal decisions, big business interests, and individual practices are all subjects of controversy. The one thing with which everyone agrees is that we all need more information.

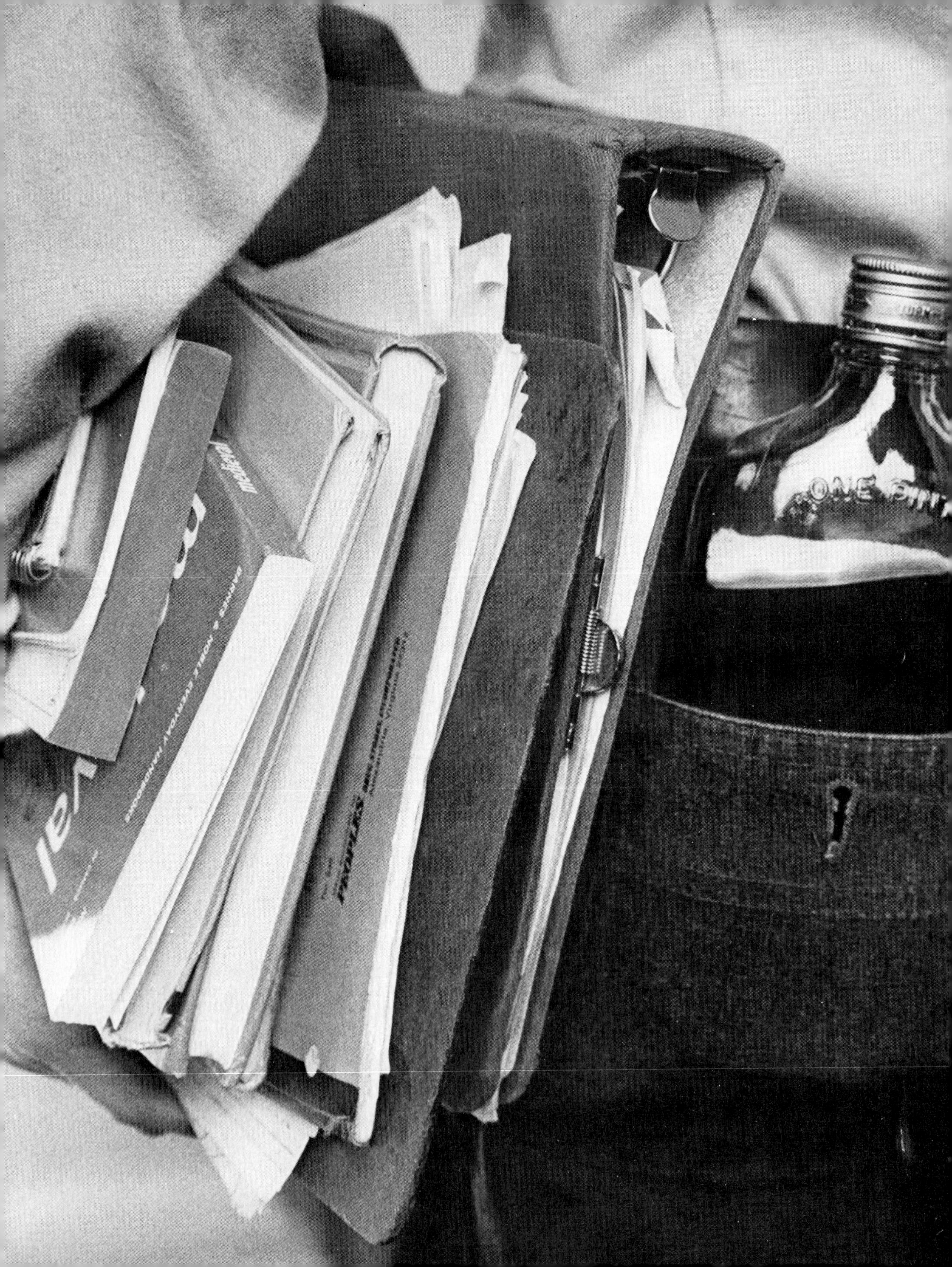
medieval
BARNES & NOBLE EVERYDAY HANDBOOKS

Chapter 9
Alcohol

KEY POINTS

- ☐ Alcohol is an important part of American life: seven out of ten Americans drink alcoholic beverages at least occasionally.
- ☐ A central nervous system depressant, alcohol produces symptoms that increase in severity as its level in the blood rises.
- ☐ Among the factors affecting the rate of the body's absorption of alcohol are the type of beverage consumed and how fast it is consumed; the drinker's body weight, general health, emotions, and expectations; and the condition of the drinker's stomach.
- ☐ Serious health problems that are related to chronic heavy drinking include cardiomyopathy (a disease of the heart muscle), ulcers, nutritional deficiencies, memory loss, lowered resistance to infection, and various cancers.
- ☐ Other alcohol-related problems include traffic and other accidents, dangerous reactions from the combination of alcohol with other drugs, the Fetal Alcohol Syndrome, and violent crime.
- ☐ Drinking responsibly means being aware of the effects of alcohol, exercising good judgment in determining when to stop drinking, and regulating one's activities while under the influence of alcohol.

IT IS OBVIOUS that alcohol commands a significant place in American society. In the media alcoholic beverages are often portrayed as an element that enhances the good life. Drinking seems to be a way to relax, to celebrate, or to have fun. In fact, for the majority of drinkers many of the relaxing and pleasant effects associated with alcohol can be enjoyed without problems or physical harm. However, for many others drinking causes tragedy. At least half of all deaths caused in traffic accidents are alcohol-related, and drinking has been involved in an enormous number of pedestrian fatalities and other deaths. For the 10 percent of all drinkers for whom alcohol is a problem, it causes a broad range of medical and social problems, including illnesses, the disruption of family life, and the inability to work efficiently.

College Students' Drinking Patterns

According to a study conducted by Toohey, Dezelsky, and Kush, alcohol is the drug of choice for college students today. The study showed that 70 to 90 percent of the students at some of the nation's largest universities presently drink to some extent and that the number of drinkers on college campuses is increasing. In addition, of the college

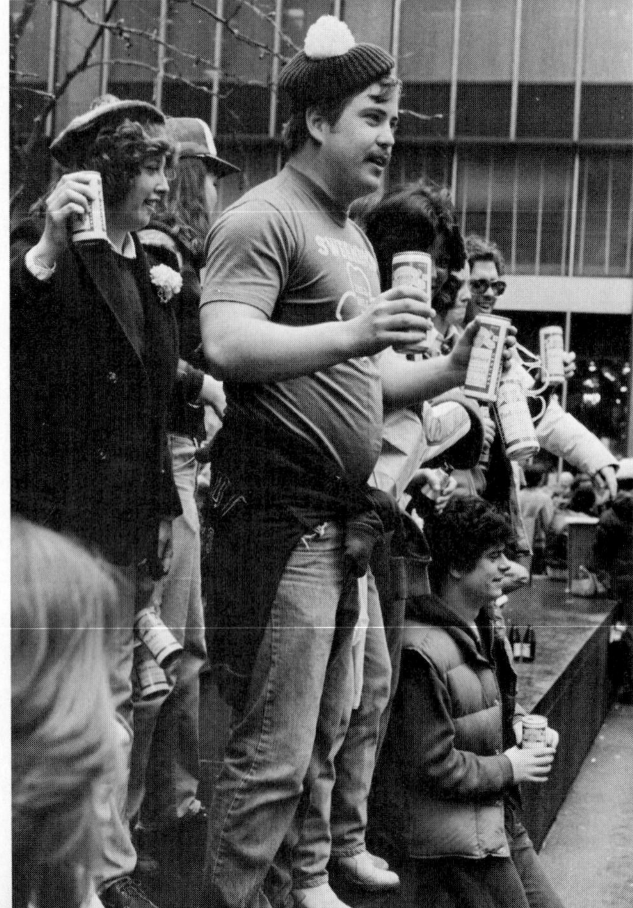

According to a recent study, it appears that most college students are "social drinkers." But even social drinking can become problem drinking if it interferes with the student's interpersonal relationships or academic life. (Photo by Marc P. Anderson)

population using alcohol, 82.7 percent consume alcohol on weekends and at parties while less than 2 percent used alcohol throughout the day.[1]

It appears that most college students are "social drinkers." This can be misleading since the patterns and amount of drinking within a social context vary from student to student. Certainly, to say that one is a "social drinker" might sound benign enough; but the frequency and amount of alcohol intake and behavior associated with drinking may be interrupting many realms of a student's life, including academic endeavors and social/interpersonal relationships. If this is occurring, the "social drinker" is now a problem drinker even in the context of drinking alcohol at parties or on weekends. (See the discussions at the end of chapter regarding problem drinking and responsible drinking.)

Measuring Alcohol Content

Ethanol, or ethyl alcohol, is the intoxicating ingredient in beers, wines, and distilled beverages. A natural substance, ethanol is a byproduct of the metabolism of yeasts. Though other kinds of alcohol are readily available, ethanol is the only one that can be completely broken down in the body. The end products of ethanol metabolism are carbon dioxide and water. However, alcohols like *methyl alcohol* (made from wood) or *isopropyl* (rubbing) *alcohol* not only may accumulate in the body but produce poisons when oxidized in the body. They therefore are very dangerous to drink.

Ethanol The intoxicating ingredient in alcoholic beverages.

Pure ethanol is a thin, lighter-than-water, colorless liquid with a strong, burning taste. The concentration of ethanol in intoxicating beverages varies widely, though beers contain the least, and **distilled or "hard" liquors** contain the most. In distilled spirits the amount of alcohol is expressed as "proof." In the United States, the percentage of alcohol in a beverage is half the proof number; 100 proof whiskey, for example, contains 50 percent alcohol by volume.

Distilled liquors "Hard" liquors.

How Much Alcohol Equals One Drink?

For purposes of discussion in this chapter, we need to know how much ethyl alcohol is in a **standard-sized drink** of beer, wine, or hard liquor. A standard serving of each of the following contains about one-half ounce of ethanol:

Standard-sized drink A serving containing ½ oz. ethanol (12 oz. beer, 4 oz. wine, 1 oz. hard liquor).

- 1 12-ounce can of beer
- 1 4-ounce glass of wine
- 1 "cocktail" or 1-ounce glass of distilled spirits

The serving size varies because beer generally contains 4 percent ethyl alcohol; wine usually contains 12 percent ethyl alcohol; while distilled, or "hard," liquors (cocktails) contain 40–50 percent alcohol, depending on the proof. If you multiply the percentage of alcohol by the number of ounces in a standard drink of beer, wine, or distilled spirits, you will come up with approximately one-half ounce of ethanol in each case. For practical purposes, remember that if the size of your drink varies in number of ounces or in percentage of alcohol, it no longer contains one-half ounce of ethanol.

Blood Alcohol Concentration (BAC)

Blood Alcohol Concentration (BAC) A measurement of alcohol absorbed by the body.

A central nervous system depressant, alcohol produces a series of symptoms that increase in severity as its level in the blood rises. The measurement of the **Blood Alcohol Concentration (BAC)** indicates how much alcohol the body has absorbed. Expressed as a percentage, the BAC is the ratio of alcohol present in the blood compared to total blood volume. Since the amount of alcohol excreted in the breath and urine is in exactly the same proportion as the concentration of alcohol in the blood, the BAC can be determined in three ways: by analyzing samples of the breath, blood, or urine. The easiest test to determine Blood Alcohol Concentration is the breathalyzer test. In most states a BAC of 0.1 percent (ten units of alcohol per ten thousand units of blood) has been established as the legal level of intoxication, but human brain functions are altered at even lower concentrations.

The Body's Response to Alcohol

Factors Affecting Alcohol Absorption

Because the body is able to metabolize alcohol and clear itself of its effects, the extent to which drinking affects an individual is determined in part by how much is ingested and how quickly the alcohol is absorbed into the bloodstream. The body's absorption of alcohol is affected by the type of drink, the way in which it is consumed, and the physical and psychological characteristics of the drinker.

Type of Beverage

Because there are other nutrients present in wine and beer, the alcohol in these beverages is absorbed more slowly than the same amount of alcohol in distilled liquor. When alcohol is served as a mixed drink with fruit juice, sugar, syrup, or water, its absorption is delayed. The presence of carbonation in a drink, however, increases the rate at which alcohol is absorbed because carbon dioxide relaxes the muscle that controls the flow of foods into the small intestine, where alcohol is absorbed more quickly than in the stomach.

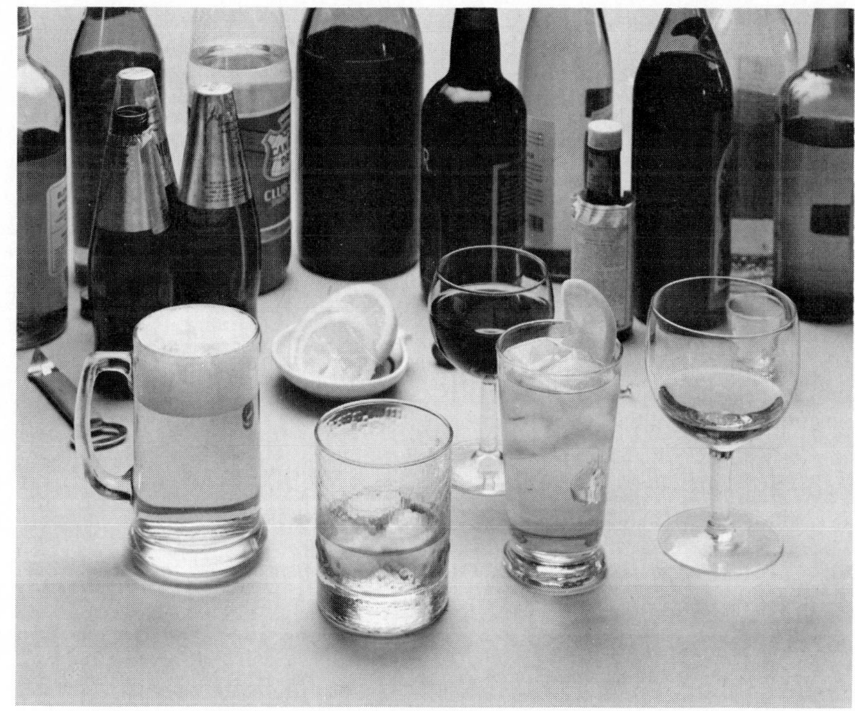

Among other factors, setting may determine whether "hard" liquor, beer, or wine will be consumed. (Photo by Don Renner/Photo Trends)

The greater its concentration in a beverage, the more rapidly alcohol is absorbed — up to a limit of about 40 percent (80 proof). Beyond this concentration, alcohol tends to be absorbed more slowly.

The Drinker's Body Weight

Because alcohol depresses the central nervous system to the extent that it is concentrated in the blood and body fluids, the same amount of alcohol will have different impact on people of different sizes and weights. Table 9–1 shows the effect of body weight on BAC.

The Drinking Rate

About one-third ounce of pure alcohol — somewhat less than the amount contained in a standard mixed drink — can be metabolized by the average person in about an hour. If someone were to sip a drink containing that concentration of alcohol over an hour's time, the individual would be unlikely to feel its effects. But the same drink consumed quickly would probably cause the first symptoms of intoxication, and these symptoms might take approximately an hour to wear off. Variations in metabolic rate and in body chemistry may also affect a drinker's reaction to alcohol.

Some people experience variations in their own responses to alcohol. After illness or when they are very tired, for example, alcohol may affect them more quickly and more noticeably.

Table 9-1 **BAC by Sex and Weight**

Ethyl alcohol (ounces)	Beverage intake (in one hour)	Blood alcohol concentration (percentages)					
		Female (100 lb)	**Male (100 lb)**	**Female (150 lb)**	**Male (150 lb)**	**Female (200 lb)**	**Male (200 lb)**
½	1 cocktail 1 glass wine 1 can beer	0.045	0.037	0.03	0.025	0.022	0.019
1	2 cocktails 2 glasses wine 2 cans beer	0.090	0.075	0.06	0.050	0.045	0.037
2	4 cocktails 4 glasses wine 4 cans beer	0.180	0.150	0.12	0.100	0.090	0.070
3	6 cocktails 6 glasses wine 6 cans beer	0.270	0.220	0.18	0.150	0.130	0.110
4	8 cocktails 8 glasses wine 8 cans beer	0.360	0.300	0.24	0.200	0.180	0.150
5	10 cocktails 10 glasses wine 10 cans beer	0.450	0.370	0.30	0.250	0.220	0.180

Source: Adapted from Ray, Oakley. *Drugs, Society and Human Behavior,* 3rd ed. (St. Louis, Mo.: C. V. Mosby Co., 1983), 168.

Food in the Drinker's Stomach

Taken on an empty stomach, alcohol is absorbed quickly, but if consumed with food or shortly after eating, it is absorbed more slowly. The chemical compositions of foods affect the rates at which they are digested. Carbohydrate foods break down relatively quickly; proteins and fats take longer. Thus, if a person eats foods containing proteins and fats before or during drinking, the rate at which alcohol enters the bloodstream will be slowed considerably.

Irritation of the Stomach

Sometimes alcohol irritates the stomach lining and causes the pylorus, the sphincter muscle between the stomach and the small intestine, to contract. This causes alcohol to remain in the stomach, where its absorption is slower than in the small intestine.

The Drinker's Emotional State

If someone is tense or upset and has a drink, the effect of the alcohol is often experienced more quickly than usual. This is because emotions like fear, anxiety, or anger affect the involuntary nervous system, which opens the pyloric valve and allows alcohol to pass into the small intestine.

Psychological and Cultural Factors

Many psychological and cultural factors seem to influence the extent to which alcohol may affect an individual. Someone celebrating with a friend might become dizzy and euphoric from a single drink. That same person at a business meeting where drinks are served might not show any reaction at all to the same quantity of alcohol. The settings and situations in which people drink, their expectations of how alcohol will affect them, their previous drinking experiences, and the customs and attitudes of their culture all influence the way they react to specific concentrations of alcohol in the blood.

Sometimes a person with little or no drinking experience will have unpleasant or extreme reactions to even moderate amounts of alcohol. This may happen because the drinker is unfamiliar with the sensations and changes in perception that alcohol produces. First-time users may become frightened or overreact because the experience is new, or they may have strong reactions because they believe this is the appropriate way to behave. As might be expected, experienced drinkers seem to adapt to the effects of alcohol. When the situation demands it, they can behave as if they are sober, even when relatively high concentrations of alcohol appear in the blood. However, these behavioral characteristics are actually masking significant changes in reaction time and other psychomotor functions. Even people with low BAC, due to inexperience and other factors can behave in a manner normally seen in people with high BAC. The responsible drinker will understand this factor and employ his or her knowledge in alcohol-related decisions, especially in deciding whether or not to drive an automobile.

Effects on Body Organs

Once alcohol is ingested and absorbed, literally every body organ will be affected, some more so than others. The body organs most affected by alcohol intake include the brain, heart, gastrointestinal tract, and liver.

The Brain

Even in small quantities alcohol disrupts the brain's ability to work. Most people are affected by even one drink. The three main areas of the brain affected by alcohol are the cerebral cortex, cerebellum, and the brain stem, or medulla.

Figure 9 – 1 shows the effects on behavior of varying BAC levels. As can be seen in the figure, when the amount of alcohol in the blood is as low as .05 percent (5 parts of alcohol per 10,000 parts of blood), a drinker experiences a sense of warmth, mild euphoria, and general well-being. This is primarily due to the effect of alcohol on the cerebral cortex.

As the BAC rises, a drinker's inhibitions and social restraints are

Amount of Beverage Consumed in one Hour	Approximate Concentration of Alcohol in the Blood	Brain Areas Affected	Effects on Behavior
2 beers 2 glasses of wine 2 cocktails	0.05%	Cerebral cortex— areas affecting judgment and controlling inhibitions	Sense of warmth, mild euphoria, sense of well-being
4 beers 4 glasses of wine 4 cocktails	0.1%	Cerebral cortex, cerebellum— areas controlling skilled physical activity	Noticeably less inhibition; slight staggering; some difficulty in speaking and dressing
8 beers 8 glasses of wine 8 cocktails	0.2%	Cerebral cortex, cerebellum— all areas concerned with physical activity, and areas controlling emotions	Cannot dress or walk without help; easily made angry or sad
12 beers 12 glasses of wine 12 cocktails	0.3%	Cerebral cortex, cerebellum— some of the areas concerned with perception	Stupor; little comprehension of what is seen or heard
16 beers 16 glasses of wine 16 cocktails	0.45%	Cerebral cortex, cerebellum, medulla— all areas concerned with perception	Coma, complete unconsciousness; automatic responses occur more slowly
24 beers 24 glasses of wine 24 cocktails	0.6%	Cerebral cortex, cerebellum, medulla— areas regulating breathing and heartbeat	Death

Figure 9-1. Effects of Alcohol Consumption on Brain Areas and Behavior.

loosened. At .2 percent there is noticeably less inhibition, a slight staggering, and some difficulty in speaking and dressing. At this BAC not only is the cerebral cortex affected but also the cerebellum. In most states, law enforcement officials feel that a driver with a .1 percent BAC is driving while intoxicated.

The cerebellum is further affected when BAC levels reach .3 percent. The individual with this BAC has little comprehension of what is seen or heard. At this point, the drinker is noticeably extremely drunk, or intoxicated. At a BAC .4 percent the drinker is in a coma, and automatic responses occur much more slowly. If the BAC rises to .6 percent the individual will die due to respiratory failure caused by the depressant effect of alcohol on the medulla.

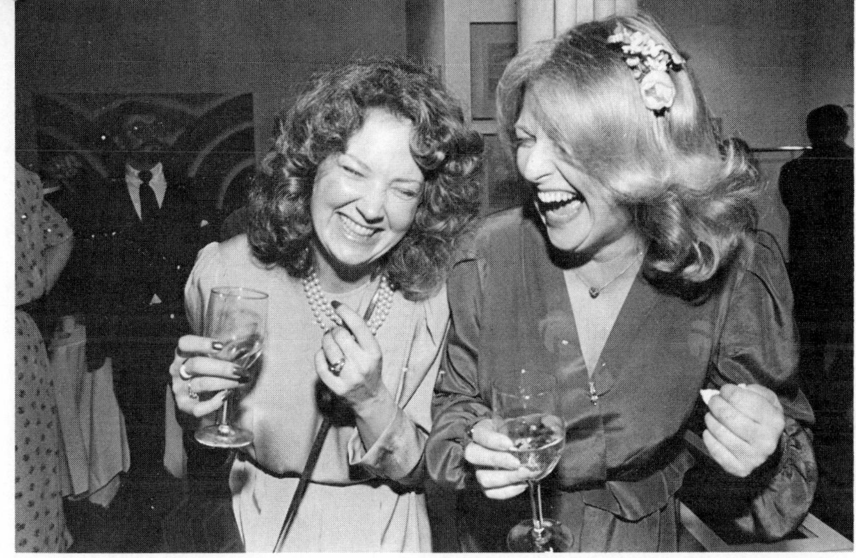

Even one drink will affect the brain's functioning, causing various behavioral changes such as lowering of inhibitions and social restraints. (Photo © Abigail Heyman/Archive Pictures, Inc.)

It should be pointed out that most individuals will "pass out" before the BAC rises to a dangerous level. However, don't rely on this: if a large enough quantity of alcohol is consumed just before a person loses consciousness, alcohol levels in the blood may continue to rise enough to depress the respiratory center of the brain.

Before reading about the effects of alcohol on other body organs, why not complete Self-Assessment Exercise 9.1 in order to determine your "Alcohol Quotient."

The Heart

Both alcohol and acetaldehyde affect the heart muscle in ways that may eventually damage it. Some people experience palpitations and other irregularities in heartbeat during or after acute intoxication. Doctors often call this the "holiday heart syndrome" because it commonly appears around holidays, times often associated with heavy drinking.

Cardiomyopathy, a condition that is a common cause of death of alcoholics, seems to be caused by the effects of alcohol or acetaldehyde on the myocardium, or middle layer of muscles in the heart walls. The affected heart becomes enlarged and swollen and its rhythm becomes disturbed, and the person's breathing becomes labored and noisy.

However, the relationship of alcohol consumption to other forms of cardiovascular disease is unclear. Some research suggests that heavy drinkers run an increased risk of developing coronary artery disease, whereas other studies show no relationship between drinking and heart disease. Yet others have shown a correlation between moderate drinking (no more than 2½ ounces of ethanol daily) and a decrease in the incidence of myocardial infarction and coronary artery disease.[2]

The Gastrointestinal Tract

Strong solutions of alcohol (40 percent and more) can damage the tissues of both esophagus and stomach by irritating them. Consump-

SELF-ASSESSMENT EXERCISE 9.1

Test Your AQ

To test your alcohol quotient (AQ), answer the following true-false questions. Check your answers below.

1. ______ Most alcoholics are skid row bums.
2. ______ Drinking black coffee, taking a cold shower, and running around the block are good ways to sober up.
3. ______ Heavy drinking shortens your life.
4. ______ You are less likely to become an alcoholic if you only drink beer.
5. ______ The more you drink, the better sex is.
6. ______ If you are depressed, a drink may cheer you up.
7. ______ More men than women are alcoholics.
8. ______ If parents drink moderately, the odds are that their children will drink moderately, too.
9. ______ A recovered alcoholic can drink socially again.
10. ______ Most alcoholics are middle-aged or older.
11. ______ You are not an alcoholic unless you have six or more drinks a day.
12. ______ The drunk-tank does not cure alcoholics.
13. ______ Alcohol is a stimulant.
14. ______ If you can hold your liquor, you will never become an alcoholic.
15. ______ People get drunk, hungover, or sick from switching drinks.
16. ______ People are friendlier when they are drunk.
17. ______ It is rude to refuse a drink.
18. ______ Alcohol warms you up.
19. ______ Nothing can be done about alcoholism unless the alcoholic wants to stop drinking.
20. ______ It is hopeless to treat alcoholism. A patient may reform for a while but will always slip back.
21. ______ Alcohol itself is the only cause of alcoholism. If it were unavailable, there would be no alcoholism.
22. ______ Only "psychological cripples" become problem drinkers and develop into alcoholics.

Answers to Test Your AQ

1. False. Only 3 to 5 percent of alcoholics in the United States are in the "skid row" category.
2. False. Coffee, a stimulant, makes a drunk person feel more alert and capable, but it does not improve his judgment or reaction time. Neither a cold shower nor running will speed up metabolism of alcohol in the body.
3. True. Chronic, heavy drinkers do not live as long as moderate drinkers or nondrinkers.
4. False. A person is as likely to become an alcoholic by drinking beer as by drinking any alcoholic beverage, because it is the alcohol in the drink that is addicting.
5. False. Sexual activity is more difficult to perform after heavy drinking.

6. True. However, the anxiety-relieving effect of alcohol lasts for only a couple of hours. Then alcohol tends to make a person feel more anxious for up to eighteen hours.

7. True. However, more women are alcoholics than you might think. Some authorities believe that nearly half the alcoholic population in the U.S. is female.

8. True. However, the highest incidence of alcoholism occurs among offspring of parents who were either alcoholics or nondrinkers.

9. False. Most experts believe that the alcoholic who attempts social drinking will almost certainly return to uncontrolled drinking.

10. True. Most alcoholics are between thirty and fifty-five, but the highest proportion of problem drinkers is among men in their early twenties.

11. False. There is no simple rule. Most experts feel that how much one drinks is not as significant as why, how, and when one drinks.

12. True. Alcoholism is an illness. We do not throw people in jail for having a heart attack or an epileptic seizure. Why the alcoholic?

13. False. Physiological, alcohol is a depressant. Alcohol may help release inhibitions against more active behaviors, but this is a temporary psychological state that passes as the nervous system becomes depressed.

14. False. Those people who appear to "hold their liquor" need to exercise special caution because they may drink indiscriminately and develop alcohol dependency.

15. False. Switching drinks, as from cocktails to beer, makes little difference. It is the *amount* of alcohol, not the source, that is related to drunkenness, illness, and hangovers.

16. True. However, they are also more depressed, more hostile, more brutal, and more suicidal. One-half of all murders and one-third of all suicides involve the use of alcohol.

17. False. Refusing a drink is no more rude than refusing a piece of pie. What is rude is trying to push a drink on someone who does not want it or should not have it.

18. False. A feeling of warmth sometimes occurs with drinking as a result of increased blood flow in the capillaries of the skin. Actually, the body loses heat and its temperature drops.

19. False. A sudden and absolute break from alcohol is often both a prerequisite and a goal of treatment, even if imposed from outside. During such periods of sobriety, the alcoholic can build his capability for control by understanding why he drinks and learning alternatives to drinking.

20. False. We do not consider treatment of tuberculosis or heart disease hopeless because the patient has recurrences. An individual with any chronic disease, including alcoholism, needs treatment.

21. False. The majority of people who use alcohol do not become alcoholics.

22. False. This is a myth. "Normal, well-adjusted" people are not immune to alcoholism.

Adapted from *Test Your Alcohol Quotient* (Washington, D.C.: Department of Health, Education, and Welfare, 1975); from Brent Q. Hafen, *Alcohol: The Crutch that Cripples* (St. Paul: West, 1977), 80–82; and from *Drinking Myths,* a publication of Operation Threshold by the Jaycees Foundation.

tion of extremely large amounts of alcohol can result in inflammation and bleeding lesions of the stomach, though the mechanisms of this damage are not well understood. Stomach and intestinal ulcers are common among chronic drinkers. Alcohol also decreases the peristaltic movements of the small intestine so that partially digested food passes more quickly through the intestinal tract. Absorption of nutrients seems to be reduced as well, which contributes to the malnutrition common among alcoholics.

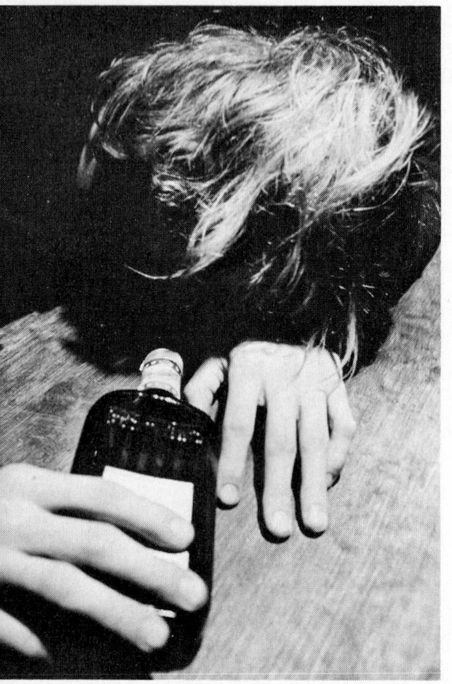

Consuming large enough quantities of alcohol will inevitably lead to death. However, the life-sustaining function in an individual will generally cause the individual to pass out before reaching that point. (Photo © Michael D. Sullivan)

The Liver

Although the liver can repair occasional damage to itself, regular heavy drinking can have lasting effect on it, and about 75 percent of all heavy drinkers experience some liver damage. Susceptibility to liver degeneration seems to be influenced by genetic and other factors. Though the exact role of drinking in liver damage is unclear, such damage seems to be produced by nutritional disturbances rather than from the direct action of alcohol or acetaldehyde on the liver itself.

The damage begins when fats accumulate in the liver, producing a condition known as fatty liver. If a person continues to drink large amounts of alcohol over a long period of time, the liver becomes inflamed, enlarged, and tender to the touch—a condition called alcoholic hepatitis. If drinking continues, the size and shape of the liver change, and liver functions become measurably impaired. As the disease advances, cells in the liver are destroyed and the most serious of liver conditions—cirrhosis—develops, in which the liver is scarred by fibrous tissue, and the drinker suffers chronic indigestion, nausea, and abdominal pain. Although at this stage damage to the liver cannot be reversed, its progress can be slowed if drinking stops and the nutritional inadequacies of the diet are corrected. However, continuing to drink with such a badly weakened liver can lead to death.

Physical Effects of Chronic Alcohol Abuse

Heavy use of alcohol over long periods of time can produce a variety of other problems, many of which are caused directly or indirectly by nutritional deficiencies produced when the empty calories of alcohol regularly replace more nutritious foods. Furthermore, drinking large quantities of alcohol usually depresses a person's appetite for other foods. For example, alcoholics may often drink a pint of whiskey a day. This amount of liquor provides about 1,200 calories, perhaps half the drinker's daily caloric needs but without the proteins, vitamins, or minerals that are needed for healthy body functioning.

Blackout Temporary amnesia due to drinking.

Because alcohol interferes with the transmission of nerve impulses in the brain, chronic drinking can cause significant losses of memory. An extreme example of this is the so-called **blackout,** an episode of heavy drinking during which the drinker, usually an alcoholic, remains conscious but cannot remember anything later. Material learned when a person is sober is harder to recall when alcohol is present in the brain tissues, and information learned either sober or under the influence of alcohol may be most easily recalled in the condition in which it was learned. Even when they are sober, chronic drinkers and alcoholics show serious impairment in certain thinking skills, including the ability to shift from one concept to another and to perceive fine details. One study suggests that even light or moderate drinking may reduce certain thinking capacities.[3]

Chronic drinkers show a lowered resistance to a variety of infections and disease conditions, including pneumonia. The mechanism by which alcohol depresses certain immune systems in the body is unclear, but some loss of immunity may be the result of alcohol altering the body's metabolism of minerals like magnesium, calcium, zinc, and iron. Alcohol also seems to inhibit the mobilization of white blood cells, one of the body's major defenses against infection.

Alcohol consumption is clearly related to the development of cancer in certain areas of the body. Heavy drinkers suffer more cancers of the mouth, pharynx, larynx, esophagus, liver, and lungs than nondrinkers. And because distilled liquors are especially irritating to the mouth and esophagus they tend to be involved in upper gastrointestinal tract cancers.

A person who both smokes and drinks runs an increased risk of developing cancer of the upper digestive or respiratory tracts. And clearly, using both alcohol and tobacco increases the risk of certain types of cancer synergistically (that is, to a greater extent than would be indicated by simply adding the separate risk factors for the two substances).

Alcohol-Related Problems

Drinking and Driving

Alcohol plays a role in about half of the 60,000 highway deaths each year. According to annual statistical estimates from the National Highway and Traffic Safety Association (NHTSA), 45 to 75 percent of the drivers at fault in fatal crashes are impaired by alcohol. Their blood alcohol levels are at or above the .10 percent legal level of intoxication.[4] In contrast, studies of drivers not at fault in fatal crashes indicate that only 7 to 12 percent have such high blood alcohol concentrations.

A person who is found with a BAC of .10 or above can be legally classified as driving under the influence (DUI) or driving while intoxicated (DWI). It is easy to see that as the blood alcohol level rises, so does the potential for a highway accident. A driver with BAC of .10 is seven times more likely to have a highway accident than a driver who has not been drinking. A driver with a BAC of .15 is 25 times more likely to have an accident. Figure 9–2 shows the relationship between the number of drinks consumed and driving ability.

MADD, SADD, and Other Organizations

As a response to the large number of accidents involving drunk drivers — and especially those accidents involving innocent children — a special California-based organization was developed known as Mothers Against Drunk Drivers (MADD). MADD now has over 80

Figure 9-2. How Alcohol Impairs Driving Ability. (Source: "Alcohol in Perspective," *Consumer Reports* 48 [July 1983]:353.)

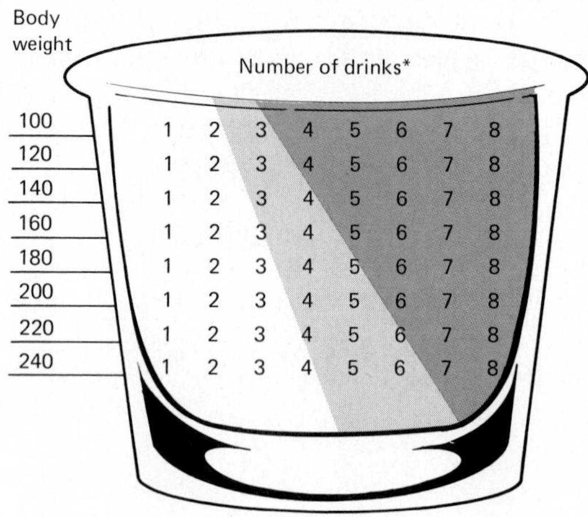

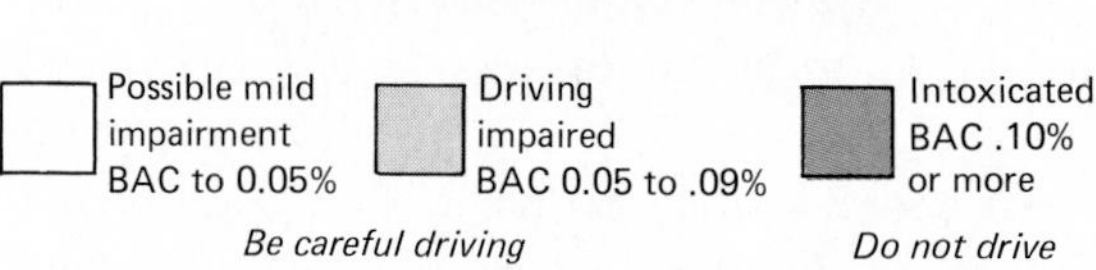

Be careful driving *Do not drive*

*In a 2-hr. period. Each drink, about 0.5 oz. alcohol: 1½ oz. 80-proof liquor, 12 oz. beer, 5 oz. table wine, or 3 oz. sherry (fortified wine).

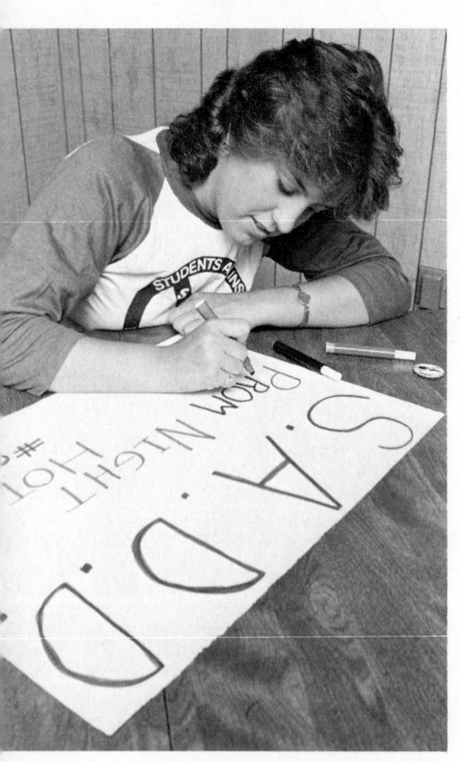

Organizations across the country, such as MADD (Mothers Against Drunk Drivers) and SADD (Students Against Drunk Drivers), are fighting to keep drunk drivers off the roads. (Photo © Frank Siteman 1983/The Picture Cube)

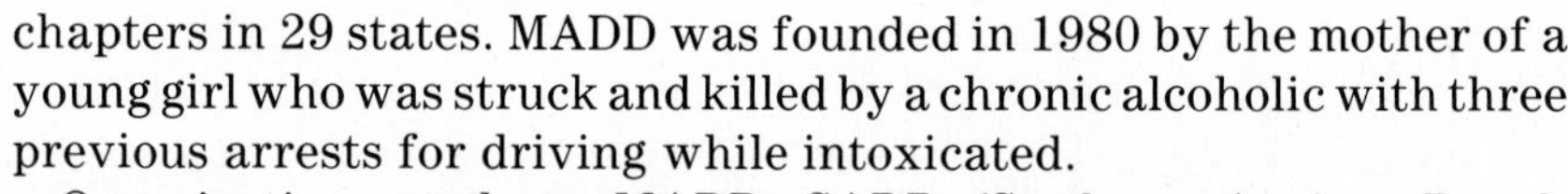

chapters in 29 states. MADD was founded in 1980 by the mother of a young girl who was struck and killed by a chronic alcoholic with three previous arrests for driving while intoxicated.

Organizations such as MADD, SADD (Students Against Drunk Drivers), and RID (Remove Intoxicated Drivers) are growing and becoming a strong political force for stiffer punishment of the drunk driver involved in an accident. Among the results of such organizational efforts has been the raising of the drinking age in many states to 21 years of age or in some cases changing the drinking age back to 21 years of age. Part of this was due to federal mandates that federal highway funds would be withheld from states having a drinking age below age 21.

There is no doubt that driving while intoxicated is a major societal problem. Therefore, it is important for one's own safety, as well as the safety of others, that the individual who makes a decision to drink be a responsible drinker.

Other Kinds of Accidents

Alcohol plays a major role in many of the accidents people have at home, at work, and at play. Heavy drinkers sustain more accidental injuries than nondrinkers. In a national survey, over four times as many regular drinkers as nondrinkers reported two or more accidents during the preceding year.[5] Not only is alcohol use often part of the cause of fires in homes and public buildings, but the effects of alcohol prevent people from responding quickly and saving themselves from severe burn injuries or even death.

Alcohol may be involved in about 7 out of 10 drownings. In addition to suffering the obvious physical impairments associated with drinking, swimmers who are intoxicated may take more risks than when sober. Also, they may be unaware of fatigue or cold that normally would serve as a signal for them to get out of the water.

Some serious birth defects may result when pregnant women persist in drinking alcoholic beverages. (Photo © Erika Stone 1984)

Drug Interaction

Whether the drugs are over-the-counter items, medications prescribed by a physician, or illicit substances, the combination of alcohol with other drugs may be dangerous. In most cases, the adverse effects of such combinations are accidental; however, some people experiment with a variety of drug combinations in order to achieve new or more intense effects.

The most dangerous drug-alcohol combinations—some of which can be lethal—are those that increase the effects of both agents. Such is the case with barbiturates, major tranquilizers, and the opiates. (See Chapter 11 for more details.) Milder tranquilizers combined with alcohol can produce unexpected levels of drowsiness, visual impairment, and reduced motor coordination as can over-the-counter antihistamines taken with alcohol.

Fetal Alcohol Syndrome

According to the National Institute on Alcohol Abuse and Alcoholism, one out of every 2,000 infants is born with birth defects caused by alcohol. **Fetal Alcohol Syndrome (FAS),** which was recognized as a disease in 1973, is a unique pattern of physical characteristics and mental impairments that may or may not appear fully developed in every FAS child. In some children there are only a few elements of the syndrome apparent; in others, certain aspects of the syndrome are severe while others are only minimally observable. (See Table 9-2 for a list of FAS characteristics.)

Fetal Alcohol Syndrome Mental and physical abnormalities of an infant due to maternal intake of alcohol during pregnancy.

Table 9-2 Fetal Alcohol Syndrome Characteristics

Fetal Alcohol Syndrome Characteristics
Growth deficiencies
Smaller head circumference
Delay in intellectual development
Possible mental deficiencies
Deformities of the facial bones, including narrow eye slits, flattened upper lips, underdeveloped mid-face
Abnormalities of the fingers or toes
Heart and brain defects

Some studies indicate that heavy drinking during the early months of pregnancy, or even prior to conception, may influence the development of the fetus; other studies have implicated moderate or even light use of alcohol by expectant mothers.[6] Furthermore, alcohol seems to contribute in some cases to the failure to become pregnant or to sustain pregnancy.

Alcohol and Crime

Although accurate information on how frequently alcohol is a factor in crimes is not available, its consumption seems to be a factor in many robberies, rapes, assaults, homicides, and suicides. In most violent crimes in which alcohol is involved, both the offender and the victim have been drinking.

Studies indicate that drinking often plays a part in violence within families, including both child and spouse abuse. In a large study on child abuse in the United States, researchers found that close to 40 percent of the parents who abused children had histories of problem drinking. Over half the violent husbands who were the subjects of another study had been problem drinkers or alcoholics.[7]

Problem Drinking

In general, problem drinking produces negative effects on the health and well-being of the drinker and on the people involved with the drinker. Problem drinkers become intoxicated frequently, sometimes to the point of blackout, and may behave in ways that normally would embarrass them. They may go to work or drive while under the influence of alcohol. Some problem drinkers get into trouble with the police or sustain injuries while they are intoxicated. A person who drinks primarily to get drunk is more likely to become a problem drinker than others.

Because 90 percent of the people who drink do not become alcoholics or problem drinkers, alcohol alone is not the cause of alcoholism. Alcoholics are people who chronically drink too much and cannot control how much they drink. Alcoholics often use alcohol in an effort to relieve anxiety or emotional pain, and many believe their lives are coming apart. The fact that alcohol induces tolerance and physical dependence undoubtedly influences its abuse. After long periods of heavy drinking, the amount of alcohol consumed no longer produces the desired effect and the drinker is thus inclined to increase the dosage. If you are concerned that you might have a drinking problem, complete Self-Assessment Exercise 9.2, "Do You Have a Drinking Problem?"

SELF-ASSESSMENT EXERCISE 9.2

Do You Have a Drinking Problem?

It isn't always easy to spot a drinking problem, especially in yourself. The problem cannot be identified by determining how many drinks you have each day, how many years you have been drinking, or how much you can hold. It is also hard to draw precise lines between social drinking, problem drinking, and alcoholism. The following test is designed to point up some specific signs that may indicate a drinking problem before the severe symptoms of alcoholism are reached.

Instructions. Check the appropriate box.

Yes	No	
☐	☐	1. Do you think about drinking often?
☐	☐	2. Do you drink more now than you used to?
☐	☐	3. Do you sometimes gulp your drinks?
☐	☐	4. Do you often take a drink to help you relax?
☐	☐	5. Do you drink often when you are alone?
☐	☐	6. Do you sometimes forget what happened while you were drinking?
☐	☐	7. Do you keep a bottle hidden somewhere—at home or perhaps at work—for a possible quick pick-me-up?
☐	☐	8. Do you need a drink to have fun?
☐	☐	9. Do you ever just start drinking without really thinking about it?
☐	☐	10. Do you drink in the morning to relieve a hangover?

Interpretation. If any of these symptoms apply to you—and especially if you have answered yes to four or more questions—you may well have an alcohol problem. This is a time to be absolutely honest with yourself. Sometimes only *you* can know how seriously alcohol is affecting your life. Often others close to you can recognize your problem as well, but they may be embarrassed to bring it up. If they do, you have all the more reason to take a hard look at what drinking may be doing to you.

Source: National Institute on Alcohol Abuse and Alcoholism.

Alcoholism

Alcoholic One who chronically drinks excessively and uncontrollably.

Many people have a specific stereotype of an **alcoholic,** or someone who is addicted to alcohol. For example, the word *alcoholic* conjures up such a mental picture as that of a "skid row" bum who carries a bottle of liquor in a brown paper bag. Since alcohol is a depressant and is so easily available and socially accepted, one can easily become dependent upon the substance. However, it is important to point out that alcoholics exist in all races, religions, and socioeconomic levels and are not confined to any stereotype.

Jellinek model Schema describing four phases of developing alcoholism.

Alcoholism is not a disease that develops quickly. Usually there are a series of progressive phases one passes through before becoming addicted to alcohol. Many different theories of alcoholism exist, and each theory usually has a listing of characteristics displayed in potential alcoholics. One of the most operational models, although it does have some limitations, is that developed by E. M. Jellinek. According to the **Jellinek model,** complete alcohol addiction results only after an individual passes through a prealcoholic phase, an early alcoholic phase, a "true" alcoholic phase, and complete addiction. The Jellinek model is pictured in Figure 9–3.

The Jellinek Model

The *prealcoholic phase* is marked by what is termed socioculturally controlled drinking, which can be interpreted simply as a drink with dinner or a drink in a social situation. Other characteristics of the

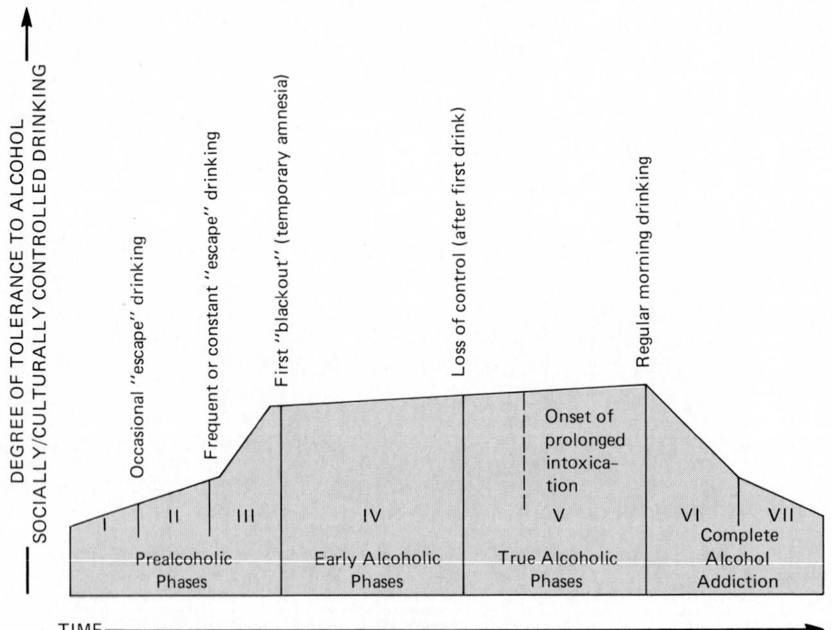

Figure 9–3. Phases of Alcoholism. (Source: Kenneth H. Jones, Louis W. Shainberg, and Curtis O. Byer, "The Phases of Alcoholism," from Instructor's Manual and Transparency Masters to *Health Science,* 5th ed. Copyright © 1985 by Harper & Row Publishers, Inc. Reprinted by permission of Harper & Row Publishers, Inc.)

prealcoholic phase include occasional escape drinking and significant episodes of escape drinking. During this time a tolerance to alcohol is developing.

The prealcoholic phase ends when the individual experiences the first **blackout,** temporary amnesia. Other characteristics of the *early alcoholic phase* include drinking secretly, being preoccupied with alcohol, having guilt feelings about drinking, rationalizing drinking behavior, and experiencing persistent remorse.

The *true alcoholic phase* is characterized by a loss of control after the first drink. In addition, the individual cannot control drinking behavior even after a moderate amount is consumed. All behavior of the individual is alcohol centered, and he or she begins to neglect proper nutrition. Usually a decrease in sexual drive begins to appear. It is often during this alcoholic phase that other persons, especially family, begin to realize that the individual has a "drinking problem."

The *complete alcohol addiction phase* is characterized by regular morning drinking, intoxication during the working hours, and mental impairment or a drug-induced psychosis. The individual can be officially classified as an alcoholic, and it is obvious that the person needs help.

A Word of Caution

The Jellinek model is useful in providing insight into a likely pattern of developing alcoholism. However, a word of caution is necessary. These phases do not apply to each and every person, nor can we classify an individual based on only a few observations of their drinking behavior. For example, a college student may have a blackout after one drinking experience. This would certainly not put him or her in the early alcoholic phase. What is necessary is that we base any ideas regarding alcoholism on patterns of behavior, not on one-time observations—and even then, only a medical professional has the qualifications to make a diagnosis of alcoholism.

Treatment for Alcoholism

There are many different kinds of services and treatment programs available to alcoholics and their families, and the manner in which alcoholics seek treatment varies from individual to individual. Some begin treatment during a period of sobriety, others during the sickness following a binge of heavy drinking, and still others during acute intoxication. Withdrawal from alcohol must be handled carefully, and medical management is often necessary.

Detoxification

A body that is continually exposed to ethanol adjusts itself so that the presence of the substance becomes an essential part of the way it functions. Abrupt withdrawal causes chronic drinkers to become ill.

The symptoms of withdrawal are caused by the body's inability to revert quickly to normal functioning without alcohol. Severe forms, called *delirium tremens,* involve hallucinations and violent shaking. Pharmaceutical drugs can, therefore, play an important part in detoxification and withdrawal. In some cases drugs that produce unpleasant reactions to alcohol are used during long-term treatment programs.

Psychotherapy and Counseling

Because the behavioral patterns of alcoholics vary tremendously, the effectiveness of different treatments seems to depend on an individual's personality and concept of alcoholism and on the support systems of family members, friends, and coworkers that are available. For some people *behavior modification therapies* seem effective. These may use a variety of techniques, including aversion experiences, assertiveness training, biofeedback, and relaxation techniques, to help alcoholics change their drinking behavior and their previous methods of coping with stress. For some alcoholics *hospital treatment* and a comprehensive follow-through program seem helpful. Hospitalization is especially appropriate for alcoholics with psychiatric disorders, like depression, or medical or surgical problems that require hospital care. Variations in treatment programs have made comparing their rates of success very difficult; nonetheless, treatment for alcoholism seems to help many people: the improvement rate for alcoholics ranges from 30 percent to 70 percent, depending upon how rehabilitation is defined.

Alcoholics Anonymous

Alcoholics Anonymous (AA) Alcoholic rehabilitation program for those willing to be helped.

Alcoholics Anonymous (AA) has perhaps the most successful approach for treating alcoholics. The membership of AA is primarily "recovering" alcoholics. Thus the alcoholic who desires help from AA has a support group of people who understand what he or she is going through.

If the individual who desires help from AA can subscribe to the twelve steps (see the box entitled "Twelve Steps of Alcoholics Anonymous"), then AA can be of help. Through these steps AA provides an alternative to alcohol use based on a faith in God, or a higher power. As with any rehabilitation, the individual must be motivated to get help and must be willing *never* to have another alcoholic beverage. If this motivation is absent, there is a high drop-out rate.

AA recognizes the importance of family and friends' support as a part of rehabilitation. Al-Anon is an AA-sponsored group for family members of alcoholics, and Al-Ateen is an AA-sponsored group for children of AA members. Both of these groups emphasize how to help the family member or friend who is an alcoholic. In essence, they help family and friends to understand the alcoholic better.

YOUR HEALTH TODAY

Twelve Steps of Alcoholics Anonymous

1. We admitted we were powerless over alcohol—that our lives had become unmanageable.
2. Came to believe that a Power greater than ourselves could restore us to sanity.
3. Made a decision to turn our will and our lives over to the care of God **as we understood Him.**
4. Made a searching and fearless moral inventory of ourselves.
5. Admitted to God, to ourselves and to another human being the exact nature of our wrongs.
6. Were entirely ready to have God remove all these defects of character.
7. Humbly asked Him to remove our shortcomings.
8. Made a list of all persons we had harmed, and became willing to make amends to them all.
9. Made direct amends to such people wherever possible, except when to do so would injure them or others.
10. Continued to take personal inventory and when we were wrong promptly admitted it.
11. Sought through prayer and meditation to improve our conscious contact with God, **as we understood Him,** praying only for knowledge of His will for us and the power to carry that out.
12. Having had a spiritual awakening as the result of these steps, we tried to carry this message to alcoholics, and to practice these principles in all our affairs.

Responsible Drinking

Exercise Good Judgment

Because people's responses to alcohol are highly individual and influenced by so many different things, it is hard to determine safe amounts for people to drink. Research suggests that the amount of alcohol one drinks is less important than when, why, and how one drinks. Most people who drink do it without harming themselves or other people. Yet because alcohol affects the brain, it is potentially dangerous. The responsible use of alcohol depends on the drinker's knowledge of its effects. A drinker must exercise good judgment in determining when to stop drinking and in deciding what activities are appropriate while certain body and brain functions are altered or impaired.

When considering whether to drink and how much, think about

LOOK, SCHOOL'S ALREADY HARD ENOUGH
WHY WOULD I WANT TO GET DRUNK AND MAKE IT WORSE?
NIAAA
FOR INFORMATION OR FOR HELP, WRITE:
NATIONAL CLEARINGHOUSE FOR ALCOHOL INFORMATION, BOX 2345, ROCKVILLE, MARYLAND 20852

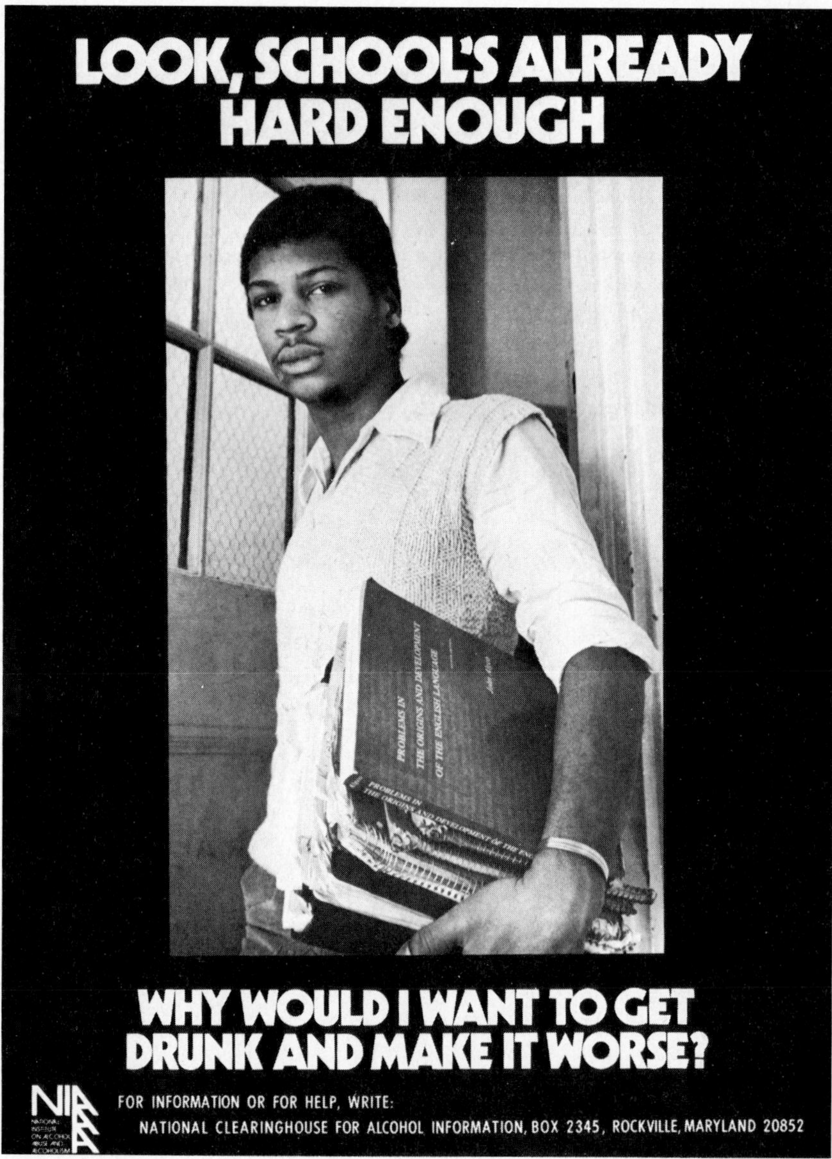

Many organizations and agencies conduct media campaigns to alert the public to the dangers of alcohol abuse. (Photo from U.S. Department of Health and Human Services, Public Health Service)

why you're drinking and what the effects on your health might be, both now and in the future. If you're drinking to have a good time and relax at a party, remember that you can still have a good time and certainly feel a lot better the next day if you don't overdo it. But, again, it will be easier to say no if you take a moment to consider the consequences of drinking too much.

Don't Mix Drinking and Driving

If you are ever in a situation in which you feel you must drive after drinking, drink even less than you consider to be safe — preferably no

YOUR HEALTH TODAY

Points to Remember for Responsible Drinkers

1. Alcohol is a drug that can cause positive and negative social, psychological, and physical effects.
2. The responsible use of alcohol can be socially, psychologically, and physically beneficial.
3. To drink or not to drink should be a personal decision. However, those who choose to drink have a responsibility not to damage themselves or society.
4. People who drink need to respect the decision of those who do not drink. Do not encourage others to drink.
5. People who serve alcoholic beverages need to contribute to a healthy drinking environment and not "push" drinks on others.
6. Intoxication is not responsible drinking.
7. There is a direct link between responsible attitudes toward drinking and alleviation of the problem of alcoholism.
8. *Don't drive* if you think you are intoxicated. Recognize that it takes time for the liver to oxidize the alcohol in your body, so you should stop alcohol intake at an appropriate time before driving.
9. Do not use alcohol as a means of escape from stress.
10. Do not mix alcohol with other drugs.

Source: National Institute of Alcohol Abuse and Alcoholism

more than a drink or two taken over more time than is necessary to metabolize it—bearing in mind that alcohol affects your judgment of your capabilities at the same time that it is diminishing them. However, it is even better to avoid driving entirely after drinking. Perhaps you could arrange with friends to take turns being the one to stay sober at parties and drive home. If no sober person is available to ride with, simply stay where you are or take a bus or taxi home; it's worth losing a little time or convenience to ensure your safety.

Don't Use Alcohol as an Escape

Be aware of how much alcohol you're consuming in your daily life. If you are drinking much, or drinking more than you used to, think about why. Is the drinking really much of a pleasure, or does it help you forget about unpleasant situations? Difficult and frustrating as it can be trying to cope with the problems we experience in life, it is more satisfying—and much better for our health—to face our problems than to seek an escape in alcohol. For a summary of the points regarding responsible drinking, see the Box entitled "Points to Remember for Responsible Drinkers."

Summary

Alcohol plays an important role in American life. For the majority of drinkers, alcohol can be enjoyed without problems. However, for many others, drinking can lead to tragedy.

Among the factors affecting an individual's drinking patterns are age, sex, place of residence, level of education, occupation, socioeconomic status, ethnicity, and religion. Although young people tend to drink less often than adults, they often consume more alcohol when they do drink. Otherwise, their patterns of alcohol use are similar to those of adults.

Ethanol, or ethyl alcohol, the intoxicating ingredient in alcoholic beverages, is a by-product of the metabolism of yeasts. Although classified as a food, it supplies only empty calories and contains no nutritional value. Alcohol is absorbed directly into the bloodstream. Within minutes after being consumed it is found in all tissues and organs of the body, and the body begins to dispose of it almost immediately.

A central nervous system depressant, alcohol produces a series of symptoms that increase in severity as its level in the blood rises. The measurement of Blood Alcohol Concentration (BAC) indicates how much alcohol the body has absorbed. Alcohol is chemically converted by the body at a rate of about one-third ounce of pure alcohol per hour, or somewhat less than an average drink.

A person consuming one or two drinks will experience a feeling of warmth, although heat loss actually increases. Even in small quantities alcohol disrupts the brain's ability to work. In small amounts alcohol is a mild sedative; in somewhat larger amounts it loosens inhibitions and social restraints. As BAC levels increase, a person suffers muscular and sensory impairment and a decrease in the ability to reason. Enough drinking may cause a person to lose consciousness; consuming a large enough quantity of alcohol to raise the BAC level to 0.50 percent before passing out may cause death.

Health problems associated with alcohol consumption include cardiomyopathy, stomach and intestinal ulcers, cirrhosis of the liver, nutritional deficiencies, memory loss, lowered resistance to infections, and various cancers. Alcohol also plays a major role in accidents. The combination of alcohol with other drugs may be dangerous, even fatal.

One out of every 2,000 infants is born with birth defects caused by alcohol. Although it is not certain what degree of drinking will produce a child suffering from Fetal Alcohol Syndrome (FAS), the surgeon general of the United States has warned that any consumption of alcohol during pregnancy may harm the fetus.

Problem drinking produces negative effects on drinkers and on the people involved with them. Defining alcoholism as a disease may discourage alcoholics from assuming reponsibility for their condition; altering alcoholic behavior seems to require the alcoholic's active, responsible participation. The effectiveness of different treatments seems to depend upon the individual's personality and concept of alcoholism and the support systems of family, friends, and coworkers.

The responsible use of alcohol depends upon the drinker's knowledge of its effects and good judgment in determining when to stop drinking and what activities are appropriate while under the influence of alcohol.

Review and Discussion

1. Discuss the factors that influence alcohol absorption.
2. Define Blood Alcohol Concentration (BAC) and describe the different effects of alcohol at different BACs.
3. Summarize the impact of heavy alcohol consumption on the major organs of the body.
4. What physical and mental abilities required for safe driving does alcohol affect?
5. What do you feel are the implications of withholding federal highway funds from states that have a legal drinking age below 21 years?
6. What is the Fetal Alcohol Syndrome?
7. Discuss current approaches to dealing with alcoholism.
8. How would you define responsible drinking? What steps can you take to avoid potentially dangerous consequences of drinking?

Further Reading

Dennison, Darwin, T. Prevet, and M. Affleck. *Alcohol and Behavior.* St Louis, Mo.: C. V. Mosby Company, 1980.
Basic coverage of alcohol as a drug, with a good discussion of the biological dimensions of alcohol. (Paperback.)

Ewing, John, and Beatrice Rouse, eds. *Drinking.* Chicago: Nelson-Hall Publishers, 1978.
A good overview of the role of alcohol in present day society, with special emphasis on sociological patterns of drinking behavior. (Paperback.)

Pattison, E. Mansell, L. Sobel, and L. C. Sobel. *Emerging Concepts of Alcohol Dependence.* New York: Springer Publishing Company, 1977.
A discussion of physiological aspects of alcohol abuse with an emphasis on alcohol dependence.

U.S. Congress, VSDHHS. *Fourth Special Report on Alcohol and Health.* Washington: USDHHS, January, 1981.
Excellent overview of alcohol consumption patterns in the United States. Also excellent source for data on alcohol-related problems.

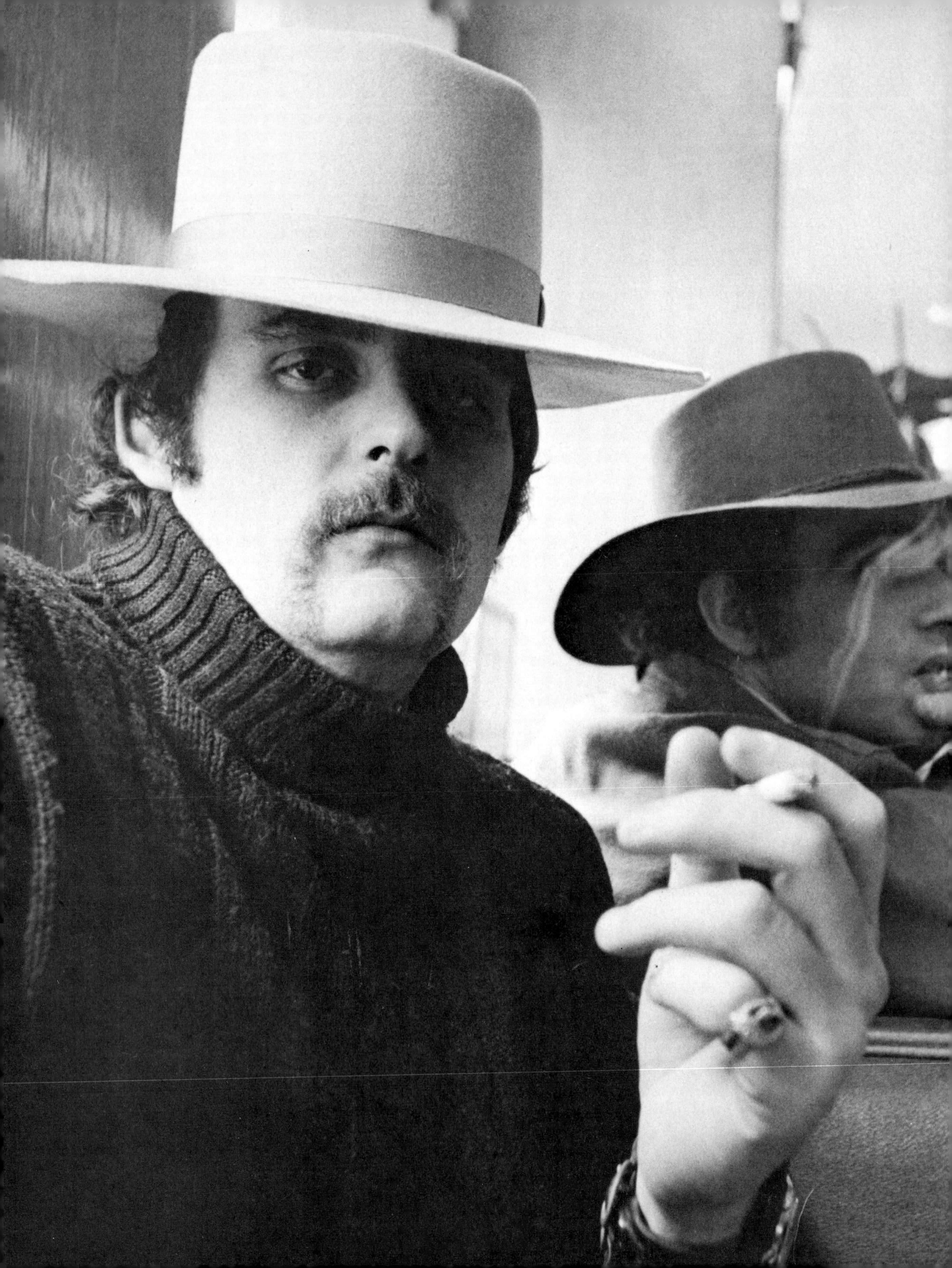

Chapter 10
Tobacco

KEY POINTS

- ☐ Despite scientific evidence that smoking is harmful to health, millions of Americans continue to smoke.
- ☐ Although smoking was initially considered a male prerogative, changes in the roles and self-images of women have contributed to their increased smoking.
- ☐ Cigarette smoke contains many substances that are harmful to health.
- ☐ The immediate physical effects of smoking include damage to the lungs and trachea, increased heart rate and blood pressure, and constriction of blood vessels.
- ☐ Smoking increases the risk of coronary heart disease, lung cancer, and lung diseases, among others.
- ☐ Sidestream smoke, the smoke in the air around a smoker, is harmful to others, a fact that has led to a growing concern for nonsmokers' rights.
- ☐ Although there are many programs designed to help people stop smoking, most of the millions of Americans who have succeeded have done it on their own.
- ☐ Tobacco and smoking are the subject of great political controversy, in which the economic interests of the tobacco industry are often opposed to the health interests of the public.

SCIENTIFIC evidence that smoking is harmful to health increases every year. Although many Americans in recent years have given up the habit or decided not to start, more than 50 million Americans continue to smoke cigarettes today. About 620 billion cigarettes are sold each year; the average adult smoker buys 206 packages of cigarettes per year. By the early 1980s Americans were spending over $15 billion on cigarettes annually, about half as much as they spend on alcohol.

In recent years most people, including many smokers, have come to believe that smoking is harmful and to consider it a form of air pollution. Legislators in the United States and in other countries have tried to limit the places where people can smoke. The most radical approach to altering a nation's smoking habits is being tried in Sweden, where the year 2000 has been set as a target date for the country to become a cigarette-free environment. The Swedish government has discouraged smoking by raising taxes on cigarettes, which now cost the equivalent of about $2.00 a pack, by banning the sale of cigarettes in vending machines, limiting advertising, and educating adults and children through medical counseling, in schools, and through the media. Nonsmokers there are also able to benefit from a monetary reward in the form of lowered life insurance costs.

According to recent reports by the U.S. surgeon general, cigarette smoking is the greatest cause of preventable illness and death in the United States. It is estimated that well over 300,000 Americans die prematurely every year because they smoked. Smoking costs Americans about $15 billion a year in medical care expenses and an estimated $25 billion in lost productivity because of illness.

While the number of cigarettes smoked by adults has decreased appreciably in recent decades, smoking among young people has not followed suit. Between 1964 and 1979 the percentage of American men who smoked dropped from 53 percent to 37.5 percent, while the percentage of women smokers showed a slight decline. However, there are now about 3.3 million regular smokers in junior and senior

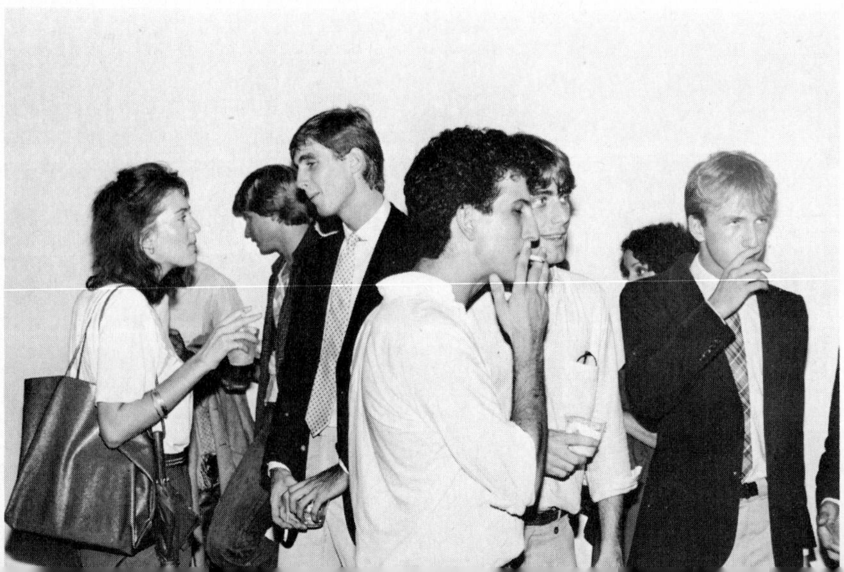

Despite warnings and increased awareness of health risk, more and more young people are becoming cigarette smokers. (Photo © Jim Anderson 1981/Woodfin Camp & Associates)

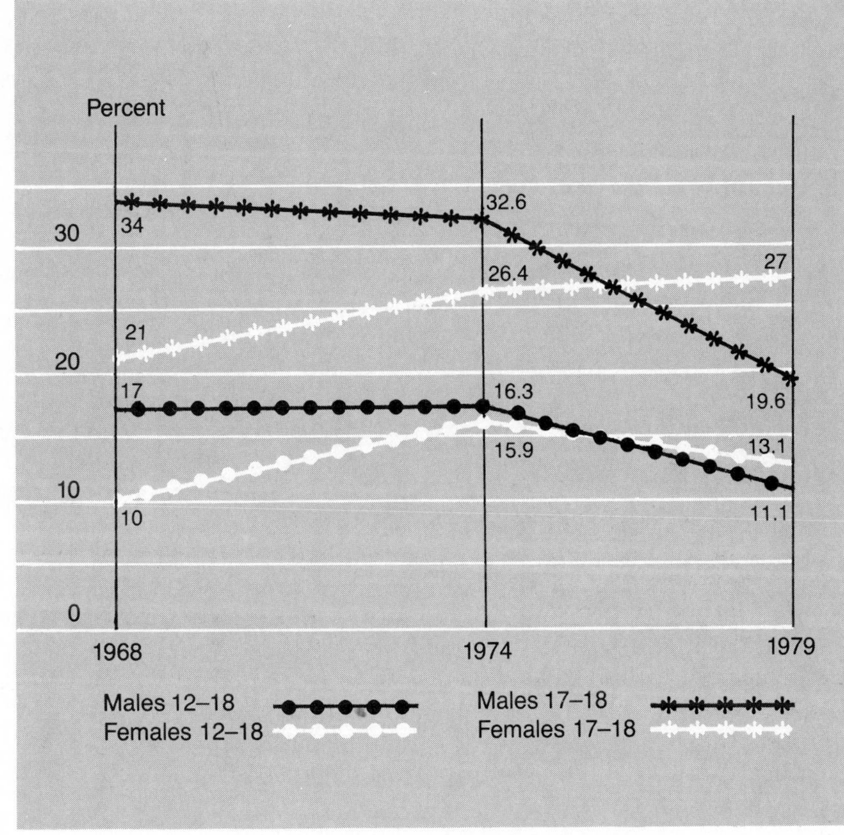

Figure 10–1. Teenage Smoking. Traditionally, smoking was a male prerogative, but in recent years the percentage of teenage girls who smoke has been greater than the percentage of teenage boys. (Source: U.S. Department of Health and Human Services, *Health: United States 1981* [Washington, D.C.: U.S. Department of Health and Human Services, 1981]:223.)

high school. Though in recent years smoking has decreased for boys between the ages of 12 and 18, among 17- and 18-year-old girls there has been a steady increase in regular smoking (see Figure 10–1). The proportion of the latter group who smoke reached nearly 30 percent during the 1970s. This increase is a concern, although the latest surveys indicate that the rate of smoking among young women has begun to level off and that it simply increased to approximate the higher smoking rates of young men.

To some health professionals the increase in young women's smoking has been alarming, partly because it has occurred despite more and more information about the negative impact of smoking on health and longevity, and partly because disease and mortality rates for smokers increase the longer they smoke. The average age at which women begin smoking has changed radically. Women who were born before 1900 rarely began smoking until they were at least 35 years old. In recent years, the median age for starting smoking has been 16. Cultural change and changes in the roles and self-images of women have probably contributed to the increases in their smoking. In fact, the advertising campaign for one brand of cigarettes aimed directly at women sums up the improvement in women's status with its slogan,

"You've come a long way, baby!" The ads go on to suggest that smoking that brand of cigarettes is the natural next step for the contemporary woman.

Ingredients in Cigarette Smoke and What They Do

A recent chemical analysis of the content of tobacco leaves and smoke has identified more than 3,000 separate substances, and *chromatographic scans* of the smoke indicate there are still many substances to be identified. About one third of the chemicals found in cigarette smoke are also found in tobacco leaves. The other smoke constituents are created when the dry leaves are lit and burned during the smoking process.

Impact of Carbon Monoxide and Other Gases

Hydrogen cyanide Gaseous component of smoke that damages respiratory lining.

Nitrogen oxide Pollutant in smoke linked to lung disease.

Carbon monoxide Toxic gas that reduces the oxygen-carrying capacity of blood.

Even though the tar and nicotine content of smoke is emphasized in the advertising campaigns of certain cigarettes, the particulate matter that includes them makes up only about 10 percent of tobacco smoke. The remaining 90 percent of the smoke consists of about a dozen gases. Some of these gases have specific impact on organs and systems in the human body. **Hydrogen cyanide,** for example, damages the lining of the airways in the bronchial tubes and lungs, and **nitrogen oxide** is involved in causing emphysema and other lung diseases. From 1 to 5 percent of the smoke in the average cigarette consists of carbon monoxide, another gas with even more powerful physiological effects than hydrogen cyanide and nitrogen oxide.

A colorless, odorless gas, **carbon monoxide** is produced when fuels or other materials are burned incompletely. Carbon monoxide is one of the gases in automobile exhaust. It has 210 times the affinity for hemoglobin that oxygen has, so it prevents the oxygen from combining with the blood's red cells. When carbon monoxide displaces oxygen in the blood it forms *carboxyhemoglobin,* which makes the walls of arteries more permeable, and produces edema or swelling from the abnormal accumulation of fluids in the tissues around the arteries. It also alters the interior walls of arteries, making them rough, which encourages the accumulation of cholesterol. If cholesterol continues to build up, the arteries become narrower and the heart must work harder to circulate blood. This condition is called atherosclerosis (see Chapter 16).

Impact of Tar and Nicotine

There are about 1 billion particles in a cubic centimeter of cigarette smoke. Very tiny and easily inhaled, these particles enter the deepest recesses of the lungs. If a smoker inhales, about 70 percent of the particulate matter is retained in the lungs. The tar and nicotine in these particles have powerful effects on the body.

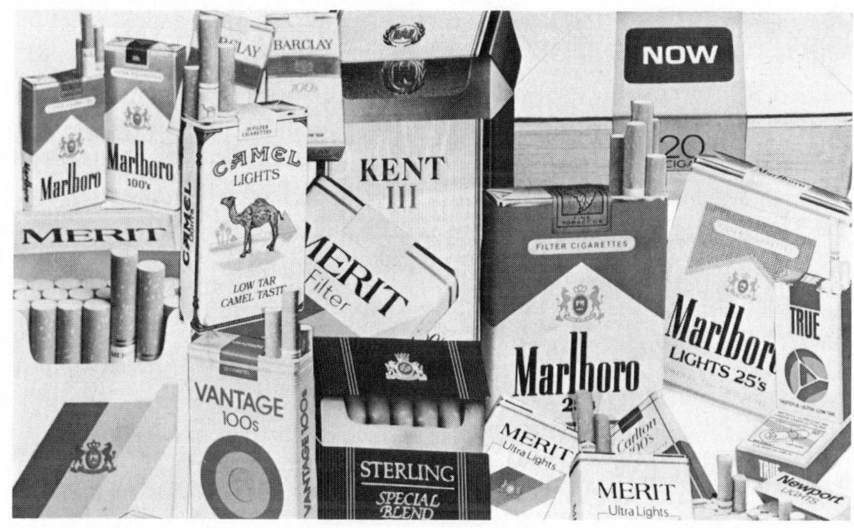

Although cigarettes all contain basically the same ingredients, various brands direct their advertising to particular audiences. (Photo by Paul Waldman)

Tar is actually a gummy mixture of hundreds of chemicals, and although there is only a minute amount of tar in each cigarette, it contains most of the cancer-causing agents in cigarette smoke. **Nicotine,** also present in the particulate matter in smoke, is a powerful chemical that affects the heart, blood vessels, digestive tract, kidneys, and nervous system. Although nicotine alone does not cause cancer, it seems to interact with other substances in the tar to produce cancerous tumors.

Tar The most carcinogenic substance in cigarettes.

Nicotine Component of tobacco smoke that affects major bodily organs.

Nicotine stimulates the adrenal glands and certain tissues in the heart, causing them to release substances that raise the blood pressure and elevate the heart rate. Because the heart muscle works harder, it requires more oxygen. However, the carbon monoxide also present in cigarette smoke displaces some of the oxygen in the blood so that there is less available. These effects of carbon monoxide and nicotine contribute to the development of heart disease and heart attacks among smokers. Some studies indicate that a program of regular exercise for smokers improves the body's mechanism for releasing oxygen from the blood even in the presence of elevated carboxyhemoglobin levels. This may help to reduce the incidence of heart disease among some smokers.

Nicotine also produces a number of changes in the digestive system. The nicotine in a cigarette has a two-stage effect on the salivary glands. When inhaled, it stimulates the glands to produce more saliva than usual, but when it is absorbed by the body, it reduces saliva production so that a smoker's mouth feels dry. Nicotine also causes the stomach to produce more acid, and it increases the activity in the small intestine. These physiological effects may be positively related to the pleasures of smoking around mealtime that many smokers report. The wide range of tar and nicotine levels present in the varieties of cigarettes now available is shown in Table 10–1.

Table 10–1 Tar[1] and Nicotine Content of One Hundred Seventy-Six (176) Varieties of Domestic Cigarettes (Shown in Increasing Order of Tar Values)

Brand	Type	Tar (mg/cig)	Nico-tine (mg/cig)
		less than	less than
Carlton	King (HP)	0.5	0.05
Carlton	King, M	1	0.1
Benson & Hedges	Reg. (HP)	1	0.1
Carlton	King	1	0.1
Tareyton Ultra Low-Tar	King, M	2	0.2
Now	King, M(HP)	2	0.2
Now	King, M	2	0.2
Now	King	2	0.2
Now	King, (HP)	2	0.2
Triumph	King, M	2	0.3
Kent III	King	3	0.3
Triumph	King	3	0.4
Iceberg 100's	100mm, M	3	0.3
Lucky 100's	100mm	4	0.3
Decade	King, M	4	0.4
Decade	King	4	0.4
True	King, M	5	0.4
True	King	5	0.4
Carlton 100's	100mm, M	5	0.4
Doral II	King, M	5	0.4
Doral II	King	5	0.5
Carlton 100's	100mm	6	0.4
Pall Mall Extra Light	King	7	0.6
L & M Lights	100mm	7	0.6
L & M Lights	King	7	0.6
Tempo	King	8	0.6
Lark Lights	King	8	0.6
Lark Lights	100mm	8	0.6
American Lights	120mm	8	0.6
Tareyton Lights	King	8	0.6
Merit	King	8	0.6
Arctic Lights	King, M	8	0.7
Kent Golden Lights	King	8	0.7
Merit	King, M	8	0.6
Real	King, M	9	0.7
Lucky Ten	King	9	0.7
Belair	100mm, M	9	0.7
Kent Golden Lights	King, M	9	0.7
Kool Super Lights	100mm, M	9	0.7
Viceroy Rich Lights	King	9	0.7
Tareyton Long Lights	100mm	9	0.7
Kool Super Lights	King, M	9	0.7
Kent Golden Lights	100mm	9	0.8
American Lights	120mm, M	9	0.8
Raleigh Lights	King	9	0.8
Parliament Lights	King	9	0.7
Raleigh Lights	100mm	9	0.8
Arctic Lights	100mm, M	9	0.8
Newport Lights	King, M	10	0.8
		less than	less than
Belair	King, M	10	0.8
Viceroy Rich Lights	100mm	10	0.8
Old Gold Lights	King	10	0.8
Real	King	10	0.9
Kent Golden Lights	100mm, M	10	0.8
Camel Lights	King	10	0.9
Parliament Lights	King, (HP)	10	0.7
Silva Thins	100mm, M	10	0.8
Merit 100's	100mm	10	0.7
Benson & Hedges Lights	100mm, M	11	0.7
Merit 100's	100mm, M	11	0.8
Vantage	King, M	11	0.8
Benson & Hedges Lights	100mm	11	0.8
Salem Long Lights	100mm, M	11	0.9
Vantage	King	11	0.8
Salem Lights	King, M	11	0.8
Multifilter	King	11	0.8
Kent	King	11	0.9
Parliament Lights 100's	100mm	12	0.8
Marlboro Lights	King	12	0.8
Marlboro Lights	100mm	12	0.8
Vantage	100mm	12	0.9
Multifilter	King, M	12	0.8
Pall Mall Lights	100mm	12	0.9
Doral	King, M	12	0.9
Silva Thins	100mm	12	1.0
Kool Milds	King, M	13	0.8
Doral	King	13	1.0
Kent	King, (HP)	13	1.0
Eve	120mm, M (HP)	13	1.0
Eve	120mm, (HP)	13	1.0
True 100's	100mm	13	0.8
Winston Lights 100's	100mm	13	1.0
Viceroy	King	13	0.9
Camel Lights	100mm	13	1.1
True 100's	100mm, M	14	0.8
Kent	100mm	14	1.0
Winston Lights	King	14	1.1
Tareyton	100mm	14	1.0
Tareyton	King	14	0.9
L & M	King, (HP)	14	0.9
Marlboro	King, M	15	0.9
Alpine	King, M	15	0.9
Kent	100mm, M	15	1.2
Virginia Slims	100mm, M	15	0.9
Eve	100mm	15	1.1
Marlboro	King, M	15	0.9
Saratoga	120mm, M (HP)	15	1.0
St. Moritz	100mm, M	15	1.1
		less than	less than
Chesterfield	King	15	0.9
L & M	King	15	1.0
Du Maurier	King, (HP)	15	1.0
Eve	100mm, M	15	1.1
Oasis	King, M	15	1.0
Virginia Slims	100mm	16	1.0
Viceroy	100mm	16	1.1
St. Moritz	100mm	16	1.1
Pall Mall	100mm, M	16	1.2
Salem	King, M	16	1.1
Newport	King, M (HP)	16	1.2
Tall	120mm, M	16	1.3
L & M	100mm	16	1.0
Kool	100mm, M	16	1.2
L & M	100mm, M	16	1.0
Long Johns	120mm, M	16	1.4
Raleigh	King	16	1.0
Kool	King, M	16	1.3
Chesterfield	101mm	16	1.1
Kool	King, M, (HP)	16	1.3
Twist	100mm, L/M	16	1.3
Raleigh	100mm	16	1.1
Benson & Hedges	100mm, M, (HP)	16	1.1
Salem	King, M, (HP)	17	1.2
Marlboro	100mm	17	1.1
Benson & Hedges	100mm, (HP)	17	1.1
Old Gold Filters	King	17	1.2
Marlboro	100mm, (HP)	17	1.1
Saratoga	120mm, (HP)	17	1.1
Galaxy	King	17	1.1
Benson & Hedges	100mm	17	1.1
Montclair	King, M	17	1.2
Newport	King, M	17	1.2
Benson & Hedges	100mm, M	17	1.1
Marlboro	King	17	1.1
Marlboro	King, (HP)	17	1.1
Lark	King	17	1.2
Long Johns	120mm	17	1.3
Max	120mm	18	1.4
Benson & Hedges	King, (HP)	18	1.4
Winston 100's	100mm	18	1.3
Max	120mm, M	18	1.4
Pall Mall	100mm	18	1.3
Philip Morris International	100mm, (HP)	18	1.1
Philip Morris International	100m, M, (HP)	18	1.1
Tall	120mm	18	1.5
Pall Mall	King	19	1.2

Brand	Type	Tar (mg/cig)	Nicotine (mg/cig)
		less than	less than
Camel	King	19	1.4
Old Gold 100's	100mm	19	1.4
Kool	reg. (NF), M	19	1.1
Winston	100mm, M	19	1.4
Lark	100mm	19	1.3
Winston	King, (HP)	19	1.4
Spring 100's	100mm, M	19	1.1
Salem	100mm, M	20	1.5
Winston	King	20	1.4
Newport	100mm, M	20	1.5
Philip Morris	reg. (NF)	21	1.3
Picayune	reg. (NF)	23	1.4
Chesterfield	reg. (NF)	23	1.4
Piedmont	reg. (NF)	23	1.3
English Ovals	reg. (NF), (HP)	23	1.8
More	120mm	23	1.8
More	120mm, M	24	1.8
Lucky Strike	reg. (NF)	24	1.4
Home Run	reg. (NF)	24	1.5
Raleigh	King, (NF)	24	1.3
Pall Mall	King, (NF)	24	1.4
Half & Half	King	24	1.8
Old Gold Straights	King, (NF)	25	1.6
Players	reg. (NF) (HP)	26	1.9
Camel	reg. (NF)	26	1.8
Philip Morris Commander	King, (NF)	27	1.7
Chesterfield	King, (NF)	28	1.7
Herbert Tareyton	King, (NF)	28	1.7
Fatima	King, (NF)	28	1.6
Bull Durham	King	28	1.9
English Ovals	King, (NF), (HP)	30	2.4

[1] TPM dry (tar)—milligrams total particulate matter less nicotine and water

NF—Non-Filter (All other brands possess filters)

M —Menthol

HP—Hard pack

Source: Federal Trade Commission; distributed by the American Cancer Society

Factors Affecting the Absorption of Substances in Smoke

Many factors affect an individual smoker's exposure to the toxic materials in tobacco smoke. These factors include the number of cigarettes a person smokes, the number of years smoking has been a habit, and variations in smoking style.

Studies indicate that smokers average about eight puffs per cigarette. When smoke is held in the mouth, nicotine and other substances can be absorbed directly through the mucus membrane there. Of course, when cigarette smoke is inhaled, more gas and particulate matter are absorbed. Some research indicates that a smoker who inhales absorbs nine times the nicotine and other substances absorbed by a smoker who simply puffs a cigarette. In addition, if a smoker inhales, the depth of the inhalation and the length of time smoke is held in the lungs help to determine how much of the chemical contents of smoke enters the body.

American Smoking Patterns Today

The growth of cigarette smoking continued nearly unabated until the surgeon general's first report on smoking and health was issued in 1964. At that time, more than 53 percent of American men and 32 percent of the women 21 years old and older smoked cigarettes. Per capita consumption, too, had reached its peak, with estimates indicating that each smoker consumed an average of 4,366 cigarettes that year.

Over the next twenty years or so, cigarette consumption decreased among adults, for several reasons. Publicity about the health risks of smoking had real impact, especially on males, who were—and still are—the greatest users. Consumption began to drop promptly after the first surgeon general's report. Laws prohibiting smoking in many public places also helped to reduce the number of cigarettes smoked each year, and the rising cost of cigarettes was still another factor. Studies have found that cigarette consumption declines 0.4 percent for every 1 percent increase.

Several factors help to determine the concentration of chemicals in the cigarette smoke itself. In cultivated tobacco, nicotine content is directly related to the amount of nitrate fertilizer applied to the plants and soil. Filters, which trap some of the tars in smoke, may actually increase the level of carbon monoxide a smoker inhales. Filters may also introduce other chemicals with the smoke. Finally, because chemicals collect in the tobacco itself as a cigarette burns, a smoker takes in higher concentrations of chemicals in puffs from a cigarette that is almost finished. Certain smoking styles are clearly more dangerous than others. Taking many puffs of each cigarette, retaining the smoke in the mouth, inhaling deeply and holding smoke in the lungs, and smoking a cigarette down to the end all increase one's exposure to toxic chemicals.

Certain differences in smoking style have been found among men and women, although these differences are gradually becoming less pronounced. Women tend to leave more of their cigarettes unsmoked and puff for less time than men; but they usually take more puffs of each cigarette, so their total contact with each is about the same as men's.

Physical Effects of Smoking on the Body

Immediate Effects

May people believe that cigarette smoking causes disease only after a person has been smoking a long time. As a result, many young people think they are immune to smoking's ill effects. To see if you already know what the effects of smoking are, complete Self-Assessment Exercise 10.1.

Smoking has an immediate negative impact on the body. Damage to the lungs and **trachea** begins with the first cigarette and increases as smoking continues. Cigarette smoke irritates the trachea and reduces the secretion of protective mucus. Furthermore, it damages the **cilia** in the respiratory tract, leaving the smoker vulnerable to infections.

Trachea Respiratory tube that conveys air to the lungs.

Cilia Small hairlike projections that sweep foreign material out of lungs.

SELF-ASSESSMENT EXERCISE 10.1

What Do You Think the Effects of Smoking Are?

PART I —

For each statement, circle the number that shows how you feel about it. Do you strongly agree, mildly agree, mildly disagree, or strongly disagree?

Important: Answer Every Question.

	Strongly Agree	Mildly Agree	Mildly Disagree	Strongly Disagree
A. Cigarette smoking is not nearly as dangerous as many other health hazards.	1	2	3	4
B. I don't smoke enough to get any of the diseases that cigarette smoking is supposed to cause.	1	2	3	4
C. If a person has already smoked for many years, it probably won't do him much good to stop.	1	2	3	4
D. It would he bard for me to give up smoking cigarettes.	1	2	3	4
E. Cigarette smoking is enough of a health hazard for something to be done about it.	4	3	2	1
F. The kind of cigarette I smoke is much less likely than other kinds to give me any of the diseases that smoking is supposed to cause.	1	2	3	4
G. As soon as a person quits smoking cigarettes he begins to recover from much of the damage that smoking has caused.	4	3	2	1
H. It would be hard for me to cut down to half the number of cigarettes I now smoke.	1	2	3	4
I. The whole problem of cigarette smoking and health is a very minor one.	1	2	3	4
J. I haven't smoked long enough to worry about the diseases that cigarette smoking is supposed to cause.	1	2	3	4
K. Quitting smoking helps a person to live longer.	4	3	2	1
L. It would be difficult for me to make any substantial change in my smoking habits.	1	2	3	4

(continued)

PART II — HOW TO SCORE:

1. Enter the numbers you have circled to the questions in the spaces below, putting the number you have circled to Question A over line A, to Question B over line B, etc.
2. Total the 3 scores across on each line to get your totals. For example, the sum of your scores over lines A, E, and I gives you your score on *Importance*—lines B, F, and J give the score on *Personal Relevance,* etc.

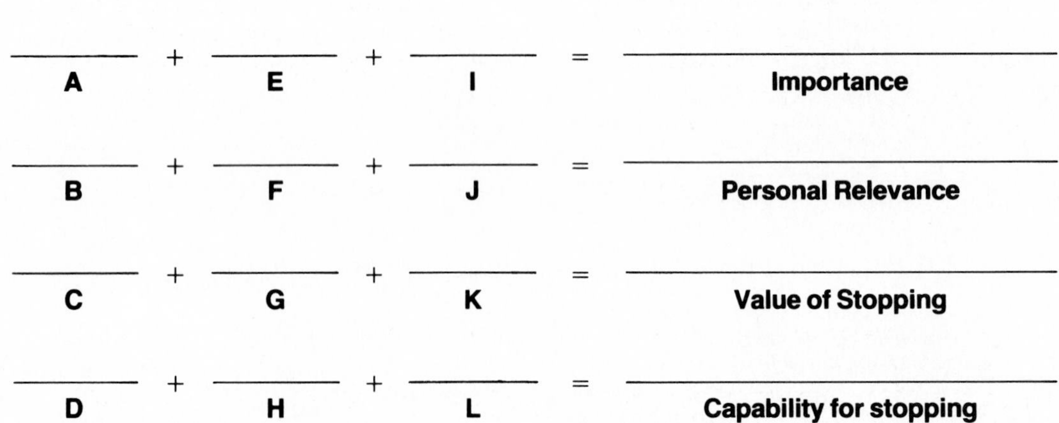

							Totals
____	+	____	+	____	=		____
A		E		I			Importance
____	+	____	+	____	=		____
B		F		J			Personal Relevance
____	+	____	+	____	=		____
C		G		K			Value of Stopping
____	+	____	+	____	=		____
D		H		L			Capability for stopping

Scores can vary from 3 to 12. Any score 9 and above is *high;* any score 6 and below is *low.* Learn from Part 2 what your scores mean.

PART III — ANSWERS:

To attempt to give up smoking you must do more than simply acknowledge that "cigarette smoking may be harmful to your health." You must be aware that smoking is an *important* problem, that it has *personal* meaning for you, that there is *value* to be gained from stopping, and that people are *capable* of stopping. This test measures the strength of your recognition of each of these factors.

If your score is 9 or above on any factor, that factor supports your desire to try to stop smoking. If your score is 6 or below, that factor will not help you, but note that you may have scored low because you lack correct information. For every factor for which you *do* have a low score, read the accompanying explanatory material with special care.

1. Importance

Cancer, heart disease, respiratory diseases—all related to smoking—are among the most serious to which man is exposed. You should not shrug off the growing evidence that they cause death and severe disability. Yet you may be doing this if your score is 6 or lower on the first part of this test.

Research has shown that one death in every three is an "extra" death among men who die between the ages of 35 and 60, because cigarette smokers have higher death rates than non-smokers. One day of every five lost from work because of illness, 1 day in every 10 spent in bed because of illness, 1 day of every 8 days of restricted activity—all are "extra," because cigarette smokers suffer more disability than nonsmokers.

2. Personal Relevance

Some smokers kid themselves into thinking: "It can't happen to me—only to the other guy." If you score 6 or below, you may be one of these people.

Your reasoning may go something like this: "I don't really smoke enough to be hurt by it. It takes two packs a day over a period of many years before harmful effects show up."

Unfortunately, this is not true. Even people who smoke less than half a pack a day show significantly higher death rates than nonsmokers. Breathing capacity can diminish after only a very few years of regular smoking. Even what used to be considered light smoking, such as half a pack a day, can be harmful.

3. Value of Stopping

Evidence shows that there are benefits to health when you give up smoking—even if you have smoked for many years. A score of 6 or lower indicates that you do not realize this.

There are real advantages in giving up smoking even for long-term smokers; people who quit before any symptoms of illness or impairment occur suffer lower death rates than those who continue to smoke, and reduce the likelihood of serious illness.

People who have had heart attacks and those with stomach ulcers and chronic respiratory diseases should definitely give up smoking. It is difficult if not impossible to control such illnesses if they do not.

4. Capability for Stopping

If your score is 6 or lower on this part of the test, you believe that it will be hard for you to quit. But you may find encouragement in the fact that over 20 million adults are now successful ex-smokers. Of these, over 100,000 doctors, well over half of those who were ever cigarette smokers, have successfully quit.

Source: U.S. Public Health Service, *Smoker's Self-Testing Kit,* Washington, D.C.: US Dept. HEW, USDHS Publ. No. 75-8716, 1975, p. 3.

Normally, the cilia, tens of millions of microscopic hairlike projections lining the respiratory tract, prevent germs and dirt from reaching the lungs. They do this by waving back and forth about 12 times a second, sweeping tiny particles back toward the throat and away from the lungs. Cigarette smoke slows the cilias' movements and interferes with the body's defense system.

After only a few weeks of regular smoking, cells in the lungs grow abnormally large, and excess mucus is secreted. A few months of smoking causes enough lung damage for scar tissue to form.

Normal heart rate and blood pressure are altered by a single cigarette. Nicotine stimulates the heart to beat faster and constricts the arteries and the blood vessels in the skin, especially in the extremities. For some smokers the result is cold, clammy hands and feet. Because of the vascular changes, the smoker's blood pressure rises.

Nicotine and the Brain

Though the exact mechanism by which nicotine reinforces a person's desire to smoke is not clearly understood, scientists believe this reinforcement takes place somewhere in the brain. Absorbed quickly, a dose of nicotine travels through the heart directly to the brain in about 7½ seconds. Nicotine remains in the blood for about 30 minutes, and because habitual smokers who use about a pack of cigarettes a day light up about every 30 or 40 minutes, some scientists believe they are trying to maintain a consistent level of nicotine in their bodies. In truly addictive smoking, only a few of the 25 or more cigarettes a day provide pleasure for the smoker. The other cigarettes smoked are to avoid the irritability and inability to concentrate that are often the symptoms of withdrawal. It is estimated that about one out of three men and one out of five women become addictive smokers.

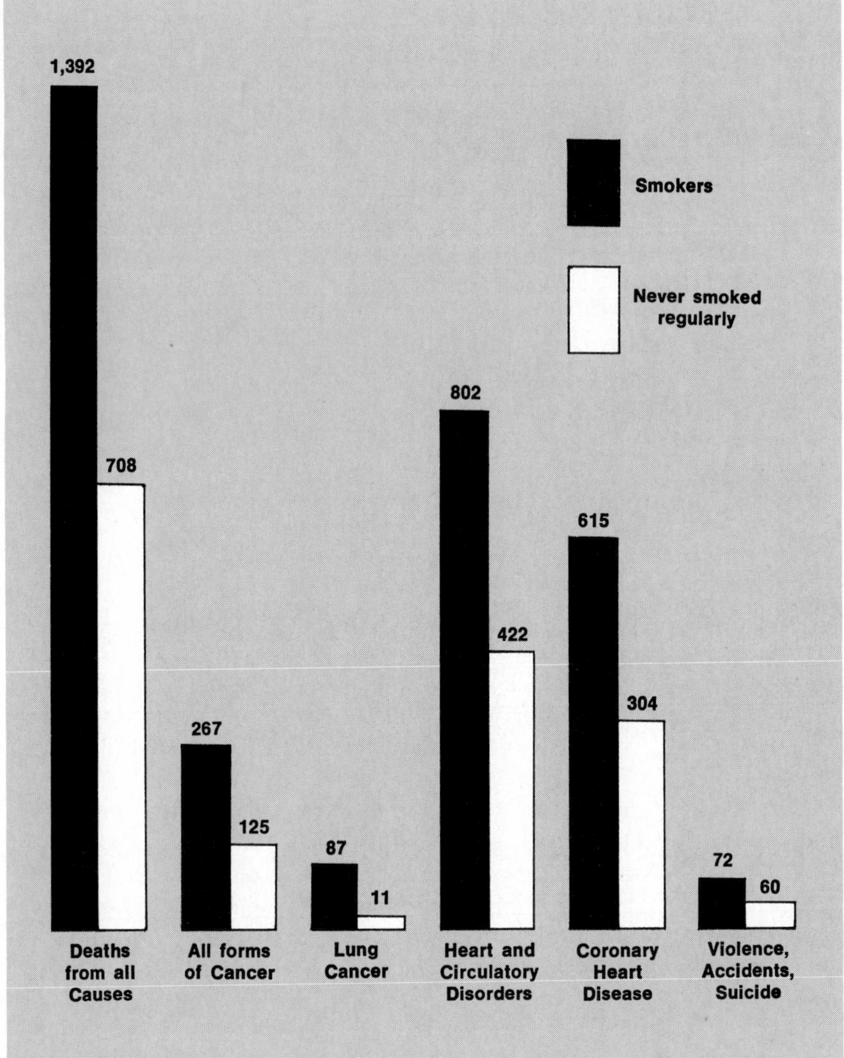

Figure 10–2. Smoking and Death Rates. These comparative rates are for male smokers aged 45–64, based on a recent study. They highlight the increased risk of premature death from smoking. Rates are in deaths per 100,000 person-years; person-years are the number of individuals multiplied by the number of years studied. (Source: U.S. Public Health Service)

Smoking cigarettes seems to cause a variety of changes in a persons's mental and emotional states. At times smoking provides a stimulation, and at times sedation. Sometimes a cigarette seems to increase a smoker's alertness and improve the ability to concentrate. Smoking can help a person to perform efficiently in tasks that demand attention. At other times tobacco may have a tranquilizing effect. Smoking can make a person feel calm and relieved from unpleasant emotions like anxiety or anger. Smoking a cigarette, most smokers report, is especially pleasant after a meal or as an accompaniment to coffee, tea, or an alcoholic beverage. The mechanisms for the variations in people's responses to cigarettes are not well understood.

Long-Term Effects

Cigarette smoking is a factor in several major causes of premature death in the United States (see Figure 10–2). The risk of disease and death increases with increasing exposure to the harmful constituents in smoke. The premature death rates for both men and women who smoke is about 70 percent higher than for nonsmokers. The largest number of smoking-related premature deaths in the United States is the result of coronary heart disease, followed by lung cancer, other cancers, and chronic lung disease. In 1978 smoking was a factor in about 346,000 premature deaths in America. Of these, 225,000 were from heart disease and stroke; 80,000 resulted from lung cancer; 22,000 were from other smoking-related cancers, such as cancer of the kidney or pancreas; and approximately 19,000 deaths were attributable to chronic lung disease.

Although many smokers using low-tar cigarettes believe the health risks to them are substantially reduced, this is not true. Premature death rates for smokers of low-tar cigarettes are only about 15 percent lower than for smokers of other kinds of cigarettes. The many cigarette-related diseases make an astounding impact on the American economy. The economic effects of cigarette-induced major illnesses are shown in Table 10–2.

Table 10–2 Costs to American Economy for Cigarette-Induced Major Illnesses, 1964–1983

Health Care Costs for Cigarette-induced Cancer	$ 56,200,000,000.00
Productivity Lost due to Cigarette-induced Cancer	$186,300,000,000.00
Subtotal—Cancer	$242,500,000,000.00
Health Care Costs for Cigarette-induced Cardiovascular Disease	$108,300,000,000.00
Productivity Lost due to Cigarette-induced Cardiovascular Disease	$265,600,000,000.00
Subtotal—Cardiovascular Disease	$373,900,000,000.00
Health Care Costs for Cigarette-induced Chronic Lung Disease	$120,000,000,000.00
Productivity Lost due to Cigarette-induced Chronic Lung Disease	$195,400,000,000.00
Subtotal—Chronic Lung Disease	$315,400,000,000.00
TOTAL COST	**$931,800,000,000.00**

Source: American Council on Science and Health, 1984.

Coronary Heart Disease

The relationship between smoking and coronary heart disease is strong and consistent. Though cigarette smoke cannot be said to be a cause of heart disease, smoking is among the important factors that increase the risk of developing this condition. Other factors include hypertension, diabetes, a sedentary life-style, and obesity. For people who smoke more than a pack of cigarettes per day, the risk of heart disease is estimated to be three times as high as for a nonsmoker. Cigarette smoking seems to be especially related to the occurrence of coronary heart disease in men between the ages of 35 and 55. Because cigarettes seem less often related to this disease among men 65 and older, cigarette smoking seems to be an aggravating factor rather than a cause.

As we have discussed, there is a strong positive relationship between the thickening of the walls of the arteries in the heart and the number of cigarettes a person smokes each day. In three out of 10 nonsmoking males between the ages of 45 to 55, some degree of fibrous thickening of the coronary arteries occurs. The incidence of artery damage increases to seven out of 10 for men who smoke less than a pack a day. When cigarette consumption exceeds two packs a day, 95 out of 100 men have some degree of coronary artery damage.

Cancer

Cigarette smoking is the most important risk factor for lung cancer. More than 75 percent of all cases of lung cancer develop among smokers. In this disease, abnormal cells grow uncontrolled in the lungs and finally crowd out the healthy tissue. (For a more detailed discussion of this and other cancers see Chapter 17.) The risk of lung cancer, like the risk of coronary heart disease, increases with the number of cigarettes smoked. Thus the risk is highest among people between 50 and 70 years old who have long-time smoking habits. Lung cancer is fatal for cigarette smokers about eight times more often than it is for nonsmokers. And for people who smoke more than two packs a day, the death rate from lung cancer rises to 20 times that for people who don't smoke at all.

Heredity seems to play a part in the development of lung cancer. Family members of someone who has had this disease have a slightly higher risk of developing it too. But when these people smoke cigarettes, the risk is even greater. Smokers who drink alcoholic beverages, especially whiskey and other drinks with a high alcohol content, are another group with a higher risk of developing lung cancer (as well as cancers of the mouth and throat). Cigarette smokers, in general, also stand a greater risk of developing cancer of the mouth or throat. In addition, cigarette smoking is associated with cancers of the bladder, kidney, and pancreas. People who smoke, for example, are twice as likely to develop bladder cancer as people who don't smoke.

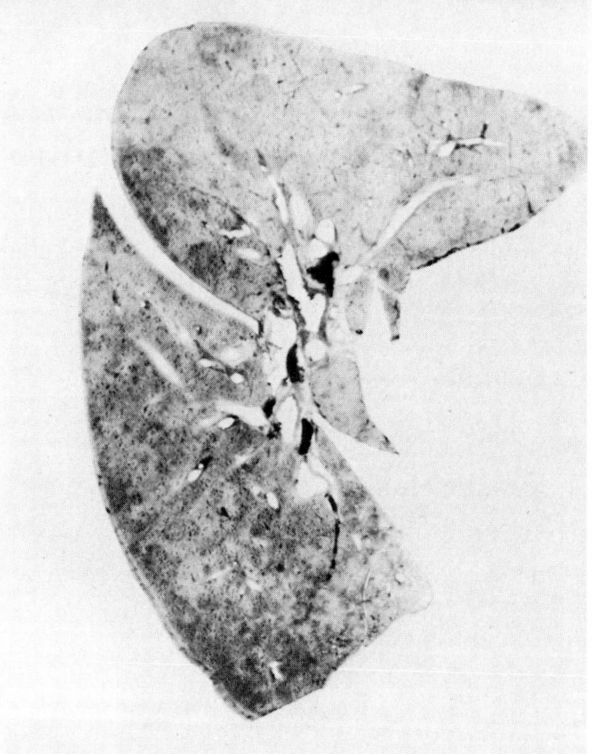

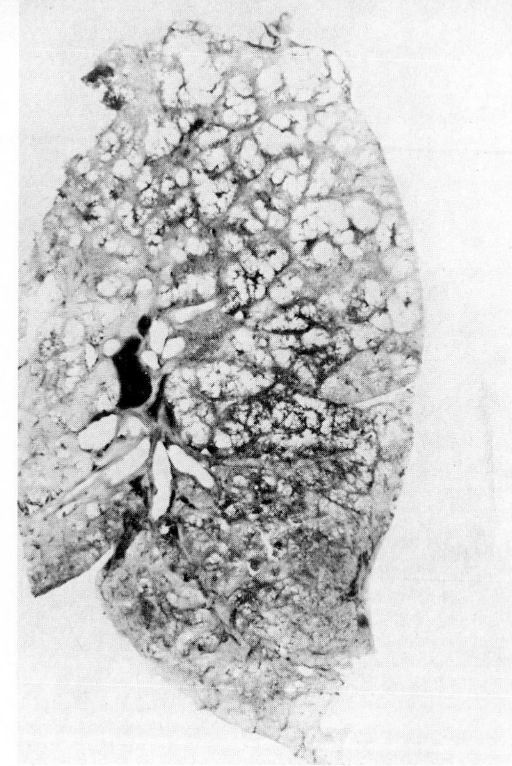

In normal lung tissue (left) the air sacs are too fine to be visible. In the lung tissue of a heavy smoker (right), greatly enlarged air sacs are abundant. (Photo courtesy of American Cancer Society)

Because inhaling is less common among pipe and cigar smokers than among people who smoke cigarettes, their risk of developing lung cancer is significantly lower, but it is greater than the risk faced by nonsmokers. They also have a higher incidence of mouth cancers and cancers of the lips and tongue than other types of smokers.

Lung Disease

Smoking is a major cause of lung diseases such as chronic bronchitis and emphysema. These diseases progress slowly, beginning with abnormalities in the lungs that may not produce symptoms for a long time. One form of lung disease is **bronchitis,** which causes increases in the mucus secretions in the respiratory tract and an increase in the frequency of coughing. If smoking continues and the damage increases, the condition becomes chronic, the airways in the respiratory tract become inflamed and constricted, and air flow is reduced. A person with chronic bronchitis feels short of breath and has occasions of painful breathing.

Bronchitis Inflammatory lung disease that increases mucus in respiratory tract.

Another type of chronic lung disease is called **emphysema.** In this disease the walls of the air sacs in the lungs tear, air becomes trapped in the sacs and the spaces between them, and the lungs become overinflated. The normal exchange of carbon dioxide for oxygen becomes disrupted. Breathing is sometimes painful for a person with emphysema, and even small physical efforts are exhausting. The heart is forced to pump harder, and it may become enlarged. A high percentage of emphysema victims are smokers, and most have been heavy smokers for many years. When a person stops smoking, the damage to

Emphysema Chronic respiratory-weakening disease that results in destructive changes in the air sacs in the lungs.

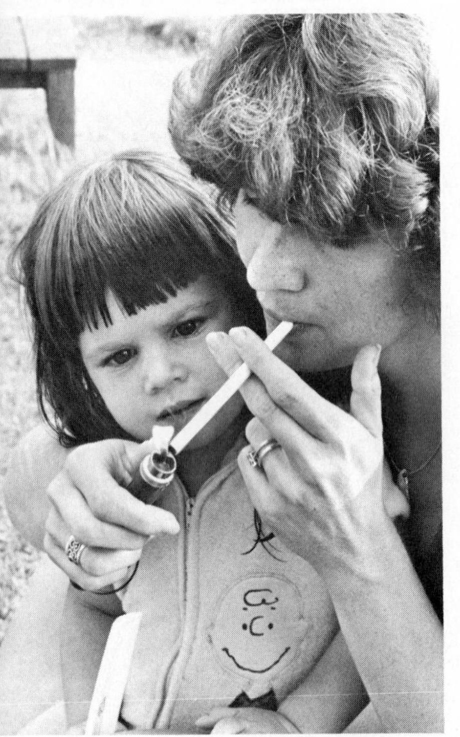

Children of parents who smoke have a greater chance of becoming smokers as adults. (Photo © Alice Kandell/ Photo Researchers, Inc.)

the lungs and respiratory tract ceases to worsen, and emphysema may be avoided.

Even when smokers do not develop advanced stages of lung disease, they have more minor upper respiratory infections and miss more days of work because of colds and sore throats than do nonsmokers. Smokers take longer to recover from respiratory illnesses, and if they must undergo surgery, they are more likely than nonsmokers to develop postoperative complications like pneumonia.

Smokers Facing Increased Health Risks

People with Stomach Ulcers

Smoking is associated with increased illness and death rates from peptic ulcers and, especially, gastric ulcers. Smoking stimulates the stomach to secrete more digestive acid and increases the activity in the small intestine. Gastric and duodenal ulcers heal slowly for smokers, and if smoking continues it tends to make these stomach conditions chronic. Smoking may even impair the process of normal digestion.

People Exposed to Toxic Materials

When people are exposed to toxic agents in their environment or on the job, smoking can act in combination with the agents and multiply the risk of illness or death. For example, asbestos workers who smoke have 92 times the risk of developing lung cancer as nonsmoking workers. For uranium miners who smoke, the risk of dying from cancer increases tenfold compared to the risk faced by their nonsmoking counterparts.

People with Circulatory Disease

Smoking is especially dangerous for people with diseases of the blood vessels in the hands, feets, arms, and legs. Because smoking constricts their already narrowed and damaged blood vessels, it increases their risk of gangrene, amputations, and even death.

Oral Contraceptive Users

Women who use oral contraceptives and also smoke increase their risk of stroke and heart disease. This is especially true for women age 35 and older. Death from strokes or heart attacks is more than three times as frequent for smokers using birth-control pills as for their nonsmoking counterparts. Among women who use oral contraceptives but do not smoke, there are 10 deaths per 100,000 users. Among those who smoke there are 33 deaths per 100,000 users. This risk is so serious that the Food and Drug Administration has revised its labeling requirement for oral contraceptives. These products all display the warning: "Women who use birth control pills should not smoke."

Pregnant Women

Cigarette smoking is harmful to pregnant women and their unborn children and has been related to premature births and associated with physical and mental impairment in the children of smoking mothers. In a study of women who smoked at least 10 cigarettes a day, doctors found damage in the subjects' maternal-fetal circulatory systems. Smoking narrows and damages the arteries in the umbilical cord connecting the developing fetus to the placenta. These arteries carry nutrients and oxygen from the placenta to the unborn child.

In some cases the capillaries in the fetus were partially blocked. Smoking reduces the flow of nutrients to the fetus, causing the newborns of smoking mothers to be smaller and weigh less than newborns of nonsmokers. Another factor in the reduced size and weight of smokers' newborns is the carbon monoxide, other gases, and toxins that cross the placenta and enter the fetal blood.

Women who smoke have more miscarriges (spontaneous abortions) and more stillbirths than women who do not, and the babies of smoking mothers are more apt to die during the first years of their lives. If a woman stops smoking before the fourth month of pregnancy, the risk of death for her child is small.

The Effects of Smoke on Nonsmokers

Sidestream Smoke

Inhalation of tobacco smoke comes primarily from two sources—mainstream and sidestream smoke. **Mainstream smoke** is the smoke that is directly inhaled and exhaled by the smoker; **sidestream smoke** (also called secondhand smoke) is the smoke that is generated by the tobacco-containing product (generally a cigarette) while it smolders in an ashtray. In recent years, nonsmokers have been concerned about inhaling sidestream smoke, and this concern is reflected in antismoking legislation

Mainstream smoke Smoke that is directly inhaled.

Sidestream smoke Smoke generated by smoldering tobacco.

The direct long-term health effects of sidestream smoke have not been fully documented. However, it has been established that nicotine and carbon monoxide are found in much higher concentrations in sidestream smoke than in mainstream smoke. Therefore, persons who suffer from chronic cardiovascular and pulmonary diseases are certainly at some risk of intensifying their conditions when exposed to sidestream smoke.

Most people say that sidestream smoke irritates their eyes, noses, and throats. People in a room where many people are smoking are found to have higher-than-normal heart rates, elevated blood pressure, and abnormally high carbon monoxide levels in their blood.

Sidestream smoke is especially harmful to babies and young children. Because they breathe faster than adults and inhale more air and more pollutants in comparison to their body weight, smoke-filled air is especially dangerous for little children. Furthermore, many of their natural defenses against lung infections have not developed. Very young children spend also more time indoors at home than people in any other age group, so it is not surprising that young children whose parents smoke at home have twice as many respiratory illnesses as other children. This may be the result of their breathing air containing tobacco smoke coupled with their parents passing on their own respiratory infections to the children.

Nonsmokers' Rights

For a long time the only American laws prohibiting smoking were designed to protect public health and safety rather than to promote personal health. For example, smoking was prohibited in places where combustible materials were used. But in recent years the number of people who believe smoking is harmful and should be restricted to fewer places has increased. In 1964, the year of the first surgeon general's report, *Smoking and Health,* only 52 percent of the people interviewed in a national survey thought smoking should be increasingly restricted. By 1975 that figure jumped to 70 percent. Even though smoking restrictions would inconvenience them at times, more than half of the smokers in the 1975 survey wanted more legal limitations on smoking. In many states smoking is prohibited in public buildings, like schools, libraries, legislative meeting rooms, and places

No Smoking
Please
smoking is
permitted only in
designated areas.
Minnesota
Clean Indoor Air Act
1975 Legislative Statute
BARBER SHOP

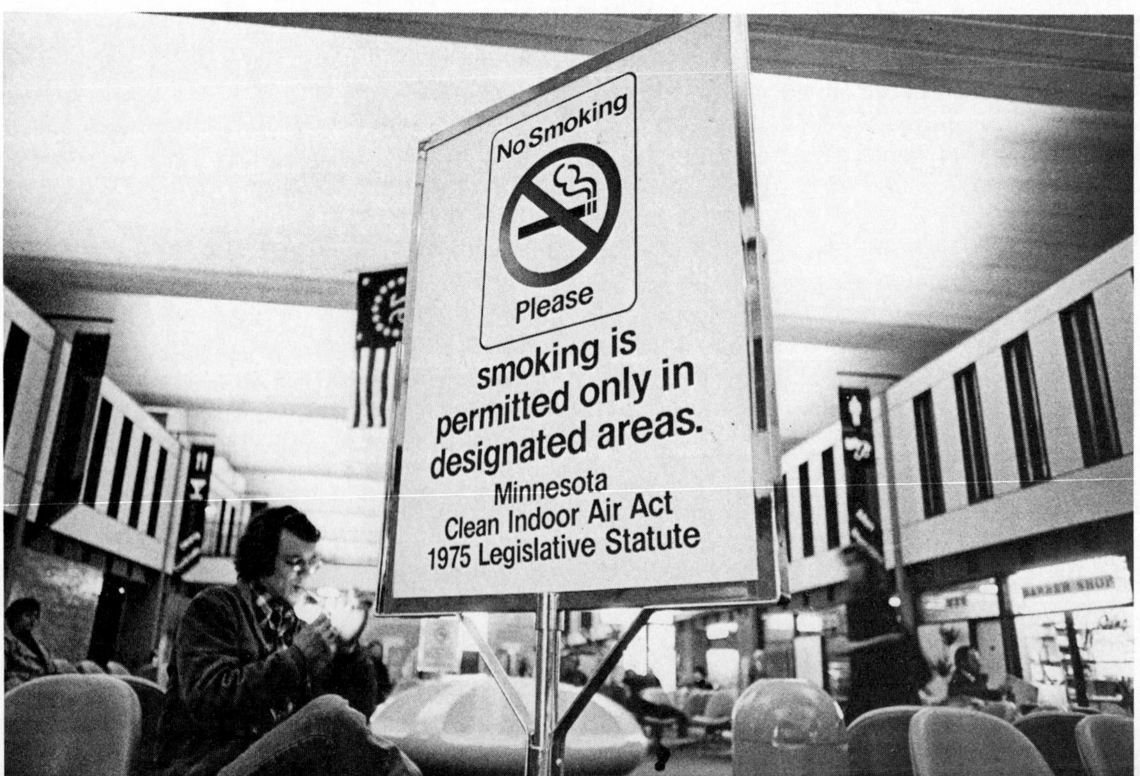

There is still a great deal of controversy surrounding the rights of smokers and nonsmokers. Recent legislation is directed at preserving nonsmokers' health by designating specific areas in public places where smoking is permitted. (Photo from Getsung/Anderson/Photo Researchers, Inc.)

of entertainment; and it is often prohibited or limited to designated areas on vehicles of public transportation. Smoking in areas where it is forbidden is a misdemeanor in some states, punishable by fines ranging from about $10 to $100.

Both the federal government and private agencies have supported the growing majority of nonsmokers. In 1978 the Department of Health, Education, and Welfare, under the leadership of Secretary Joseph A. Califano, Jr., mounted a special attack on smoking in America, including studies of the nonsmoking population and the health risks they face from secondhand smoke. Action for Smoking and Health (ASH) is a private organization that calls itself "the legal-action arm of the nonsmoking community." ASH is a nonsmokers' lobby working to promote further restrictions on tobacco use and to protect nonsmokers' rights.

People Who Smoke (and Those Who Quit)

Young People and Smoking

Young people try smoking because they are curious, because they think smoking is grown-up, because their parents or friends smoke, or because smoking is frowned upon or forbidden and therefore more attractive. Parental behavior influences children in many areas, and smoking is no exception. Children of parents who smoke are likely to emulate them. If both parents are smokers, a teenager is more than twice as likely to smoke as one whose parents do not smoke. Peer group behavior and gaining acceptance are very important, especially among younger adolescents. Teenagers often begin smoking in order to conform. When close friends or a group of friends are smokers, a teenager is more likely to use cigarettes than one whose friends are nonsmokers.

In the last decade the marked increase in the number of older teenage girls who smoke has prompted a number of studies. According to a report from the surgeon general, teenage girls who smoke tend to be more sociable and more rebellious than their nonsmoking counterparts. Smokers spent more time with their friends, used marijuana and drank alcoholic beverages more often, and reported more sexual experience than teenage girls who did not smoke. More than twice as many girls who smoked said they disliked school, and their grades were lower. They tended to get Cs or Ds, while the nonsmoking girls usually got As and Bs.

Smokeless Tobacco

In recent years the use of smokeless tobacco, or chewing tobacco, has become popular, especially among young Americans. Tobacco manufacturers have undertaken an extensive campaign to promote the use of smokeless tobacco. There is evidence that the campaign is succeeding — sales of smokeless tobacco are increasing at the rate of 11 percent per year, and it is now estimated that there are 22 million users of smokeless tobacco in the United States.

Advertisements for smokeless tobacco imply that the use of smokeless tobacco is less harmful than smoking. This may be true with respect to the development of lung cancer. However, smokeless tobacco acts as an irritant on oral mucosa and causes it to develop a white, wrinkled, and thickened appearance. In 3 to 5 percent of cases this can result in oral cancer.[1] The magnitude of the risk of oral cancer will become clearer as the results of various studies become available in the near future.

Types of Smokers

Whether or not smokers are successful in quitting is related to the reasons they smoke.

1. Pleasure smokers, who usually smoke to enhance their experience of good times, tend not to have a hard time quitting, though they often need to find an appropriate substitute for smoking.
2. Other smokers get satisfaction from the physical manipulation of cigarettes, lighters, matches, and ashtrays. The rituals of lighting up and tending to their cigarettes are soothing to them. For these people, a stone, an interesting key ring, or some other pleasant-to-touch substitute can make quitting easier.
3. A third group of smokers tend to smoke for the lift it gives them. They use cigarettes to help them stay alert or to start the morning or new tasks. For them physical activity, like jogging, calisthenics, or walking helps them to quit. Changing their early morning routines to include exercise or a shower helps them learn to do without that first cigarette they crave.
4. Finally, there is a fourth group of smokers who smoke to feel better about things or to relieve tension. The majority of all smokers and the majority of female smokers are in this group, though reasons for that are not well understood. These smokers must relearn how to cope with upsetting situations. Charting the cigarettes they smoke during the quitting process helps them to become conscious of the emotions that seem to stimulate smoking for them. Thinking through and even listing alternative ways of solving the difficulties in each cigarette-stimulating situation can help these smokers recognize more effective ways of coping.

If you are currently a smoker, why not complete Self-Assessment Exercise 10.2, "Why Do You Smoke?" This will give you an indication of the major reasons you smoke.

SELF-ASSESSMENT EXERCISE 10.2

Why Do You Smoke?

PART I — QUESTIONS

Here are some statements made by people to describe what they get out of smoking cigarettes. How *often* do you feel this way when smoking them? Circle one number for each statement.

Important: Answer Every Question.

	Always	Frequently	Occasionally	Seldom	Never
A. I smoke cigarettes in order to keep myself from slowing down.	5	4	3	2	1
B. Handling a cigarette is part of the enjoyment of smoking it.	5	4	3	2	1
C. Smoking cigarettes is pleasant and relaxing.	5	4	3	2	1
D. I light up a cigarette when I feel angry about something.	5	4	3	2	1
E. When I have run out of cigarettes I find it almost unbearable until I can get them.	5	4	3	2	1
F. I smoke cigarettes automatically without even being aware of it.	5	4	3	2	1
G. I smoke cigarettes to stimulate me, to perk myself up.	5	4	3	2	1
H. Part of the enjoyment of smoking a cigarette comes from the steps I take to light up.	5	4	3	2	1
I. I find cigarettes pleasurable.	5	4	3	2	1
J. When I feel uncomfortable or upset about something, I light up a cigarette.	5	4	3	2	1
K. I am very much aware of the fact when I am not smoking a cigarette.	5	4	3	2	1
L. I light up a cigarette without realizing I still have one burning in the ashtray.	5	4	3	2	1
M. I smoke cigarettes to give me a "lift."	5	4	3	2	1
N. When I smoke a cigarette, part of the enjoyment is watching the smoke as I exhale it.	5	4	3	2	1

(continued)

O. I want a cigarette most when I am comfortable and relaxed.	5	4	3	2	1
P. When I feel "blue" or want to take my mind off cares and worries, I smoke cigarettes.	5	4	3	2	1
Q. I get a real gnawing hunger for a cigarette when I haven't smoked for a while.	5	4	3	2	1
R. I've found a cigarette in my mouth and didn't remember putting it there.	5	4	3	2	1

PART II — HOW TO SCORE:

1. Enter the numbers you have circled to the Test questions in the spaces below, putting the number you have circled to Question A over line A, to question B over line B, etc.
2. Total the 3 scores on each line to get your totals. For example, the sum of your scores over lines A, G, and M gives you your score on *Stimulation*—lines B, H, and N give the score on *Handling,* etc.

							Totals
______	+	______	+	______	=	______	
A		**G**		**M**		**Stimulation**	
______	+	______	+	______	=	______	
B		**H**		**N**		**Handling**	
______	+	______	+	______	=	______	
C		**I**		**O**		**Pleasurable Relaxation**	
______	+	______	+	______	=	______	
D		**J**		**P**		**Crutch: Tension Reduction**	
______	+	______	+	______	=	______	
E		**K**		**Q**		**Craving: Psychological Addiction**	
______	+	______	+	______	=	______	
F		**L**		**R**		**Habit**	

Scores can vary from 3 to 15. Any score 11 and above is *high;* any score 7 and below is *low.* Learn from Part 2 what your scores mean.

PART III — ANSWERS:

1. Stimulation

If you score high or fairly high on this factor, it means that you are one of those smokers who is stimulated by the cigarette—you feel that it helps wake you up, organize your energies, and keep you going. If you try to give up smoking, you may want a safe substitute, a *brisk* walk or moderate exercise, for example, whenever you feel the urge to smoke.

2. Handling

Handling things can be satisfying, but there are many ways to keep your hands busy without lighting up or playing with a cigarette. Why not toy with a pen or pencil? Or try doodling. Or play with a coin, a piece of jewelry, or some other harmless object.

There are plastic cigarettes to play with, or you might even use a real cigarette if you can trust yourself not to light it.

3. Accentuation of Pleasure—Pleasurable Relaxation

It is not always easy to find out whether you use the cigarette to feel *good,* that is, get real, honest pleasure out of smoking (Factor 3) or to keep from feeling so *bad* (Factor 4). About two-thirds of smokers score high or fairly high on *accentuation of pleasure,* and about half of those also score as high or higher on *reduction of negative feelings.*

Those who do get real pleasure out of smoking often find that an honest consideration of the harmful effects of their habit is enough to help them quit. They substitute eating, drinking, social activities, and physical activities—within reasonable bounds—and find they do not seriously miss their cigarettes.

4. Reduction of Negative Feelings, or "Crutch"

Many smokers use the cigarette as a kind of crutch in moments of stress or discomfort, and on occasion it may work; the cigarette is sometimes used as a tranquilizer. But the heavy smoker, the person who tries to handle severe personal problems by smoking many times a day, is apt to discover that cigarettes do not help him deal with his problems effectively.

When it comes to quitting, this kind of smoker may find it easy to stop when everything is going well, but may be tempted to start again in a time of crisis. Again, physical exertion, eating, drinking, or social activity—in moderation—may serve as useful substitutes for cigarettes, even in times of tension. The choice of a substitute depends on what will achieve the same effect without having any appreciable risk.

5. "Craving" or Psychological Addiction

Quitting smoking is difficult for the person who scores high on this factor, that of *psychological addiction.* For him, the craving for the next cigarette begins to build up the moment he puts one out, so tapering off is not likely to work. He must go "cold turkey."

it may be helpful for him to smoke more than usual for a day or two, so that the taste for cigarettes is spoiled, and then isolate himself completely from cigarettes until the craving is gone. Giving up cigarettes may be so difficult and cause so much discomfort that once he does quit, he will find it easy to resist the temptation to go back to smoking because he knows that some day he will have to go through the same agony again.

6. Habit

This kind of smoker is no longer getting much satisfaction from his cigarettes. He just lights them frequently without even realizing he is doing so. He may find it easy to quit and stay off if he can break the habit patterns he has built up. Cutting down gradually may be quite effective if there is a change in the way the cigarettes are smoked and the conditions under which they are smoked. They key to success is becoming *aware* of each cigarette you

(continued)

smoke. This can be done by asking yourself, "Do I really want this cigarette?" You may be surprised at how many you do not want.

If you do not score high on any of the six factors, chances are that you do not smoke very much or have not been smoking for very many years. If so, giving up smoking—and staying off—should be easy.

If you score high on several categories, you apparently get several kinds of satisfaction from smoking and will have to find several solutions. Certain combinations of scores may indicate that giving up smoking will be especially difficult. Those who score high on both Factor 4 and Factor 5, *reduction of negative feelings* and *craving,* may have a particularly hard time in going off smoking and in staying off. However, there are ways to do it; many smokers represented by this combination have been able to quit.

Others who score high on Factors 4 and 5 may find it useful to change their patterns of smoking and cut down at the same time. They can try to smoke fewer cigarettes, smoke them only half-way down, use low-tar-and-nicotine cigarettes, and inhale less often and less deeply. After several months of this temporary solution, they may find it easier to stop completely.

You must make two important decisions: (1) whether to try to do without the satisfactions you get from smoking or find an appropriate, less hazardous substitute, and (2) whether to try to cut out cigarettes all at once, or taper off.

Your scores should guide you in making both of these decisions.

Source: U.S. Public Health Service, *Smoker's Self-Testing Kit,* Washington, D.C.: US Dept. HEW, USPHS Publication No. 75-8716, 1975, p. 4.

Some Problems of Quitting

Many people try to give up cigarettes but start smoking again because they don't feel the positive health consequences of not smoking. To them, the loss of the pleasure of smoking seems too high a price for the vague, intangible health gains. Not smoking diminishes the risk of sickness and death but does not offer clear or dramatic improvements in a person's health. It takes ten years for the risk of lung cancer to be reduced to the same level of risk of someone who has never smoked, and it may be months before a former smoker's lungs clear and heal enough for improvement to be noticed.

Within 12 hours of a smoker's last cigarette, the carbon monoxide level in the blood decreases dramatically, but unfortunately this sign of returning health cannot be felt. Gradually, coughing and sputum production decrease, and shortness of breath diminishes. Some people who quit smoking report that they are more sensitive to the taste of food, that they need less sleep, and that they feel more alert and alive in the morning. But it is unclear whether these results are caused by the absence of cigarettes, by the psychological boost quitters sometimes get from setting goals for themselves, or by the life-style changes people make during the quitting process. But when positive gains are experienced, people are more likely to stay with their resolve and resist smoking. Some smokers plan positive, tangible rewards for every few weeks in which they meet their nonsmoking goals. The first 90 days without cigarettes are the hardest, and the greatest return to smoking occurs within that time.

Motives and Strategies for Quitting

Smokers today are more aware than ever before of the health risks they are incurring, and they are experiencing more pressure to quit from their friends and families. Some would like to stop smoking to set a good example for their children or for young people they know; others would like to feel more in control of themselves and want to change aspects of their life-styles that are harmful to their health. For still others, the expense of smoking has become a burden. Smoking one pack of cigarettes each day costs about $270 a year.

There are many different approaches to quitting the cigarette habit. Because of variations in the ways they are evaluated and the lack of long-term follow-up studies, it is hard to compare their effectiveness. Many support-group smoking cessation programs are available throughout the country. Some are sponsored by profit-making

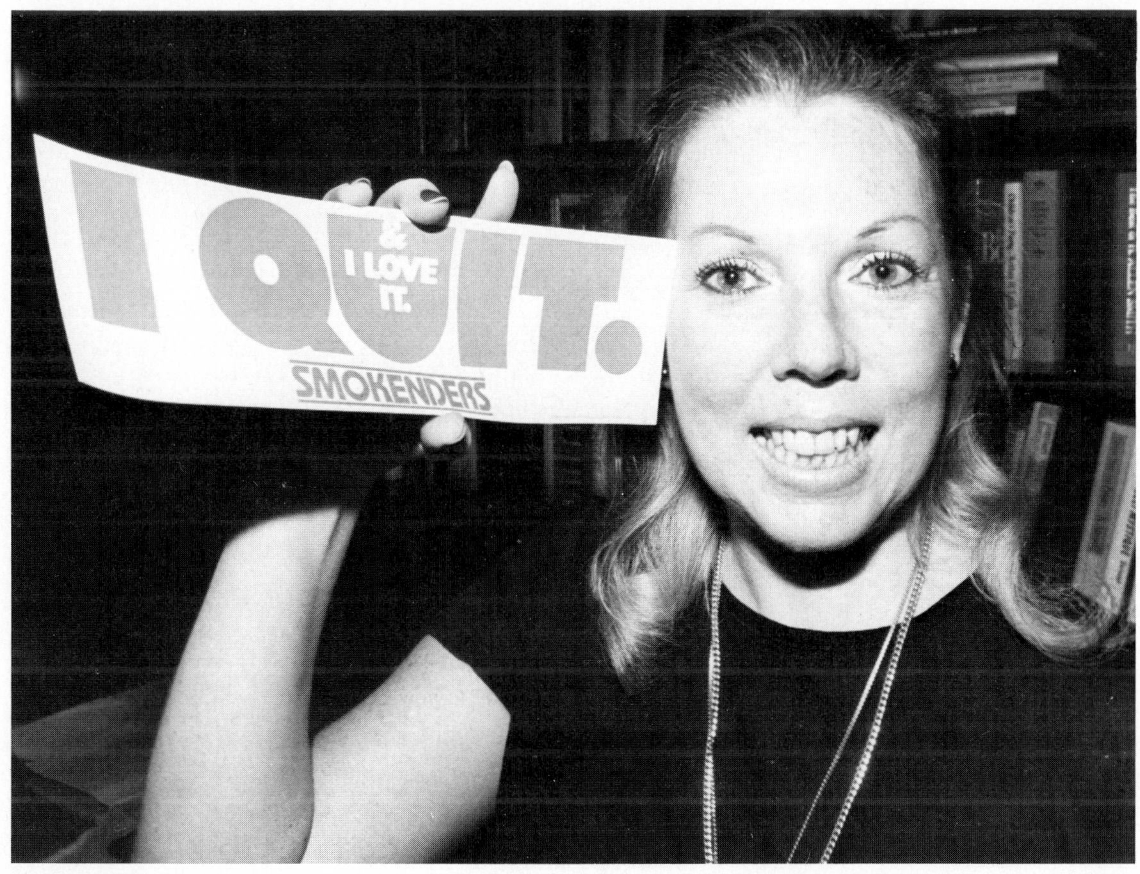

Increasing interest in leading a healthy life prompts many people to give up smoking on their own or with the group support offered at "quit smoking" clinics such as SmokEnders. (Photo from United Press International)

corporations, like SmokEnders; others are sponsored by voluntary health agencies, like the American Cancer Society or the American Heart Association. Still others are sponsored by health professionals in local communities.

Most support groups offer the quitting smoker positive reinforcement through the interaction of group members and counseling of physicians, psychiatrists, therapists, and ex-smokers. Smokers usually examine their own smoking patterns and learn several methods of quitting. After they choose a method that seems appropriate, they help each other and the members in their group with phone calls and other kinds of support. Some smokers go to physicians who have devised ways of helping people quit. Certain businesses and corporations have five-day plans during which they provide various services and incentives for their employees who stop smoking. Still other smokers use a series of special filters that gradually reduce the amount of tar and nicotine in their cigarettes. Other people use acupuncture, hypnosis, behavior modification strategies, or aversion therapy.

By far the largest proportion of people who stop smoking do so on their own. According to the National Center for Health Statistics, about 29 million Americans stopped smoking between 1964 and 1975, and 95 percent of them quit on their own.[2] As a result of this trend many organizations have developed packets of self-help materials, manuals, or workbooks designed to help people examine their reasons for smoking, become aware of and record each cigarette they smoke, and gradually eliminate certain cigarettes from their daily routines. To help smoking become a conscious behavior, many of these programs recommend that smokers wrap each pack of cigarettes in a piece of paper secured with a rubber band, thereby forcing themselves to make each cigarette a conscious decision. Rising earlier and setting aside regular time for exercise are often suggested as well. (See Table 10–3 for a synopsis of some smoking-cessation strategies.)

Nicorette

Recently a new drug that might help cigarette smokers quit the habit has been made available in the United States. The drug, called Nicorette, was developed by a Swedish company and has been used in Europe for a long time.

Nicorette is a chewing gum, available only by prescription. A full prescription contains 96 squares of gum, with each square supplying a two-milligram dose of nicotine. This is equivalent to the amount of nicotine in two strong cigarettes. According to the directions, an individual square of gum should be chewed for 20 to 30 minutes. As one chews the gum, small amounts of nicotine, released gradually, help in curbing the urge to smoke a cigarette.

Table 10-3 A Selection of Smoking Cessation Strategies and Programs

Name of Program/ Strategy	Source	Description of Strategy/Program
Freedom from Smoking in 20 Days	American Lung Association	Strategies to help cope with situations that precede smoking behavior, includes choosing rewards for not smoking and relaxation techniques.
Quit-Smoking Clinic	American Lung Association	Seven-session clinic that includes extensive use of behavior modification techniques and group support.
Great American Smokeout	American Cancer Society	More of a national promotional anti-smoking campaign than a smoking cessation strategy. The American Cancer Society selects one day in November of each year as a target day for smokers to quit. In conjunction with the target date, educational messages about the health hazards associated with smoking are part of a massive educational campaign.
I Quit Kit	American Cancer Society	Self-monitoring activities that are designed to help the smoker stop smoking in one week.
Fresh Start	American Cancer Society	Four one-hour group sessions in which a therapist uses psychotherapeutic group counseling approaches to help a group (8–18 people) of smokers stop smoking.
Schick Program	Schick Centers for the Control of Smoking (25 smoking centers located in the U.S.)	Schick program consists of five-day conditioning sessions that include the use of "electro-stimulus" conditioning techniques.
Smokeless System	American Health Foundation	Program stresses use of a conditioning system to make smoking difficult and unpleasant, thereby decreasing the frequency of smoking until the smoker has stopped.
Five Day Smoking Cessation Program	Seventh Day Adventist Churches	Stop-smoking program includes lectures by a physician-clergy team, use of multimedia methods, and group interaction strategies.
Nicotine Chewing Gum	Nicorette; Distributed by Merrell Dow Pharmaceutical, Inc.	Prescription chewing gum that contains nicotine. Use of gum satisfies the urge to smoke in some smokers.
SmokEnders	SmokEnders Clinics (30 clinics located throughout the U.S.)	Program consists of nine two-hour weekly sessions. Group therapy techniques are employed with emphasis on within-group reinforcement.

Between March and July 1984 hundreds of thousands of prescriptions for Nicorette were written. Some physicians refuse to write prescriptions for Nicorette since data on the long-term effects of its use have not been documented.

One of the big drawbacks to quitting smoking is the experience of withdrawal effects, including irritability, restlessness, and difficulty in concentration. Nicorette may not be a panacea; but if it helps to reduce the withdrawal symptoms, then perhaps millions of smokers who otherwise would not quit will be able to give up the habit.

Which Smoking-Cessation Program Is Best for You?

This is a difficult question to answer since there is so much individual variation in smoking behavior and so much individual variation in responsiveness to stop-smoking strategies. In 1983 the American Lung Association suggested that smokers should ask the following questions regarding the stop-smoking program in which they are interested:

- Does the program offer a variety of components to address cessation and its maintenance?
- Is the program sponsored by a recognized educational, public health, medical, or civic organization? If hypnosis is being used, is it being provided by a licensed or certified professional in psychology, psychiatry, or social work? If rapid smoking or nicotine gum is being used, is appropriate medical back-up available for screening before treatment is started or for referral during treatment if necessary?
- In looking over the program, does it give me a positive feeling and does it appear to meet my needs as I perceive them?

Answers to these questions will help the particular smoker select a suitable program. However, the bottom line is that whatever the program selected, the smoker must still want to quit smoking, otherwise any benefits derived from the program will probably be short-lived.

Government and Smoking

The federal government's policies on tobacco are inconsistent. On the one hand, tobacco is an important product in the U.S. economy; on the other, its negative effects have severe impact on American citizens and the total costs of health care in the country.

The U.S. Department of Agriculture continues to support tobacco farming and the manufacture of cigarettes. Because the representatives of tobacco states form a powerful faction, large numbers of antismoking measures have been introduced in Congress since 1966, but no major legislation in this field has been passed. In Congress, more bills favoring the tobacco industry are introduced and passed into law than bills and laws to support the public's health.

YOUR HEALTH TODAY

House Version of New Cigarette Warnings

Surgeon General's Warning:
Smoking Causes LUNG CANCER, HEART DISEASE and EMPHYSEMA.

Surgeon General's Warning:
Quitting Smoking Now Greatly Reduces Serious Health Risk.

Surgeon General's Warning:
Smoking by Pregnant Women May Result in Fetal Injury and Premature Birth.

Surgeon General's Warning:
Cigarette Smoke Contains Carbon Monoxide

Source: From National Interagency Council on Smoking and Health, *Smoking and Health Reporter,* Vol. 1, No. 4, July 1984, p. 4.

However, a number of state senators and representatives and governmental organizations have been instrumental in limiting cigarette advertising and smoking in public places, as well as promoting public education about the health hazards of smoking. In 1964, for example, the Federal Trade Commission ordered health warnings to appear on all packages of cigarettes sold in this country. The Federal Communication Commission's ruling in 1967 that radio and television stations broadcast public-service antismoking announcements to balance cigarette advertisements had a substantial effect on Americans' smoking habits, and in 1970 cigarette commercials on radio and television were banned. Recently, the House approved stronger warnings on cigarette packages (see the box entitled "House Version of New Cigarette Warnings").

Success on the state level has also been mixed. State antismoking laws have sometimes been poorly written, resulting in confusion and lack of enforcement. Guidelines for local laws have been clarified with the help of voluntary health organizations like the American Lung Association. One of the most successful and comprehensive antismoking laws has been enacted in the state of Minnesota. The Clean Indoor Air Act is based on the state's policy of protecting the environment and public health and comfort. Smoking in public places is limited to designated areas. Violators are guilty of misdemeanors, and state or local boards of health or any affected party may initiate court action against repeated violators.

Summary

Despite scientific evidence that smoking is harmful to health, more than 50 million Americans continue to smoke. After the publication of *Smoking and Health: A Report to the Surgeon General* in 1964, which pointed out the health hazards of smoking, the percentage of smokers declined, and by 1975 smokers were a minority in the U.S. population. The exception to the pattern is teenage girls, who are smoking more than ever before.

Cigarette smoke contains more than 3,000 separate substances, many of which are harmful to health. Hydrogen cyanide damages the lining of the bronchial tubes and lungs, and nitrogen oxide is a cause of lung disease. Carbon monoxide, by displacing oxygen from the blood, contributes to the development of heart disease. The tars in cigarettes contain cancer-causing substances.

Smoking styles affect the absorption of smoke. Taking many puffs on each cigarette, retaining smoke in the mouth or lungs, and smoking a cigarette down to the end all increase a smoker's exposure.

Smoking has an immediate effect on the body. It irritates the trachea and damages the cilia in the respiratory tract. Cells in the lungs grow abnormally large and excess mucus is secreted. Normal heart rate and blood pressure are altered.

Long-term effects of smoking include increased risk of death from several diseases. There is a strong relationships between smoking and coronary heart disease, particularly in men between the ages of 35 and 55. About 75 percent of all cases of lung cancer are found in smokers, and smoking is also associated with cancer of the mouth and throat and even of the bladder, kidney, and pancreas.

Certain groups of people face particularly great health risks from smoking. These include people with stomach ulcers, workers exposed to toxic materials, people with circulatory disease, oral contraceptive users, and pregnant women.

Smokers are not the only ones affected by smoking. Secondhand smoke is harmful to others as well, and many groups are advocating legislation to restrict smoking in public places.

The smoking habit is related to several factors, including dependency on nicotine, positive associations of smoking with pleasant events, and fear of withdrawal.

Quitting smoking has important consequences for improving health, but often these benefits are not dramatic enough to provide sufficient motivation. Many people have joined special programs, and special self-help materials are available from many organizations. Nicorette is now being used in the United States at a method to quit smoking.

Governmental policies are often inconsistent, supporting the production of tobacco but attempting to discourage people from smoking. Recently the House approved stronger cigarette warning labels.

Review and Discussion

1. What are the current trends of smoking in the United States by age group and sex?
2. Describe the effect of cigarette smoke on the body, with particular attention to the effect of carbon monoxide.
3. What are the immediate physical effects of smoking a cigarette?
4. Select two serious diseases and describe the role of cigarette smoking in increasing the risk of contracting them.
5. Name five categories of people who face greater than average health risks from smoking.
6. What health problems are associated with second-hand smoke?
7. Why is stopping smoking such a difficult task for most people?
8. Describe at least five techniques that could help a person quit smoking.
9. Discuss the advantages of using Nicorette, as a method to stop smoking.
10. How does the federal government encourage tobacco use and growth of the tobacco industry?
11. What types of legislation controlling smoking have been enacted? What additional laws do you think there should be?

Further Reading

Danaher, Brian, and Edward Lichtenstein. *Become An Ex-Smoker.* Englewood Cliffs, N.J.: Prentice-Hall, Inc., 1978.
Practical guide to smoking cessation. Excellent examples of effective stop-smoking techniques. (Paperback.)

U.S. Department of Health, Education and Welfare. *Bibliography on Smoking and Health.* Washington, D.C.: U.S. Government Printing Office, 1981.
A comprehensive annotated bibliography on smoking and health issues.

U.S. Department of Health, Education and Welfare. *Smoking and Health: A Report to the Surgeon General.* Washington, D.C.: U.S. Government Printing Office, 1979.
The definitive document on smoking and health. Surveys all the literature on smoking and summarizes key finding in practical terms. (Paperback.)

U.S. Department of Health and Human Services. *The Health Consequences of Smoking for Women.* Washington, D.C.: U.S. Department of Health and Human Services, 1980.
Excellent summary of key relationships between smoking and its impact on women. Good discussion of special risks during pregnancy. (Paperback.)

U.S. Department of Health and Human Services. *Smoking Programs for Youth.* Bethesda, Md.: National Cancer Institute, 1980.
Good overview of smoking and youth. Emphasis on programming implications for this special target group. (Paperback.)

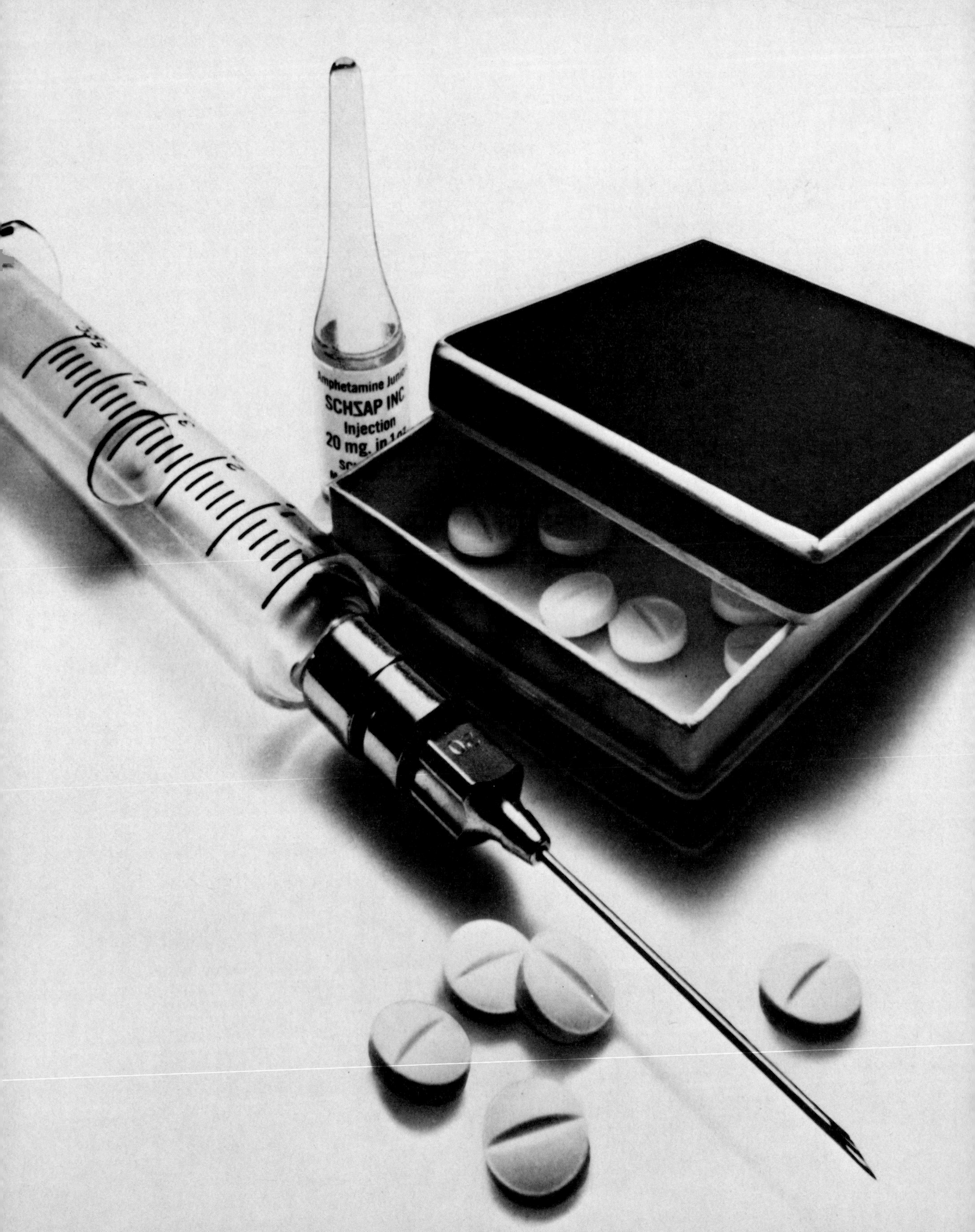
SCHZAP INC
Injection

Chapter 11
Drugs

KEY POINTS

- Drugs are substances that alter physical or mental functions when taken into the body.
- Drugs are used for a variety of reasons.
- The chronic inappropriate use of drugs is called drug abuse.
- Drugs produce their effects by altering the production, release, action, metabolism, or reabsorption of specific chemicals involved in the transmission of impulses between neurons in the brain.
- The pharmacological action of a drug, the mind-set of the user, and the setting are among the factors that determine how an individual will respond to the drug.
- A drug user's body adapts to the drug, and if administration of the drug is stopped suddenly, the user may become physically ill; this reaction is called the withdrawal syndrome.
- There are two kinds of drug dependence—physical and psychological.
- Psychoactive drugs may be classified according to their major observable effects: as depressants (including narcotic analgesics, sedative hypnotics, minor tranquilizers, and major tranquilizers), stimulants, or hallucinogens.
- Means of help for addicts include narcotic antagonists, therapeutic communities, and methadone maintenance programs.

BROADLY defined, **drugs** are substances that alter physical or mental functions when taken into the body. Most drugs are used to prevent or cure illness or to relieve pain. However, throughout history people in almost every society have also found or made drugs to alter their moods and perceptions. Many of the drugs known to the ancients are still in use today. In our own hemisphere more than 2,000 years ago, the Aztecs prepared and drank a kind of tea to induce hallucinations during religious ceremonies. Chemical analysis of the vinelike leaves they used indicates that they contained a substance related to LSD. The use of consciousness-altering drugs for the purpose of enhancing experience, relaxing, or temporarily escaping from reality was common in many civilizations, and it has become a widespread practice in our society today.

Drug Substance that alters physical or mental functions.

Many Americans overuse all kinds of drugs. From the moment they enter medical school, the men and women who become our physicians are barraged with literature from pharmaceutical companies vying for their attention and future business. Some critics of American health care suggest that both doctors and patients think first of a chemical or pharmacological solution for almost every problem instead of approaching the problem in some other way. The very nature of the American marketplace has helped to create a drug-conscious population. The public is continually exposed, for instance, to the competing claims of different drugs products; advertisements urge consumers to try over-the-counter drugs to relieve every imaginable condition from headaches to constipation. And though many people do not think of coffee, cigarettes, and alcoholic beverages as

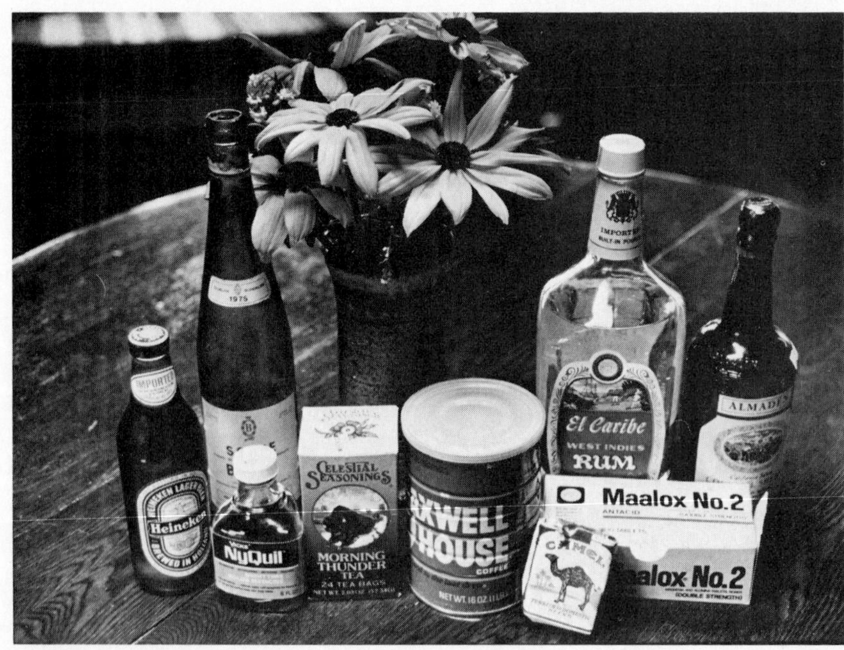

Although people do not think of coffee, cigarettes, and alcoholic beverages as drugs, their effects over the long term can sometimes be as harmful as the stronger prescription and "street" drugs. (Photo by Peter Simon/Stock, Boston)

psychoactive, or mood-altering, **drugs,** these substances do have significant effects on the human body via the central nervous system (CNS). These are not the only psychoactive drugs, of course, and we will discuss many of the more potent ones throughout this chapter.

Psychoactive drugs Drugs that alter mental processes.

The Use, Misuse, and Abuse of Drugs

When used for medical reasons, drugs can be helpful and even lifesaving. Aspirin used in moderation to relieve headache is an example of the analgesic, or pain-relieving, use of a drug. Taking prescribed antibiotics when you have a serious infection will help the body overcome the infection, and in some cases would save your life.

Either taking prescribed or over-the-counter (OTC) drugs in excess of recommended doses or taking them more often than recommended, constitutes **drug misuse.** Taking prescribed medication without consulting a physician (for example, using up an old prescription or someone else's prescription) is another case of misuse. Similarly, if you *occasionally* use a drug for some purpose other than its intended one—to feel euphoric, perhaps, instead of to kill pain—this also is considered misuse.

Drug misuse Taking prescribed medication without consulting a physician.

Chronically using a drug for a reason for which it was not intended, however, is called **drug abuse.** People are often impelled to take mood-altering drugs to escape stressful conditions that assail them in daily life. These drugs range from LSD and marijuana to painkillers, cocaine, and alcohol. However, unless drug abusers in the meantime are taking action to deal with their problems—and drug use may actually interfere with taking such action—the stressful conditions will remain unchanged. The user will continue to rely on drugs, although the escape they offer is fleeting and illusory, and thus will become fixed in a repetitive behavior pattern.

Drug abuse Chronic use of a drug for a purpose it is not intended.

Tolerance, a physical adaptation that causes certain drugs to become less effective with repeated use, also elicits abuse, since a person using a tolerance-inducing drug must take larger and larger doses to obtain a desired effect. **Physical dependence,** like the old term *addiction,* involves drug tolerance and the appearance of withdrawal symptoms if drug use is suddenly stopped. The distinction between physical and psychological dependence is necessary because they may occur separately. **Psychological dependence** is the emotional attachment to the drug's effects and even to the process of administering or taking a substance. Could drugs be causing a problem in your life? Complete Self-Assessment Exercise 11.1 and find out.

Tolerance Physical adaptation to repeated use of a certain drug.

Physical dependence The state in which one experiences withdrawal symptoms upon discontinuance of a drug.

Psychological dependence Emotional attachment to a particular drug.

Reasons for Drug Use and Abuse

People give many reasons for using all kinds of psychoactive drugs. Hallucinogens like LSD and marijuana are especially appealing to

SELF-ASSESSMENT EXERCISE 11.1

Does Your Drug Use Behavior Cause Problems in Your Life?

It is often difficult to determine if the use of drugs (prescription, OTC, alcohol, nicotine, caffeine, or even illicit drugs) is causing problems in a person's life. Most of the time people don't realize that problems they experience can be attributed to their drug use behavior. Your responses to the following series of questions will help you to determine if certain drugs are causing problems in your life.

PART I: Write in the names of drugs (alcohol, nicotine, prescription, OTC, etc.) that you use on a regular basis.

1. ______________________ 4. ______________________

2. ______________________ 5. ______________________

3. ______________________

PART II: For *each* drug you listed in Part 1, circle "yes" or "no" to the following questions.

YES NO **1.** Do you feel that your day is "not complete" unless you take this drug?

YES NO **2.** Do you find yourself thinking a lot about using this drug?

YES NO **3.** Does using this drug modify your mood or behavior to the point that you could cause an accident?

YES NO **4.** Do you neglect normal duties or responsibilities in order to take this drug?

YES NO **5.** Does use of this drug ever interfere with the quality of your interpersonal relationships?

YES NO **6.** Do you ever lie to other people about using this drug?

YES NO **7.** Do you ever lie to other people about the amount of this drug that you use?

YES NO **8.** Does use of this drug ever keep you from doing something you would like to do?

YES NO **9.** Does the use of this drug interefere with memory, awareness, or reasoning?

YES NO **10.** Does the money spent in order to use this drug cause you some financial difficulties

Interpretation: If you circled Yes to any *one* of the above questions with respect to any of the drugs you use as listed in Part I, then you should seriously consider talking to someone about your drug use behavior. Chances are that the drug is causing—or has the potential for causing—problems in your life.

people who believe such substances can help them achieve a better understanding of themselves or who hope to enhance their creativity. Other people use these and other psychoactive drugs hoping to avoid feeling powerless and ineffective in a complicated world. Still others use drugs in an attempt to establish their identity as members of a peer group or subculture and to feel a sense of belonging when regional, family, and religious ties have become weak. Other reasons for drug use, misuse, or abuse are listed in the box entitled "Reasons for Drug Use, Misuse, or Abuse." If you are interested in discovering the many alternatives to drug use, see the box entitled "Alternatives to Drug Use."

OTC and Prescription Drugs

About 175 million Americans regularly drink coffee, close to 100 million drink alcoholic beverages, and about 50 million smoke tobacco. In most areas of the country these are socially accepted, legal drugs, even though smoking cigarettes and drinking alcoholic beverages cause more illness and death every year than use of all other mood-altering drugs combined. These and other legal drugs are purchased over-the-counter, the largest channel of drug distribution in the United States. Psychoactive drugs sold on the OTC market include diet aids, cough syrups, tranquilizers, and sleep aids.

Most barbiturates, sedative-hypnotics, minor tranquilizers, antidepressive drugs, and amphetamines are purchased through the prescription market. Drugs sold in this way require the written or verbal order of a physician. OTC and prescription drugs combined cost Americans more than $16 billion a year, and more than a quarter of the drugs bought through these channels are psychoactive.

Illegal Drugs

Drugs purchased on the black market include marijuana, LSD and other hallucinogens, illegally manufactured alcohol, and vast quantities of prescription drugs that have been diverted from their normal channels of distribution. These are often referred to as *street drugs.* Another important source of psychoactive drugs for many people is the informal "gray market" of friends and associates who provide drugs that are normally prescribed by physicians.

The use of psychoactive drugs is extensive. Some estimates suggest that more than half of all Americans over the age of 13 have tried at least one mind-altering drug other than coffee, cigarettes, or alcoholic beverages. Annual surveys of drug use by high school seniors indicate that most have at least tried marijuana and that many use it on a regular basis. A variety of other illegal drugs are used in varying degrees, although alcohol and tobacco are the most widely used drugs among young adults (see Figure 11–1).

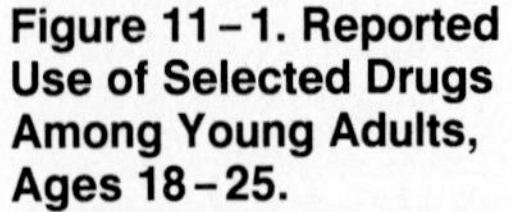

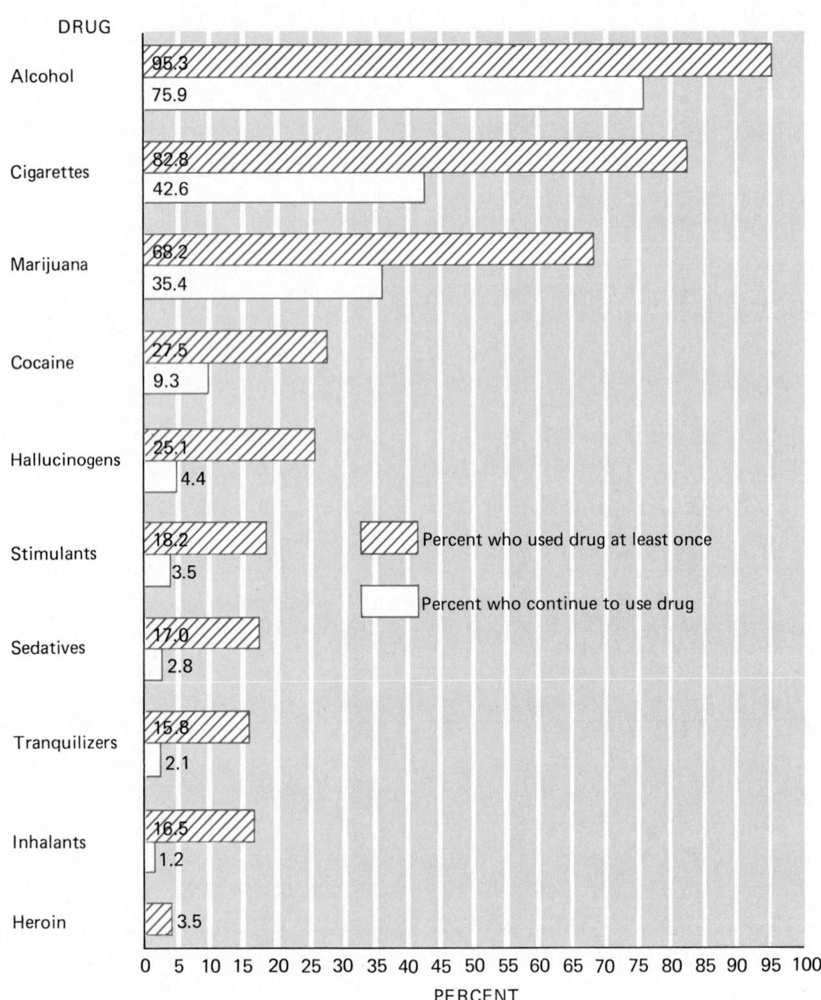

Figure 11–1. Reported Use of Selected Drugs Among Young Adults, Ages 18–25. (Source: National Institute on Drug Abuse, *National Survey on Drug Abuse: Main Findings, 1979* [Washington, D.C.: USDHHS, 1980].)

Factors Influencing Drug Effects

Pharmacological Action

Pharmacological action A drug's scientifically tested effects.

Any discussion of the effects of drugs is complicated by several factors. First, a single drug often causes multiple effects in more than one part of the brain. Second, different doses of the same drug produce a variety of effects. Finally, drug effects are not constant and entirely predictable, because the substances are acting on the brain and nervous system of a unique individual, and the effects can vary considerably from one person to another. Therefore, the **pharmacological action** of a drug (its scientifically tested effects) is only one of the factors that determines how an individual will react to a drug on a given occasion.

YOUR HEALTH TODAY

Reasons for Drug Use, Misuse, or Abuse

- Desire for physical satisfaction
- Physical relaxation
- Relief from sickness
- Desire for more energy
- Desire to stimulate senses
- Sexual stimulation
- Relief from psychological problems
- Relief from bad moods
- Relief from anxiety
- To gain peer acceptance
- To solve personal problems
- To promote social change
- To escape boredom
- To study better
- To improve creativity

Set and Setting

Besides the pharmacological action of a drug, two other factors, called set and setting, are especially important in determining the effects of mood-changing drugs. **Set** is an individual's personality and expectations about what a drug will do, and **setting** is the physical and social environment in which a drug is taken.

Set An individual's perceptions and expectations of a drug's effect.

Setting Physical and social environment in which a drug is taken.

Studies have indicated that the more a drug alters the user's perceptions and emotions, the greater the importance of setting. If amphetamines, which are central nervous system stimulants, are admin-

YOUR HEALTH TODAY

Alternatives to Drug Use

- Relaxation exercises
- Recreational activities
- Mental or intellectual hobbies
- Change of peer groups
- Participation in community activities
- Participation in political activities
- Physical exercises
- Change of dietary patterns
- Increased interest in work activities
- Increased interest in religious activities

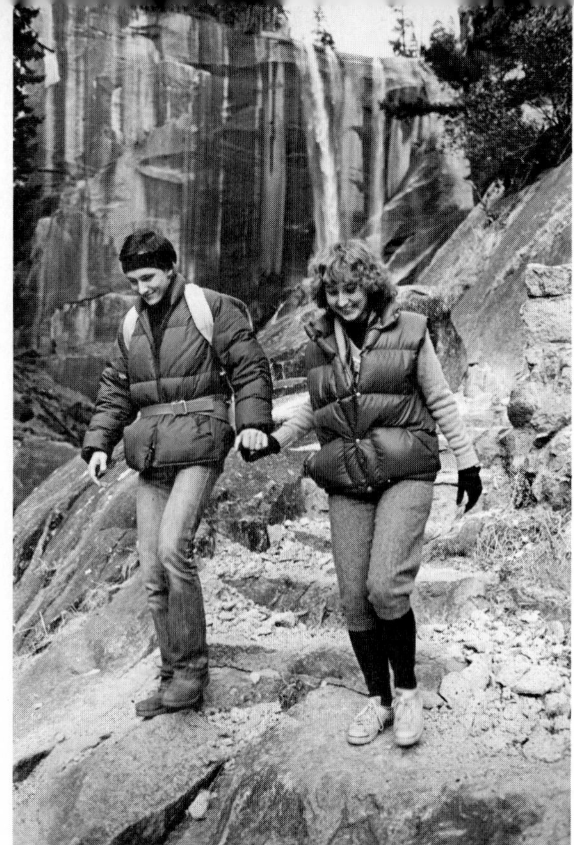

Often people take drugs to relieve tensions or stress, or just as an escape. However, there are many stimulating alternative activities a person can become involved in. (Photo © Peter Menzel/Stock, Boston)

istered in a restful setting to persons who have been told the drugs will induce relaxation and drowsiness, the drugs can actually produce measurable depression of the nervous system — the opposite of their pharmacological effect. Expectations about the effects a drug will produce exert a powerful influence in determining how someone responds to it.

In laboratory experiments to determine the effectiveness of new or established drugs, subjects are often divided into two groups. Without knowing which group is which, one set of subjects will receive the drug being tested, and the other will receive a pharmacologically inactive substance, or **placebo,** like milk sugar or saline. Placebos in such research have produced not only the desirable effects of certain drugs but have also produced side effects like skin rashes, nausea, and dizziness. Most drug researchers and physicians have come to recognize the *placebo effect,* in which people experience certain effects because they expect to experience them, as convincing evidence that the workings of the mind and the body are inseparable and that illness must be treated both psychologically and physically.

Placebo Inactive substance that the user falsely expects to act as a drug.

Other Factors Affecting an Individual's Response

Besides set and setting, a number of other factors affect an individual's reaction to any drug. These factors are related to qualities of the drug, the size of the dose, the way it is administered, and the physical condition of the user.

Size of the Dose

With most drugs larger doses simply intensify the effects produced by smaller amounts, as might be expected. But some other drugs have entirely different effects at different dose levels. Atropine, for example, can slow a heart that is beating too rapidly when the drug is administered in small doses. In larger doses, it can be used to increase heart rate in patients whose hearts are pumping too slowly.

Purity of the Drug

Many illegal psychoactive drugs are "cut," or mixed, with other, less expensive substances. Heroin, for example, is usually cut to a very small proportion of the substance with which it is mixed, and when heroin of unusual strength appears unexpectedly on the street, users may overdose by accident. The substances with which any drug is mixed, of course, may themselves have pharmacological effects and thus alter a person's response to the original drug.

Biological Variables

People's age, sex, weight, and physical condition affect their individual reaction to a drug. Since the effects of most drugs are related to their chemical concentration in the blood, the impact of a certain amount of the drug will naturally vary according to the size and weight of the person taking it. Furthermore, a drug is likely to have greater effect on a person who is tired or run-down than on one who is healthy and robust. In addition, a dose of barbiturates taken at midday, for example, may have less effect than the same dose taken late at night when the body's systems are in a fatigued state.

Development of Tolerance

When people take a tolerance-inducing drug for a long time and at sufficient dosages, their reactions to another dose of the same drug, or a dose of a related drug, will usually be less than the reactions of those who have never used the drug before.

Contents of the Stomach

The presence of food or other substances in the stomach can affect the way the drug enters the bloodstream when taken orally. Tetracycline, an antibiotic, is rendered ineffective by the presence of milk or dairy products, for example. And when drugs prepared in time-release capsules are taken with alcohol, they enter the bloodstream all at once instead of at intervals.

Drug Interactions

Certain drugs taken together produce very different pharmacological actions than they would if they were taken singly. Particularly dangerous are drug interactions characterized by **potentiation,** or **synergism**—that is, the increasing of the effects of a drug by another

Potentiation Increased effect of certain drugs in combination.

Synergism Augmented action of one substance upon the activity of another.

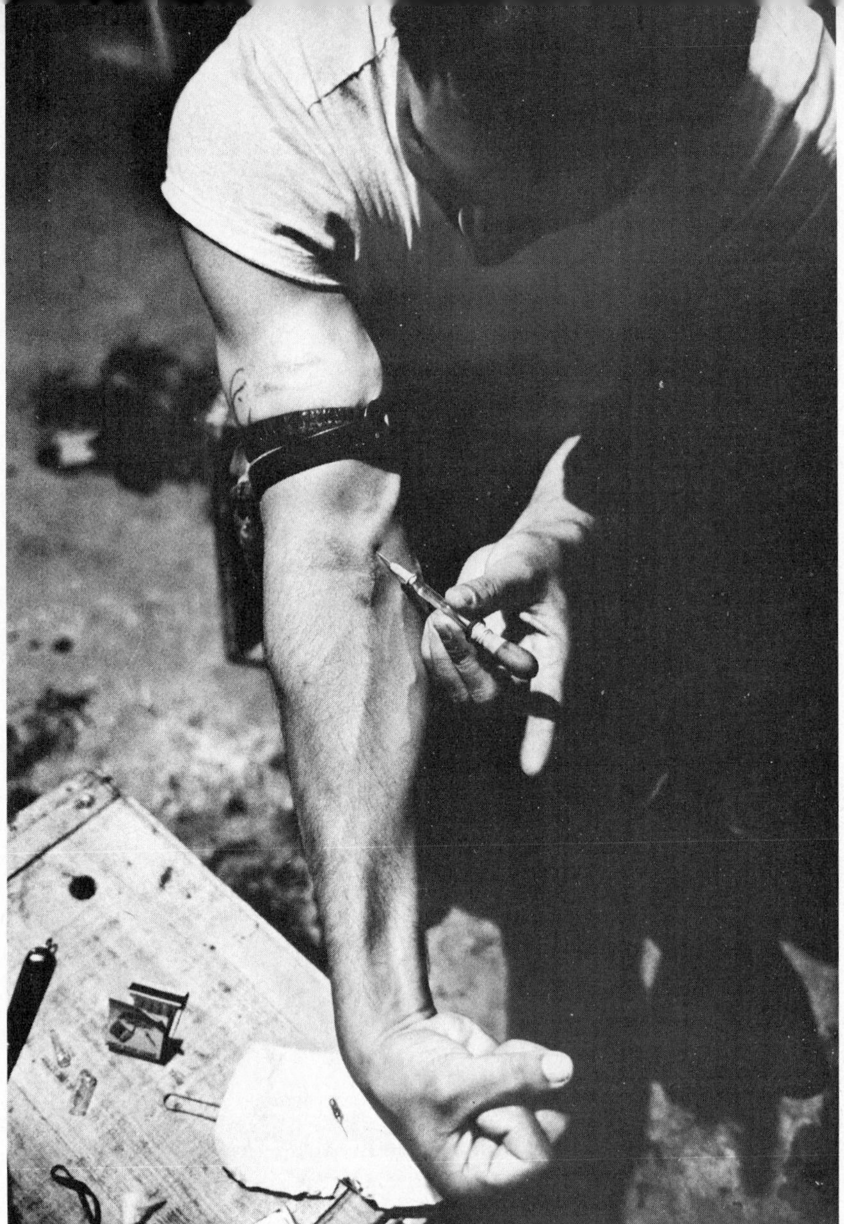

The way in which a drug is taken can affect how a person will react to it. Here the victim mainlines heroin, a highly addictive opium product. (Photo © Bob Combs/Rapho/Photo Researchers, Inc.)

agent taken at the same time. Alcohol can potentiate the effects of OTC drugs like antihistamines or tranquilizers, causing such severe drowsiness that driving a car or operating machinery becomes dangerous. Potentiation of drugs can also work positively: when used in combination, certain antibiotics have increased effectiveness against infection.

Inhibition Interference with the metabolism of a drug.

Antagonism Drug used to counteract symptoms of another drug.

Sometimes a substance inhibits the metabolism of another drug or displaces the other drug from its receptor sites, so that a person experiences the effects of only one of the chemical substances in the body. Such an interaction is called **inhibition.** One example is the inhibiting of the effectiveness of oral contraceptives by barbiturates.

In another sort of interaction, called **antagonism,** one drug nullifies the effect of another by causing the body to react in a certain way. For example, a person who regularly drinks alcoholic beverages may find that the tranquilizing effects of drugs like Valium, Librium, or Miltown are reduced. The nicotine in cigarettes also seems to enhance the metabolism of certain drugs, and smokers tend to get less pain relief than nonsmokers from analgesics like Talwin or Darvon.

Route of Administration

The way a drug is taken affects its total impact on the user and the duration of its effects. For example, morphine injected under the skin (subcutaneously) produces a maximum pain-relieving effect in 30 to 60 minutes, although its effectiveness dissipates rapidly. Injected into a vein, however, morphine's peak effect occurs sooner and is greater. Taken by mouth, it has only 20 to 30 percent of the pain-relieving effect on the same dose of the drug injected under the skin.

Varieties of Psychoactive Drugs

Classifying the varieties of psychoactive drugs is not a simple matter. The legal classification of **narcotics,** established in 1914, is confusing because not all the drugs in this group are narcotic, or sleep-inducing, in nature. Although opium and its derivatives, morphine, heroin, and codeine, are the true narcotics in this group, their synthetic equivalents, such as Percodan, methadone, and Demerol (a milder pain-reliever), are appropriately included in the legal classification. But cocaine and marijuana, substances that have been legally classified as narcotics, are very unlike those drugs in chemical makeup and in the effects they produce, and furthermore, they are extremely different from each other.

Narcotics Opiate derivatives used for pain relief.

For many years drugs were classified according to their potential for leading to **addiction,** or repeated compulsive use thought to be caused by physical adaptations in the user's body. These adaptations produced tolerance and a characteristic illness when drug use was stopped abruptly. **Withdrawal syndrome,** as this reaction was called, is now believed to occur as a result of the body's efforts to function as normally as possible in the continued presence of a drug. Though the exact mechanism of the body's adjustment is not fully understood, it appears to be metabolic in nature. If the administration of the drug is stopped suddenly after the adaptation has occurred, the user becomes physically ill. Current theories of drug action suggest that this happens because the body cannot reverse its adaptation quickly enough when the drug is no longer in the system. In most cases, withdrawal can be reversed with the readministration of the addictive drug or administration of one that produces similar effects.

Addiction Repeated, compulsive use of a drug.

Withdrawal syndrome Physical illness upon discontinuing use of an addictive drug.

The most useful means of classifying psychoactive drugs is according to their major observable effects. In the discussion that follows,

Table 11–1 Types of Psychoactive Drugs

Drug Category	Drug Action*	Specific Drugs
Depressants	depress central nervous system	
narcotic analgesics, or opiates	reduce pain, induce sleep	morphine, codeine, Percodan, Dilaudid, methadone, Demerol, heroin
sedative-hypnotics	act as calming agents, induce sleep	barbiturates, methaqualone (Quaaludes)
minor tranquilizers	reduce anxiety, relieve tension	Valium, meprobamates (Miltown and Equanil), Librium
major tranquilizers	reduce psychotic symptoms	Compazine, Thorazine, Stelazine
Stimulants	stimulate central nervous system	caffeine, cocaine, amphetamines (Benzedrine, Dexedrine, methamphetamine)
Hallucinogens	alter mood and behavior, induce illusions and hallucinations (to a degree varying greatly from one drug to another)	marijuana (?), peyote, mescaline, psilocybin, LSD, PCP (angel dust), deliriants (glue, cleaning fluids, nitrous oxide)

* Note: Individual effects of specific drugs may vary widely.

Depressants Drugs that lower muscular and nervous activity.

Stimulants Drugs that heighten activity of the central nervous system.

Hallucinogens Drugs capable of causing a false perception of sights, sounds, and feelings.

we use three main categories: **depressants** (which tend to depress the central nervous system), **stimulants** (which tend to stimulate the central nervous system), and **hallucinogens** (mind-altering drugs used recreationally). Depressants are divided into four subcategories: narcotic analgesics or opiates (pain-killing, and sleep-inducing drugs), sedative-hypnotics (calming agents and sleep-inducing drugs), minor tranquilizers (antianxiety agents), and major tranquilizers (antipsychotic drugs). (For a convenient summary of the different types of psychoactive drugs, see Table 11–1).

Among the three main categories, the hallucinogens are the drugs with the greatest diversity in their effects. They include drugs that produce relatively mild effects, like marijuana (often not classified as a hallucinogen), and drugs with powerful, long-lasting effects, like phencyclidine hydrochloride (PCP).

In general, drugs play an important role in people's lives, especially in terms of the costs in time and money. In order to determine what role drugs play in your life, complete Self-Assessment Exercise 11.2, entitled "What Role Do Drugs Play In Your Life?"

SELF-ASSESSMENT EXERCISE 11.2

What Role Do Drugs Play in Your Life?

1. Identify the psychoactive substances that are a regular part of your life. Indicate how much of each substance you use and how often. Calculate the expense of your drug use both in the cost of the drug and in the time involved obtaining and/or preparing it. (Alcohol and nicotine are not included.)

Drug	How Much?	How Often?	Expense (Money)	Expense (Time)
Coffee/tea				
Cola Drinks				
Barbiturates				
Heroin/PCP				
Cocaine/or tranquilizers				
Marijuana				
Sleeping Pills				
Over-the-counter medicines				

Source: Walter D. Sorochan, *Promoting Your Health,* New York, John S. Wiley, 1981, p. 238. Reprinted by permission of the author.

Depressants

Narcotic Analgesics or Opiates

Narcotic analgesics are a form of depressant made from opium or a synthetic equivalent. The narcotic analgesics used medically today include the opium-based drugs morphine, codeine, Percodan, Dilaudid, and the synthetic equivalents, methadone and Demerol. The natural opiates and the still-illegal drug heroin are made from components of the sap of the opium poppy.

The narcotic, pain-relieving effects of opium have been known for thousands of years. Popular for centuries in China, the practice of smoking opium was brought to the United States by immigrants during the nineteenth century. Soon opium became a common ingredient in many patented medicines. In 1806 morphine was isolated from crude opium, and by the time of the Civil War, opium and its alkaloids were used extensively to relieve the pains of wounded soldiers. During the late nineteenth century, American physicians prescribed morphine regularly to treat asthma, persistent coughs, and numerous other complaints, and by the beginning of the twentieth century, estimates suggest that one out of every 400 Americans was addicted to the drug. In 1880 a new wonder drug, heroin, was derived from morphine. Physicians at first believed that heroin was not addictive and recommended this new drug as a cure for their morphine-dependent patients.

Pure heroin was slightly more than three times the pain-relieving effects of morphine, but because it quickly breaks down into morphine in the body, its pharmacological action is similar to morphine's. Prepared for the street user, heroin is mixed with such substances as quinine, a plant product once used to treat malaria; strychnine, a poison; and milk sugar. Other substances sometimes mixed with heroin include cornstarch, flour, and talc, which can cause dangerous or fatal clots when injected into the bloodstream.

The Effect of Opiates. *Opiates* are central nervous system depressants that exert their effects on certain areas of the thalamus, cerebral cortex, and parts of the spinal cord, but how they work is not entirely understood. A person using morphine remains sensitive even to a light touch, so it appears that morphine drugs do not block the transmission of sensory or pain impulses through the nerves. Rather, morphine may have some effect on the part of the brain that interprets pain messages. Morphine produces drowsiness and a kind of mental clouding, lethargy, and, in large doses, unconsciousness. Opiate-induced sleep is deep and dreamless, lacking in normal periods of REM, or rapid eye movements, which are associated with dreaming. All of the opiates depress the activities of the gastrointestinal tract and reduce the secretions of the stomach, liver, and pancreas. Because they reduce intestinal activity, opiates like paregoric, a mixture of opium, alcohol, and camphor, have been used to treat dysentery and diarrhea. Occasionally, morphine stimulates a reflex center in the brain and causes nausea and vomiting. Opiates depress respiratory function and suppress the cough reflex as well. Codeine, an alkaloid that makes up about 5 percent of crude opium, is about one-twelfth as effective as morphine for relieving pain, but it is a better cough suppressant.

Dependence on Narcotics. A number of factors contribute to an individual's developing physical and psychological dependence on opiates, or narcotics. First, some opiates are chemically more likely to induce physical dependence than others. For example, heroin and morphine are more likely to induce physical dependence than codeine. Second, the amount of drug in each dose and the number of times it is administered also influence the development of dependence. The more often a drug is used, the more likely the user is to become physically dependent upon it. Third, the way a drug is taken may also be a factor, in part because the pharmacological action of drugs increases when the substance is administered in certain ways, and also because the repetitious, almost ritualized activities associated with preparing and administering a drug may become important psychologically to the user. Preparing heroin, filling a syringe and injecting it, is more dependency-inducing, for example, than swallowing a pill. Finally, though there is probably no specific drug-dependent personality type, the individual's response to drugs, ability to handle stress, quality of self-image, and other characteristics probably have much to do with the development of dependence.

Because opiates cross the placental barrier, infants born to women who have used these drugs during pregnancy may be born physically drug-dependent, and they must be medically treated in order to avoid life-threatening withdrawal symptoms. *Narcotic antagonists*, or drugs that reverse the effects of narcotics, are an effective means of reversing the respiratory and other symptoms of withdrawal syndrome in newborns.

Barbiturates and Other Sedative-Hypnotics

Barbiturates have been used medically since 1903, and some of them, including Seconal and phenobarbital, are frequently prescribed today. All are derivatives of barbituric acid, a chemical compound discovered in 1864 by Adolf von Baeyer, a German organic chemist.

Barbiturates are especially effective on the central nervous system (CNS) but also affect every level of physical functioning down to the workings of individual cells. Barbiturates do not prevent or relieve pain. Their CNS effects range from mild sedation to coma, depending upon the size of the dose and route of administration. As calming agents, or **sedatives,** those drugs at low dosages produce relaxation by reducing stimuli to the CNS, but unlike some other depressants, they do not cause a significant loss of alertness. Used as **hypnotics,** at higher dosages, barbiturates induce sleep but decrease the time spent in REM (rapid eye movement) sleep, during which most dreaming occurs. Research has indicated that anxiety and irritability may result from being frequently deprived of dreaming sleep. Thus, the use of barbiturates as sleeping aids may actually deprive a person of a quality of sleep that is important for good health.

Sedatives Drugs that have a calming effect.

Hypnotics Sleep-inducing drugs.

Barbiturates, usually taken as capsules, are often associated with dependence and abuse because they induce tolerance. The barbiturate high, less dramatic than the euphoric effects of many psychoactive drugs, is generally characterized by peaceful, calm feelings. To an observer, barbiturate intoxication, actually a state of moderate poisoning, is similar to intoxication by alcohol. The symptoms include slurred speech, poor reflexes, and lowering of inhibitions.

Severe barbiturate poisoning may result in coma, dangerous respiratory depression, and a number of other complications. Because barbiturates do not stimulate vomiting, an overdose is more likely to be fatal than is an overdose of alcohol. When combined, however, these two substances have a potentiating effect and may cause death by severely depressing the respiratory center in the brain. They should never be used together.

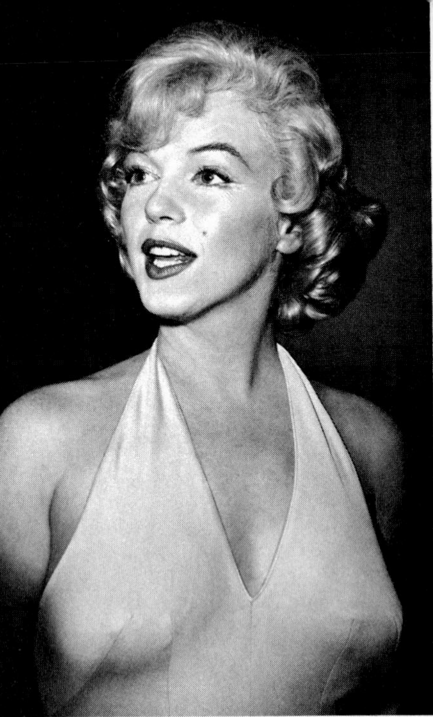

An increased tolerance for barbiturates may have caused the death of movie actress Marilyn Monroe. (Photo from Photo Trends)

Tolerance to the sedative and hypnotic effects of barbiturates develops slowly, eliciting the use of larger and larger doses; but the amount of a lethal dose remains relatively constant. Thus, the risk of fatal overdose becomes greatly increased in tolerant individuals. When barbiturates are used habitually at high doses, withdrawal may be severe and even life-threatening. Withdrawal from barbiturates is unlike "kicking" any other drug; it is very dangerous and may even be fatal without medical supervision.

It has been estimated that barbiturates cause more deaths than all other drugs combined. They are involved in thousands of suicides or accidental deaths every year, many of which are believed to be caused by the unexpected potentiation of these drugs with alcohol or the additive effects they produce when used with other CNS depressants. Powerful drugs, barbiturates are not easily cleared from the tissues; the half-life of most barbiturates is more than 24 hours.

Another danger of regular barbiturate use is the development of cross-tolerance to tranquilizers, alcohol, antidepressants, and some other drugs. This means that the body is automatically tolerant to the effects of drugs the individual may never have used before, and that larger-than-normal doses will be required to produce their pharmacological effects.

Methaqualone. A nonbarbiturate sedative-hypnotic, *methaqualone (Quaalude)* was thought to be a nonaddicting and safer substitute for barbiturates when it was introduced in 1965. But it has since become evident that Quaaludes—which became popular because of their inhibition-releasing and euphoric qualities—may induce tolerance and lead to both physical and psychological dependence. Though its depressant effects are not as strong as those of the barbiturates, methaqualone may also cause death from overdose. It is dangerously potentiated in effects when taken with alcohol, and it greatly reduces REM sleep.

Minor Tranquilizers (Antianxiety Agents)

Minor tranquilizers Drugs used to treat persistent anxiety.

The **minor tranquilizers,** which are used primarily for the treatment of severe or persistent anxiety, were introduced in the 1950s and steadily grew in popularity, which reached a peak in 1975 when nearly 100 million prescriptions for these drugs were written by American physicians. Nearly 60 percent of these were for Valium, which has become the most widely prescribed drug in America.

Minor tranquilizers can relieve tension and calm people for whom anxiety and stress have become problems. They are especially effective in allaying physical symptoms associated with anxiety, such as dizziness, choking sensations, or heat palpitations. Valium helps to induce sleep by reducing tension and has been prescribed as a muscle relaxant, though its effectiveness in this area may not be significant. Valium is also used as an anticonvulsant for certain kinds of epileptic seizures and as an aid to allay withdrawal symptoms related to alcohol or barbiturate abuse. All of the minor tranquilizers, however, produce physical sedation—not unlike the barbiturates—accompanied by drowsiness and impairment of the reflexes and motor skills one might use in driving.

Unlike the meprobamate tranquilizers (Miltown and Equanil), Valium used alone, even in large doses, does not produce fatal respiratory depression. Valium is a somewhat more benign drug than the meprobamates, and the sleep it induces is more normal, including more periods of REM sleep than that induced by Miltown or Equanil. At high doses (3,200 mg meprobamate per day for 30 days or more), Miltown or Equanil can induce severe barbiturate-type withdrawal syndrome characterized by convulsions and hallucinations.

The widespread use of minor tranquilizers in America has prompted some critics to suggest that people may be abusing these drugs or using them in maladaptive ways, rather than confronting the sources of their anxiety and learning to cope with them. How much anxiety is tolerable or even productive in a person's life varies with the individual and is difficult for both physicians and patients to judge. Some experts on drug use recommend short-term, closely monitored use of minor tranquilizers when they appear to be needed.

The minor tranquilizers have a dangerous potentiating effect with other CNS depressants like alcohol and barbiturates and should not be combined with these drugs. And some minor tranquilizers seem to be associated with birth defects, especially if they are used during the early months of pregnancy. Preliminary studies indicate that Librium and the meprobamates especially should be avoided at that time.

Major Tranquilizers (Antipsychotic Drugs)

Major tranquilizers are used to treat serious mental illness, and though they produce their effects in the brain and nervous system, they generally are not used recreationally. Three well-known antipsychotic drugs are *Compazine, Thorazine,* and *Stelazine.* These substances act to calm patients, reducing periods of hallucinations or delusions, and are often used to help prepare hospital patients for some form of psychotherapy. Though the antipsychotics take time to become effective (concentrations of them apparently must build up in the tissues) and may produce some troubling side effects, they represent a major breakthrough in the treatment of people who are mentally ill.

Major tranquilizers Drugs used to treat serious mental illness.

Stimulants

Caffeine

Caffeine is the most popular stimulant and is consumed in enormous quantities every day in the United States. Americans are said to use more than 100 billion doses of caffeine each year, some of it in the estimated three cups of coffee consumed per day by every American over the age of 14. At least 25 percent of all Americans over age 17 drink six or more cups of coffee or tea each day. Caffeine is an ingredient in other popular foods and drinks as well, though its presence may be less well known. Here are a few examples of everyday foods and beverages, together with a rough estimate of the amount of caffeine, in milligrams, that each contains:

6 oz. cup of coffee . . . . .100–150 mg caffeine
12 oz. can of cola . . . . .up to 72 mg caffeine
6 oz. cup of tea. . . . . .50–60 mg caffeine
1¹⁄₁₆ oz. bar of chocolate . . . . .20 mg caffeine
one typical dose, OTC stimulants . . . . .100 mg caffeine
(such as NoDoz)

Caffeine is a powerful central nervous system stimulant that can affect the brain at many different levels. Caffeine stimulates the cortex to produce clearer thinking and increased alertness as well as improved coordination. It also affects the portions of the brain and spinal cord that control the respiratory and cardiovascular systems. The presence of caffeine in the body stimulates increased respiration and the dilation of the coronary arteries. Blood pressure rises slightly, and the muscles of the heart contract more forcefully, increasing the organ's efficiency and at the same time causing the heart to require more oxygen. Caffeine may stimulate secretion of the stomach enzyme pepsin, and if no other food is present in the stomach, the natural oils in coffee and the pepsin can interact to irritate the stomach lining.

Doses of more than 250 milligrams of caffeine per day are considered excessive for an adult by some researchers, though it is clear that millions of Americans consume far more than that. Children's consumption of caffeine, which may cause such symptoms as anxiety, irritability, and upset stomachs, should be even more carefully limited. Because caffeine stimulates the release of excitatory hormones, it should be limited or eliminated in the diets of cardiac and older patients and those with unusual sensitivity to any stimulant. Research has suggested that the consumption of coffee may increase the risk of developing cancer of the pancreas. It is also thought possible that consuming caffeine during pregnancy may contribute to the development of birth defects.

Regular use of caffeine induces tolerance and may cause mild withdrawal symptoms, such as restlessness, headaches, or inability to concentrate. At high doses of several hundred milligrams, caffeine can cause heartbeat irregularities, muscular tremors, or convulsions.

Cocaine

Cocaine is a plant product made from the leaves of *Erythroxylon coca*, a woody shrub indigenous to Bolivia and Peru. In America, cocaine appeared in many of the patent medicines and tonics of the late nineteenth and early twentieth centuries, among them the original Coca-Cola. This product still uses coca leaves—though without their psychoactive chemicals—for flavoring. In 1914, cocaine was legally classified, taxed, and restricted as a narcotic under the Harrison Act, and for many years traffic in the drug continued underground without much notice. But in the early 1970s cocaine began to appear again among other drugs that were smuggled into the country, and its popularity grew.

Cocaine may be snorted, blown into the back of the mouth and throat, smoked in cigarettes, or injected. Locally irritating, frequent snorting of cocaine can cause nasal irritations and a runny or stuffed-up nose or even perforate the septum, the central partition in the nose. Cocaine produces an amphetamine-like euphoria, intense pleasure, and a sense of physical power. It increases the pulse and respiratory rates, raises the blood pressure and body temperature, and dilates the pupils of the eyes. Large doses or chronic use can cause auditory and visual hallucinations, aggressive behavior, agitated depression, panic reactions, or paranoid delusions.

Although once thought to be lethal only rarely, cocaine has recently been implicated in numerous deaths.[1] When cocaine is injected—alone or in combination with an opiate such as heroin—toxic levels in the blood can kill the user almost immediately. Smoking, or "freebasing," cocaine is another extremely dangerous method of ingestion. Repeated use of cocaine in any form, although it may not kill, produces nervousness and anxiety at a level that can lead users to take opiates to counter these effects. A double dependency often results.

Though cocaine does not appear to produce tolerance or physical dependence, users frequently develop an intense psychological involvement with the drug. Even infrequent users report that the elation of using cocaine is often followed by depression, nervousness, or anxiety. Anyone having problems with cocaine abuse can call the toll-free number 800—COCAINE for information regarding professional help.

Amphetamines

Amphetamines, first used medically during the 1930s, are strong central nervous system stimulants with effects similar to those of the natural catecholamines like epinephrine (adrenaline). Among the medical purposes for which amphetamines have been used since the 1930s are keeping patients with narcolepsy from falling asleep at inappropriate times and, paradoxically, calming down hyperactive children. Until the passage of the drug control amendments by Congress in 1965, the use and distribution of amphetamines were unregulated.

Amphetamines increase blood pressure, respiration, and muscle tension; slow down digestion (thus depressing the appetite); and cause the user to feel wakeful, alert, and often excited or euphoric. Among their unpleasant side effects are headaches, heart palpitations, insomnia, irritability, and anxiety; users may experience depression when the effects of the drug wear off.

Amphetamines have frequently been used by those who wish to keep themselves awake for longer periods than normal, including truck drivers on long hauls and students studying for exams. Such persons are, in effect, buying time, but the quality of the time they get seems to be inferior to natural wakefulness. Persons who stay awake by taking amphetamines may feel not only alert but also confident in their abilities as a result of the mood-elevating qualities of the drug; but, despite this physical alertness, judgment and reasoning abilities are impaired.

Another widespread use of amphetamines—principally Dexedrine, Benzedrine, and methamphetamine—is in attempts to lose weight. However, although amphetamines do indeed reduce the appetite, they have at best only slight, short-term effects and are not significant in maintaining permanent weight loss.

A particularly dangerous form of amphetamine abuse is taking high doses, usually of methamphetamine ("speed"), by injection, which produces an intense, euphoric rush. "Speedfreaks" typically maintain their high by taking a number of injections over a period of several hours.

Marijuana

Marijuana may be classified as a mild hallucinogen, though it does not produce many of the effects associated with these drugs and may create its effects in completely different ways. Some consider marijuana to be better classified as a sedative-hypnotic, since some of its characteristic effects are like those of sedatives.

Marijuana, the dried leaves and stems of the *Cannabis sativa* plant, is usually smoked but is sometimes eaten. Hashish, the resin scraped from the flowering tops of the plant, can be taken in the same ways.

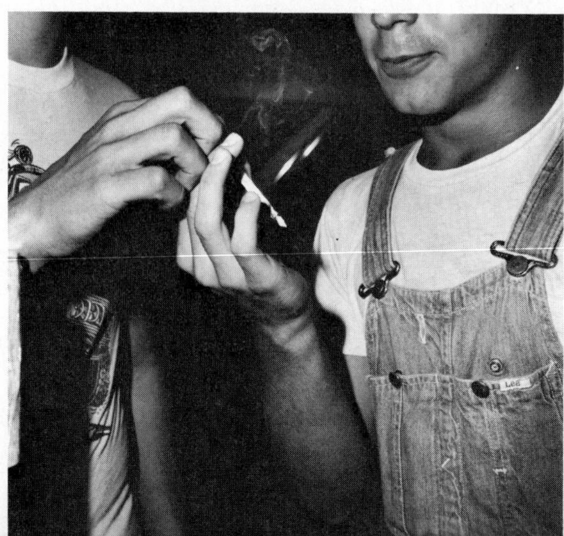

The legalization of marijuana is still a highly controversial issue. The popularity of this drug may be due to its availability. (Photo by Joseph Szabo/Photo Researchers, Inc.)

Although cannabis contains a number of other psychoactive chemicals, tetrahydrocannabinol (called THC) has been shown to be the primary ingredient responsible for the drug's mood-altering effects. Hash oil, a liquid concentrate sometimes applied to cigarettes and smoked, contains an even higher concentration of THC.

Despite the fact that it is generally illegal, marijuana is the third most popular recreational drug in America. Relatively mild, it produces its maximum effects about one-half hour after it is smoked. These effects may last from three to five hours. When it is eaten, the effects of marijuana are delayed several hours, but they are more persistent and may last as long as twenty-four hours. The mood-altering effects of marijuana are heavily dependent on a user's expectations and the setting in which the drug is used. In a positive, supportive setting, most users feel an increased sense of well-being, often accompanied by laughter and heightened sensitivity to colors, textures, tastes, and sound patterns. At high doses, marijuana induces sleep.

Smoking marijuana rarely produces strong negative reactions, though such reactions are more likely when the substance is eaten or when it is taken in stronger forms. But occasionally, when users have had no previous drug experience or are anxious or ambivalent about using the drug, panic reactions, toxic psychosis, or depression may occur.

Marijuana causes a moderate increase in heart rate, dilates the blood vessels in the eyes, and reduces the pressure of the fluids within the eyes (which has led to its medical use in treating glaucoma). It also produces bronchodilation (expansion of the lung's air passages). After smoking marijuana, a person's visual acuity decreases and the eyes' ability to recover from glare is impaired. Furthermore, reaction time is slowed. These effects cause significant impairment of driving performance while under the influence of marijuana.

To date, there is no reliable evidence that marijuana causes organic damage, though regular smoking irritates the throat and bronchial tubes. One joint of marijuana contains about four times as much tar as many of the low-tar, low-nicotine cigarettes on the market today, but so far there are no long-term studies to demonstrate whether years of marijuana smoking increase a user's risk of developing cancer. Because marijuana increases the heart rate from 30 to 60 percent and temporarily decreases the contractile strength of the heart, it can be harmful to people with heart conditions, but for others the impact on the heart of years of smoking marijuana regularly is unknown.

The half-life of THC is about fifty-six hours, and traces may continue to be found in the urine for up to eight days; therefore, smoking marijuana only once a week is enough to keep the body continually exposed to the drug. The body's retention of THC lends support to the existence of the phenomenon of *reverse-tolerance* that many users describe. Regular users appear to be more sensitive to marijuana than sporadic users or people who have never tried the drug before. It is possible that after THC has accumulated in the body's tissues, a user may require only a small additional amount to produce the drug's psychoactive effects.

Hallucinogens

Hallucinogenic drugs (some of which are also known as *psychedelics*) distort sensory input and alter a person's mood or perceptions, sometimes to the point of severely distorting experiences, inducing hallucinations.

Peyote and Mescaline

Peyote was among the consciousness-altering drugs used by the Aztecs, and its use has long been an integral part of worship for Indians in certain parts of Mexico and the American Southwest. In 1965, American Indians of the Native American Church won affirmation from the U.S. Supreme Court of their right to use peyote as a sacrament. Peyote, the dry, brown, bitter-tasting buttons of the peyote cactus, is taken by chewing or sucking. Its psychoactive chemicals first produce a state of peacefulness and enhanced sensitivity and then a period of excitation, usually accompanied by visual hallucinations. Peyote may also cause nausea and vomiting.

Mescaline, one of several alkaloids in peyote cactus, is about 50 times more potent than peyote, and its effects are similar to those produced by LSD. Most street mescaline is not the natural product isolated from the peyote cactus, but LSD, sometimes combined with amphetamines or other drugs. Mescaline appears in powdered or liquid form and may be sold in gelatin capsules, and it is usually taken orally.

Psilocybin

The practice of eating hallucinogenic mushrooms is an ancient one and has occurred in many parts of the world. In 1958 a chemical from a small marsh mushroom indigenous to Mexico was isolated by Dr. Albert Hofmann, who also discovered the hallucinogenic effects of lysergic acid. *Psilocybin* and another derivative of the *Psilocybe mexicana* mushroom called psilocin are sold on the street as powders or liquids and are similar in effects to mescaline.

"Magic mushrooms" are also available on the street; most often, however, these are simply ordinary mushrooms that have been impregnated with LSD or other drugs.

LSD (Lysergic Acid Diethylamide)

In 1938 a derivative of lysergic acid was synthesized by Dr. Albert Hofmann in a pharmaceutical laboratory near Basel, Switzerland. Some five years later when Hofmann was handling the substance, he accidentally absorbed some of it. He deliberately took more of the drug a few days later and described in his journal what we have come to know as an *LSD* trip.

LSD is usually swallowed in a solution or put in some ingestible substance like an aspirin or a sugar cube. It may also be put on a tiny piece of paper or cloth (a "tab") and placed under the tongue. A tiny dose—100 to 200 micrograms—is enough to produce all of the drug effects of this extremely powerful substance. The major effects of LSD are produced almost entirely on the central nervous system, and they last from 8 to 12 hours. Users experience intensely altered sensory impressions, and the sense of time becomes distorted. Normal personal boundaries seem to disintegrate, and those using LSD may feel both inside and outside themselves. Similarly, intense and opposite emotions may be felt at the same time. Often the user has seemingly special insights or a sense of renewal. Users may find their heightened sensory experiences and strong emotions to be frightening or overwhelming. In people who are mentally unstable, LSD may precipitate panic reactions or psychotic breakdowns, though in many instances "bad trips" can be alleviated by supportive, gentle talk.

LSD seems to induce tolerance quickly—in some users, after taking it for only three days in a row—but sensitivity to the drug returns after a few days of abstinence. LSD is not known to induce either physical or psychological dependence. Claims that the drug causes chromosomal damage or birth defects have not so far been substantiated. Cross-tolerance occurs among LSD, mescaline, and psilocybin, which are chemically similar, but not for drugs like PCP or STP.

PCP

Phencyclidine hydrochloride, also known as *PCP* or "angel dust," may be the most dangerous illicit drug on the market today because its effects are unpredictable and often extreme. Introduced in 1963 as an anesthetic, PCP produced such varied and troubling side effects that its use was discontinued two years later. In recent years, for reasons that are unclear, PCP has become popular as a street drug. Some estimates suggest that as many as 7 million Americans, many of them affluent suburban young people, have used PCP.

Easily synthesized, PCP can be taken in tablet, capsule, or powdered form. Sprinkled on low grade marijuana, dried parsley, or mint leaves, it is smoked by the user. Like other street drugs, PCP is often misrepresented by sellers and sold as other drugs, especially THC, amphetamines, LSD, or cocaine.

PCP elevates the heart rate and blood pressure to a moderate extent and produces powerful effects on the central nervous system. At low doses PCP's effects resemble those of barbiturate intoxication; it induces euphoria and relaxation and enhances a user's sensitivity to certain stimuli. At higher doses its effects may become very unpleasant. The user may feel estranged from people and surroundings and experience extremely distorted sensory impulses, such as auditory hallucinations. PCP users may fear death or imminent disaster and become extremely agitated. At other times, users may have delusions of extraordinary power, leading them to act in bizarre ways or to become aggressive. Self-destructive and violent behavior has been associated with the drug. The long-lasting (usually from 8 to 12 hours) and intense effects of this drug may be difficult even for experienced users to handle. High doses may be lethal, causing death from convulsions or from extreme depression of the respiratory center in the brain.

Inhalants

People who enjoy hallucinations and disorientation sometimes inhale petroleum distillates, like glue, or volatile solvents, such as cleaning fluids. Unlike street drugs, inhalants such as these are sometimes popular with children primarily because they are accessible and inexpensive. Though the effects these substances produce may be considered pleasant by the user, they are actually the brain's response to poisoning, and repeated use of these substances may cause structural damage within the brain and spinal cord. Petroleum distillates are also frequently damaging to the liver, especially when taken with alcohol.

Some drug users also try inhaling general anesthetics like ether and nitrous oxide. Little is known about the ways in which these substances induce their effects, even though millions of people have been anesthetized under medical supervision. Most anesthetics that are inhaled are cleared from the body by the liver and exhaled in the breath. Although nitrous oxide ("laughing gas") may be harmless when inhaled at low concentrations, inhaling the pure substance can cause anoxia (a lack of oxygen in the body tissues) and resultant brain damage, and may even lead to death from heart failure.

Help for the Drug Dependent

In recent years a number of approaches to helping drug-dependent people, and especially narcotics addicts, have been tried, including the use of narcotic antagonists, substances with a high affinity for the receptor-sites where opiates are bound.

According to the *receptor-site* theory, which explains how and why drugs exert their effects on only certain parts of the body, there are receptor cells or cell-surfaces, specific to their particular tissues or organs, located at different places throughout the body. These receptor-sites are designed to receive body chemicals like hormones and catecholamines but can also receive the molecules of certain drugs

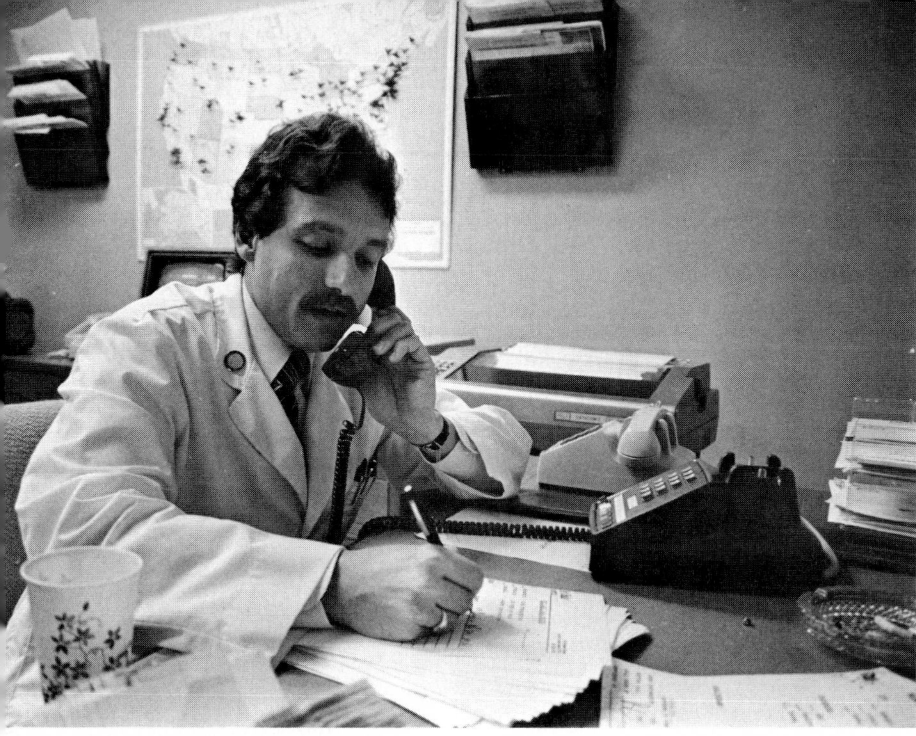

In the United States, special telephone "hot lines" have been set up to receive calls from people with drug abuse problems and from their families. Shown here is Dr. Mark Gold, founder of the (800)-COCAINE hot line, which offers telephone counseling regarding drug abuse of any kind. (Photo by Tannenbaum/Sygma)

which somehow fit the sites in size, shape, and chemical-electrical characteristics.

Narcotic antagonists can be used to counteract and reverse the symptoms of overdoses, and they can be used by addicts wanting to overcome their craving for heroin. Some narcotic antagonists produce no narcotic effects in the body, and others produce some effects. But all can be administered in sufficient doses to prevent a true narcotic from having an effect, so that the antagonist acts as a blocking agent. Some antagonists, administered at sufficient doses, can actually drive the molecules of a narcotic away from the receptor-site and reverse the body's response to the drug. Narcotic antagonists are an effective means of reversing the respiratory depression and other symptoms of the withdrawal syndrome in newborns.

Therapeutic Communities

Another approach to helping drug-dependent people has been the development of **therapeutic communities.** Initially modeled after Alcoholics Anonymous, these communities treat drug addiction as a personality disorder and strive to help drug abusers rebuild their personalities so that they are more effective and more self-actualizing. Most therapeutic communities have the goal of returning the addict to the outside world with the strength and resources he or she needs to remain drug-free. Some groups, however, believe that for the patients, ongoing life as productive members within the safety and support systems the communities provide is an appropriate goal and more likely to be successful.

Therapeutic community Form of rehabilitation based on group therapy and support.

Addicts entering therapeutic communities usually live there for a period lasting from a month or two to a few years. Addicts must abide by the rules, remaining drug-free and behaving appropriately in order to raise their status and prove their responsibility. Intensive group therapy, in which community members confront each other about their behavior and attitudes, and the highly structured system of rewards and punishments within the typical therapeutic community are designed to help addicts develop personal responsibility and effective ways of coping with stress.

Most therapeutic communities are residential; therefore, they are expensive, and the number of addicts they can treat is limited. Because they provide a sheltered setting, emphasizing mutual support and a high level of idealism, critics suggest that such communities do not prepare addicts for the life they must face outside. Furthermore, there are many problems in evaluating the success of therapeutic communities. These range from differences in the ways one may calculate their assets and their costs to the lack of long-term follow-up studies of the people who have "completed" such programs. Most observers estimate that only a relatively small percentage of the people who have gone through the programs in therapeutic communities succeed in remaining drug-free after a year or two.

Methadone Maintenance

Methadone maintenance Heroin treatment programs that use an opiate substitute called methadone.

Still another response to the problem of opiate addiction is **methadone maintenance** programs. Begun in 1964, methadone maintenance involves the substitution for opiates of an addictive but legal drug administered regularly in a clinic setting. Methadone, taken orally, is an effective pharmacological substitute, is cheap (about a dime per dose), is long-acting (it may be taken once every day or two), and does not produce the euphoria or sedation associated with heroin or morphine. Though it is possible that addicts may be maintained perpetually on methadone with few side effects, the goal of most methadone maintenance programs is to enable patients to withdraw eventually from methadone and then to live drug-free.

To enter methadone programs, addicts are screened and must prove their history of drug dependence and their inability to stop using drugs without some form of help. Under supervision in clinics, addicts regularly receive doses of methadone adjusted to match their habits. Certain ancillary services, including psychological or employment counseling, are usually offered as well.

Methadone maintenance programs have been criticized on a number of grounds. Though methadone costs themselves are low, the costs of maintaining clinics are high and sometimes have been escalated by mismanagement and dishonesty. Furthermore, physical dependence on methadone may be more difficult to break than dependence on heroin. The urge to take narcotics again seems to reappear in most people who withdraw from methadone, and although some people can live with this "narcotics hunger" and not use drugs, for others it means a return to narcotic abuse. When low doses of methadone are maintained in order to minimize opiate dependence and the potential problems associated with any long-term drug use, addicts discover they can use other drugs like amphetamines, alcohol, and marijuana to get high and may continue to do so, eliciting criticism from those who believe that any recreational drug use is dangerous.

However, for addicts who have voluntarily undergone withdrawal, the success rate may be relatively high. One program in Connecticut, for example, estimated that 68 percent of volunteers who had undergone withdrawal remained drug-free after having been followed for as long as 19½ months.

University, College, and Community Agencies

It must be reemphasized that an individual can have problems with literally any drug. The best indicator of a drug problem is when use of the drug is interfering or beginning to interfere with a person's life, including interpersonal relationships and academic work. The university or college environment, including the community, usually has a number of good resources that can be used if a student or other member of the university community is experiencing problems with a drug. These resources vary from university to university, college to college, or community to community, but generally the following organizations can be found in most university and college environments.

1. Student Health Services (university or college)
2. Psychological Counseling Centers (university or college)
3. Health Education Departments (university or college)
4. Community Hospitals, including emergency rooms
5. Community Crisis Centers, Substance Abuse Centers
6. Local or County Health Departments
7. Specific Drug- or Substance-Abuse Health Agencies, (e.g. Alcoholics Anonymous)
8. Community Mental Health Centers

Each of these organizations usually provides specialized services, but they can at least act as a referral agency for people with a potential drug problem. If a student or other member of the university community is having problems involving any kind of drug(s) then perhaps a good place to start in an attempt to deal with the problem is to call or visit any of the above agencies.

Summary

Drugs may be misused often, in particular, when people rely upon them as a means of escaping problems in life. The chronic inappropriate use of drugs may be termed drug abuse. Some drugs, such as those that induce tolerance — a physical adaptation that causes a drug to be less effective with repeated use — tend to elicit misuse. Psychoactive drugs, which affect the central nervous system, include coffee, cigarettes, and alcoholic beverages — the most popular drugs in America. People give many reasons for using psychoactive drugs: searching for personal meaning; trying to avoid feeling powerless; attempting to establish identity with peers and feel a sense of belonging.

Drugs produce their effects by altering the production, release, action, metabolism, or reabsorption of specific chemicals involved in the transmission of impulses between neurons in the brain. Besides the pharmacological action of a drug, set and setting determine how an individual will respond to it. Other factors affecting response to a drug include the purity of the drug, the size of the dose, how it is administered, and the physical condition of the user. Among the interactions of drugs taken together that produce different — often more dangerous — effects than when taken alone are potentiation, inhibition, and antagonism. Drugs may be taken by ingestion, inhalation, or injection; through body orifices; or by absorption.

According to the receptor-site theory, which explains how and why drugs exert their effects on only certain parts of the body, receptor sites located at different places throughout the body, which are designed to receive body chemicals, can also receive the molecules of certain drugs. Enzymes and processes in the body chemically alter and eliminate drugs in much the same ways as food is metabolized. The half-life of a drug is the period of time required for the body to reduce the initial peak concentration of the drug in the blood by one-half. Drugs may be excreted from the body in urine, feces, breath, perspiration, breast milk, and vomit.

For many years drugs were classified according to their potential for leading to addiction, thought to be caused by physical adaptations in the user's body producing tolerance and a characteristic illness, called withdrawal syndrome, when drug use was stopped. Today two kinds of drug dependence are recognized — physical and psychological — which may occur separately.

Psychoactive drugs may be classified according to their major observable effects as depressants, including narcotic analgesics or opiates, sedative-hypnotics, minor tranquilizers, and major tranquilizers; as stimulants; or as hallucinogens. The various drugs in these categories may differ widely in their effects. Among the factors contributing to an individual's developing physical or psychological dependence on narcotics are the nature of the drug, the amount of drug in each dose and frequency of use, the way the drug is taken, and characteristics of the individual. Means of help for narcotics and other addicts include narcotic antagonists, therapeutic communities, and methadone maintenance programs.

Review and Discussion

1. What are some of the reasons that people take drugs?

2. Discuss the difference between physical and psychological dependence.

3. Define the terms "set" and "setting." Discuss how set and setting affect the drug-taking experience.

4. Define the terms "potentiation," "inhibition," and "antagonism." Provide an example of each of these drug interactions.

5. Identify drugs derived from opium.

6. What means of help are available for people dependent on narcotics?

7. Discuss the pros and cons of methadone maintenance.

8. Compare and contrast the similarities and differences between tolerance, addiction, and withdrawal from barbiturates, alcohol, and heroin.

9. Compare the physiological effects of caffeine and amphetamines.

10. To what extent is marijuana smoke similar to cigarette smoke in its effects on the respiratory system? What are some other effects of marijuana?

11. Discuss the reasons why PCP may be the most dangerous illegal drug on the market today.

12. Identify some alternatives to drug use, misuse, and abuse.

Further Reading

Duncan, D., and R. Gold. *Drugs and the Whole Person.* New York: John Wiley and Sons, 1982.
Basic coverage of drug use and misuse, well researched and up-to-date. (Paperback.)

Dusek, Dorothy, and Daniel Girdano. *Drugs.* Reading, Mass.: Addison-Wesley Publishing Co., Inc., 1980.
An interesting approach to drug education, with a very strong section on the motivation of drug users.

Julien, Robert. *A Primer of Drug Action.* San Francisco: W. H. Freeman and Company, 1978.
Very good overview of the physiological action of drugs. (Paperback.)

Liska, K. *Drugs and the Human Body.* New York: Macmillan Publishing Company, Inc., 1981.
An analysis of physiological and psychological aspects of drug use, with implications for society. (Paperback.)

Ray, Oakley. *Drugs, Society, and Human Behavior.* 3rd ed. St. Louis, Mo.: C. V. Mosby Company, 1983.
Excellent, comprehensive coverage of all drug categories. Special emphasis given to historical and behavioral perspectives on drug use, misuse, and abuse.

Part IV
Personal Health

"The first wealth is health."
Ralph Waldo Emerson

The World Health Organization defines health as "a state of complete physical, mental, and social well-being, not merely the absence of disease or infirmity." Personal health is the individual's endeavor to achieve such a goal. It is the concept of self-determined wellness, and it is no secret that a key factor in such a program is self-control. The following three chapters reflect this personal responsibility. Chapter 12, "Physical Fitness," examines the current boom in keeping the body at the optimum level of performance through jogging, cycling, tennis, swimming, and related aerobic exercises. "Nutrition," Chapter 13, provides reasons and guides for proper nourishment. "Weight Control," Chapter 14, concerns itself not only with the problems of overweight and underweight, but also with how to maintain the weight that is right for you.

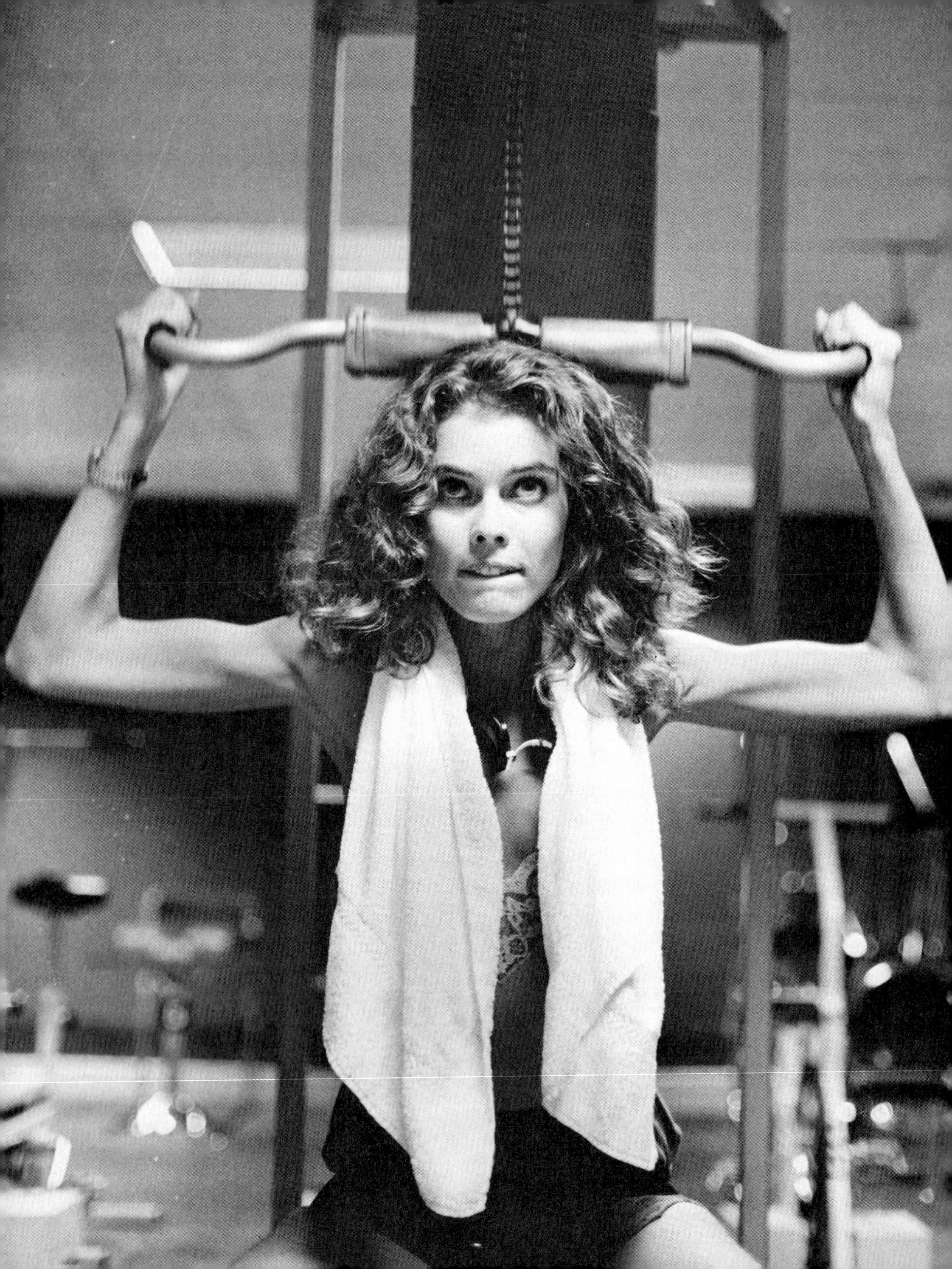

Chapter 12
Physical Fitness

KEY POINTS

- ☐ Physical fitness is the ability to meet all the ordinary demands of life without becoming tired and to respond to extra demands when necessary.
- ☐ Major components of physical fitness include muscular strength and endurance, cardiorespiratory endurance (the ability of the circulatory and respiratory systems to provide oxygen), flexibility, and body composition.
- ☐ The most important components of physical fitness for everyone include cardiorespiratory endurance and flexibility.
- ☐ An individual physical fitness program should include aerobic exercise (exercise to improve cardiorespiratory endurance); and each exercise session should include a warm-up and cool-down period.
- ☐ Benefits of physical exercise include improved functioning of vital organ systems, decreased risks of certain diseases, and an increased sense of psychological well-being.

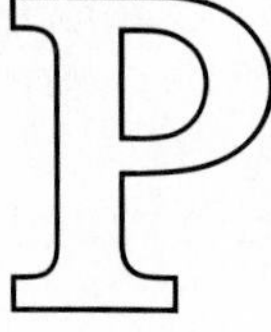HYSICAL fitness means more than well-developed muscles. It means feeling good and full of vigor—and showing it. It means not only being able to meet all of the ordinary and daily physical demands on the body without becoming tired but also being able to respond to extra demands—for example, in strenuous activities or in emergencies—without experiencing undue stress.

Keeping yourself physically fit is your personal responsibility. People can advise you on how to achieve fitness and can even prescribe specific and effective programs, but you can become physically fit only through your own efforts. Keeping fit is a remarkable preventive medicine that contributes to both physical and mental well-being.

In the 1960s a fitness boom hit the nation and is still with us. People have become concerned about taking care of themselves; they have taken charge of maintaining their own health, rather than making unreasonable demands of physicians or a paternalistic government. Millions have become involved in physical fitness programs. Not all go at it in the same way, but all are conscientiously working toward the same goal—becoming fit. They smoke less, or not at all. They watch their diets. They exercise. They patronize privately operated exercise clubs and buy athletic equipment, supporting a business estimated to take in some $30 billion a year. Only a few years ago the few people following such regimens with enthusiasm were called health nuts, but now physical fitness is an accepted part of American life.

All of this is good. People unquestionably feel better. But are they healthier, and living longer, more active lives? The physical fitness movement has not been with us long enough yet to provide the wealth of supporting statistics necessary for making such a proclamation, but the evidence is impressively favorable. Physical fitness seems to be a means for attaining optimum wellness because it contributes not only to physiological well-being, but also to a person's psychological and social well-being.

Health Benefits of Regular Exercise

Although the immediate effect of any exercise is stress on those parts of the body involved, when the exercise is continued in a program, the body adapts. It becomes stronger, functions more efficiently, and has greater endurance. The physically fit person is able to withstand greater amounts of physical and emotional stress than the person who is not fit.

Physical Benefits

When an individual engages in physical activity, the entire body benefits. The broader the range of activity in which the individual engages, the greater the benefit received. Studies indicate that the individual who exercises on a regular basis is able to perform daily activities more efficiently than an individual who does not exercise regularly.

Although all of the body systems are stimulated with regular physical exercise, the cardiovascular and respiratory systems—perhaps the two most important systems in physical fitness—receive the greatest benefit.

Psychological and Social Benefits

Almost everyone who begins a physical fitness program reports feeling much better within a few weeks. Although most people who have been sedentary start their exercise programs with some specific goal, such as losing weight, this original purpose generally becomes less important after they experience the sheer joy of being fit. They are getting the physical benefits, but they feel a tremendous psychological boost as well.

It is doubtful that the millions of Americans participating in physical fitness programs now would be disciplined enough to continue

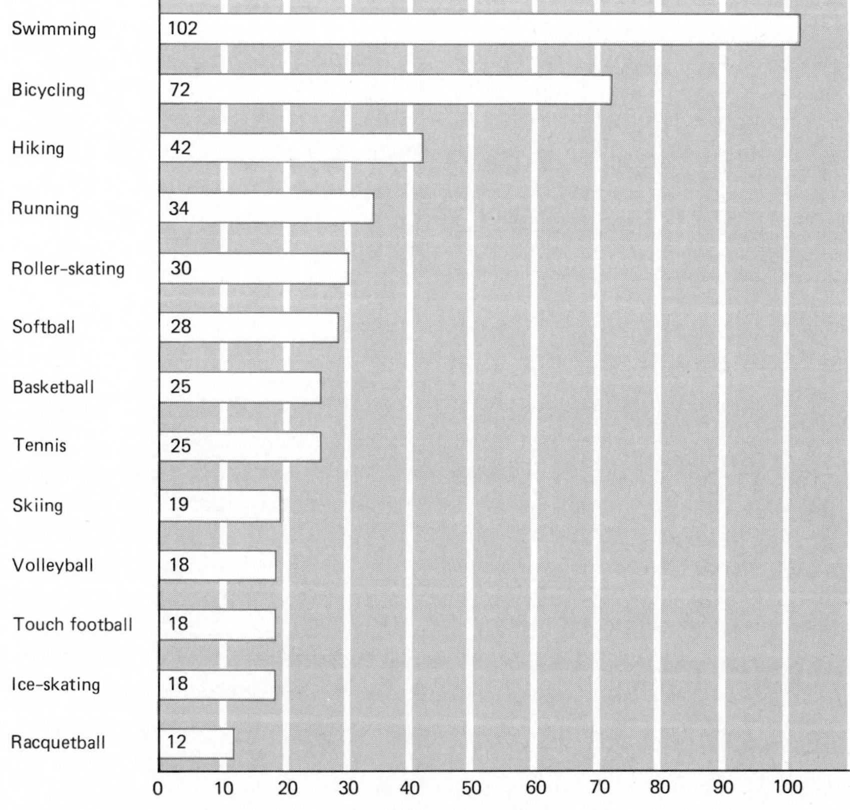

Figure 12-1. Recreational Activities of Americans.
Although millions of Americans participate annually in recreational activities, not all recreational activities contribute to aerobic fitness. (Source: Data from the President's Council on Physical Fitness and Sports, 1984.)

were it not for the exhilaration that comes from the physical activity. They feel fulfilled and more capable of coping with life's problems. Tensions, depressions, feelings of inadequacy, and worries may diminish. These changes are an effect of exercise that some doctors explain as resulting from an increase in the body's production of **norepinephrine,** a hormone known to reduce anxieties while at the same time bringing about greater alertness and responsiveness. After a physical fitness program begins to have these effects, the regular exercise routine becomes an essential part of life.

Norepinephrine Anxiety-reducing hormone produced during exercise.

As physical fitness and positive attitudes increase, social relationships also tend to improve. People who are physically active often become more confident and outgoing, do better work, and get greater pleasure from their association with other people. In addition, many people perform their exercise activities in groups or with partners. This can strengthen old social ties and help form new ones. However, it must be remembered that recreational activities, though enjoyable, may not contribute a great deal to fitness. Softball, for example, is a very good recreational activity but does not contribute much to overall fitness.

Components of Physical Fitness

The popular image of physical fitness is too often restricted to highly developed muscles, but muscular strength is only one component of physical fitness. Cardiorespiratory endurance is in fact more important for building total fitness. The three remaining components of physical fitness are muscular endurance, flexibility, and body composition.

Cardiorespiratory Endurance

The efficient use of the heart, blood vessels, and lungs over prolonged periods of activity is called **cardiorespiratory endurance.** Exercises that build this kind of endurance are called **aerobic exercise** because they increase the utilization of oxygen transported by the heart and respiratory systems to the muscles. By engaging in aerobic activities such as hiking, running, walking, and bicycling on a regular basis, people can increase their lung capacity and improve their breathing ability, thus being able to take in greater amounts of oxygen per minute but at a slower breathing rate.

Cardiorespiratory endurance Efficient use of heart and lungs during strenuous exercise.

Aerobic exercise Exercise that increases cardiovascular endurance.

Correlated with improved respiratory ability is the more efficient operation of the heart and circulatory system. Aerobic exercise helps strengthen the heart so that it delivers more blood with each beat and benefits from longer rests between beats. Another result of this kind of exercise is that as much as twenty times more blood is delivered to

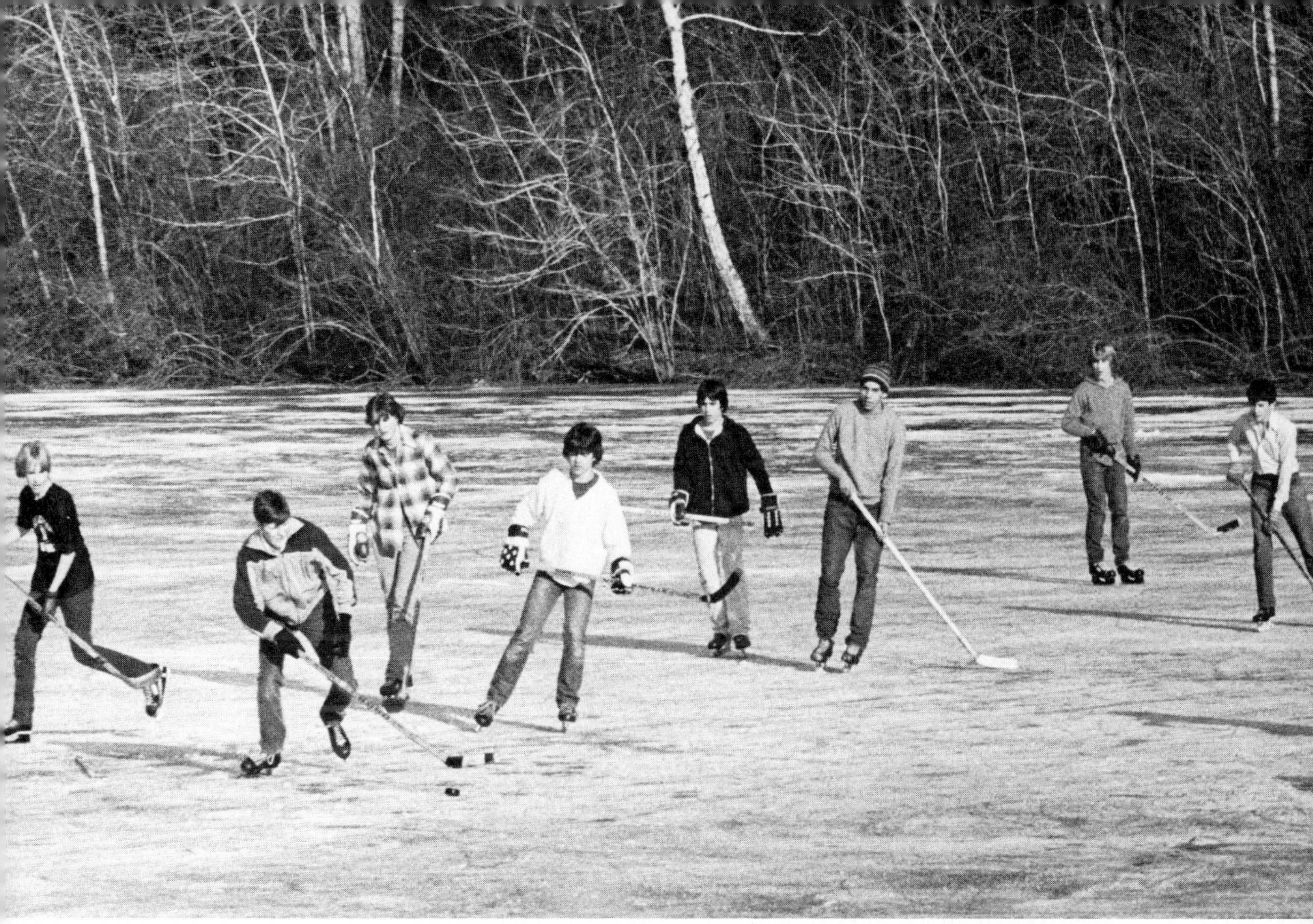

Physical fitness is not simply a question of strength. Endurance, flexibility, and body composition are essential as well, as these hockey players would testify. (Photo © Marjorie Pickens 1982))

muscles throughout the body. Over a period of time, these muscles develop more capillaries to aid in the efficient exchange of carbon dioxide for oxygen.

The greater efficiency with which the entire cardiorespiratory system functions is thought to be a major weapon against the nation's number one killer: cardiovascular disease.

Muscular Strength

The capacity to exert force against a resistance — for example, to lift weights — is called **strength.** Exercises done primarily to build muscles are called **anaerobic exercises** because they do not get their energy directly from oxygen but rather from power stored in the muscles. By regularly exercising to build strength, the size of the muscle fibers and the ability of the individual to apply force increase. If the muscles are not used, they no longer perform as well as they once did in meeting the demands of everyday living. In the past, people often excused reduced muscular ability as part of a natural aging process. Today it is recognized that muscles begin to atrophy or waste away mainly from lack of use. Good muscular fitness is attained by regular exercise combined with a good diet.

Strength Ability to exert force against a resistance.

Anaerobic Condition when oxygen demand exceeds supply.

Anaerobic exercises Exercises done to build the power stored in muscles.

Muscular Endurance

Muscular endurance Capacity of muscles to sustain force over a period of time.

The capacity of a muscle or group of muscles to sustain force over a period of time or to contract repeatedly, such as when doing push-ups or sit-ups, is called **muscular endurance.** To the extent that muscular strength is involved in muscular endurance, exercises such as push-ups and sit-ups are primarily anaerobic in nature.

Flexibility

Flexibility Range of movement within a joint and its specified muscle group.

The ability to move, twist, and bend is called **flexibility.** It is closely connected with muscular fitness but involves the joints, skin, and connective tissue as well as the muscles. Flexibility is typically greatest in young children and decreases with age. Loss of flexibility is minimized by training programs, with a resultant reduction in lower-back problems, better posture, and less muscle soreness in general.

Body Composition

Body composition The comparative amounts of body tissue, muscle, bone, and fat.

Lean body weight Body weight consisting of body tissue, muscle, bone, and fat.

Metabolism Chemical and physical bodily processes.

Body composition is a measure of two elements: lean and fat. **Lean body weight** consists of the body's bones, muscles, connective tissues, and vital organs. The remainder of the body's weight is fat. Some of this fat is essential, supplying the fuel for regular body **metabolism;** fat deposits also form protective cushions around most vital organs and occur in a layer just beneath the skin. But excessive fat stored in the body is responsible for obesity—a condition that is not only detrimental to good physical fitness, but also leads to general lethargy and greater susceptibility to diseases, cardiovascular diseases among them (see Chapter 16). Obesity can generally be controlled through a combination of exercise and diet (see Chapter 14).

Assessing Your Fitness

Many people don't know their current level of physical fitness. In Self-Assessment Exercise 12.1 are listed some basic tests that will give you a rough estimate of your fitness in at least one area in each of the five categories: cardiorespiratory endurance, muscular strength, muscular endurance, flexibility, and body composition.

A word of warning: If you find while doing any of these tests that you become dizzy or short of breath, you should slow down or stop. Any activity that exceeds what is normal for you can conceivably bring on these reactions. Extreme fatigue after any exercise means that you must start at a lower level of activity and work up to a higher level. For example, a brisk walk for five minutes can be a good start for some people; they can extend their walk and later add more vigorous exercises. The ability to do more and exercise longer comes surprisingly fast.

SELF-ASSESSMENT EXERCISE 12.1

A Quick Reference Test for Physical Fitness

Test	Purpose	Fitness Component	Procedure	Scoring
Ruler	Identify abdominal fat	Body composition	Lie on your back, flat on the floor. Place a ruler across your abdomen at the midline (across the pelvis).	The ruler should touch the pelvic bone on both sides without touching the abdomen.
Pinch	Identify body fat	Body composition	Use the thumb and index finger to take a deep pinch of skin and fat from four sites: upper thigh, back of upper leg, back of upper arm (right arm), and the abdomen, 1" to the right of the navel.	If you pinch 1" or more at any of the four sites, you need to lose some body fat.
Push-up (Women)	Upper body strength	Muscular strength & endurance	Lie flat on your stomach on the floor. Place your hands at shoulder width, palms flat on the floor and elbows bent. Keeping the knees on the floor, the back straight, and the toes on the floor, push yourself upward, then lower yourself until your chin touches the floor and repeat the movement.	Do five to pass.
Push-up (Men)	Upper body strength	Muscular strength & endurance	Follow the same basic procedure as for the women, only keep the knees off the floor and keep the back and legs in alignment as the exercise is repeated.	Do five to pass.
Toe-touch	Flexibility of the trunk	Flexibility	From a sitting position, knees locked, arms extended above the head, bend forward and touch the toes and hold for 3 seconds.	Do one to pass.
Sit-up	Abdominal endurance	Muscular strength & endurance; flexibility	Lie on the floor on a mat with your knees bent at a 90° angle, feet flat on the floor, heels 12"–18" from your buttocks. Cross your arms over your chest by putting your hands on opposite shoulders. A partner holds your feet flat on the floor, or you can put them under a heavy object that won't toppple. Arms must remain touching the chest; and slowly curl up to a sitting position until the elbows touch the thighs.	In 60 seconds, women should be able to do 20 and men should be able to do 30.

(Continued)

Test	Purpose	Fitness Component	Procedure	Scoring
Leg-raise	Abdominal endurance	Muscular strength & endurance	Lie on the floor, flat on your back. Keep your feet together and raise them 6"–10" off the floor. Hold for 10 seconds. Don't do this if you have back problems!	Do one to pass.
1.5 Mile Walk-run	Aerobic endurance (Cardio-respiratory endurance)	Cardio-respiratory endurance	On a measured course or track, run or walk 1.5 miles. Time how long it takes to complete the 1.5 miles	Age: 13–19 / 20–29 Men Poor 13:51 / 15:00 Fair 11:29 / 13:00 Good 10:11 / 11:15 Women Poor 17:05 / 18:45 Fair 15:40 / 17:12 Good 13:30 / 14:42

Source: Adapted from AAHPERD, *Health Related Physical Fitness Test* (Reston, Va. The Alliance, 1980); from Bud Getchell, *Being Fit* (New York: John Wiley & Sons, 1982); from G. B. Dintiman, S. E. Stone, J. C. Pennington, and R. G. Davis, *Discovering Lifetime Fitness* (St. Paul, Minn.: West Publishing Company, 1984); and from Kenneth H. Cooper, *Aerobics Program for Total Well-Being* (New York: M. Evans and Company, Inc., 1982).

The Exercise Session

The exercise session should consist of three parts: (1) the warm-up, (2) the exercise activity, and (3) the cool-down.

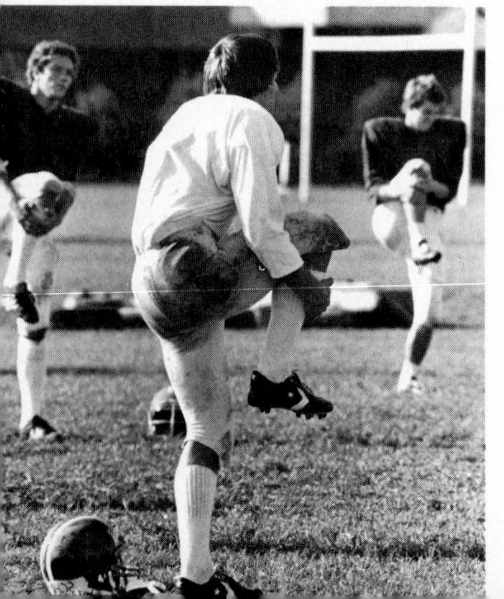

It is important to warm up before beginning any exercise. In preparation for a competition, athletes often do flexibility exercises. (Photo © Phyllis Graber Jensen/Stock, Boston)

The Warm-Up and Cool-Down

How do you know when the warm-up exercises have been sufficient to get you ready for more vigorous activity? The name of the exercise really gives the answer, for you literally feel "warmed up" to the extent that you may begin to sweat. Outdoors or in cool or cold weather, this will take longer than indoors or on a warm day. A period of five to ten minutes is generally enough. The cool-down exercises are important because they slow down the body by degrees to reduce the breathing and heart rate to normal again. The warm-up and cool-down segments of the exercise session should be planned as a part of the flexibility segment of the total fitness program. We will discuss flexibility exercises in the next section.

The Exercise Activity

When planning an exercise routine, the following principles should be considered: **specificity, intensity, duration,** and **frequency.**

Specificity

Not all people are physically "unfit" in the same area. After taking the tests in Self-Assessment Exercise 12.1, you should have some idea of the specific areas of physical fitness (**specificity**) on which you need to work. For example, a person with poor muscular strength and endurance would choose exercises that attended to those two components of total fitness. If on the other hand, you found that your time on the 1.5 mile run was not up to par for your sex and age level, or if you got "winded" easily, you probably lack **aerobic fitness** and need to concentrate on developing cardiorespiratory endurance. We will discuss some exercises for aerobic fitness, for muscular strength and endurance, and for flexibility in the next section of this chapter. Body composition can be altered through attention to weight control, good nutrition, and any exercise activity—mainly aerobic—that burns calories.

Specificity Exercises that work a specific muscle group.

Aerobic fitness Body's ability to meet oxygen needs.

Regardless of the area of fitness in which you choose specifically to concentrate, you will not want to neglect others. In fact, you probably will not be able to neglect any given area since many of these areas are interdependent. Aerobic exercises, for example, help develop muscular strength and endurance. And you may get muscle cramps while running (for cardiorespiratory endurance) or lifting weights (for muscular strength and endurance) if you have not done stretches (for flexibility) beforehand.

Intensity

Intensity of exercise refers to how hard the heart must work to reach a rate wherein cardiorespiratory benefit will occur. Although the most scientific means of determining exercise intensity levels involves measuring the amount of oxygen the person uses during the exercise session, **exercise physiologists** have suggested other methods that use only the heart rate as a good basic guideline for most persons.

Intensity A measure of the heart's exertion during exercise.

Exercise physiologist Specialist in the effects of exercise on the body.

Exercise specialists suggest that exercises should be strenuous enough to require the heart to beat between 70 and 90 percent of its maximum rate, depending on the individual's level of fitness. If the exercises do not demand more than 60 percent of the maximum heart rate, they give little or no benefit. One way of determining your target heart rate, or training zone, is presented in Table 12–1. According to the American College of Sports Medicine this method tends to underestimate target heart rate by about 15 percent, so the calculated target heart rate must be adjusted upward by 15 percent in order to determine the intensity level of exercise that will produce cardiorespiratory benefit. There are other ways to determine your training target heart rate, but regardless of the formula you use, duration and frequency of exercise are two other important variables that must be considered.

Table 12–1 Determining Your Maximum Heart Rate and Aerobic Fitness Target Heart Rate

To determine maximum heart rate, subtract your age from 220. For a twenty-year-old individual, for example, the maximum heart rate is 200 (220 − 20), and for beneficial effects, the individual should exercise at a heart rate that is 70–90 percent of this maximum heart rate, plus 15 percent correction factor.

Maximum Heart Rate (MHR)

220 − ______ = ______
(Your Age) (Your MHR)

Aerobic Fitness Target Heart Rate (AFTHR)

For Beginners:

_____ × .70 = ______
(MHR) (Intensity)

______ × ______ = ______
(Intensity) (Correction Factor) (Corrected Intensity)

______ + ______ = ______
(Corrected Intensity) (Intensity) (AFTHR)

For Intermediates: The calculation is exactly the same as for beginners except that the intensity factor is .75.

For Advanced: The calculation is exactly the same as for beginners except that the intensity factor is set at 80 to 90 percent, depending upon the degree of fitness of the individual.

You can determine heart rate by taking your pulse. To do this, you press lightly on your neck just under the jawbone and beside the Adam's apple. (Use your fingers rather than your thumb, which also has a detectable pulse.) After several minutes of exercising, take your pulse for ten seconds and then multiply by six to determine the number of beats per minute. If your pulse is below your AFTHR, you should exercise harder until your pulse reaches the AFTHR and then sustain the exercise at that level for a minimum of fifteen minutes.

Duration

Duration Length of time of an exercise session.

How long should you exercise each session to derive the most cardiorespiratory benefit possible? The time that should be spent in each exercise session, or **duration,** depends greatly on the intensity of the exercise (the higher the intensity level, the shorter the duration to derive essentially the same benefit). For cardiorespiratory benefit to occur, it is important that the intensity of the exercise be maintained throughout the exercise period. If you are just initiating an exercise program, you should not begin with an extremely strenuous workout. It probably took you several months or years to get out of shape, and you will not regain your past fitness in a week or two of strenuous exercise. In all likelihood, you will develop sore muscles, and that might cause you to discontinue your exercise program. Such exercises as walking or swimming for the beginner, or jogging, cross-country skiing, ice skating, cycling, or roller skating for more advanced persons can generally be maintained at a given intensity level for the entire exercise session. Remember, the more fit the individual, the intensity level of the exercise or the duration of the exercise session —or both—should be increased to derive maximum cardiorespiratory benefit.

Frequency

How often (**frequency**) should you exercise in order to get results? Exercise physiologists suggest that to maintain aerobic fitness—which will be discussed more thoroughly later in this chapter—you need to exercise a minimum of 15 minutes, three times per week. To increase your aerobic fitness, or as you become more fit, you should exercise four to five times per week for a minimum of 20 to 30 minutes each session.

Frequency Number of exercise sessions per week for an individual.

Preexercise Precautions

Be sure you are fit enough to start a physical fitness program. If you are young and active, you are probably very much ready. Exceptions are people who have diagnosed illnesses and who are advised by their physician not to engage in strenuous exercises. If you have been mostly inactive or sedentary for several years—and especially if you are in your late 20s or older—get a physical examination first just to make certain everything is all right. The examination will reassure you that whatever discomforts you may experience initially after exercising are not because there is something wrong with you but

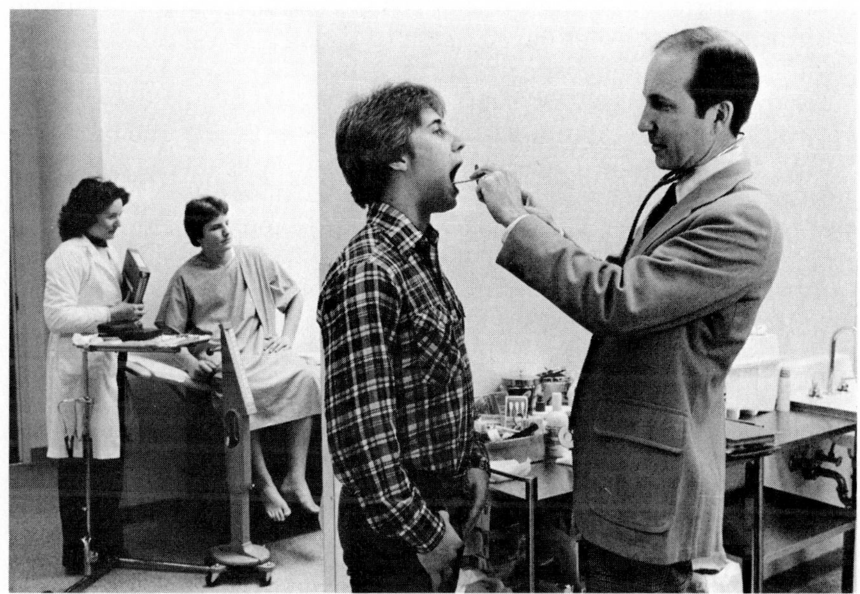

Before beginning a program of exercise, it is always wise to have a complete medical examination. (Photo by Meri Houtchens-Kitchens/ The Picture Cube)

because you are putting muscles to work that have not been used for a long time.

Electrocardiogram Examination to monitor heart functioning.

Stress Test A maximum exercise test to determine cardiovascular fitness.

If you have been inactive for a long period of time, a complete examination of your heart is advisable before you start a physical fitness program. This should include an ECG, or **electrocardiogram,** which checks your heart's performance during both rest and exercise. If there are abnormalities, they are most likely to become evident during exertion or immediately afterward. In the exam, electrodes are attached to different parts of the body so the physician or medical technician can monitor the functioning of each part of the heart. In a **stress test,** commonly given on a motorized treadmill or a stationary bicycle, the person exercises to the point that the heart is beating near its estimated maximum (as determined by age and other factors). The testing continues during the rest and recovery.

The value of these tests is that even unsuspected heart abnormalities that would make exercising a risk can be discovered. They also provide an opportunity to make an accurate check of aerobic power. People learn from these tests precisely how fit—or unfit—they are. Additional tests during their physical fitness programs give them an indication of their progress.

Just as an automobile is warmed up before it is driven and just as a body is warmed up with preliminary exercises before vigorous exercises are started, physical fitness programs should be started slowly and with caution. No one should attempt vigorous exercises without being sure they can be done without danger.

How Quickly Do Results Come?

Most people note improvements of 10 percent or more during the first month after initiating an exercise program. Within six or eight months they seem to reach a plateau. After that, improvements come more slowly, but only by continuing the exercise program can the built-up aerobic power and attendant good feelings be maintained. Gains can be lost in only a few weeks or months. Some people do manage to reduce their number of exercise sessions per week to one or two, but most want to increase them. Once they feel good, they opt for the chance to feel still better. They no longer think of exercise only as a means of achieving fitness; now they consider their particular kind of exercise enjoyable in itself.

What Kind of Exercise?

Compared with no exercise, any kind of exercise is an improvement, since it will at least help increase circulation and put some muscles into motion. But as we have already discussed, exercises can also be

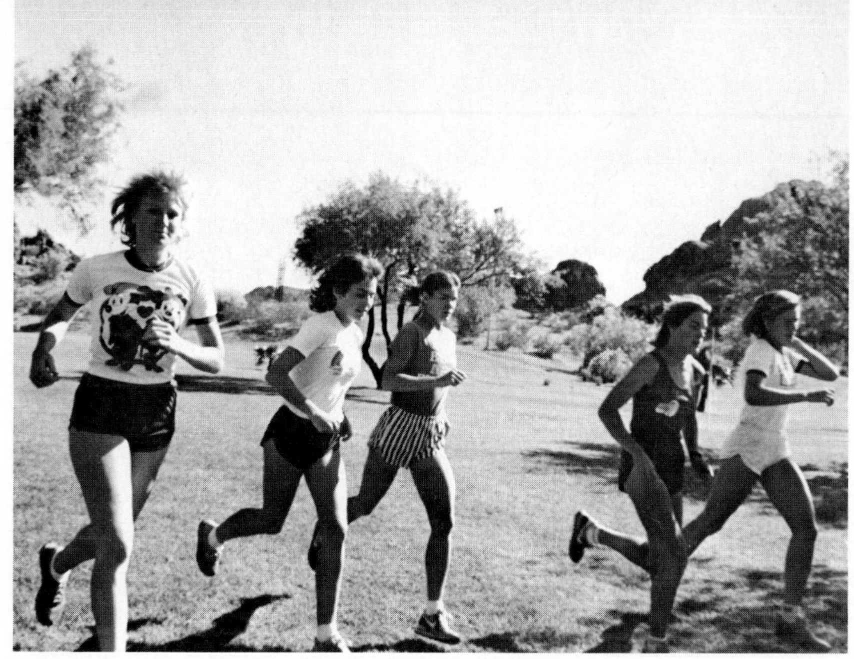

Jogging has become an extremely popular way to build cardiorespiratory endurance. (Photo by Laurel Eisenberg)

very specific in their effect. In this section we will discuss exercises for the various components of physical fitness: those that increase cardiorespiratory endurance, those that develop muscular strength and endurance, and those that increase flexibility.

Exercises for Cardiorespiratory Endurance

Although many kinds of exercise increase aerobic power, some do not. Golf, for example, contributes little to aerobic power—and virtually none if a cart is driven around the course: the greatest benefit from golfing is the walking. Whether on the golf course or elsewhere, brisk daily walks do contribute to building aerobic power. Other exercises that help develop cardiorespiratory endurance and that can be continued for long periods without discomfort are jogging, bicycling, swimming, aerobic dance, hiking, and skipping rope.

Each kind of exercise, in fact, has its special appeal to those who participate. Investigate a variety and try several. The choice is yours to make, and it may depend on where you live, what you enjoy doing, the time you can spare, and the equipment or facility needed. The specific kind of exercise—as long as it is aerobic—is really not as important as its type. To be effective, it must require exertion and involve your whole body. It is best also to select something you know you will enjoy for many years.

Jogging

Jogging is popular partly because of its versatility. People of any age can jog, and they can go at whatever speed they wish. They can also pick the time of day they like best and jog for as long as fits their schedule. The only equipment absolutely necessary is a good pair of shoes and comfortable socks. These can be purchased at any sporting goods store and in many shoe stores. With long underwear, gloves, a windbreaker, and a knit hat, some joggers keep at it even in zero-degree weather.

There are good running techniques. You will learn some of these by talking to and watching other joggers who have been running for a long while. It is most important from the start to use the proper foot action. Let your foot come down on its heel, then rock forward to push off with the ball of your foot. This is least tiring and least jolting. Your back should be nearly straight and your head held up. Keep your arms up and bent at the elbows. Avoid vigorous swinging. Use a comfortable stride of average length. You will undoubtedly develop a rhythm naturally that makes the jogging easy and fun.

Bicycling

Bicycling has several advantages. For one, you can go places on a bicycle. You can use the bicycle for training exercise while at the same time commuting to work, shopping, picking up the mail, or doing whatever you might otherwise do by automobile. You can ride alone and go at the speed that suits you best, or you can ride with other people. And while you are enjoying the ride, you are also building your fitness.

For short-distance rides around town, a three-speed bicycle may be adequate for your needs, but if you intend to take longer rides, you will appreciate a 10- or 12-speed vehicle. Speed on a bicycle is different from speed in a motorized vehicle. Nothing changes on the bicycle when you shift into a higher speed except the gear ratio. You still supply the power that determines how fast you go. The different speeds on a bicycle are used to enable you to maintain the same pedaling power, or expenditure of energy, whether you are going up or down hills or along level ground and whether you are pedaling into the wind or have it at your back. The gears make it possible for you to get the amount of exercise you want from your bicycling.

Swimming

Another popular aerobic exercise, probably the most widely pursued of all the forms, is swimming. Most people have access to swimming facilities, at least from time to time, and no special equipment is necessary to enjoy the sport. Swimming is an excellent all-around exercise in which most of the body's muscles come into play, and it can help increase lung capacity and cardiac output. A variety of strokes and fitness exercises can be done while swimming to further increase the health benefit of the sport.

Aerobic Dance

Aerobic dance has nearly unlimited potential for increasing aerobic endurance. This type dance requires continual movements that combine dance steps, running, jumping, and calesthenics. When an indi-

YOUR HEALTH TODAY

So You Want to Join a Fitness Center?

As more and more people join the exercise movement, so too a growing number of people are getting into the business of providing a place for exercise. Many of the people who are advertising their health spa or fitness center are not qualified to conduct such a program. Further, the staff that is hired often is not qualified to conduct exercise sessions nor to develop a program of fitness for you. Since licensing requirements have not been developed for persons working in this type of establishment, the uninformed individual may be misled and can, in fact, injure rather than improve her or his health.

Here are some timely questions you should consider prior to joining a health spa or fitness center.

- Is the staff qualified? Do they have special training in physical education, exercise physiology, nutrition, or a related field? Is this training from a recognized college or university?
- Is the center run by a competent medical advisor? Is there a medical advisor on the staff?
- What are the safety precautions that have been taken by the establishment? Is there someone always present who knows cardiopulmonary resuscitation? Is a preenrollment physical examination a requirement for membership? Is first-aid equipment readily available? Is there an insurance policy that is available for members, and who is the company that carries the policy? Is there a written emergency policy?
- Is the equipment in the establishment well maintained? Is it equipment that is generally "known" or is it something that the owners have devised? Is the equipment designed for the "complete" workout, or is it limited in scope?
- Does the staff promise quick results with little effort? (See Chapter 19 for more on this issue.) Is quick weight loss advocated, or is a more gradual approach suggested? Do the staff members advocate the use of a special diet for which you have to purchase pills or some other implement that is available only at the establishment?

Regardless of the responses to these questions, the best indicator is a visit to the establishment. Even then, proceed with caution.

vidual engages in aerobic dance, it takes a relatively short time to reach the aerobic fitness target heart rate. This type of activity is generally quite enjoyable because of the social aspect involved; and since the activity is maintained for a rather lengthy period, the cardiorespiratory benefits of training for at least 20 minutes are usually reached and surpassed. Many spas and fitness centers include aerobic dance as a part of the exercise classes they offer because of its great popularity.

Hiking

Many people enjoy hiking, but hiking is an activity that generally requires a fair degree of muscular strength and aerobic endurance. Depending upon the terrain, the elevation, the size of the individual, the speed at which the individual is moving, and whether or not the person is carrying a backpack, the amount of strength and endurance will be greater than or less than that required in other forms of aerobic activity. Further, for the exercise to be beneficial, the intensity of the exercise should be maintained throughout the duration of the exercise session. This is often difficult to do when hiking. For aerobic fitness to be improved by hiking, the individual should travel at the rate of one mile every 15 minutes (4 MPH).

Skipping Rope

Skipping, or jumping, rope is a good alternative for those who have no good place to jog or walk. A jump rope can even be taken on trips for use in motel or hotel rooms. As with jogging, the pace is up to the individual. Ten minutes of skipping rope can be equivalent to half an hour of jogging, but the individual should have a good degree of fitness prior to using skipping rope as a primary means of developing cardiorespiratory endurance.

Exercises for Muscular Strength and Endurance

Biceps big enough to brag about may boost the ego, but they are not an assurance of good general health. Strong muscles are needed for performing daily work chores and for being able to enjoy tennis, jogging, and similar sports, but only a generalized strength is necessary.

While push-ups and sit-ups will develop upper body and abdominal strength and endurance, resistance exercises with weights or strength machines are required for building strength in specific muscles. Most aerobic exercises will build leg strength in sufficient amounts, but few strength exercises will develop aerobic fitness.

A good general fitness exercise program, including the warm-up and cool-down phases, aids in developing the total muscle strength sufficient for most needs and pleasures of everyday living. Exceptional strength in a particular set of muscles, or in all of them, may be needed for some kinds of work or sports, but most people need only moderate strength. More important for the average person is endurance, which is the ability to continue activities without tiring.

Overloading Working a muscle harder than usual.

Hypertrophy Increased size in muscle fibers.

Muscles develop strength when the muscle fibers in a muscle increase in size. By causing a muscle to work harder than normal (**overloading**), the fibers **hypertrophy,** or get larger, and this is what gives the individual more strength.

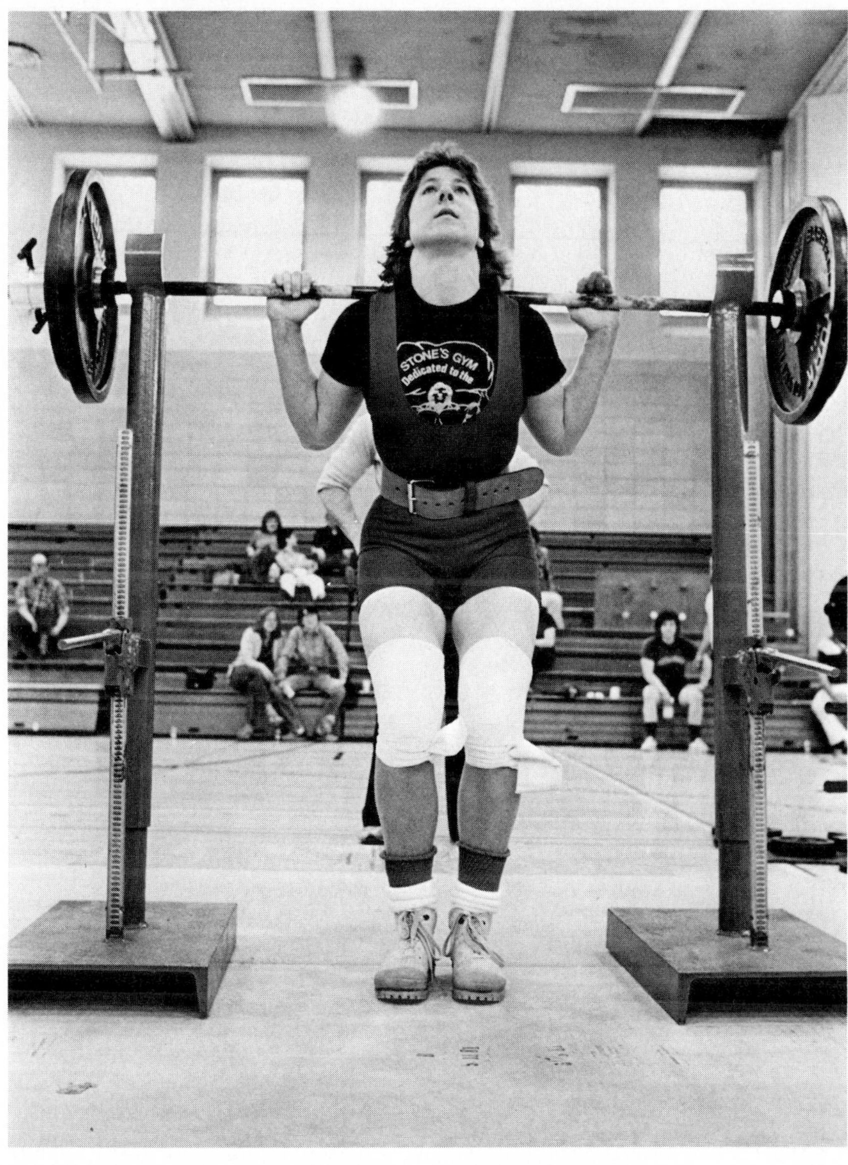

In lifting weights of any kind, it is important to keep the back straight, use a belt, and let the legs do most of the work. (Photo © 1982 Sarah Putnam/The Picture Cube)

In general, lifting heavy weights with fewer repetitions tends to build strength, while lifting lighter weights with more repetitions tends to build endurance.

Isotonic Lifting movable objects or weights.

Isometric Application of force against an immovable object.

Isokinetic Exertion of maximal force throughout a range of motion.

Isotonic, Isometric, and Isokinetic Exercises. Muscular strength and endurance can be developed **isotonically** (lifting movable objects or weights) or **isometrically** (applying force against an immovable object). Most recently, **isokinetic** exercise (exertion of maximal force throughout a range of motion) has been receiving a great deal of attention. Since isokinetic exercise requires fairly expensive equip-

YOUR HEALTH TODAY

Women and Exercise

Myths about the harmful effects of exercise on women abound. Several of these—and the facts—are included here.

- *Weight training is detrimental for women.* Weight training helps strengthen muscles and helps firm the body. Although muscle definition will improve, the reason for this is primarily because the fat tissue in the area has been somewhat depleted. When the "fat suit" disappears, the "muscle suit" can reappear.
- *Women shouldn't exercise during their menstrual flow.* Olympic medals have been won by women during all phases of the menstrual cycle. There is no evidence indicating that exercise should be discontinued during menstruation. If you have dysmenorrhea (painful menstruation), you should see a physician and you might reduce the intensity and duration of your exercise activity; but don't completely abandon it unless your physician orders it.
- *Women who exercise become more masculine.* This myth has been perpetuated throughout the ages. Hormonal influences keep the female feminine and the male masculine. All one needs to do is attend a swimming or gymnastics meet to realize that exercise may, in fact, increase femininity.
- *Women who are pregnant should not exercise.* Although the literature is sparse, researchers in this field state that if a woman exercised prior to pregnancy, there is no major reason (barring complications of the pregnancy) that she should discontinue her regular exercise routine, though perhaps at a somewhat reduced intensity. Naturally, certain exercises should be done with caution (i.e., uneven parallel bar routines, horseback riding, etc.) It is not a good idea to begin a strenuous exercise program if you have not exercised regularly prior to becoming pregnant; however, moderate exercise may prove beneficial to your subsequent delivery.

ment such as may be found in fitness centers, health clubs, or spas, this form of exercise is not available to most individuals.

Sit-ups. Sit-ups strengthen stomach muscles. The procedure for doing a sit-up is presented in Self-Assessment Exercise 12.1. When you begin your exercise program, two or three sit-ups may be all you can do, or should attempt. You will feel the effects in your stomach muscles not only immediately, but also the next day. As your muscles get stronger and gain endurance, you will be able to do ten or more without soreness.

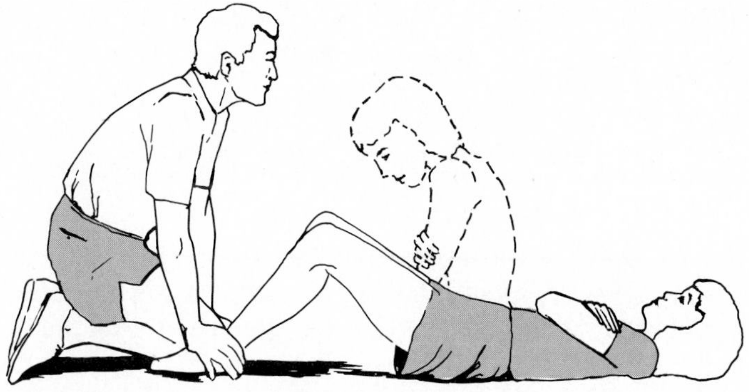

Figure 12-2.
Sit-ups help build abdominal strength and endurance and help increase trunk flexibility.

Starter Push-ups. For an easy starter push-up that will loosen your back, get on your hands and knees on the floor. Keep your arms slightly out at the sides of your body and then by bending your elbows lower the front of your body until your chest touches the floor. Keep the rear of your body elevated. Repeat this half a dozen times or more.

Full Push-ups. You can move from the previous exercise to full push-ups as described in Self-Assessment Exercise 12.1. This may not be an easy exercise at first, but as you get in better condition, you should be able to do ten or more push-ups with no difficulty. Push-ups will do much to strengthen the muscles of your arms and shoulders.

These exercises can also be done as a part of the flexibility segment of your exercise routine.

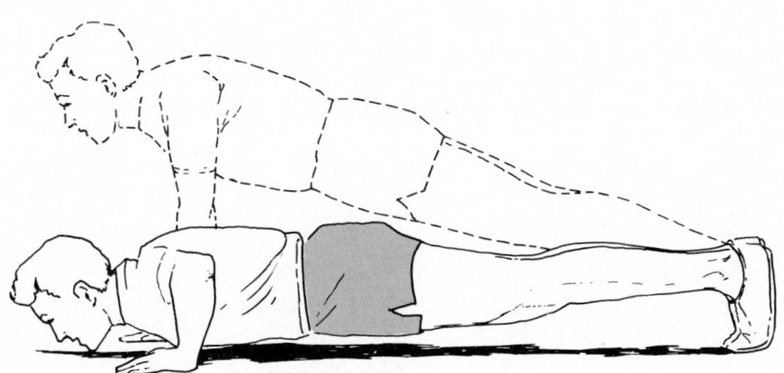

Figure 12-3.
Push-ups are a way to build upper body strength and endurance.

Flexibility Exercises

Before a takeoff, airplanes are taxied to the end of the runway, where the pilots warm up the engines. Circulating fuel and oil through the system and getting the motor prepared to respond without strain to the demands that will be made will cause an engine to operate smoothly and without strain. Wise athletes warm up their bodies for the same reason. They get the blood circulating and limber their muscles and joints to get ready for action.

Flexibility exercises are actually stretching exercises and are used both for warming up and cooling down. The flexibility exercises should be started slowly and smoothly. Avoid jerky motions or bouncing motions, since these can result in muscle strains and tears, especially if the individual has not warmed up sufficiently. Get to the full stretching position by degrees. If you go too fast, you may get the opposite effect from what is wanted—a tightening. And just because joints move freely does not necessarily mean the body is sufficiently warmed up. The muscles controlling the movement of these joints need to be limbered too so that undue stress is not put on tendons and ligaments when the more vigorous exercises are started. Flexibility exercises tend to limber the muscles.

Here are some good stretching exercises.

- Roll onto you back. Grab one leg below the knee with both hands and pull your knee up to your chest. Hold it there until the muscles in your back no longer feel pulled. Then repeat this with the other leg. Finally pull both legs up at the same time. Repeat this sequence at least three times.

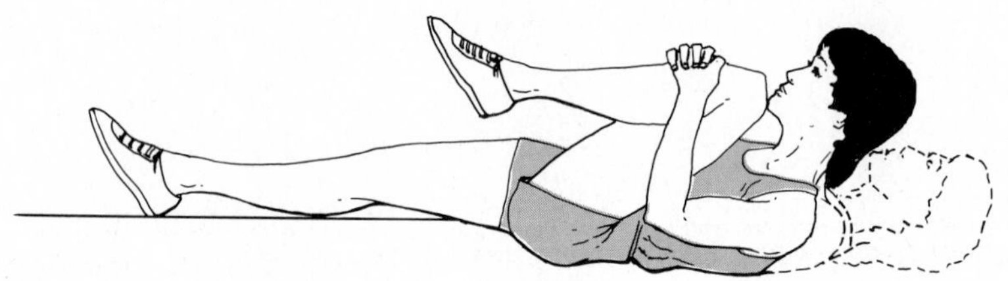

Figure 12–4. Stretching the low back is a good way to help alleviate low back pain.

- A familiar stretch is to sit with your feet slightly apart, one knee bent, and one knee kept straight. Then bend forward—slowly and very cautiously at first—twist, and reach for the outside of one shoe with the tips of your fingers. Stay in this position for a few seconds, then sit upright again. Repeat this half a dozen times. (On the first bend your fingers may be several inches from

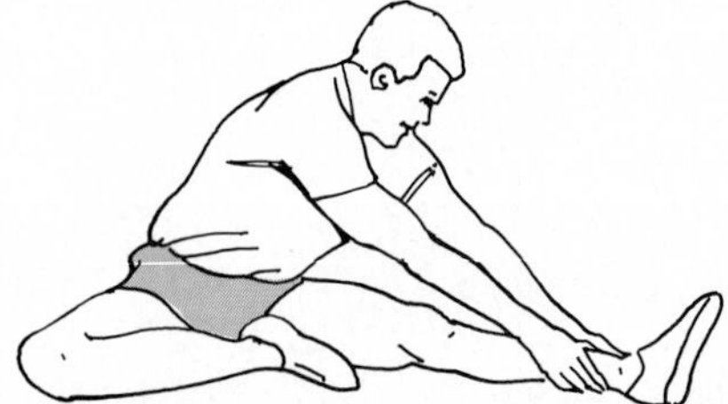

Figure 12–5. Doing a toe touch from a sitting position helps stretch the low back as well as the muscles along the back of the leg. One should not do a standing toe touch because of possible strain on the low back.

your toe, but after several bends they will probably touch it easily.) With this exercise, you stretch the muscles in your back and legs. Do this both to the right and left sides.

- For another back-limbering exercise, stand straight with your legs slightly apart and your arms hanging down at your sides. Then bend slowly as far as you can to the right, letting your hand slide down the side of your leg. Hold this position for several seconds, then return to an upright stance. Now repeat, but this time bending to the left. Repeat half a dozen times.

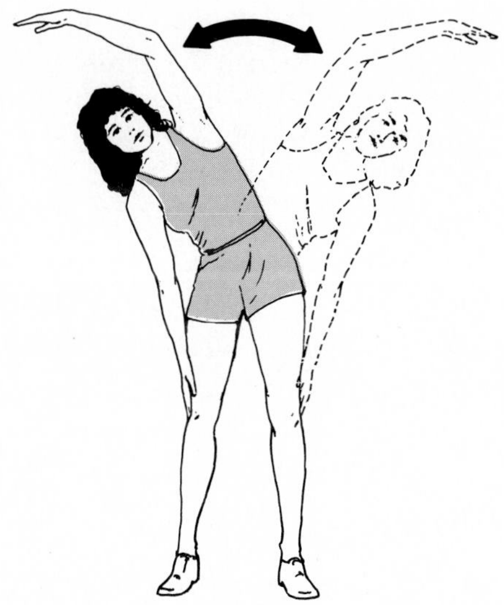

Figure 12-6. It is important to stretch the side muscles when warming up.

Figure 12-7. It is important not to neglect the shoulders and upper chest when stretching and warming up.

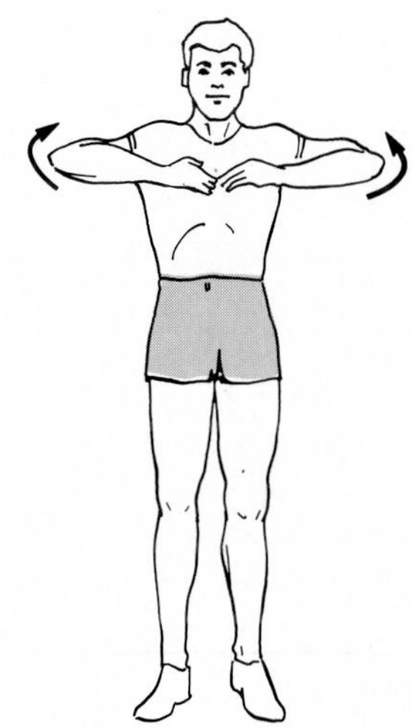

- Still another back stretch is done by putting your hands on your hips, then bending forward at the waist. Keep your legs slightly spread, and then slowly turn your body to the right and hold it there for a count of four. Return to an upright position, then bend forward again and turn to the left. Repeat this three or four times for each side.
- For stretching shoulder muscles gently, hold your arms up at shoulder level with your elbows bent inward. Then pull your arms back and forth as though slowly rowing a boat. Repeat this at least ten times.
- Another good arm exercise is done by extending your arms outwards and then rotating them, making six-inch circles with your hands. Rotate them about ten times in one direction, then the same number of times in the opposite direction. Repeat at least two times. Now lift one arm high above your head and keep the other at your side. Swing your arms so that first one and then the other is lifted. Continue swinging your arms in this way until each arm has been lifted a dozen times or more.

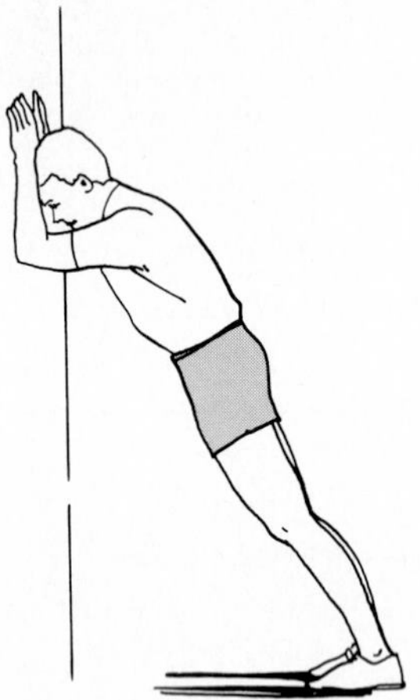

Figure 12–8.
The Achilles tendon and the hamstrings in the back of the leg must be stretched when warming up.

- Too often we ignore the calf and Achilles tendon when we are stretching. Stand in front of and about an arm's length away from a wall. The feet are flat on the floor and the knees are kept straight. Place the hands on the wall and slowly lean forward, bending your elbows but keeping your body straight. Continue leaning forward until you feel a stretching sensation in the calf and Achilles tendon. Hold the position for five to ten seconds and then slowly push backward to the starting position. Do this at least a half-dozen times.
- The upper thigh is another area that is often neglected in the warm-up. To stretch the upper thigh (quadriceps), stand erect and bend the left knee and lift the left foot directly toward the buttocks. Grasp the ankle with the left hand and try to touch the buttocks with the heel. There should be a stretching sensation in the upper thigh. You should use the wall for balance when you do this exercise. Repeat the exercise using the right knee and foot. Hold the exercise for five to ten seconds and repeat each side at least a half-dozen times.

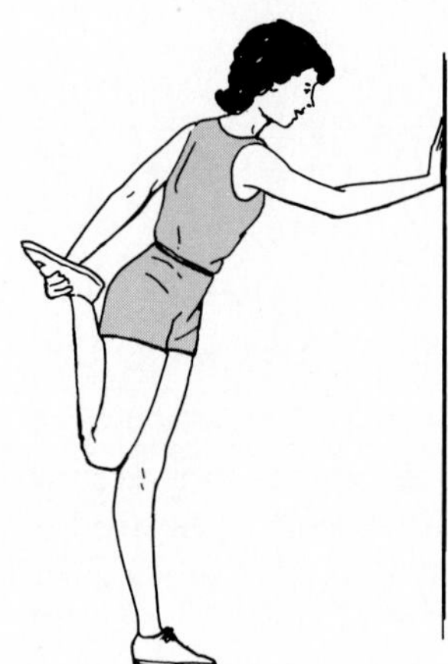

Figure 12–9.
Be sure to have good support when doing this exercise to stretch the quadriceps and upper thigh.

These are just a few of the exercises that can be used for warm-up and cool-down periods. It is not necessary to do all of them, but do make selections that exercise all parts of your body. If you see people doing other kinds of warm-up exercises, ask what benefits they get from them. You may want to give them a try if they will help in your particular fitness program. Some stretching or warm-up exercises are more effective than others for particular kinds of physical activity.

All of these are simple exercises, but until you are sure of your strength and flexibility, do not overdo. Be cautious. Bending over to touch the toes, for example, is harmless for most people, but for people who have been sedentary for years or for those with existing back problems, this is an exercise that can cause trouble. It is possible to get pains that are not at first identified with the back-stretching exercise. Flexibility is important for general fitness, but the degree of flexibility that athletes need is not necessary for everyone.

Motivation

No one starts a physical fitness program without good intentions of continuing, but it is sadly true that only about half of those who start are still exercising after a year. The professionals in the physical education field are greatly concerned about this high dropout rate and why it occurs.

People typically get into a physical fitness program to lose weight or to improve their general health. Fewer people start simply because they expect to enjoy themselves. Those who keep at it apparently do so because they derive personal or social pleasures from the activity or, in the case of sports, because they are driven by the spirit of competition. A third and very significant reason is that they feel good and want to continue the kind of life-style that has brought them this change.

You can avoid becoming a victim of the high dropout rate by making wise choices at the start. If jogging has absolutely no appeal to you and you are convinced even after a few tries that it would never be enjoyable, do not jog. If bicycling does excite you, then get a bicycle and start pedaling your way to aerobic fitness. You may end up pedaling from coast to coast, and along the way, you would encounter a surprising number of people of all ages doing exactly the same thing. If you get your greatest pleasure from competition, maybe your only consideration should be a competitive sport such as tennis.

If you are essentially a loner, do not feel compelled to join a group. But if you thrive on companionship, you may find that a partner, or a group, is the answer to keeping you involved in whatever activity you have selected. However you decide to go about it, make your physical fitness training program something you look forward to with enthusiasm and excitement. It should not be a self-imposed sentence to drudgery.

You might try keeping a few notes and statistics that will remind you later of your outlook on life and your physical condition when you started the program. Update the notes and other data regularly. After a few months you will have a clearer picture of why you are involved in an exercise program and also of the benefits you are getting.

Summary

Physical fitness is the ability to meet all of the ordinary and daily physical demands on the body without becoming tired and also being able to respond to extra demands when necessary.

The idea of physical fitness is a relatively new idea. For centuries people survived by physical exertion, but with modern labor-saving devices and changing life-styles, people became sedentary and less fit. During the 1960s, a new interest in physical fitness swept the nation, and millions of people became involved in various forms of fitness programs.

The main components of physical fitness are cardiorespiratory endurance, muscular strength and endurance, flexibility, and body composition. Cardiorespiratory endurance is a measure of how much oxygen is delivered to the tissues of the body and of how efficiently it is used. Strength is the capacity to exert force. Muscles require exercise to maintain strength. Endurance is the ability to exert force for a sustained period of time. Flexibility, or the degree of movement possible, involves joints, skin, and connective tissue as well as the muscles. Body composition is a measure of two components, lean and fat.

For most people the two most important fitness components are cardiorespiratory endurance and flexibility. Aerobic exercises are designed to increase lung capacity and circulatory efficiency. Running, swimming, and other exercises that require prolonged effort are effective in improving aerobic capacity.

Flexibility exercises are stretching exercises, and there are many different types that are effective. They should be begun slowly and cautiously, however, to avoid strain.

Each aerobic fitness exercise session should include a warm-up, a vigorous exercise activity, and a cool-down period. Jogging, skipping rope, and bicycling, among many others, are excellent forms of aerobic exercise.

It is recommended that people who have been inactive for several years or who are in their late twenties or older check with their doctor before undertaking a strenuous exercise program.

Motivation remains a problem in physical fitness programs: only about half of those who start are still exercising a year later. It is essential, therefore, to plan a program that takes your individual preferences into account.

Review and Discussion

1. Why is physical fitness a personal responsibility?
2. What improvements does exercise provide in the functioning of the circulatory and respiratory systems?
3. What are some other health benefits of physical exercise?
4. What are the five major components of physical fitness?
5. What components of physical fitness are most important for most people?
6. Demonstrate eight flexibility exercises.
7. What are the three parts of an aerobic exercise session? How often and how long should a person exercise?
8. Describe several types of aerobic exercise.
9. What precautions should be taken before beginning a strenuous exercise program?
10. Do you think you are getting enough exercise now? What physical fitness exercises do you think would be right for you?

Further Reading

Bailey, Covert. *Fit or Fat?* Boston: Houghton Mifflin Company, 1978.
The author describes how to attain fitness through nutrition and aerobic exercise and how to become a "better butter burner." (Paperback)

Cooper, Kenneth H. *The Aerobics Way.* New York: Bantam Books, 1978.
The author describes his system of aerobic exercise and provides a method for measuring individual progress. (Paperback)

Dintiman, George B., Stephen E. Stone, Jude C. Pennington, and Robert G. Davis. *Discovering Lifetime Fitness.* St. Paul, Minn.: West Publishing Company, 1984.
A basic text that contains key concepts of exercise and weight control. (Paperback)

Fixx, James. *The Complete Book of Running.* New York: Random House, 1977.
A well-illustrated description of the techniques of running.

Getchell, Bud. *Physical Fitness: A Way of Life,* 3d edition. New York: John Wiley & Sons, 1983.
A well-illustrated book designed to provide the basics of physical fitness. (Paperback)

Gilmore, C. P. *Exercising for Fitness.* Alexandria, Va.: Time-Life Books, 1981.
A good introductory guide to exercise programs.

Katz, Jane, with Nancy P. Bruning. *Swimming for Total Fitness.* New York: Doubleday & Company, 1981.
A complete guide to swimming as a form of aerobic exercise. (Paperback)

Root, Leon, and Thomas Kiernan. *Oh, My Aching Back!* New York: New American Library, 1975.
A guide to relief of backaches, with useful exercises that can help you guard against back pain in the future. (Paperback)

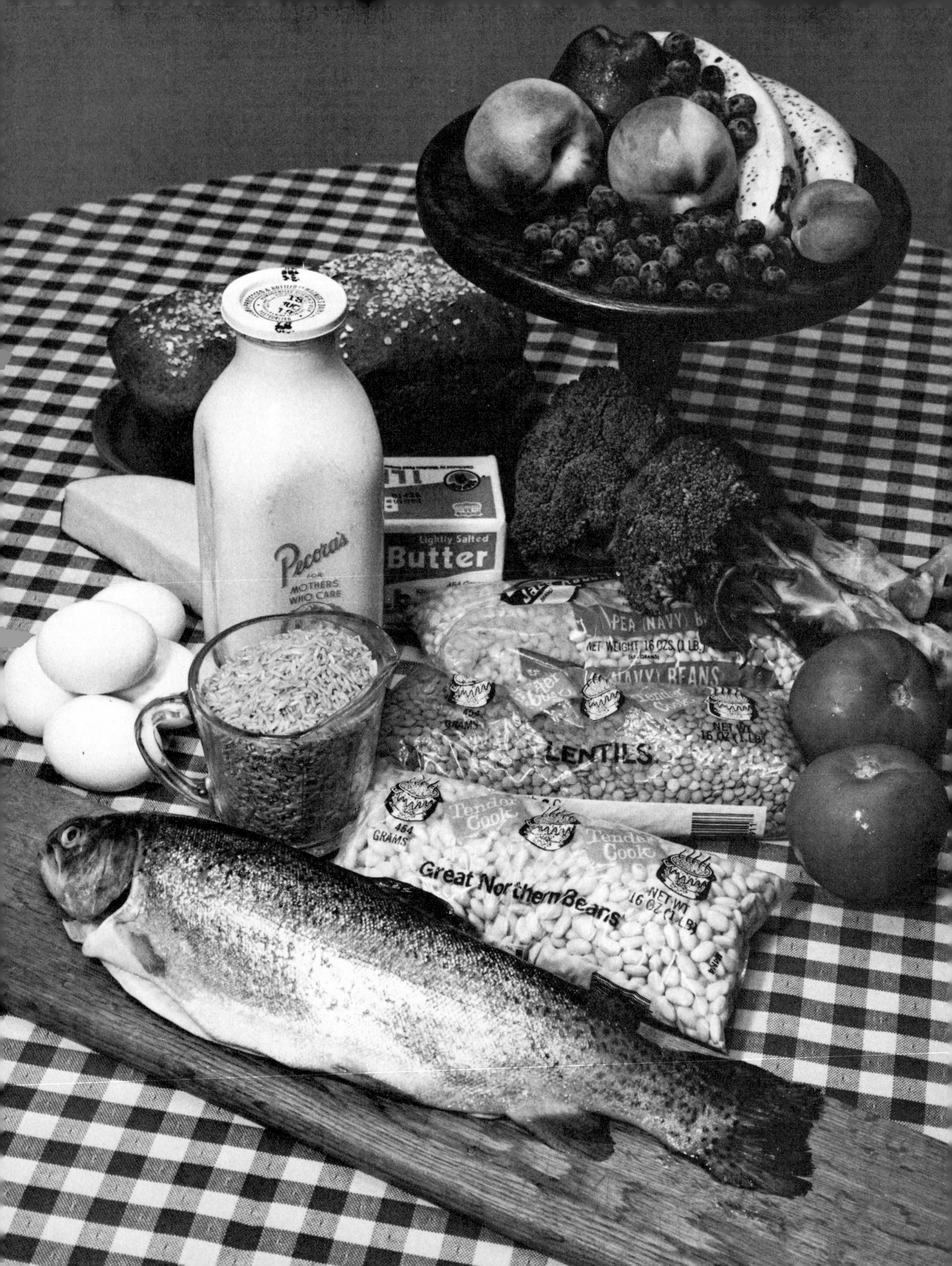
Pecora's
FOR
MOTHERS
WHO CARE
Lightly Salted
Butter
NET WEIGHT 16 OZS. (1 LB.)
454
GRAMS
LENTILS
NET WT
16 OZ (1 LB)
Tender
Cook
Great Northern Beans

Chapter 13
Nutrition

KEY POINTS

- ☐ Only in the last decade has nutrition emerged as a subject of wide concern.
- ☐ Recommended Dietary Allowances (RDA), first established in 1941 and revised every four to six years since then, measure the nutritional needs of people according to age, weight, and sex.
- ☐ Recommended Daily Allowances (U.S. RDA), devised by the Food and Drug Administration, are the legal standard for labeling the nutrient content of food.
- ☐ The basic, or "leader," nutrients are representative of six classes: carbohydrates, fats, proteins, vitamins, minerals, and water.
- ☐ Nutritionists have classified foods into groups according to the primary contributions they make in the diet. The basic food groups are meats and meat substitutes; dairy products; fruits and vegetables; grains and cereals; and fats, sweets, and alcohol.
- ☐ Research and adequate diet have eradicated many of the deficiency diseases. The new frontier is diet therapy applied to the chronic diseases of mankind, many of which are fostered by the individual's life-style.
- ☐ Infants, children, and adolescents, as well as the elderly, have special nutritional needs. Athletes, for the most part, do not need a special diet.

IT WAS a series of discoveries in the 1970s that generated first concern, then wide public interest, in nutrition. Reports began circulating about the harmful substances in food: pesticides and fertilizers from the farm, cancer-producing hormones in cattle feed, fish polluted by industrial waste. In the laboratory, megadoses of many substances induced cancer in rats.

In reaction, people began to turn away from processed foods. Some resorted to health food stores and "organic" foods. Others became vegetarians, in the belief that this posed less of a threat of consuming quantities of toxic pollutants. Convinced that all natural goodness had been processed out of food and restored with synthetics, Americans began to read food labels and condemn all additives and dyes, no matter how benign or natural.

Interest in nutrition received another boost from the growing wellness movement. Good nutrition was fundamental to the idea that health was not simply the absence of disease but a continual process of attaining greater personal well-being. "We must stop trying to buy health with our dollars," said one early leader, "and start earning it with our behaviors."

Nutrition can be defined as "the science of food as it relates to optimal health and performance." In the past, nutritionists confined themselves to taking inventory of the kinds and amounts of food eaten. Now the greatest needs in nutrition, in addition to ongoing research, are education and communication. A solid background in the basics of good nutrition is essential for understanding functioning of the human body. In this chapter you will be given a strong foundation upon which to build a nutrition program that will contribute to your personal well-being. Do you feel comfortable with your current level of knowledge about nutrition? Why not test your "Nutrition Quotient" by completing Self-Assessment Exercise 13.1.

SELF-ASSESSMENT EXERCISE 13.1

What's Your NQ (Nutrition Quotient)?

In the space provided, indicate whether you think the item is true or false.

	True	False
1. Fiber is considered one of the basic nutrients.	____	____
2. Vegetables are generally considered high-quality protein sources.	____	____
3. It's okay to skip breakfast as long as you take a vitamin pill each day.	____	____

	True	False
4. A meal that includes fish, cottage cheese, coffee and cake would be considered well-balanced.	____	____
5. Foods such as bee's honey and wheat germ have unusual nutritional benefit.	____	____
6. Processing of foods generally adversely affects their nutritional value.	____	____
7. The danger of pesticides to consumers of foods is greater than the value of using them for food production.	____	____
8. Eating a variety of foods each day ensures good nutrition.	____	____
9. Fats can be eliminated from the diets without serious health effects resulting.	____	____
10. Getting more of one nutrient can compensate for not getting enough of another nutrient.	____	____
11. The elderly need fewer vitamins than younger persons.	____	____
12. The caloric value of a gram of carbohydrate is greater than a gram of protein.	____	____
13. Growing foods using chemical fertilizers detracts from the nutritional value of foods.	____	____
14. Low-serum cholesterol has been found to be associated with heart disease.	____	____
15. Vegetables grown in nutrient-poor soil will lack vitamins and minerals necessary for good nutrition.	____	____
16. Saturated fats are found primarily in vegetable oils.	____	____
17. Large doses of Vitamin C will prevent colds.	____	____
18. Buying sugar-coated cereals is economically and nutritionally sound since the sugar is already added to them.	____	____
19. If your weight is in the normal range, your nutritional status would be considered good.	____	____
20. The essential amino acids can be made by the body.	____	____

Scoring: All of the above items are false. Give yourself one point for each item you got correct. If you score 18 or above, congratulations—you have a good knowledge of some of the basic nutritional misconceptions held by many people. If you score 15–17, you have some basic information about nutritional misconceptions, but you may hold some misconceptions that could adversely affect your health. If you scored between 12–14, you tend to hold more nutritional misconceptions than many individuals and should be careful about how you select foods. If you scored below 12, you should carefully reevaluate the knowledge you have about nutrition, for your decisions in this area could have serious consequences for your health.

Dietary Guidelines

In December 1977 the Senate Select Committee on Nutrition, chaired by Senator George McGovern, published its Dietary Goals, which took a tough stand on American dietary practices. Since then, four other major agencies, including the surgeon general's office, have come out with policy statements that are in accord for the most part. The most recent recommendations are the Dietary Guidelines set by the United States Department of Agriculture (USDA) and the Department of Health and Human Services (DHHS). These recommendations are a step ahead of the McGovern committee goals because they reflect the belief that nutrition can have a beneficial effect in preventing disease. They were formulated to take into consideration the risk that many people have of developing heart disease, diabetes, high blood pressure, or cancer. Briefly stated, the guidelines are:

1. Eat a variety of foods.
2. Maintain an ideal weight.
3. Avoid excesses of fat, saturated fat, and cholesterol.
4. Eat foods with adequate starch and fiber.
5. Avoid excessive amounts of sugar.
6. Avoid excessive amounts of sodium (salt).
7. Consume alcohol only in moderation.

These simple but prudent guidelines were intended to complement the earlier recommendations of several governmental bodies.

Recommended Dietary Allowance (RDA)

Recommended Dietary Allowances (RDAs) General guideline for nutritional requirements.

The nutritional standards of the **Recommended Dietary Allowances** were first established in 1941 by the Food and Nutrition Board of the National Research Council of the Academy of Sciences. For the purposes of national defense at the outset of America's entry into World War II, the country needed to measure the nutritional needs of groups of people. Since then the RDAs have been revised every five years to keep pace with new research.

Recommended Daily Allowance (U.S. RDA)

U.S. Recommended Daily Allowances (U.S. RDAs) Legal standard for labeling the nutritional value of foods.

Devised by the Food and Drug Administration as an aid to consumers, the **Recommended Daily Allowances** (U.S. RDAs) are a simplified version of the Recommended Dietary Allowances (RDAs) set by the Food and Nutrition Board in 1968. These recommendations represent the highest nutrient recommendations for males and nonpregnant or nonlactating females who are over four years of age (somewhat different standards exist for persons under four years of

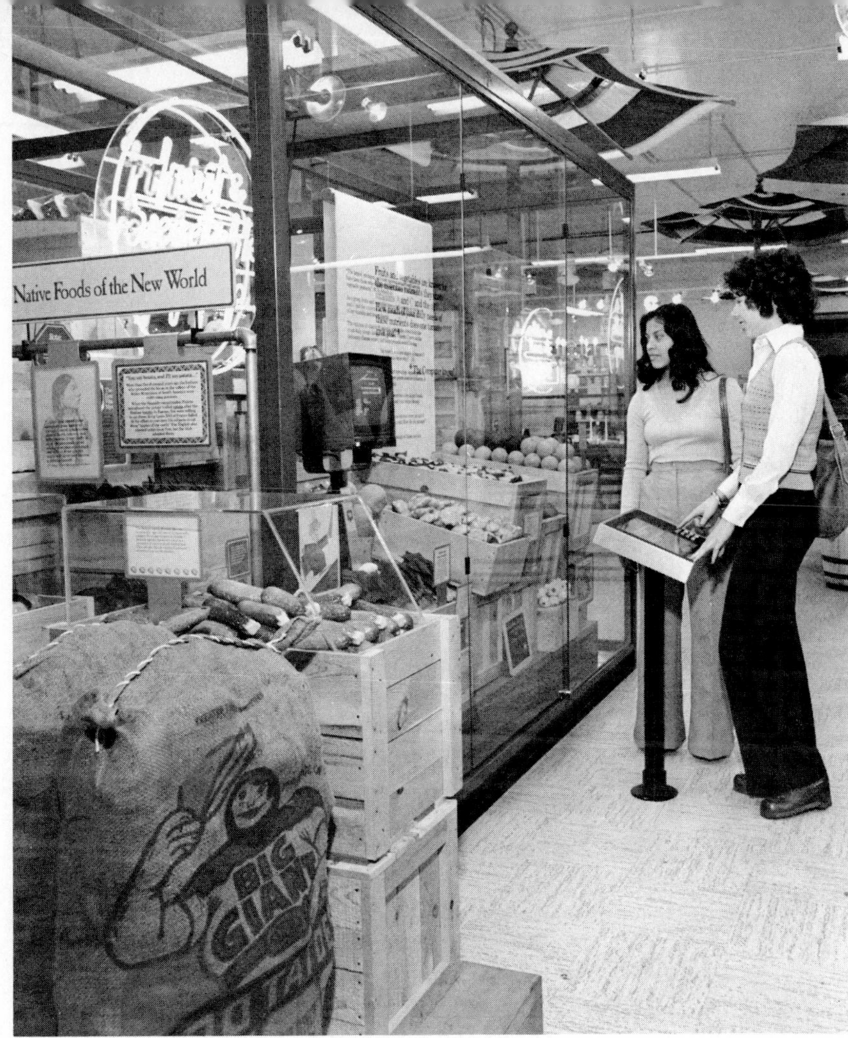

The Food for Life exhibit at Chicago's Museum of Science and Industry. Education of the public is among the greatest needs in the field of nutrition today. (Photo by Paul Waldman)

age). In 1975 the U.S. RDAs became the legal standard for labeling the nutrient content of food. It is important to remember that these are not specific standards but rather recommendations for healthy, not ill, individuals. These recommendations are not intended to be the minimal amounts of nutrients that are needed to keep people from showing signs of deficiency disease; however, they are set high enough to surpass the nutrient needs of as much as 98 percent of the population of healthy persons.

Certain nutrient contents of some 350 different foods must be listed on the package if the products contain anything other than the "standards of identity," or basic ingredients, for the product. The labels must list ten "leader" nutrients and any vitamin and mineral additives. The **leader nutrients** are protein, carbohydrate, fat, vitamins A and C, thiamin, riboflavin, niacin, calcium, and iron. If these nutrients are present in the diet in appropriate amounts, it is probable that the rest are being supplied (see Figure 13–1 and Table 13–1). If the manufacturer chooses to do so, 12 other vitamins and minerals may also be listed.

Leader nutrients Basic nutrients. the amount of which must be specified on labels.

Figure 13-1. The Body's Basic Needs.

NUTRIENT	Important Sources of Nutrient
Protein	Meat, Poultry, Fish Dried Beans and Peas Egg, Cheese, Milk 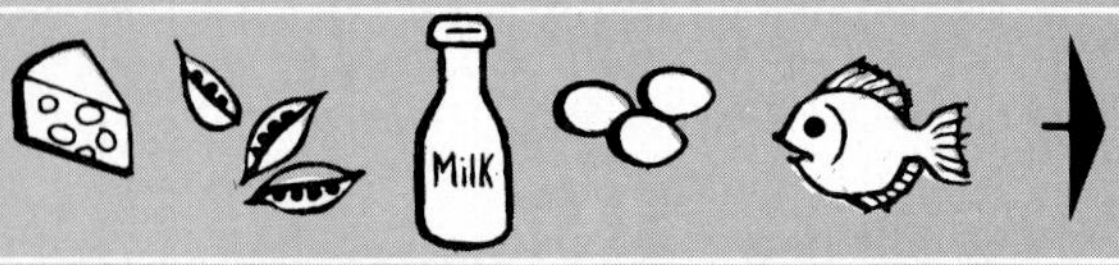
Carbohydrate	Cereal, Potatoes Dried Beans Corn Bread Sugar 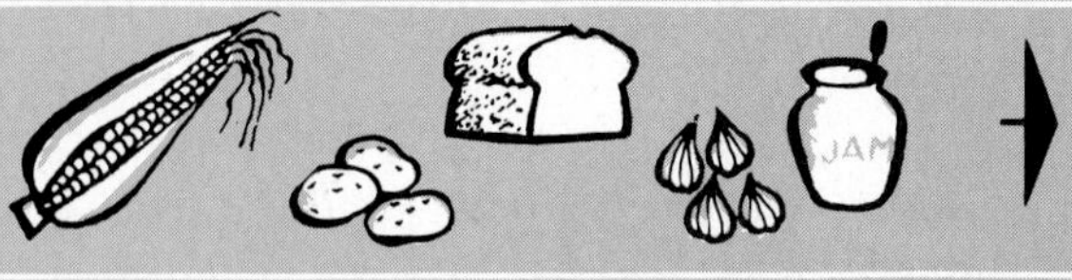
Fat	Shortening, Oil, Butter Margarine, Salad Dressing Sausages 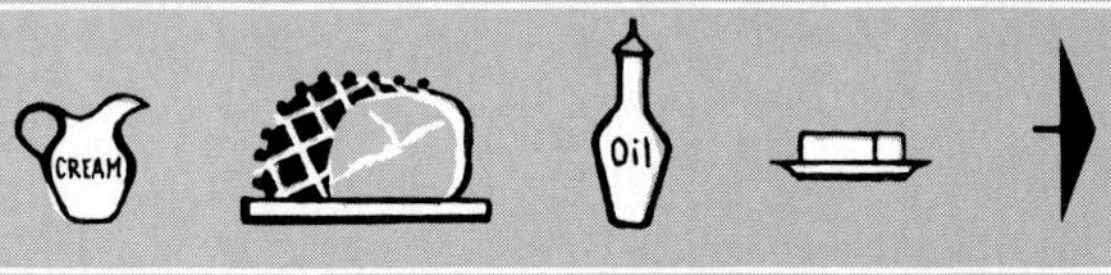
Vitamin A	Liver Carrots, Greens Sweet Potatoes Butter, Margarine 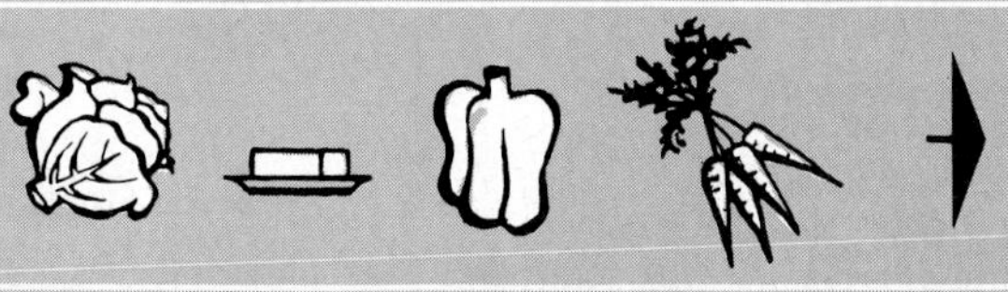
Vitamin C (ascorbic acid)	Broccoli Orange, Grapefruit Papaya, Mango Strawberries 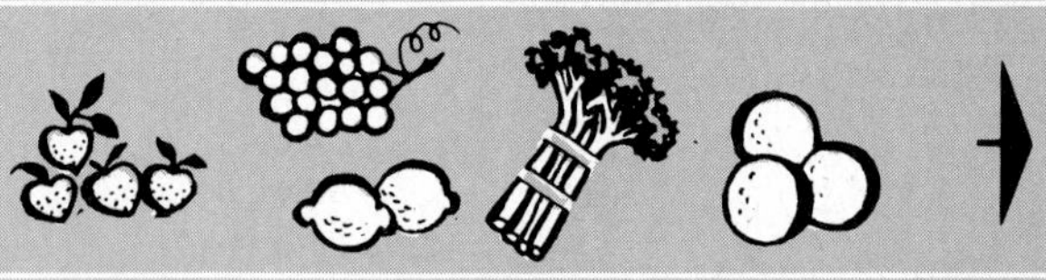
Thiamin (vitamin B_1)	Lean Pork Nuts Fortified Cereal Products 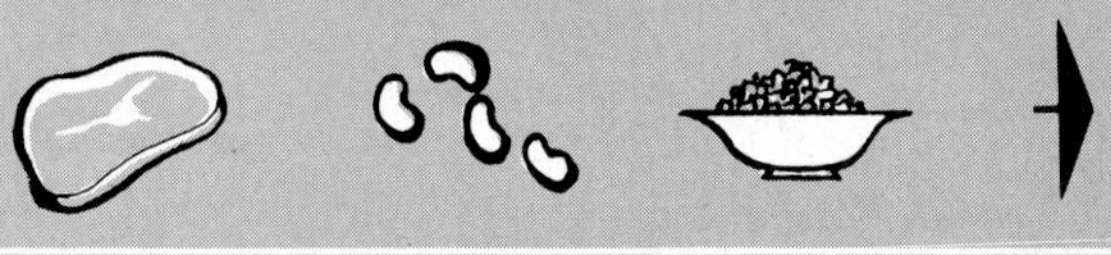
Riboflavin (vitamin B_2)	Liver Milk, Yogurt Cottage Cheese 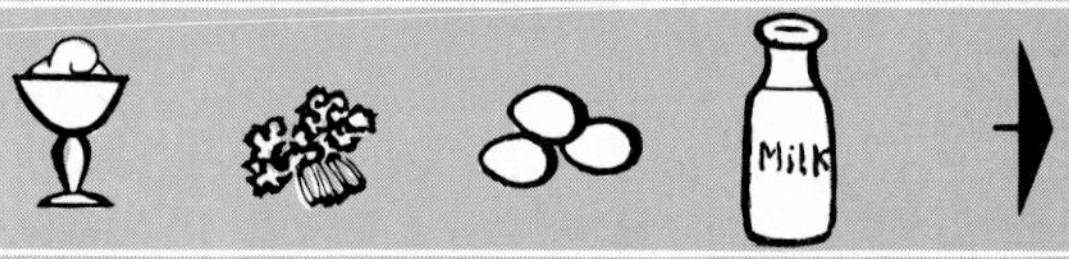
Niacin	Liver Meat, Poultry, Fish Peanuts Fortified Cereal Products 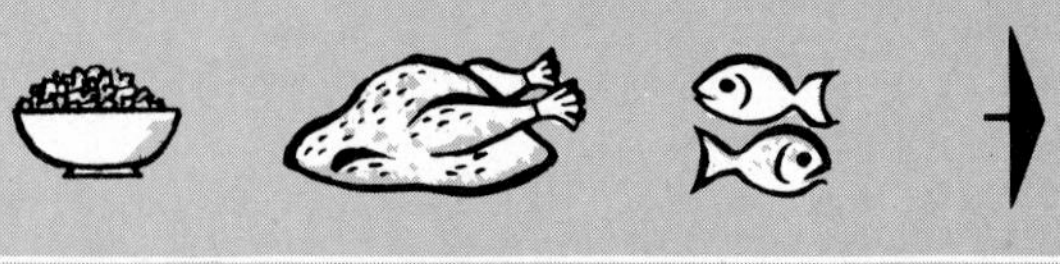
Calcium	Milk, Yogurt, Cheese Sardines and Salmon with Bones Collard, Kale, Mustard, and Turnip Greens 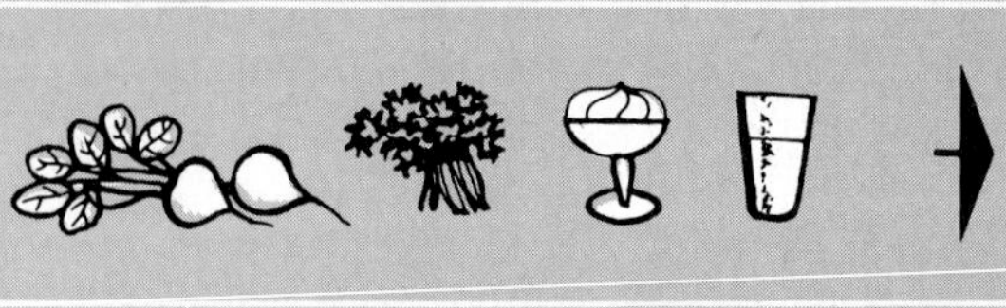
Iron	Enriched Farina Prune Juice Liver Dried Beans and Peas Red Meat 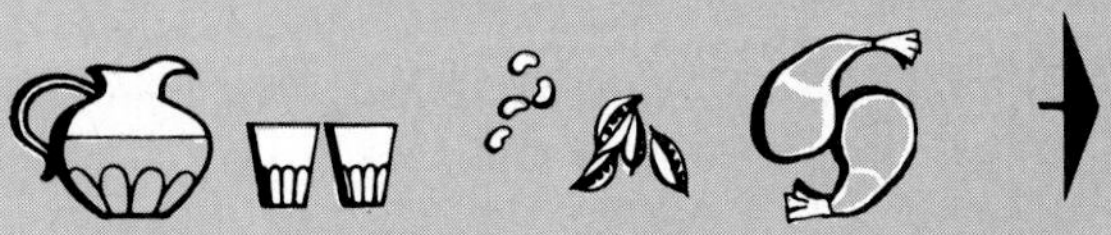

Some Major Physiological Functions

Provide Energy	Build and Maintain Body Cells	Regulate Body Processes
Supplies 4 calories per gram.	Constitutes part of the structure of every cell, such as muscle, blood, and bone; supports growth and maintains healthy body cells.	Constitutes part of enzymes, some hormones and body fluids, and antibodies that increase resistance to infection.
Supplies 4 calories per gram. Major source of energy for central nervous system.	Supplies energy so protein can be used for growth and maintenance of body cells.	Unrefined products supply fiber—complex carbohydrates in fruits, vegetables, and whole grains—for regular elimination. Assists in fat utilization.
Supplies 9 calories per gram.	Constitutes part of the structure of every cell. Supplies essential fatty acids.	Provides and carries fat-soluble vitamins (A, D, E, and K).
	Assists formation and maintenance of skin and mucous membranes that line body cavities and tracts, such as nasal passages and intestinal tract, thus increasing resistance to infection.	Functions in visual processes and forms visual purple, thus promoting healthy eye tissues and eye adaptation in dim light.
	Forms cementing substances, such as collagen, that hold body cells together, thus strengthening blood vessels, hastening healing of wounds and bones, and increasing resistance to infection.	Aids in utilization of iron.
Aids in utilization of energy.		Functions as part of a coenzyme to promote the utilization of carbohydrate. Promotes normal appetite. Contributes to normal functioning of nervous system.
Aids in utilization of energy.		Functions as part of a coenzyme in the production of energy within body cells. Promotes healthy skin, and clear vision.
Aids in utilization of energy.		Functions as part of a coenzyme in fat synthesis, tissue respiration, and utilization of carbohydrate. Promotes healthy skin and nerves. Aids digestion and fosters normal appetite.
	Combines with other minerals within a protein framework to give structure and strength to bones and teeth.	Assists in blood clotting. Functions in normal muscle contraction and relaxation and normal nerve transmission.
Aids in utilization of energy.	Combines with protein to form hemoglobin, the red substance in blood that carries oxygen to and carbon dioxide from the cells. Prevents nutritional anemia and its accompanying fatigue. Increases resistance to infection.	Functions as part of enzymes involved in tissue respiration.

Source: © 1977 National Dairy Council, Rosemont, Ill. 60018.

Table 13-1 U.S. Recommended Daily Allowances*

Protein†	45 g‡
Vitamin A†	5,000 IU§
Vitamin C (ascorbic acid)†	60 mg
Thiamin (vitamin B_1)†	1.5 mg
Riboflavin (vitamin B_2)†	1.7 mg
Niacin†	20 mg
Calcium†	1.0 g
Iron†	18 mg
Vitamin D	400 IU§
Vitamin E	30 IU§
Vitamin B_6	2.0 mg
Folic acid (folacin)	0.4 mg
Vitamin B_{12}	0.006 mg
Phosphorus	1.0 g
Iodine	0.15 mg
Magnesium	400 mg
Zinc	15 mg
Copper	2 mg
Biotin	0.3 mg
Pantothenic acid	10 mg

* U.S. RDAs for adults and children 4 years and older.

† These, along with carbohydrates and fats, are the 10 "leader" nutrients.

‡ Figure refers to animal protein. Since proteins in plants are lower in quality, it would take 65 g of plant protein to meet the U.S. RDA for protein.

§ An IU is an International Unit, an agreed-upon international standard amount that will produce a particular biological effect.

Source: U.S. Food and Drug Administration.

The amount of each nutrient is listed on the label according to the percentage it represents of the U.S. RDA. A 100 percent U.S. RDA rating is more than enough for most people because the RDA standards include a margin of safety and because the FDA usually took the highest RDA value within each category in determining the U.S. RDA. Generally speaking, daily intake of each nutrient should approach 100 percent of the U.S. RDA.

Consumers can also use the ingredients listed on the label to determine the relative amounts of the various nutrients in a product. Although only protein, carbohydrate, and fat are listed by weight at the top of the label, the ingredient list also provides clues. The contents of the product are listed in descending order by weight. The ingredient that makes up the largest part of the product is listed first. If your cereal lists sugar in any form before the grains, you have a good idea of its nutritional content.

Basic Nutrients

Exactly what substances and quantities are included in the U.S. RDAs?

The leader nutrients are representative of six classes, or categories, of **essential nutrients:** carbohydrates, fats, proteins, vitamins, minerals, and water. To function properly, the body must have some of each regularly. It cannot, for example, operate on carbohydrates alone, protein alone, or even on only four or five. The nutrients interact with each other, and all must be present in the right amounts. Eating a variety of foods is the only way to ensure good nutrition (see Figure 13–2).

Essential nutrients Nutrients vital to proper bodily functions.

The Function of Food

In the body, food performs three functions:

1. Provides materials to build, repair, and maintain body tissues.
2. Supplies substances that help regulate body processes.
3. Furnishes fuel needed for energy.

If calorie input surpasses energy output, overweight results (see Chapter 14, "Weight Control"). This energy imbalance troubles many Americans, particularly as they grow older. With advancing age, calorie intake often remains high while physical activity decreases. The

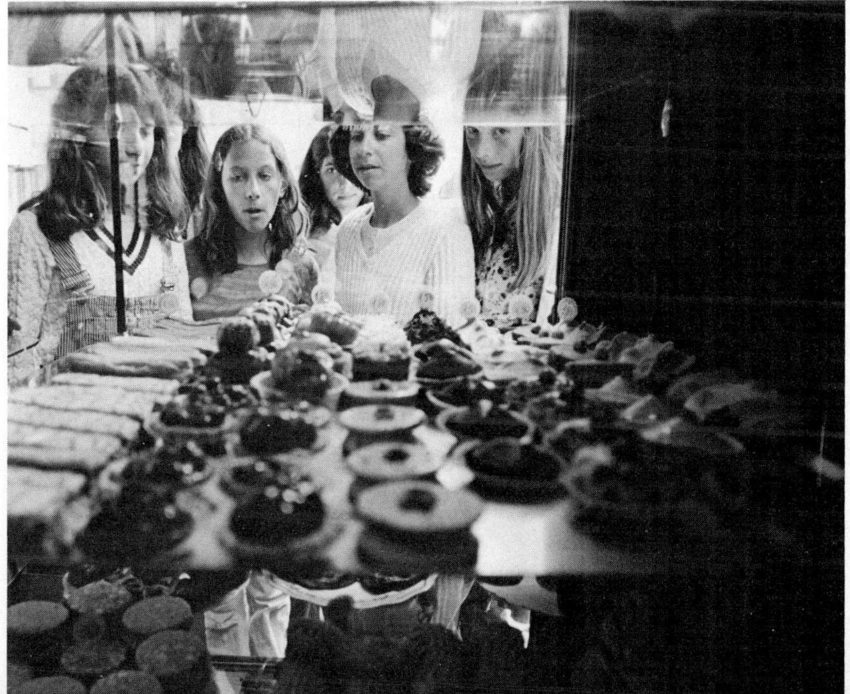

We are often confronted with choices about the type of snacks we will consume. The American passion for sweets, such as the baked goods shown here, has alarmed many nutritionists. (Photo by Carol Wolinsky/Stock, Boston)

Foods in This Group Include
Meats and Meat Substitutes
Beef, pork, veal, lamb, fish, poultry, eggs, organ meats, cheeses, dry beans, lentils, peas, and nuts
Dairy
MILK
Milk, yogurt, natural and processed cheeses, ice cream, ice milk, and food products made with milk
Fruits and Vegetables
All fruits and vegetables (fresh, canned, frozen, dried, and juices)
Grains
Whole-grain or enriched white flour, pasta, rice, and cereal products
CALORIC EXTRAS: The following foods have relatively little nutritional value besides calories. Therefore, no specific amount is recommended, and they should be added to your diet according to your caloric allowance: butter, margarine, shortening,

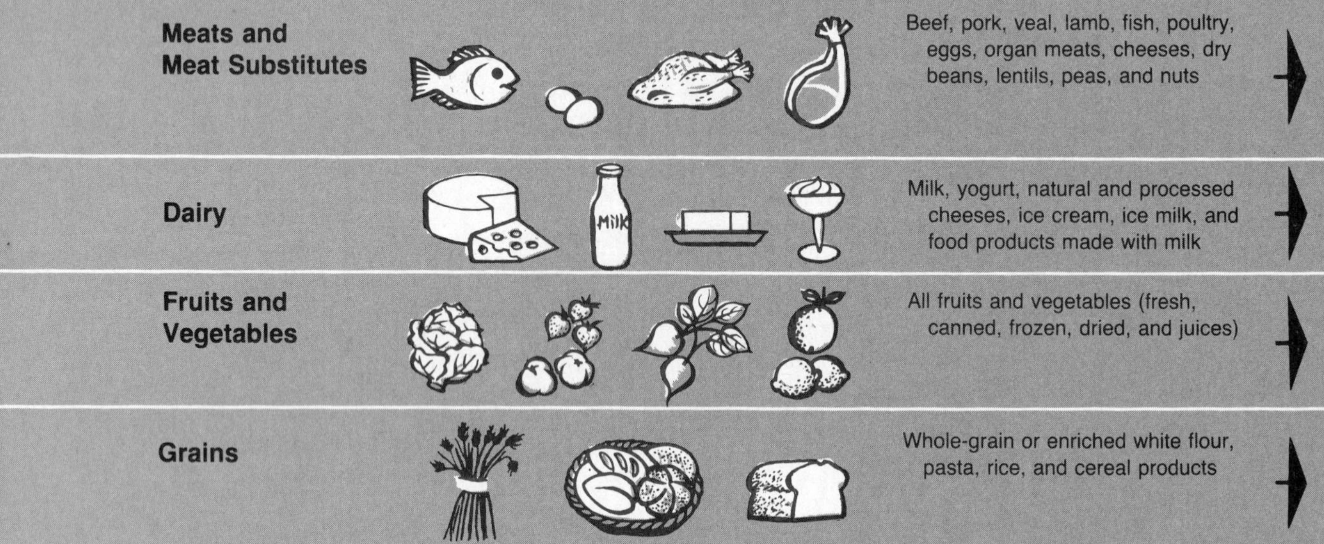

Figure 13-2. Basic Food Groups.

results of deficiencies and imbalances in the first two areas of function listed are less apparent but just as serious.

Carbohydrates

Carbohydrates Essential nutrients composed of sugars and starches.

At present, Americans derive about half of their caloric requirements from **carbohydrates** — sugars and starches — which are an excellent energy source. The McGovern Committee recommended that we increase our consumption of complex carbohydrates (potatoes and whole-grain breads, for instance) from 46 to 58 percent of our total energy intake and limit to 10 percent our consumption of refined carbohydrates. Thus most of us should reduce our refined and processed sugar intake by 50 percent while doubling our intake of "natural sugars." This would tend to increase our intake of both dietary fiber and many vitamins and minerals.

Natural sugars are found in fruits and their juices. Starches, which are simply more complex forms of sugars, are found mainly in whole grains, beans, and green vegetables.

Nutritionists have become alarmed at the percentage of sugar in the American diet. Since 1900 it has increased from 31 percent to 50 percent. Our per capita consumption is estimated at more than 130

Major Nutrients Supplied	Recommended Servings	One Serving Equals
Protein, fat, niacin, iron, thiamin, vitamin B_{12}, vitamin E, phosphorus, copper	Adults, children, and teenagers—2; pregnant and nursing women—3	2 ounces cooked meat, fish, or poultry; 2 eggs; 1 cup cooked dry beans, peas, or lentils; ½ cup nuts or 4 tablespoons peanut butter; 2 ounces hard cheese; ½ cup cottage cheese; 2 cups milk may be substituted for 1 meat serving
Protein, fat, calcium, riboflavin, vitamins A and D, magnesium, zinc	Children—3; teenagers—4; adults—2; pregnant and nursing women—4	1 cup milk or yogurt; 1 ounce cheese; ½ cup cottage cheese; ½ cup ice cream; 1 cup milk-based product (pudding, soup, or beverage)
Carbohydrate, water, vitamins A and C, iron, magnesium	Everyone—4 (including 1 citrus fruit daily and 1 deep green or yellow vegetable every other day)	1 cup cut-up raw fruit or vegetable; 1 medium apple, banana, orange, tomato, or potato; ½ melon or grapefruit; ½ cup cooked vegetable or fruit; ½ cup fruit or vegetable juice
Carbohydrate, fat, protein, thiamin, niacin, vitamin E, calcium, iron, phosphorus, magnesium, zinc, copper	Everyone—4	1 slice bread; 1 ounce dry cereal; 1 roll or muffin; 1 pancake or waffle; ½ cup rice, pasta, or cooked cereal

oils, dressings, condiments, sugars, candies, syrups, jams, unenriched refined grain products, sweetened desserts and pastries, soft drinks, and presweetened fruit drinks.

Source: *U.S. Department of Agriculture.*

pounds of refined sugar a year. This refined sugar comes from such things as desserts, food additives, and processed foods like bread and luncheon meats. Soft drinks have assumed the number one position as the beverage of choice of Americans (replacing coffee), and the average American consumes 410 cans or bottles of soft drinks per year.

The problem is that although a sugar-laden food does provide energy, it lacks other needed nutrients. In addition, sugar reduces appetite, so people can feel satisfied though they are not being properly nourished. Frequent high intake of sugar can lead to diabetes, dental cavities, and obesity. Obesity itself can lead to a wide range of diseases, including cardiovascular disease (see Chapter 16).

The Body's Need for Carbohydrates

Although many people feel that eliminating carbohydrates from the diet is a good way to lose weight, it should be stressed that approximately 125 milligrams of carbohydrates are needed daily in order to effectively burn the fat that is stored in the body. It is generally agreed that we should consume from 50 to 100 grams of carbohydrate each day (the equivalent of four servings of breads, cereals, rice, or pasta) if we are to obtain enough fuel for our daily activities. It should also be pointed out that, in general, carbohydrates provide the cheapest source of fuel for our bodies and that if we do not take in enough, we don't burn fat. This contributes to the storage of the fat that would normally be used during daily activity and can lead to obesity (see Chapter 14).

Fiber

Fiber (roughage) Indigestible carbohydrates that aid elimination of wastes.

Not all carbohydrates are digestible. Cellulose, the main constituent of wood, cannot be digested by man. Even termites are unable to digest cellulose and must depend on one-celled animals, protozoa, in the gut to perform this function for them. However, some of the largely indigestible carbohydrates contribute to what is called roughage, or dietary **fiber,** that is needed in the diet. Fiber appears to delay stomach emptying and promote regular elimination of undigested wastes by making the solid waste bulkier and softer. Scientists are still investigating the role of fiber in the diet and in the treatment or prevention of such disorders as diverticulosis, colon cancer, overweight, constipation, the lowering of blood cholesterol levels, and hemorrhoids. Whole-grain cereals and breads, fruits and vegetables (raw or barely cooked), and legumes are good fiber sources.

Proteins

Protein Essential nutrients that consist of 22 amino acids.

Amino acids The 22 "building blocks" of protein.

More than half of our body mass is **protein.** Skin, hair, nails, blood, muscles, and organs all contain unique protein configuratons. Proteins consist of 22 small units called **amino acids,** 20 of which are needed to carry on such basic body functions as maintenance and repair of body tissues, production of hemoglobin, antibody formation, and enzyme and hormone production.

Essential amino acids The nine protein units that the body cannot produce by itself.

Most amino acids can be made by the body, but nine (ten in children) must be ingested daily since they cannot be synthesized by the body. These nine are called the **essential amino acids** and must be present in the body in the correct amounts at the same time in order for the body to function properly. Thus, although some experts think it is important to space protein intake in such a manner as to provide a steady, constant supply at intervals throughout the day, it is important to consume foods containing the nine essential amino acids at one time to assure all of them are present simultaneously in the body.

Complete proteins Foods containing all the essential amino acids.

Incomplete proteins Proteins lacking some amino acid.

Foods containing all the essential amino acids are called **complete proteins.** Most animal proteins (fish, poultry, eggs, and milk products) fall into this category. Plant proteins such as in grains, legumes, and some fruits contain fewer of the essential amino acids and thus are called **incomplete proteins.** This has implications for people who prefer vegetarian diets, for it is necessary to combine several of these low-quality protein sources at the same time to ensure simultaneous intake of the essential amino acids (see Your Health Today, "So You Want to Be a Vegetarian?").

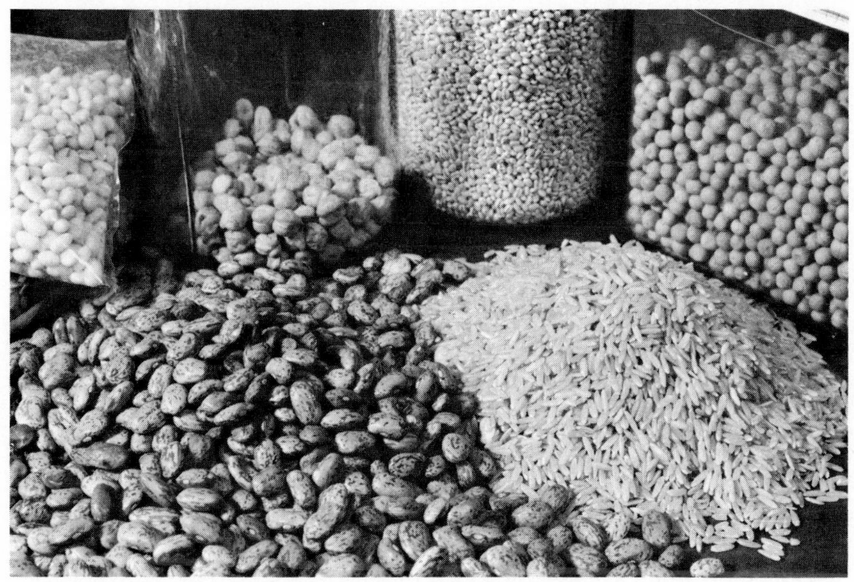

In Spanish-American cuisine rice and beans are used extensively. The nutrients in the two complement each other to help produce a balanced diet. (Photo by Paul Waldman)

How Much Protein Is Needed?

According to the National Research Council of the Academy of Science, approximately 0.9 grams (28 grams equals one ounce) of protein per kilogram (2.2 pounds) of body weight is needed in order to meet the body's daily requirements. In the 15 to 65 age group, most males need approximately 54 grams of protein per day, and most females need 45 grams of protein per day. However, we generally consume approximately 100 grams per day, 70 percent of which are from animal sources. Since protein is not stored in the body, this excess consumption is converted to fat, and the extra nitrogen that is produced is excreted in the urine. This excess has implications in terms of fat consumption, kidney problems, and coronary heart disease. You can estimate your protein needs by dividing your body weight by three. It would be wise to increase your consumption of flour and cereal grain products in order to meet your daily protein requirement.

Fat

Fat is an essential component in a balanced diet. It is a concentrated, high-energy nutrient that contains more than twice as many calories per weight unit than carbohydrates or proteins do. This caloric energy is stored for use when the body's energy needs exceed caloric intake. While no definite dietary requirements have been established for fat, most nutritionists recommend a reduction from the present levels, 40 to 45 percent of the calorie content of the American diet, to 25 to 30 percent.

Fat A concentrated, high-energy nutrient.

Glycerol A liquid formed by the hydrolysis of fat.

Triglyceride Consists of one molecule of glycerol and three molecules of fatty acid.

Fats consist of fatty acids and **glycerol,** a clear, colorless, syrupy liquid formed by the hydrolysis of fat. When three molecules of fatty acid combine with one molecule of glycerol, the combination is called a **triglyceride.** A high level of triglycerides in the body can predispose a person to the development of cardiovascular disease (see Chapter 16).

Saturated and Unsaturated Fats

Saturated fats Fats that contain more cholesterol and fatty acid.

Unsaturated fats Fats that occur primarily in vegetable oils.

Fats are classified as saturated or unsaturated, based upon the type of fatty acids that are present. **Saturated fats** are hard at room temperature and occur in both animal and vegetable fats, though primarily in animal fats. Nutritionists, physicians, and researchers have linked saturated fats with the development of arteriosclerosis and the subsequent development of cardiovascular disease (see Chapter 16).

Unsaturated fats, or those fats that occur primarily in vegetable oils, are further divided into two categories—*monounsaturated,* or semisolid, fats, such as those found in olive oil, and *polyunsaturated* fats found in corn, peanut, and soybean oils, to mention a few. The unsaturated fats are liquid at room temperature. These fats are usually oils and are found in fish as well as in plant sources. The one exception is coconut oil, which is a highly saturated fat.

Fat-soluble vitamins The vitamins that can be stored in the human body (A, D, E, and K).

Fats are important from the standpoint of satiety, palatability, and flavor of foods. Since fats are not digested quickly, we tend to feel full longer after consuming them (satiety). Fats also add to the taste of the foods we eat (palatability and flavor). Fats must be present in the intestines if we are to absorb and use the **fat-soluble vitamins** (A, D, E, and K). They also provide protective padding for vital organs, especially the kidneys, and are a source of linoleic acid, an essential fatty acid vital to the normal functioning of nearly all the body's cells. This essential fatty acid can be obtained in a single tablespoon of nearly any unsaturated oil each day. Diets with as much as 10 to 15 percent of the calories supplied by polyunsaturated fats frequently lead to a lowering of blood cholesterol levels. To avoid possible health problems as a result of not getting enough fats, an individual should not drastically change his or her diet to reduce fat levels without the advice of a physician or professional nutritionist.

Fats must combine with water-soluble protein to travel in the bloodstream. In the course of investigating these compound molecules, known as the lipoproteins, scientists found that one type, the high-density lipoproteins (HDL), is associated with decreased risk of cardiovascular disease. Because polyunsaturated fats appear to increase HDL activity, some authorities recommended that a certain percentage of polyunsaturates be included in the diet.

Cholesterol

Cholesterol Substance found in saturated fat of animal origin.

Cholesterol is a substance found in saturated fat that occurs only in foods of animal origin. However, it is so important that the body can manufacture all it needs. The problem is that our diets too often

YOUR HEALTH TODAY

So You Want to Be a Vegetarian?

In recent years, a great deal of interest has been generated about vegetarianism. Vegetarianism means that the individual does not consume flesh foods (meat, poultry, and fish). Pure vegetarians eat only fruits and vegetables. Those who consume dairy products as well as fruits and vegetables are called lacto-vegetarians; and if they also consume eggs and dairy products, they are called ovo-lacto-vegetarians. One other group, called vegans, use no animal products at all, including such items as wool, leather, and silk.

If ovo-lacto vegetarians consume a wide variety of foods in sufficient quantity to maintain their weight and promote normal growth in children, they will probably obtain an adequate supply of the necessary nutrients. On the other hand, those who follow a pure vegetarian diet may find that their diet is low in certain nutrients unless they take special care in planning to meet these requirements. The nutrients likely to be lacking in a pure vegetarian diet are calcium, riboflavin, and vitamin B_{12}. For children and pregnant women, vitamin D also may be lacking.

If well planned, the vegetarian diet can be quite nutritious. The basic foods included are grains and cereals, breads, pasta, beans, peas, nuts, seeds, fruits, and vegetables. Milk, cheese, and eggs are also included in the ovo-lacto-vegetarian diet. Oil, butter, honey, molasses, or sugar may also be used in small amounts.

To be sure that all the essential amino acids are present, complementary protein combinations should be used. Such combinations might include rice and beans, corn and beans, sunflower seeds and peanuts, rice and sesame seeds, or other such combinations. A good rule of thumb is to combine grains with legumes, seeds with legumes, or any plant protein with a high-quality animal protein such as milk. If animal products are not consumed, adequate vegetable protein can be obtained by combining corn with the legumes, a plant family that includes chick-peas (garbanzo beans), soybeans, black-eyed peas, lentils, kidney beans, pinto beans, and peanuts.

It is particularly important for pure vegetarians to consume a food that has been fortified with vitamin B_{12} since this essential vitamin occurs only in animal foods. A lack of vitamin B_{12} can, over time, result in severe neurological damage. This same caution of being sure the food is fortified holds for vitamin D as well.

There are advantages to the vegetarian diet, since researchers have found that vegetarians are seldom overweight and usually have low cholesterol levels. If you are contemplating becoming a vegetarian, you would be wise to consult with a nutritionist and do a lot of reading in scientifically accurate publications to be sure that you are getting enough of the essential nutrients for good health.

contain a great deal of animal fat. This results in having excess cholesterol present in the bloodstream. When this occurs, the cholesterol will form deposits (**plaque**) on the arterial walls, harden, and cause the arteries to lose their elasticity, a condition called arteriosclerosis (discussed in Chapter 16).

Plaque Deposits that form in arterial lining or on teeth.

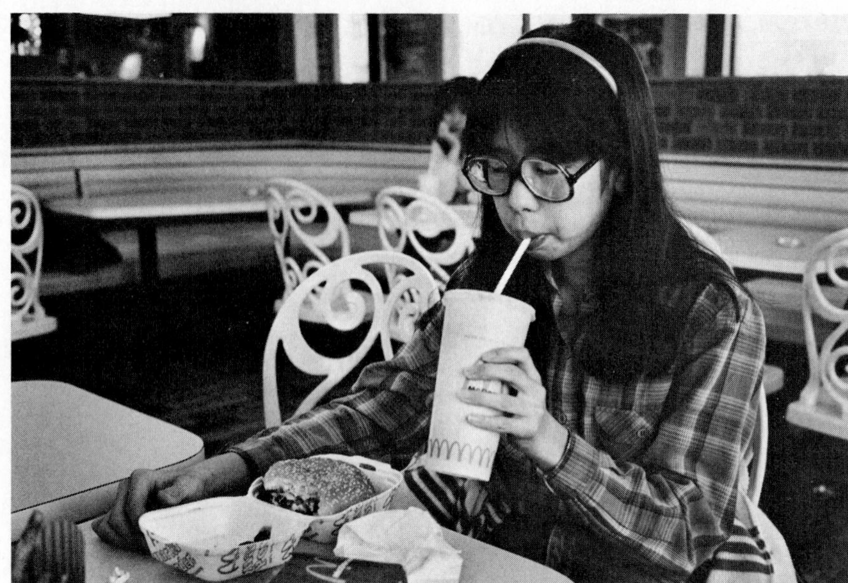

Most people are aware of their need for a balanced diet, and although this food may be available to them, many people will choose to eat less nutritious foods. (Photo © Jean-Claude Lejeune/ Stock, Boston)

Cholesterol is a structural component of cell membranes and is necessary for the normal development of brain tissue. It is also the chief constituent that makes the skin impervious to water. When cholesterol is broken down by the liver, bile salts, necessary for the digestion of fats, are produced. Many of the body's hormones require cholesterol for their production, and another compound (7-dehydrocholesterol) necessary for the body to produce vitamin D is synthesized from it. Thus, cholesterol is important, but, if consumed in excess in the diet, can result in health problems.

Vitamins

Vitamins Nutritional catalysts that facilitate metabolic processes in the body.

Of all the nutrients, **vitamins** are unquestionably the most discussed. Yet many misconceptions remain. Some people seem to regard them as a magic elixir for instant health. Many believe that two or three vitamin pills multiply the benefits of one. The fact is that vitamins are not a substitute for a nutritious diet. They are not nutrients themselves, since they do not supply energy, but they are important catalysts that facilitate the metabolic processes in the body.

Coenzymes Substances that work with enzymes to carry out their functions.

Water-soluble vitamins Easily destroyed vitamins that are not stored in the body.

Vitamins are organic compounds needed in small amounts to assist in processing other nutrients and to participate in the formation of blood cells, hormones, genetic material, and nervous system chemicals. Often they work with enzymes to carry out their functions and are called **coenzymes.** Classified as **water-** or **fat-soluble,** about 14 vitamins are recognized as essential. Each serves a specific need in the human body that cannot be filled by any other substance. A substantial deficiency in any one of them produces unique symptoms of disease (see Table 13–2).

Table 13-2 Vitamins: Their Sources, Functions, Effects of Deficiency, and Adverse Effects

Vitamin	Selected Food Sources	Functions	Deficiency Symptoms	Adverse Effects—Megadoses
		Fat-soluble Vitamins		
A	liver, butter, carrots, sweet potatoes, melons, yellow corn, peaches, apricots	growth, vision	weakening of body tissues, poor night vision, failure of bones to grow in length, lower resistance to infection	irritability, swelling of long bones, dry, itchy skin
D	egg yolk, milk, liver, butterfat	bone calcification	rickets	abnormal calcium levels, loss of appetite, retarded growth
E	salad oils, shortening, liver, beans, whole grains	protect vitamin A & carotene from destruction by oxidation	not noted, but possibly anemia	none noted
K	green leafy vegetables, liver, soybean oil, cauliflower	produce prothrombin needed for blood clotting	prolonged blood-clotting or coagulation time	jaundice
		Water-soluble Vitamins		
B_1 (Thiamin)	pork, wheat germ, dried beans, nuts	efficient use of carbohydrates	nausea, loss of appetite, constipation, depression beri-beri	none noted
B_2 (Riboflavin)	liver, milk, dark green leafy vegetables, cheese	release energy in the cells	eruptions of skin, eyes, mouth, growth retardation	none noted
B_6 (Pyridoxine)	liver, meats, poultry, nuts	metabolism of amino acids & use of fatty acids	convulsions in infants, greasy dermatitis, inflamed mouth with facial rash in adults	none noted
Niacin	liver, meats, poultry, fish	release of energy from carbohydrates, fats, & proteins	several diarrhea, sore GI tract, skin disease	itching and flushed skin, abnormal heartbeat, gastrointestinal ulcers
Pantothenic acid	liver, peanuts, wheat, bran, eggs, chicken, broccoli	carbohydrate metabolism, as well as for fats & proteins, formation of cholesterol	fatigue, insomnia, abdominal pain, numbness of hands & feet	possible diarrhea and water retention

(Continued)

Table 13-2 Vitamins: Their Sources, Functions, Effects of Deficiency, and Adverse Effects

Vitamin	Selected Food Sources	Functions	Deficiency Symptoms	Adverse Effects—Megadoses
		Water-soluble Vitamins		
Folacin	liver, dried beans, dark green leafy vegetables, orange juice, cereals	formation of red blood cells & DNA & RNA	anemia, toxemia in pregnancy, sore, red tongue, irritability, hostility, retarded production of white blood cells	can hide anemia due to B_{12} deficiency
B_{12}	animal foods, liver, meats, poultry, fish, eggs, milk	synthesis of DNA & RNA, normal growth maintenance of nerve tissue, normal formation of blood	numbness of hands & feet, anemia, poor coordination, severe mental disturbances, spinal cord degeneration	none noted
Biotin	liver, dried beans, whole grains, some fresh vegetables	removal or addition of CO_2 in metabolism of proteins & carbohydrates	dermatitis, hardening of skin, muscle pain, nausea, loss of appetite	none noted
Choline	egg yolk, whole grains, legumes, wheat germ, meats	fat metabolism, normal nerve functioning	fatty liver deposits	none noted
C (Ascorbic acid)	citrus fruits, fresh vegetables	healthy gum tissue, collagen formation, tooth formation	bleeding gums, scurvy, sore joints, poor healing of cuts	none noted

Doses and Megadoses

Megadoses Unusually large doses, often of vitamins.

The quantities of vitamins required for good health are so small that the measure used for them is thousandths of a gram, or milligrams. Yet there continues to be interest in **megadoses** of vitamins, self-prescribed for a variety of ills. It is only in rare instances that healthy people who eat balanced meals need vitamin supplementation, let alone need to consume massive doses of vitamins. Americans spend $300 to $500 million annually on unnecessary vitamin supplements, some taking as much as 10 to 1,000 times the Recommended Daily Allowance with the unfounded hope of improving health or performance.

When excessive amounts of the water-soluble vitamins are consumed, the amounts not needed by the body are excreted, generally in the urine. Since fat-soluble vitamins can be stored in body tissue, an excessive intake of these vitamins may result in a toxic level in the body, and disease states may occur. If a person eats a well-balanced diet, the variety of foods included will furnish the essential vitamins in sufficient quantity that supplementation is not needed.

Minerals

Some inorganic elements, or **minerals,** are essential nutrients. Calcium, phosphorus, potassium, sulfur, sodium, and magnesium are called **macrominerals** because they are needed in relatively large amounts, more than 10 milligrams every day. Iodine, iron, and zinc are among the 13 **trace elements,** so called because they are needed in barely traceable amounts. (See Table 13–3 for a list of the macrominerals and trace elements.)

Minerals Inorganic elements needed for basic body metabolism.

Macrominerals Minerals needed in the body in large amounts.

Trace elements Chemical elements needed in minute amounts for normal metabolism.

Like vitamins, minerals do not supply calories. They are utilized in the body in the same inorganic form they take in nature, as described in a chemistry Table of Elements. We could use the iron in nails if we could eat them. Most minerals — iron is an exception — are excreted after they have served their function. All must be replaced constantly. The best way to get them is in a good diet. Although they are not as unstable as vitamins during cooking, some are water-soluble and will cook out. So urgent is our need for these dietary elements — though often in the smallest amounts — that some believe it motivates a craving for unnatural foods like clay, dirt, laundry starch, or lead paint chips.

"Organic" Foods

There is no evidence that **organic foods** are richer in minerals or any other nutrient than foods fertilized with synthetic compounds. Nor are they free from contamination by mold, bacteria, natural toxins, or heavy metal pollutants like mercury. The nutrient content of a plant is determined by its species, and if its needs are supplied, it will grow well. Plants do not need nutrients in the organic form of manure or compost but in the inorganic form found in synthetic fertilizers. Further, if "organic" crops are fertilized with manure and compost from local sources, all will reflect any regional soil deficiencies, as well as any pesticides used in previous years. Because the health food industry is not regulated, the consumer cannot be assured that the "organic" foods, with their higher price stickers, were grown in the way stated in the claims.

Organic foods Food grown without artificial chemical fertilizers.

Water

Water is also one of the essential nutrients; only oxygen is more fundamental to life. About 45–60 percent of the healthy young body's weight is water. A 1 percent loss signals thirst; a 10 percent loss causes spastic muscles and incapacitating weakness; a 22 percent

Table 13–3 **Minerals**

	Sources	Functions	Deficiencies
		Macrominerals	
Calcium	Milk and dairy products; also legumes, nuts, and leafy vegetables.	Of critical importance to bones and teeth for the regeneration of new bone cells; in the blood it helps maintain normal heartbeat, blood clotting, transmission of nerve impulses, cellular osmosis, and enzyme activity.	Can cause bone abnormalities, muscle spasms, osteoporosis, heart arrythmias; slows blood clotting.
Phosphorus	Protein-rich foods and cereal products.	Takes part in nearly every body function; 80% in bones and teeth; the rest is needed in cell reproduction, protein synthesis, transmission of hereditary traits within cells, transportation of lipids, and oxidation of carbohydrates.	Uncommon, but can result from a strictly vegetarian diet.
Magnesium	Central component of chlorophyll; found in whole grains, nuts, dark green leafy vegetables.	Activates enzymes that convert sugar into energy; maintains structure of RNA and DNA; promotes protein synthesis; regulates body temperature; enables muscles and nerves to contract.	Indicated by nervousness, excitability, and depression.
Sodium	Most from sodium chloride (salt).	Balance and control of body fluids; helps in transmitting nerve impulses and in maintaining the acid-base balance in the body.	Can cause weakness, muscle cramps, lassitude, vomiting, low blood pressure.
Potassium	Lean meats, milk (but not cheese), and many fruits.	Necessary for the growth of all lean body tissues or whenever muscle is broken down from starvation, injury, or protein deficiency.	Symptoms include fatigue and weakness or paralysis of muscles and finally cessation of the heart muscle.
		Trace Elements	
Iron	Organ meats and lean meats; lesser amounts are found in fortified cereals, legumes, nuts, eggs, and dried fruit.	Most combines with protein in the bone marrow to make hemoglobin; the rest is stored in the liver, spleen, and bone marrow.	Characterized by anemia and fatigue.
Iodine	Potassium iodine added to common salt.	Necessary to form thyroid hormones that determine the body's metabolism rate and govern reproduction.	Can cause goiter.
Zinc	Most comes from animal protein, but oysters and wheat germ are excellent sources.	Essential in humans for the growth of genital organs, prevention of anemia, wound healing, and prevention of dwarfism. Also for formation of RNA, DNA, hormones that trigger the menstrual cycle, and insulin.	Results in severely retarded growth in the young; fewer litters, deformed offspring in lab animals.

loss is fatal. Water is the solvent that transports nutrients through the body and carries away the wastes. It must be present as the fluid medium for digestion and in all body chemical reactions.

Water loss from the kidneys, lungs, and skin must be replaced daily. Five or six glasses a day, coupled with the water from solid food, is sufficient for most adults, but infants and children need more. More may be needed in hot weather, after strenuous work or exercise, or to combat a fever. Water also supplies minerals. "Hard" water may supply them in significant quantities. When water is softened chemically, the calcium and magnesium are replaced by sodium.

Major Food Groups

Often such guidelines as the U.S. RDAs tend to complicate rather than simplify diet selection. In an attempt to simplify the process, the basic four food groups (which in the past were variously designated the basic eleven, the basic nine, and then the basic seven[1]) were developed. Foods were assigned to each group based upon their primary nutritional contribution to the total diet (see Figure 13–2). Recently, a fifth group (fats, sweets, and alcohol) has been receiving recognition. Unfortunately, the recommendations for the number of servings per day do not take into account the calories needed by the individual or contained in the foods within each group. Consumers would be wise to select foods from the four basic food groups after determining their caloric needs and only then add foods from "group five" if the caloric value of the foods from the other groups is insufficient to meet these needs.

Meat and Meat Products

Including the red meats (beef, veal, pork, lamb, mutton, goat, and game animals), poultry, game birds, shellfish, fish, eggs, nuts, beans, peas, and other legumes, this group's primary contribution to nutrition is protein (particularly the essential amino acids). In addition, iron, phosphorus, the B vitamins, and the fat-soluble vitamins are supplied. It should be noted that vitamin B_{12}, not available from plant sources, is supplied in this group.

Dairy Products

In addition to being an excellent source of protein, milk and milk products supply calcium, phosphorus, vitamin A, and riboflavin. Most milk is also fortified with 400 IU of vitamin D per quart. Cheese and other dairy products are comparable sources of the same nutrients. Three ounces of cheese contain roughly the same nutritive value as a pint of milk.

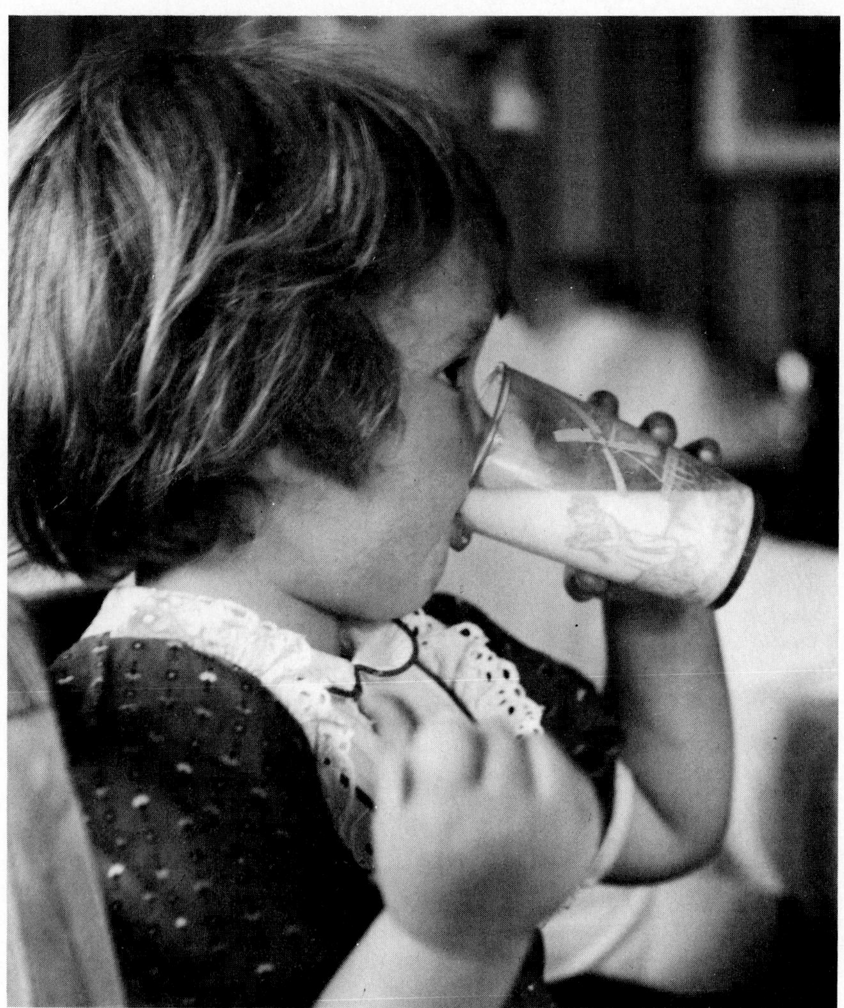

Children are not the only ones who need milk. Milk is an excellent source of essential minerals for people of all ages. (Photo © Marjorie Pickens 1982)

Grains and Cereals

Rice, wheat, corn, oats, rye, barley, and millet—these are the grains that feed the world. In some countries, they provide 80 percent of the food energy. Cereal grains consist mainly of carbohydrates. Small amounts of incomplete proteins, vitamins, and minerals are concentrated primarily in the hulls, and they are often lost in milling and processing. To increase nutritive value, most flours and cereals are now enriched, or "fortified," by the addition of these nutrients.

Vegetables and Fruits

This food group contributes 100 percent of the body's vitamin C requirement as well as up to 60 percent of the requirement for vitamin A. It should be noted that although white potatoes have been much maligned as being fattening, this is primarily because they are served heaped with butter or sour cream. In fact, the potato contributes small amounts of protein, vitamin C, iron, thiamin, potassium, and other soil-derived minerals, which vary from region to region. This group also provides dietary fiber, and prunes and figs are valued as natural laxatives.

Fats, Sweets, and Alcohol

Essential fatty acids, calories, and instant energy are supplied by this new group. Nutritionists agree that the amount of sugar we consume should be reduced. The wise consumer will read the label carefully and look for "hidden" sugar such as that found as an additive in almost all processed foods (including ketchup, crackers, soups, cereals, peanut butter, boullion cubes, and salad dressing).

Alcohol supplies little more than pure calories. However, it has been suggested that moderate amounts of alcohol, if planned as part of the diet, may not be overly detrimental to health (see Chapter 9).

Special Dietary Requirements

Some population groups need special diets or need to pay particular attention to certain aspects of diet. Among the healthy population, this is true of the young, athletes, the aging, and pregnant and lactating women. Most disease states impose special nutritional needs or require the avoidance of certain foods.

Diseases

When an individual is ill, the physician may suggest dietary changes. In fact, the patient may be referred to a dietitian. These individuals are specially trained to develop diets that take into consideration the special nutritional needs of the ill individual. Nutritional soundness, flexibility, and patient preference are primary considerations in planning special diets for the ill. Both the family and the patient must be educated about the importance of following the new regimen.

Infants, Children, and Adolescents

Only within this century have the special nutritional needs of infants begun to be established. Confusion was still widespread when this generation of college students was in its infancy: breast-feeding was at an all-time low; some newborns were fed whole cow's milk;

some breast-fed babies were switched to cow's milk at three months; solids were often introduced as early as one month. With much new information available it is important for new parents to follow their physician's recommendations and to seek advice from such groups as the La Leche League regarding infant nutrition and breast-feeding.

Children and adolescents need a high caloric intake because they are so active and new body tissue is being formed. Between the ages of 2 and 12, growth is a gradual process, but it speeds up just before puberty. Care should be taken not to "overfeed" children and adolescents. Family eating patterns and behavior are instrumental in promoting good nutrition. Regular meals, pleasant conversation, and the right foods lay the groundwork for good health and good habits in individual members.

Athletes

The debate over the most energizing diet for athletes is at least as old as the ancient Greek Olympics. The Greek belief that excess protein replenishes muscle tissue "lost" in exertion is still held—erroneously—by some today. The fact is that athletes do not need an overall diet that differs from the carefully chosen normal diet. Certain kinds of exercise impose additional requirements of specific nutrients, but these are usually satisfied because athletes eat more of everything than do less active people.

Weight lifters, for example, being bigger and heavier than runners, need more protein to replenish muscle mass. Endurance runners need to increase their carbohydrate intake several days before an event to build up glycogen stores in the muscles. This "carbohydrate loading" is not necessary in sports unless the activity is strenuous and lasts more than an hour. The body has enough fatty acids and glucose available to fuel light and moderate exercise. A regular meal, eaten at least 2½ hours before the activity, is sufficient for most athletic endeavors. In training it has been found that frequent moderate-sized meals are more energy-efficient than a few big ones.

Training itself has been found to do more than strengthen muscles. It also sets up more efficient metabolic processes by increasing oxygen uptake and improving the body's ability to utilize high-energy fat.

Except as noted, athletes should adhere to a regular diet. Additional protein is required only when new muscle tissue is being formed: by growing young athletes, by adults taking up weight lifting, by football or soccer players recovering from frequent muscle injuries.

The nutrient most apt to be neglected by athletes is water, which should ideally be replaced at the rate it is lost. It is wise to drink fluids a few hours before the event. Since much more fluid than salt is lost in sweat, salt tablets are not only unnecessary but contraindicated. Fruit juices or commercial drinks like Gatorade can restore electrolyte balance.

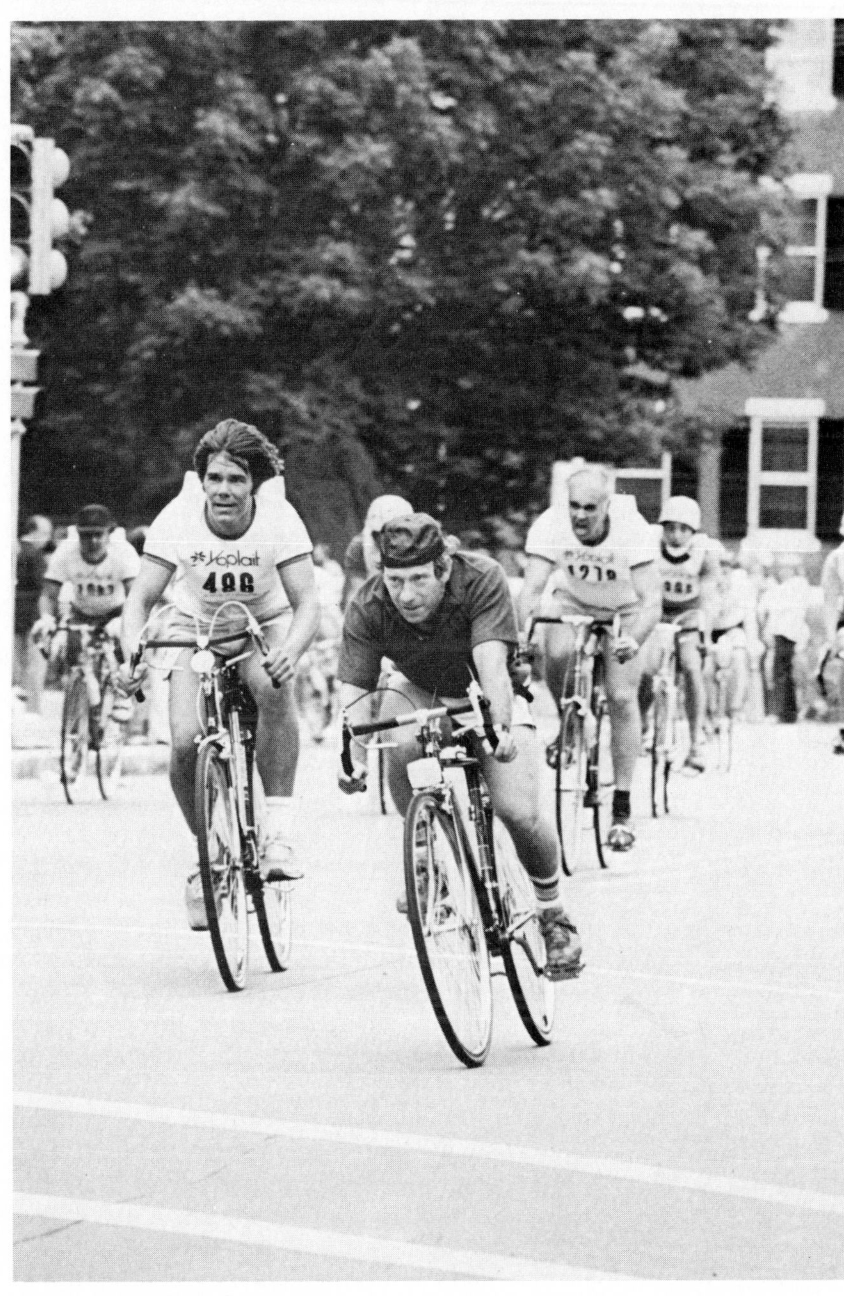

Athletes should be sure they eat a balanced diet that includes plenty of water. (Photo © Susan Lapides 1981/Design Conceptions)

The Older Generation

The elderly have essentially the same needs as any mature adult, but some physical changes and changes in life circumstances must be taken into consideration in designing a geriatric diet. Few older people have a full set of teeth. Dentures, even if they are cosmetically perfect, often do not function well enough to permit chewing all foods comfortably. Consequently, older people tend to turn to softer foods or to bolt down foods that need more chewing. Both approaches can cause problems. Eating ill-chewed food may result in discomfort because digestion is no longer optimal. A soft diet excludes essential foods in the basic food groups—the meats, fruits, and vegetables.

What kind of diet promotes a healthy old age? First the calorie count must be calculated for the ideal body weight, taking into consideration slowed metabolism and decreased activity. Many may need to cut down on their intake of carbohydrates to prevent weight gain, as obesity makes them susceptible to other disorders. The requirements for protein, vitamins, and minerals are identical to younger adults', but fulfilling them on a smaller total food intake may be difficult. In the United States deficiencies of calcium, iron, and vitamins A, B, and C are the most frequently seen. Any attempt to effect a change in the habits of the elderly must be introduced gradually, and must accommodate the individual's preferences and disabilities.

Pregnancy and Lactation

Pregnant and lactating women are nourishing two people, and their diets need special attention. A pregnant woman who has had a good diet encounters few problems. The only change necessary is to increase the allowances of the essential nutrients.

If the woman has not formed good habits and is poorly nourished at the start, deficiencies will be aggravated. The developing baby may be undernourished, and shortages in the mother's body can drop to critical levels. Overweight is no assurance of adequate nutrition—for mother or baby. Many obese people have nutritional deficiencies. Women in general are more prone to them than men because of a lower total food intake, but chronic self-imposed reducing diets are a contributing factor. Studies show that poorly nourished mothers have more miscarriages, stillbirths, premature babies, and complications at delivery than well-nourished mothers.

The issue of weight gain in pregnancy is controversial. A gain of 24–28 pounds is usual, but slender women may need to gain more. One study of 10,000 births showed that a higher maternal weight gain resulted in higher birth weight, lower incidence of prematurity, and better first-year growth. Other studies suggest an increase of toxemia in obese pregnant women, which causes obstetricians and nutritionists to worry about gains in excess of the average. Reducing diets should not be undertaken in pregnancy. In general, a pregnant woman under a physician's care, on a simple, wholesome diet, can be assured that healthy tissue is formed in her baby at a progressive rate and that her own health will remain good.

Milk is of special importance for the nursing mother. She should drink roughly as much as she secretes. This probably means adding

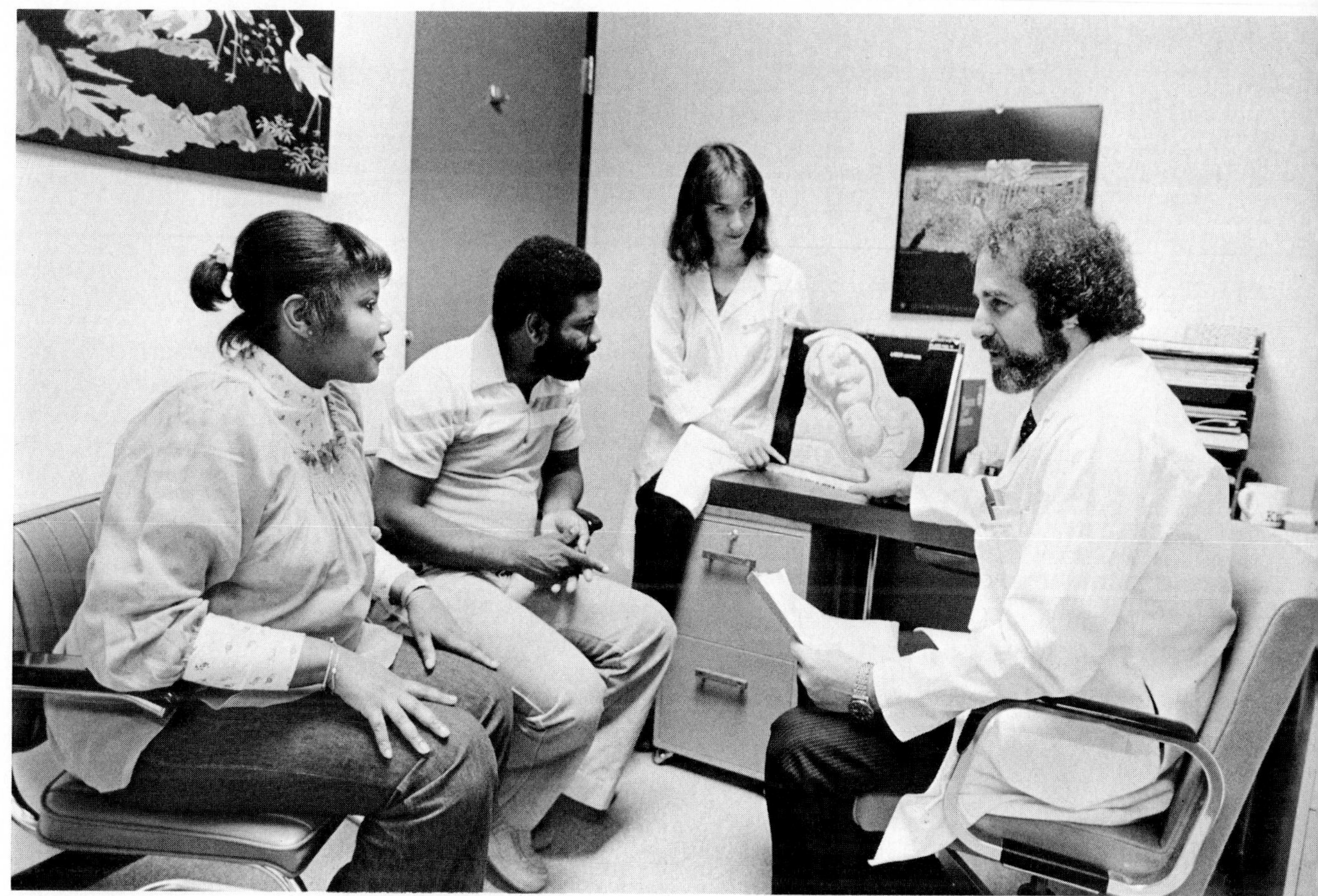

It is important for pregnant women and their spouses to understand the basics of good nutrition. A healthy mother has a much greater chance of producing a healthy baby. (Photo © Donald Dietz, 1981/Stock, Boston)

another pint to bring her milk intake to 1½ quarts. Additional carbohydrates and generous portions of vegetables and fruits, especially citrus, will fill her increased energy and vitamin needs.

Almost everything eaten is assimilated into breast milk—from alcohol, aspirin, and laxatives to oral contraceptives. All such substances should be taken only with the consent of a physician.

Good Food and Dental Health

About 90 percent of the children in the United States have tooth decay before they are five years old, and their dental problems continue. An estimated 96 percent of all high school students have tooth decay, and few people reach the age of 60 with all their natural teeth. Many have lost most of them before the age of 40. National dental bills total about $7 billion annually.

Nutrition plays a significant part in the development of the teeth even before the child is born. Calcium and phosphorus are essential building blocks, and their absorption is aided by vitamin D. Vitamins C and A are catalysts for proper calcification and enamel formation. Healthy baby teeth are necessary for speech development, proper eating, and the orderly positioning of the permanent teeth.

Dental Caries

Caries Dental cavities.

Most dental disorders fall into two major categories: caries (decay) and periodontal (gum) disease. **Caries** is a word from the Greek meaning "rottenness." It is the technical term for cavities, which are the primary cause of tooth loss before the age of 35. The decay is caused by bacteria living on the teeth as a gelatinous coating called plaque. These bacteria thrive when sticky, particularly sugary, foods are allowed to stay on the tooth surface. Teeth are especially vulnerable to caries two to four years after they come in, because that is the period when the enamel is maturing. Unfortunately, that is also the period when young humans are inclined to eat too many sweets.

Eventually it may be possible to prevent tooth decay with an antibacterial vaccination, but at this time the best weapons we have are good nutrition, avoidance of sugar, and good dental hygiene. Regular dental checkups can detect and stop caries early.

The trace element fluoride, either in toothpaste or as one part per million in drinking water, has been proven to reduce caries, particularly if it is present in the first year of life. Fluoride accumulates in the tooth enamel and makes it less subject to the bacteria-produced acid. Amounts in excess of two parts per million in water can cause mottled teeth in children under the age of six. As of 1975 only about 50 percent of the American population had the advantage of fluoridated water.

Brushing after every meal is best, but brushing before bed is especially important. During the sleep period there is less saliva in the mouth; therefore, there are fewer of the salivary secretions that buffer the bacterial acids. Dental floss helps eliminate food and plaque between the teeth.

Periodontal Disease

Periodontal disease Disease involving the gums.

Plaque Deposits that form in the lining of the arteries or on the teeth.

Periodontal disease (involving the gums) is the major cause of tooth loss after the age of 35. Poor oral hygiene appears to be the primary cause. **Plaque** buildup close to the gums creates inflammation and infection, which can progress to loosen the gum fibers and eventually destroy the supporting bone. There is some evidence that vitamins A and E and protein and magnesium deficiencies affect periodontal disease, but the studies have not been consistent or conclusive.

Dental disease can be controlled—even prevented in some—with the methods available to us. We know that dietary sugar is the single most aggravating factor. We know that timing and frequency of sweet-eating determines the rate of decay: snacking on sweets between meals produces more caries than mealtime sweets only. We know that the longer the sugar remains on the teeth, the greater the destruction it will cause. (Thus, chewing gum and caramels are worse than soft drinks.) It only remains for us to practice what is preached.

Eating with Dental Health in Mind

Naturally a well-balanced diet will also promote good dental health. However, the American Dental Association recommends that you give consideration to three major principles: Limit your snacks; avoid snacks that contain sugars; and choose reasonable snacks. By following these three rules on snacking, you can greatly enhance your own dental health, and you might influence others to follow your lead.

Summary

Nutrition became a controversial issue only during the 1970s when reports began circulating about harmful substances in food. Interest in good nutrition has grown rapidly since then. But many still suffer from malnutrition—faulty or poor nutrition.

Various governmental groups have established dietary standards, and the Food and Drug Administration has devised Recommended Daily Allowances, which became the standard for nutrient labeling. The ten "leader" nutrients and any vitamins and mineral allowances must be listed.

The six classes of essential nutrients are carbohydrates, fats, proteins, vitamins, minerals, and water.

Carbohydrates are sugars and starches. Nutritionists have become concerned over the increasing use of sugar, which provides energy but lacks other needed nutrients. Fiber appears to be important in the digestive process.

Proteins are made up of amino acids. Of the 20 amino acids the body needs, 9—called essential amino acids—must be ingested daily. Most animal proteins provide all of the essential amino acids, but plant proteins contain fewer.

Although fat is an essential component in a balanced diet, most nutritionists recommend a reduction in present levels of use and avoidance of excessive saturated fat and cholesterol. Diets, however, should not be drastically changed to reduce fat levels without professional advice, since fats contain essential nutrients.

Vitamins are not nutrients themselves but catalysts that facilitate metabolic processes and vitamin deficiencies can produce various diseases. Excess water-soluble vitamins are eliminated from the body, thus many of the vitamin supplements Americans consume are simply excreted. Essential vitamins include vitamins A, C, D, E, and K, and the B-complex vitamins.

Minerals are divided into the macrominerals—calcium, phosphorus, potassium, sulfur, sodium, chlorine, and magnesium—and the 13 trace elements, which include iodine, iron, and zinc.

Water is the solvent that transports nutrients through the body and carries away wastes. Five or six glasses a day are sufficient for most adults, but infants and children need more.

Nutritionists have also classified foods into groups according to the primary nutritional contributions they make in the diet. These include meat and meat substitutes; dairy products, grains and cereals; vegetables and fruits; and fats, sweets, and alcohol.

Nutritional needs vary considerably from individual to individual. Remember that it takes a variety of foods to supply all the requirements for good health.

Special diets are required by the young, athletes, the aging, and pregnant and lactating women. In addition, patients suffering from a wide range of diseases must follow special diets.

Good food is an important factor in dental health. The best protection against tooth decay is good nutrition, avoidance of sugar, good dental hygiene, and careful selection of snacks.

Review and Discussion

1. What are the seven recommendations for nutrition in the USDA Dietary Guidelines?
2. What information is a food label required by law to carry?
3. What are the three basic functions of food in the body?
4. Name the six classes of essential nutrients. What functions do they serve in maintaining health?
5. Describe the dangers of increased sugar consumption.
6. What are the benefits and dangers of vitamin supplements?
7. What health problems are associated with mineral deficiencies?
8. What are the major food groups? What nutritional contributions do they make?
9. What servings of the various food groups should be included in the normal diet?
10. Describe the role of nutrition in dental health.

Further Reading

Allen, Robert F., with Shirley Linde. *Lifegain.* New York, Appleton-Century-Crofts, 1981.
The practical aspects of good nutrition and a variety of programs designed for various needs.

Katch, Frank, and William McArdle. *Nutrition, Weight Control, and Exercise,* 2nd ed. Philadelphia: Lea and Febiger, 1983.
Links proper nutrition and exercise as both relate to weight control. Describes not only nutrition and metabolism but also caloric cost of foods and exercise. (Paperback)

Kuschmann, John D., director. *Nutrition Almanac.* New York, McGraw-Hill, 1979.
A revised edition of a nutrition classic for the general reader. (Hardcover and Paperback)

Miller, S., and J. A. Miller. *Food for Thought.* Englewood Cliffs, N.J., Prentice-Hall, Inc., 1979.
A survey in the field of nutrition for the reader who wants both facts and philosophy. (Hardcover and Paperback)

National Dairy Council. *Nutrition Source Book.* Rosemont, Ill., 1978.
A nutrition source which not only serves as an encyclopedia of nutrition, but also lists basic food groups and sample diets. Additional information on calories, shopping wisely, and recommended daily requirements. (Paperback)

USDA-DHHS. *Nutrition and Your Health, Dietary Guidelines for Americans.* Washington, D.C., 1980.
Among the best of the government publications on this topic. (Paperback)

Williams, Eleanor R., and Mary Alice Caliendo. *Nutrition: Principles, Issues, and Applications.* New York: McGraw-Hill Book Company, 1984.
A basic text, written in easy-to-understand terms, that deals with the common-sense approach to nutrition. Numerous controversial nutritional issues are presented from several viewpoints.

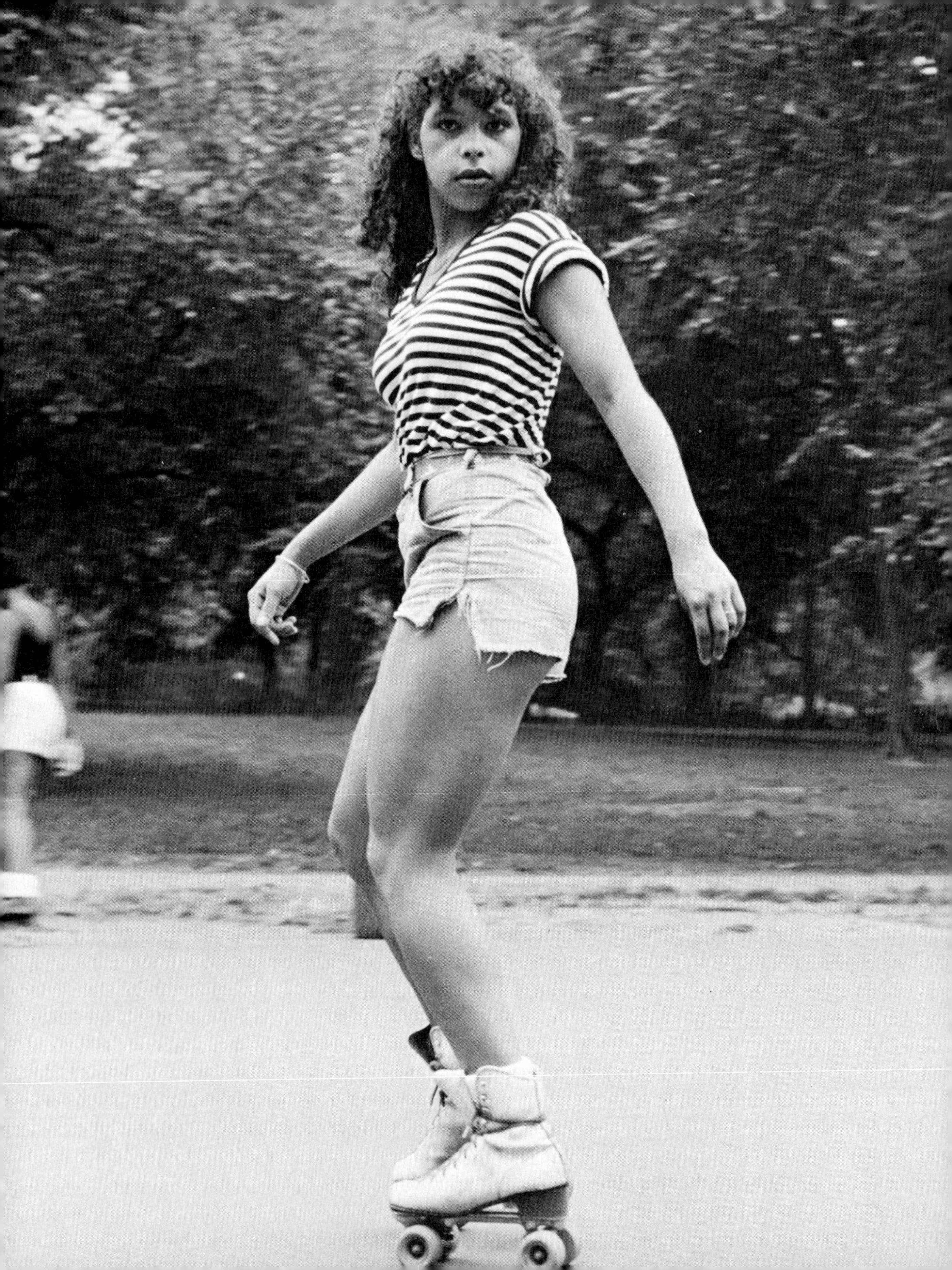

Chapter 14
Weight Control

KEY POINTS

- Weight control is one of the most important aspects of preventive medicine today.
- Charts can be consulted to find the ideal body weight for people of different ages, heights, and body builds.
- Obesity is defined as an excess amount of fatty, or adipose, tissue.
- The body has two types of fat: essential fats, its temporary reserves, and storage fat, excesses beyond the body's requirements.
- There are two kinds of obesity: hyperplasia, the result of an increased number of fat cells, and hypertrophy, larger amounts of fats in a normal number of cells.
- To lose a pound, a person must use up 3,500 calories.
- Fad diets and gimmicks generally do not work and may be hazardous to your health.
- A combination of calorie reduction and moderate physical exercise is the best way to achieve weight loss.

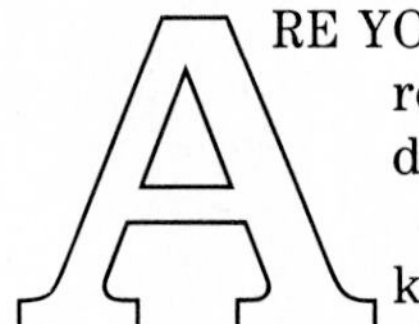

RE YOU overweight? Is it possible to be overweight but not fat? Does it really matter whether you are fat or thin? If you are fat, what can you do about it? Or are you underweight? What is normal?

Weight interests everybody. Putting weight on, taking it off, or keeping it as it is — these are basic concerns of millions of Americans, for a "just right" weight is closely correlated with feeling good, looking good, and having vitality. And while we can relate our weights to ideal standards, comparing ourselves to the statistical averages, weight is nevertheless an individual matter.

Some people watch their weight primarily for social reasons. Not only is fat no longer a symbol of good health but by today's standards it is considered a hindrance to physical attractiveness, as is underweight. Overweight people may have problems, either real or imaginary; being very fat can be embarrassing. Even being only slightly overweight may affect personal self-esteem to a damaging extent, for having a good self-image is important to emotional well-being.

Physicians now view weight-watching as one of the most important aspects of preventive medicine, which tries to avoid illness by keeping people healthy.

Weight and Health

Estimates put the number of overweight Americans at roughly 25 percent of the population. Obesity appears to be one of the curses of affluence, and it is rated by the American Medical Association as the nation's most severe health problem.

Some moderately overweight people are described as "plump," and by some appraisals, as pleasingly so. For these individuals, carrying their extra weight rarely causes the physical difficulties and inconveniences that it does for those who are grossly overweight. But being overweight to any degree may bring on disorders that create health problems. Mortality rates among the overweight are significantly higher than among those with normal weights in the same age group. Insurance companies are keenly aware of the various hazards of obesity and rank "overweight" among their high-risk categories. The companies can produce the statistics to support their reasons for doing so.

Overweight people are prone to fatigue and lack of energy. This sort of lethargy feeds on itself, progressing from a seemingly innocuous indulgence to take it easy to an actual inability to be active. The "do nothing," flabby person is unfortunately a realistic stereotype. And as pounds are added — even before the label of "fat person" becomes appropriate — health problems increase.

Among the diseases commonly associated with being overweight is

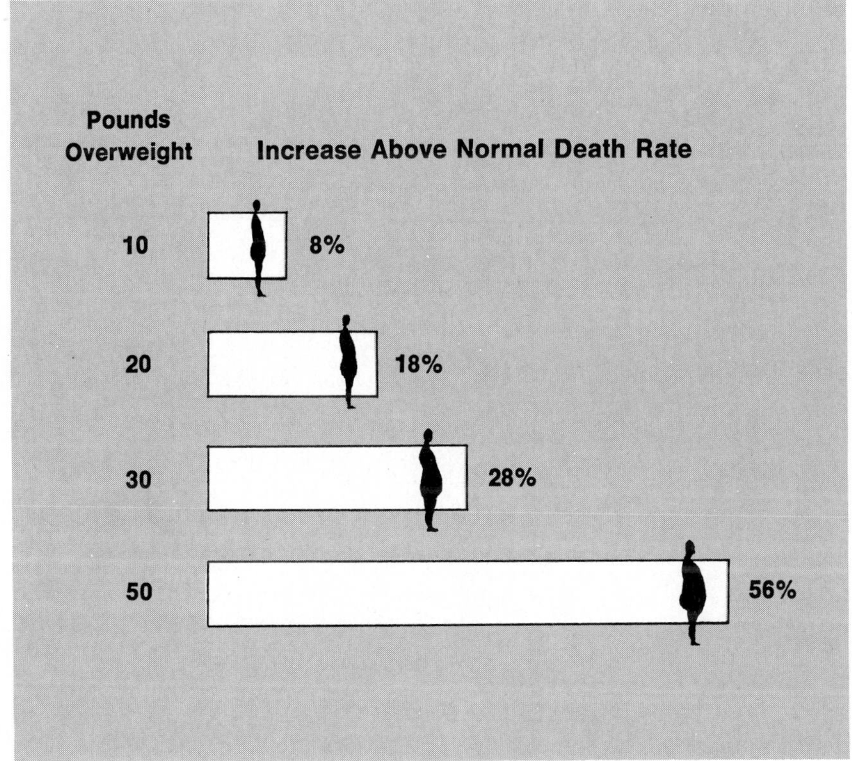

Figure 14-1. Effect of Overweight on Death Rate.
Death rates are significantly higher among the overweight than among people with normal weights. (Source: Michael H. K. Irwin, *Overweight—A Problem for Millions* [New York: Public Affairs Pamphlets, 1973]: 12.)

hypertension, or high blood pressure. Fatty deposits in and around arteries narrow the artery channels and restrict the flow of blood, resulting in a buildup of pressure. This condition is called *atherosclerosis* (see Chapter 16). If protracted, atherosclerosis can eventually cause a rupturing of blood vessels, manifested as strokes, which can cause circulatory and neurological impairments. The overweight, of course, have significantly higher levels of cholesterol, which contribute to forming the restricting and clogging layers in the blood vessels. High cholesterol levels are associated with arteriosclerosis, coronary heart disease, and other cardiovascular diseases. Diabetes, digestive tract disorders, respiratory ailments, gallbladder and kidney diseases, some kinds of cancer, and types of arthritis—these conditions as well as others occur more often among the overweight than among those who maintain desirable weights.

The Right Weight for You

How do you know if you are overweight? For most people, this is not a difficult question to answer. They can tell by a look at their body in a mirror, by a comparison of themselves to other people, and by how they feel (see Self-Assessment Exercise 14.1).

SELF-ASSESSMENT EXERCISE 14.1

Quick Reference Guide to Obesity

1. Is my waist bigger than my chest?
2. Can I pinch more than one inch of fat at my waistline? (At the level of the naval)
3. When I lie down, does my stomach protrude above my chest?

If your response was "Yes" to any of these three questions, you may well be obese and you should seriously consider going on a diet. Remember, before going on a diet, you should check with your physician.

To find out more precisely where you fit in the scale of normal weights for people of your height and body build, check the Metropolitan Height and Weight Table (Table 14–1). For most people, their weight at age 20 is close to the desirable or ideal weight that should be maintained throughout their life. Charts are not personalized. They do not give the absolute optimum weight for you as an individual, but they are excellent guides. If your weight suggests that you may be either overweight or underweight, you may want a more precise measurement. This can be done by a physician, nutritionist, or other professional technician.

Determining the Proportion of Fat to Lean

The two most common and practical methods used for determining the amount of fat in the body are underwater weighing and skinfold measurements.

Underwater Weighing. In underwater weighing, a person is weighed first out of water and then is submerged in water. In the usual method of underwater weighing, the person being weighed sits in a tank of water in a special chair attached to a scale. Air is exhaled from the lungs, and then the head is placed under the water briefly. The scale is read at this time. Because fat tends to buoy up a body in water (it is lighter than lean tissue), a comparison can be made between a person's weight out of the water and a person's weight under water. The difference between the two weights gives the **specific density** of the individual. From this the percentage of total body fat for the individual can be calculated. Normal fat content for young men is 15 percent and for young women, 22 percent.

Specific density Weight measurement used to determine percentage of body fat.

Table 14-1 1983 Metropolitan Height and Weight Table

Men*					Women†				
Height Feet	Height Inches	Small Frame	Medium Frame	Large Frame	Height Feet	Height Inches	Small Frame	Medium Frame	Large Frame
5	2	128–134	131–141	138–150	4	10	102–111	109–121	118–131
5	3	130–136	133–143	140–153	4	11	103–113	111–123	120–134
5	4	132–138	135–145	142–156	5	0	104–115	113–126	122–137
5	5	134–140	137–148	144–160	5	1	106–118	115–129	125–140
5	6	136–142	139–151	146–164	5	2	108–121	118–132	128–143
5	7	138–145	142–154	149–168	5	3	111–124	121–135	131–147
5	8	140–148	145–157	152–172	5	4	114–127	124–138	134–151
5	9	142–151	148–160	155–176	5	5	117–130	127–141	137–155
5	10	144–154	151–163	158–180	5	6	120–133	130–144	140–159
5	11	146–157	154–166	161–184	5	7	123–136	133–147	143–163
6	0	149–160	157–170	164–188	5	8	126–139	136–150	146–167
6	1	152–164	160–174	168–192	5	9	129–142	139–153	149–170
6	2	155–168	164–178	172–197	5	10	132–145	142–156	152–173
6	3	158–172	167–182	176–202	5	11	135–148	145–159	155–176
6	4	162–176	171–187	181–207	6	0	138–151	148–162	158–179

* Weights at ages 25–59 based on lowest mortality. Weight in pounds according to frame (in indoor clothing weighing 5 lbs., shoes with 1″ heels).

† Weights at ages 25–59 based on lowest mortality. Weight in pounds according to frame (in indoor clothing weighing 3 lbs., shoes with 1″ heels).

Source: Metropolitan Life Insurance Company, New York; adapted from *1979 Build Study* (Society of Actuaries and Association of Life Insurance Medical Directors of America, 1980).

Skinfold Measurement. Determining the amount of body fat by skinfold measurements is another common technique. It is estimated that about half of the body fat lies just under the skin. Here is an easy though nonscientific way of measuring this fat. With your thumb and index finger, pinch together the skin on the underside of your upper arm. If the thickness is an inch or more, you may have too much fat. The more precise and scientific method involves using special instruments called calipers that measure the skinfold thickness in millimeters. Measurements are usually taken in six areas of the body. The usual six are (1) at the midway of the triceps muscle; (2) on the back of the shoulder blade; (3) at the naval, one inch to the right; (4) just above the hip bone; (5) on the front of the thigh; and (6) over the hamstring muscle. These measurements, taken by a physician or a qualified technician, are usually made on the right side of the body (the differences between the right and left side of the body are minimal). The amount of flesh pulled together and the degree of pressure applied may differ depending on the technician, but this is not enough to alter the final results appreciably. A table is consulted that gives the amount of body fat based on skinfold measurements. The table

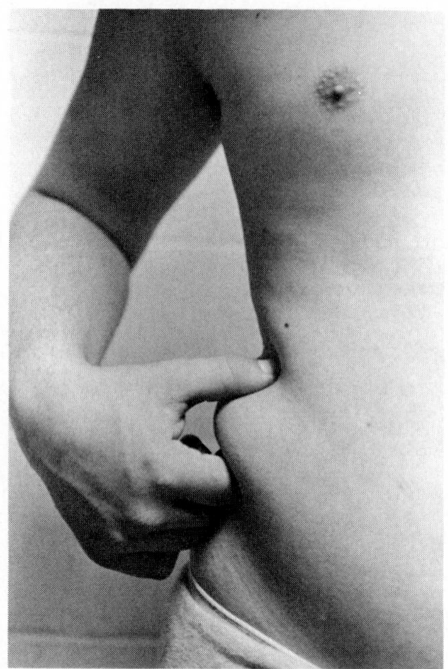
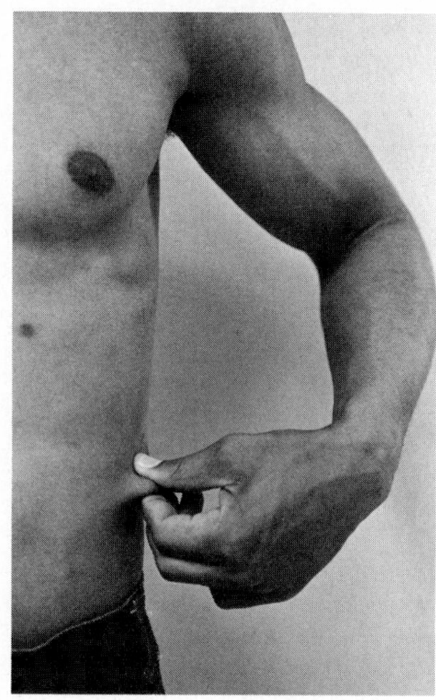

According to the pinch test, which of these people is overweight? (Photos by Philip Jon Bailey/Stock, Boston)

allows for the differences between males and females and is made in age categories with ten-year spans.

Overweight Versus Fat

Obesity Condition when over 30% of body weight is fat.

Adipose tissue Fatty tissue.

Obese is synonymous with fat. Very simply, **obesity** means that a person is carrying an excess of fatty, or adipose, tissue. Usually, obese people are overweight, sometimes excessively so, but it is also true that obese persons may be underweight. Any person who has 30 percent or more of their total body weight as **adipose tissue** is considered obese, regardless of his or her total body weight.

Underweight people may or may not be suffering from malnutrition; the two words are not synonymous. Malnutrition literally translated means "bad nutrition," but the underweight person may follow good nutritional guidelines and still not be assimilating enough nutrients to satisfy bodily needs. The cause may be some physiological disorder or a disease that prevents the utilization of the nutrients. Being underweight can actually cause as many health problems as being overweight, and in neither condition is a person's vigor at its optimum.

Research conducted a few years ago by Dr. Ancel Keys, a noted Minneapolis physiologist, showed that an astonishing 20 percent of the underweight men he studied were among the top third in the amount of fatty tissue in their bodies. On the other hand, some of the men in the top 20 percent of the overweight category were among the lower third in the amount of fat in their bodies. This was particularly true of those who use their muscles in their work. These men utilized their fat as a fuel, and their extra weight was primarily lean or solid body tissue. Overweight thus means that a person weighs more than average or normal, and an overweight person may or may not be fat.

Research has been done on football players who not uncommonly are overweight but have little fat. Their weight is in the greater development of muscles. These studies and others called attention to the fact that the old weight charts did not take into account the quality of a person's weight. Neither did they consider the size of a person's frame—whether small, medium, or large. Currently used charts do take account of differences in the person's frame; in addition, the weights overlap from one category to the next to make allowance for those people who are "in-betweens."

Kinds of Body Fat

Fat is one of the basic foods supplying body energy. In normal amounts, fat gives the body its desirable and attractive contours. In excess, it can become ugly flab.

Two types of fat are found in the body: essential fat and storage fat. **Essential fat**—kept in a number of places in the body, such as the liver, spleen, lungs, heart, kidneys, intestines, bone marrow, and some areas of the spinal cord and brain—serves as a temporary reserve that is drawn on to take care of needs in normal body functions. Excesses of fat beyond the body's usual requirements become the **storage fat** that builds up as adipose, or fatty, tissue in many parts of the body. This is the type of fat that forms layers between the muscles and the skin and over internal organs, and other vital parts. These cushions do have some protective value, but this storage fat also contributes to obesity.

Essential fat Temporary fat reserves for normal body needs.

Storage fat Fat in excess of the body's usual requirements.

Researchers have determined what they call the reference man and woman. These hypothetical individuals are the "ideals," so to speak, their measurements arrived at from the compilations of many studies to determine desirable weights. Individuals can compare measurements to these reference figures to learn how closely they match what is considered normal. There are substantial differences between the sexes. The reference man's body, for example, contains 3 percent essential fat and 12 percent stored fat—a total of 15 percent. In contrast, the reference woman's body consists of 10 percent essential fat and 12 percent stored fat, making a total of 22 percent. This higher percentage of fat in women is related to their childbearing function and to the attendant glands and hormones.

Types of Obesity: Hyperplasia and Hypertrophy

Hyperplasia Abnormal increase in number of fat cells.

Hypertrophy Abnormal increase in amount of fat stored in a stable number of cells.

Two types of obesity are recognized. One is called **hyperplasia;** the other is termed **hypertrophy.**

Hyperplasia results from an exceptionally large number of fat cells. This increase in the number of cells occurs only during the early years of life. Some of the increase takes place during the last three months before birth. More occurs during the first year of life and again in the rapid-growth years from age 9–13. An increase in the number of fat cells does not occur in adults, but the large number of cells built up earlier in life can remain high.

In *hypertrophy,* the number of fat cells is normal, but each cell contains larger amounts of the neutral fats, which are the usual type stored in the body. Control of obesity due to hypertrophy is much easier than is control of fat that results from hyperplasia.

In a normal, or nonobese, person, the number of fat cells is estimated at about 27 billion, but in an obese person, the number of fat cells may be from 40 to 100 billion. In exceptional cases, the number may be more than 200 billion. In other words, in cases of obesity due to hyperplasia, fat is deposited in from two to four times more cells than in a nonobese person. In the average nonobese person, the amount of fat in the body generally accounts for about 23 to 33 pounds of the total body weight. In an obese person, this may be 200 pounds or more. Only the size of the fat cells changes, not their number. Each fat cell in an obese person contains at least a third more fat than does a fat cell in a nonobese person. Each fat cell may consist of up to 90 percent fat. It has been suggested by some physiologists that it is these cells, particularly when their fat is depleted, that send chemical messengers through the body demanding more input and thus triggering the overeating habit.

About 50 percent of people who are fat as adults were fat as children. A very low percentage—roughly 3.5 percent—of those who are fat as adults manage to lose weight and achieve what is normal or ideal for their height and age. The extent to which obesity is controllable is still not fully determined, but it is evident from studies that the regulation of body weight is most effective if it is started at a young age. Furthermore, the regulation of quality and quantity of food by dieting appears to be no more important than exercise or physical activity in preventing the buildup of fat cells during the adolescent years.

What Causes Obesity?

Obesity certainly involves the taking in of more calories than are utilized, but that does not explain its underlying cause. For comparison, consider a person who drinks too much alcohol and becomes inebriated. This does not explain what stresses or other social or physiological factors triggered the person's desire for the alcohol.

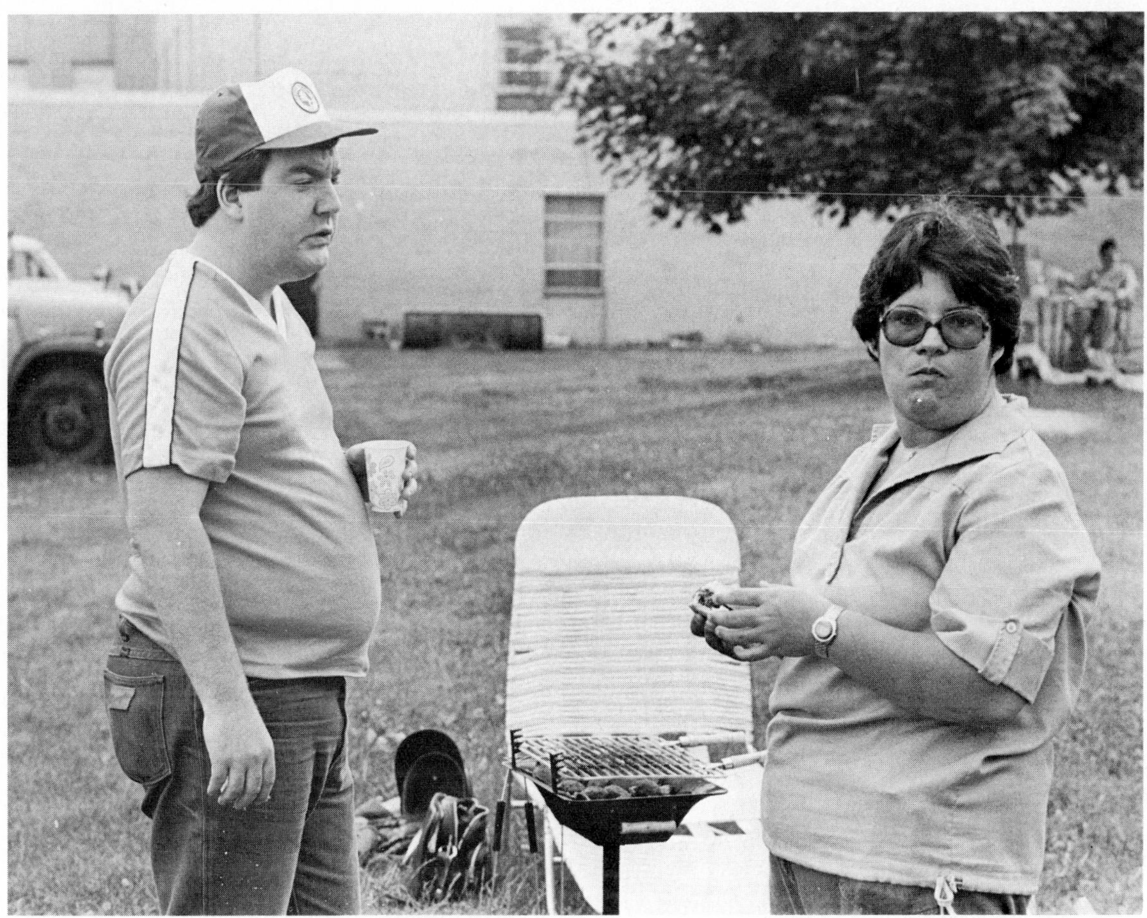

Eating habits established early in childhood can lead to obesity later in life. (Photo © Mike Rizza/the Picture Cube)

Current studies on the causes of obesity have narrowed the focus to two factors: environmental and medical.

Lack of Physical Activity

The environmental factor indicates that the onset of obesity is due mainly to a lack of exercise and general physical activity. Studies of hundreds of children have demonstrated that about 75 percent of the obese boys and an even higher percentage of the obese girls did not engage in sufficient physical activity to forestall the buildup of fat. These children, who are rarely active in sports, are the sedentaries. Their intake of calories may not be significantly higher than that of other children their age, but a larger percentage of what they take in is not utilized. More of it becomes stored as fat.

Physiologist Jean Mayer and fellow researchers first proved this in experiments with rats. Normally inactive and confined to cages, the rats were given treadmills for increasing periods of time each day.

When the rats exercised for no more than an hour a day, they did not eat more food than usual—they ate less than usual—and their weight decreased. When the hours of exercise were extended to six, the rats ate more than they did when engaging in little exercise, but their weight remained about the same. With more than six hours of exercise, the rats again ate less food than they did with no exercise, and they lost weight in large amounts. Allowed to overeat without exercise, the rats gained large amounts of weight, becoming obese. If given only a sustaining diet, these obese rats voluntarily became more active even as they lost weight. In summary, both small and large amounts of exercise were directly related to a smaller intake of food. Lack of exercise, in contrast, led to more eating and resulted in correspondingly large gains in weight.

These same observations were then carried over to humans. Findings indicate that very sedentary people eat more, use fewer calories, and become obese. Those who are moderately active eat less and have a lower body weight. As one example, in a study of obese and normal-weight high school girls, the obese girls were less than half as active as were those with normal weight, although they generally ate less food. These results have been confirmed by a number of similar investigations.

Lowering of Metabolism

Style of living thus appears to be a major cause of obesity, and being sedentary is a major contributor. This shows up clearly with increasing age. "Creeping obesity" is a term that has been used for the slow and steady weight increase that is common with age. The average weight addition may not be great, generally not more than three pounds in a year. But over a ten-year period, such a weight gain adds up to 30 pounds! What explains the commonness of "creeping obesity"? A major reason is decreased physical activity—the same factor that causes weight increases in some young people. This is further compounded by a lowering of metabolism that customarily occurs at a rate of 3 percent every ten years in people over the age of 30. People continue to take in as much food as they did in their earlier years, but they use fewer calories per day. The extra amount is "banked" in the body as fat. It is very difficult for people to admit that they are not as active as they were in younger years.

Heredity and Glandular Disturbances

Some medical causes of obesity have been pinpointed as well. Heredity is one factor. Some people do inherit from one or both parents a tendency to store excess amounts of fat. However, in many cases, heredity is used as a convenient excuse for something that could be avoided. Obesity may also be induced by glandular disturbances and imbalances that can be brought on by injury, surgery, disease, or other changes that alter the glandular control of normal body chemistry. These are rare cases, however.

The Set-point Theory of Obesity

Currently many researchers are turning to a new theory of weight gain or loss, called the **set-point theory.** This theory maintains that a person's body will "set" the percentage of body fat it will store. If the caloric intake is higher than needed, the excess will be burned off as metabolic heat. If the intake is not high enough according to a person's set point, the person will want to continue to eat even if it leads to overweight and obesity.

Set-point theory Theory that a body "sets" the percentage of body fat it stores.

Is there any way to create a long-term change in your set point? One way seems to be through aerobic exercise that is vigorous enough to raise your heartbeat to 75 to 80 percent of maximum (see Chapter 12 for a detailed explanation). This may be difficult, however, if you are already obese. Recent evidence points to a diet high in carbohydrates as another way to lower the set point, but the experimental evidence is not yet complete.

The set-point theory may explain why many people seem to have a yo-yo weight loss and gain pattern on crash and other fad diets. A drastic reduction in caloric intake will temporarily lower the set point. However, when the normal caloric intake is resumed, the body goes back to the original set point (and sometimes higher). Thus the individual experiences a weight gain.

The Physiology of Weight Control

When we use the term **calorie,** we are usually referring to what is actually a **kilogram calorie** (also called kcalories, kilocalories, or large calories). One pound of weight is roughly equal to 3,500 calories. In other words, if you store 3,500 calories as fat, you gain 1 pound in body weight. Or you can lose a pound of fat by utilizing 3,500 calories. This makes the gaining and losing of pounds a very simple mathematical equation, but for some people it is extremely difficult to translate into practice. Once obesity has set in, it is not easy to reverse. A loss of 350 calories in fat every day, however, adds up to an impressive 36 pounds in a year.

Calorie A degree of heat.

Kilogram calorie Degree of heat used to measure energy produced from food.

You can lower the calories in your diet without affecting its quality, for dieting does not have to be an ordeal. It may also help if you realize that a simple modification of your present diet may be all that is needed to give you the necessary calorie reduction. Meals should be regular, and portions should be smaller. It is better to eat half a dozen small meals every day than to eat only one big meal. Remember that skipped meals do not necessarily contribute to a loss of weight. In fact, the contrary has been observed. When meals are skipped, there is a loss of needed energy and increased hunger, and when an extra-large meal is then eaten, more of the calories are deposited as fat rather than utilized to supply energy needs. Being satisfied with less food at each meal, but utilizing the calories rather than storing them, is wiser and can become a good habit in the same way that for many people, eating more than necessary is a bad habit. Changing your food habits is easier, of course, when you want to attain a specific goal and when you can begin to see the results (see Self-Assessment Exercise 14.2).

Should You Lose Weight? If So, How?

Americans spend some $15 billion a year on exercise equipment and diet programs that are sold with guarantees to lead to weight losses. For most people, of course, losing weight is primarily a matter of cosmetics. They are convinced that looking better and feeling good go together. Psychologically, this is true. But unfortunately, most people spend more money trying to lose weight than it costs them to buy the food that caused the weight gain. In addition, there are some who insist on losing weight when it is not necessary or even advisable for them to do so.

Consider entering a weight-loss program only if you weigh about 15 percent more than the desirable weight indicated for you on a height-weight chart. You can be especially concerned if your weight is escalating steadily. If so, you should check with a physician. For males, if an accurate measurement of fat versus lean indicates that the fat in your body accounts for more than 20 percent of your weight, you definitely have a weight problem that needs attention. For females, the figure is 30 percent.

Do not try to lose a lot of weight rapidly. It is safer for your health to hold the loss to one or one-and-a-half pounds per week. A more rapid weight loss will cause general weakness and will increase your susceptibility to disease. You will probably also become irritable and depressed; therefore, go slowly. Watch your calorie intake. Keep in mind the very important figure of 3,500 calories. As noted earlier, for every 3,500 calories not utilized in your body, you are adding one pound of weight. Common sense then becomes the most important criterion in weight-loss programs. Do not be misled by advertisements that guarantee large and rapid weight losses: they can be dangerous.

Many aids to weight loss are on the market. However, the simplest way to lose weight is to cut your calorie intake, eat nutritious foods, and exercise. (See page 367.) (Photo by Don Renner)

How many calories do you need every day? To get a rough estimate, multiply your weight by 15. Most males need 2,500–2,700 calories; females generally need 1,800–2,000. If weight is a problem, intakes of more calories per day than necessary supply the reserves that accumulate as fat.

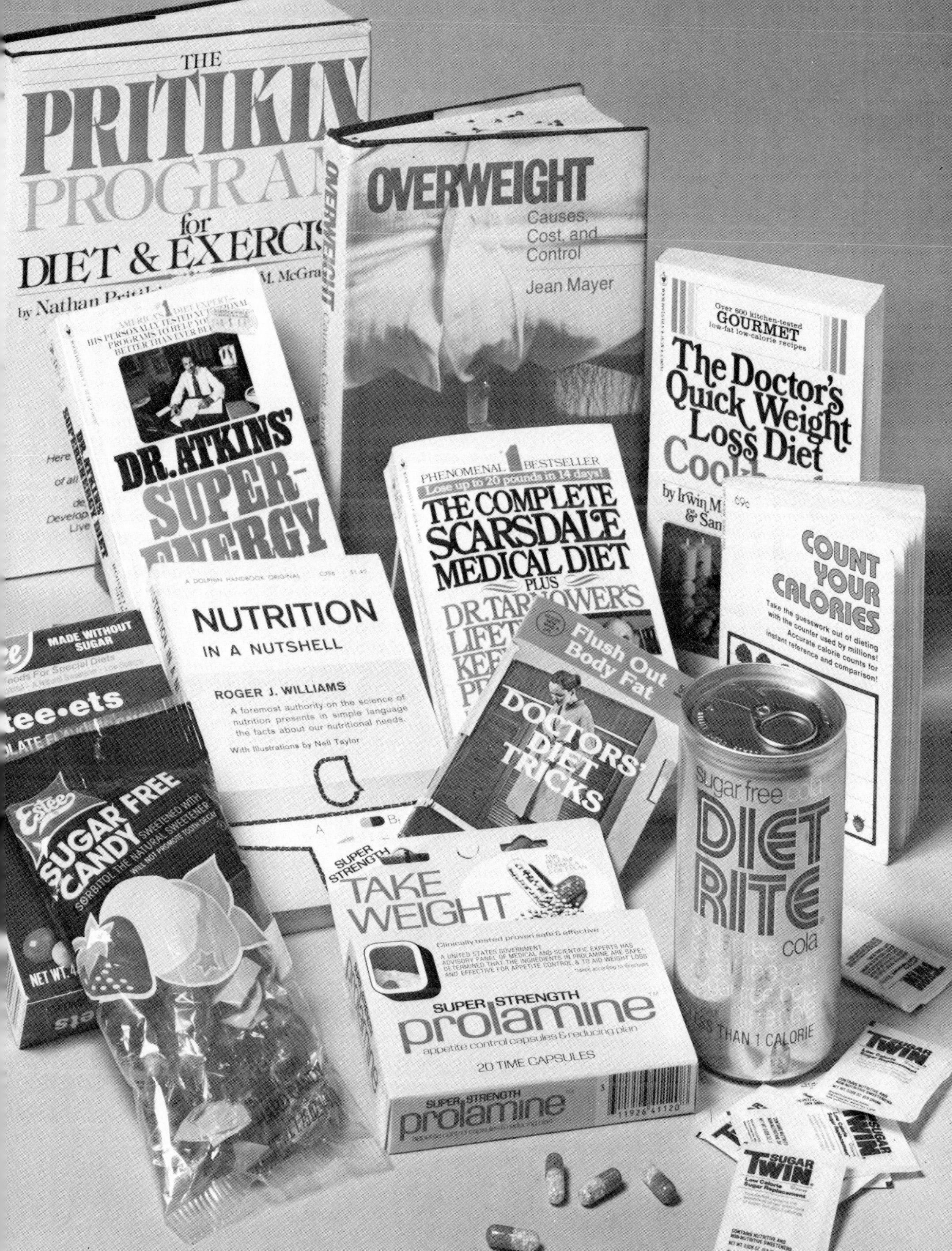
THE PRITIKIN PROGRAM for DIET & EXERCISE
OVERWEIGHT
Causes, Cost, and Control
Jean Mayer
DR. ATKINS' SUPER-ENERGY
Over 600 kitchen-tested GOURMET low-fat low-calorie recipes
The Doctor's Quick Weight Loss Diet Cookbook
PHENOMENAL #1 BESTSELLER
Lose up to 20 pounds in 14 days!
THE COMPLETE SCARSDALE MEDICAL DIET
PLUS
DR. TARNOWER'S
A DOLPHIN HANDBOOK ORIGINAL
NUTRITION IN A NUTSHELL
ROGER J. WILLIAMS
A foremost authority on the science of nutrition presents in simple language the facts about our nutritional needs.
With Illustrations by Nell Taylor
COUNT YOUR CALORIES
Take the guesswork out of dieting with the counter used by millions! Accurate calorie counts for instant reference and comparison!
Flush Out Body Fat
DOCTORS' DIET TRICKS
MADE WITHOUT SUGAR
tee•ets
Estee
SUGAR FREE CANDY
SWEETENED WITH SORBITOL THE NATURAL SWEETENER
WILL NOT PROMOTE TOOTH DECAY
SUPER STRENGTH
TAKE WEIGHT
Clinically tested proven safe & effective
SUPER STRENGTH
prolamine
appetite control capsules & reducing plan
20 TIME CAPSULES
sugar free cola
DIET RITE
sugar free cola
LESS THAN 1 CALORIE
SUGAR TWIN
Low Calorie Sugar Replacement

SELF-ASSESSMENT EXERCISE 14.2

How Do You Eat?

Answer each of the following ten items by placing the letter of your response in the space provided.

1. The quantity of food I put on my spoon or fork is usually (a) large (b) small. _______
2. I generally tend to chew my food (a) slowly (b) rapidly. _______
3. I usually (a) put one bite of food after another into my mouth (b) wait between bites. _______
4. I usually (a) eat so fast I don't have time to enjoy my food (b) eat slowly enough to enjoy it thoroughly. _______
5. I usually (a) eat all the food in front of me (b) stop eating when I am full even though there may be more food on my plate. _______
6. After I have eaten I (a) sit around the table (b) leave the table. _______
7. After I have finished the main course, I (a) leave the left leftovers on the table (b) clear the table before having a cup of coffee, tea, or other beverage. _______
8. When it comes to snacking, I generally snack (a) frequently, (more than three times per day) (b) occasionally. _______
9. When I snack I usually have (a) large quantities (e.g., a sandwich and a piece of cake) (b) small quantities. _______
10. I generally prefer as a snack food (a) cookies or other sweets or potato chips (b) celery, carrots, or fresh fruits. _______

Scoring

Total the number of *b* responses you made. If you have 6 or more, you probably have fairly good control over your eating and snacking. If you have fewer than 6 *b* responses, you might be well advised to review your eating patterns.

Source: From the book *Take It Off and Keep It Off by* D. Balfour Jeffrey and Roger C. Katz. © 1977 by Prentice-Hall, Inc. Published by Prentice-Hall, Inc., Englewood Cliffs, NJ 07632

Losing as much as a pound a day while at the same time maintaining normal body functions is not possible, even with fasting. An extremely overweight person can, of course, survive for extended periods of time by utilizing the energy stored as fat. For most people,

YOUR HEALTH TODAY

Dos and Don'ts for Good Eating

Do	Don't
Eat less fat	Eat candy
Eat less sugar	Drink soft drinks
Eat more fruits	Eat cakes and other sweets
Eat more fish	Eat fatty meats such as bacon
Drink skim milk	Add salt and sugar to foods
Eat more cereals	
Eat more vegetables	
Eat lean meats	

however, the advisable and ultimate weapons against weight increases are a lowered intake of calories plus an increase in exercise. Neither should be entered into as crash programs. Weight losses should be gradual and steady, not dramatic and rapid. If you make drastic attempts to reduce weight—other than by gradual reduction in calorie intake or increase in physical activity—you should do so only under the supervision of a physician. In general, you should not lose more than two pounds per week.

Even with no change, or only moderate changes, in diet, regular exercise programs can reduce weight significantly. In one study, overweight college-age women lost more than 5 pounds each in 2 months with only a combination of jogging and walking for one hour a day, four times a week. Furthermore, skinfold measurements revealed that the weight loss in pure fatty tissue was greater than the loss of lean or solid body tissue. In some of the women, in fact, there was even an increase in nonfat body tissue at the same time that a general loss in body weight occurred. This point is important. In diet programs that depend primarily on fasting or a reduction of calorie intake, much of the loss of weight is due to a loss of body fluids or of lean or solid body tissue. This kind of weight loss is not desirable. In fasting programs, in fact, studies have shown that as much as 45 percent of the weight lost is in only the lean body tissues.

Exercise programs, plus moderate but not drastic dieting, appear to be an excellent method of weight reduction for those who are only moderately overweight (as much as 30 percent above the normal for their height and weight). People who are more overweight than this should not attempt reducing programs without medical supervision. Exercise, for example, can do severe damage to the heart and blood vessels or put excessive strain on supporting tissues that are already

YOUR HEALTH TODAY

Tips for Losing Weight

1. Avoid situations that create hunger for you.
2. Don't eat snacks or other meals while watching television.
3. Keep fattening foods out of reach.
4. Cut down on high-sugar snacks.
5. Eat slowly at meals, don't rush and gulp.
6. Keep a record of what you eat.
7. Keep a record of how much weight you lose.
8. Establish and write down your weight-loss goals. Be sure to include both long- and short-range goals.
9. Don't shop for food when you are hungry.
10. Prepare your own meals instead of eating out.
11. Lose weight gradually.
12. Do not be discouraged if the loss seems to come slowly.
13. Be careful to eat nutritious and well-balanced meals every day.
14. Make your cutbacks in the carbohydrates and fats, not the fruits and vegetables.
15. Try to walk whenever you can.
16. Exercise regularly.

burdened by the extra weight. For these people, exercises must be carefully selected and then monitored.

Doesn't exercise increase the appetite and thus trigger more eating, resulting in weight gains that are equal to the losses? Not necessarily. It may happen in some cases, but most studies show that with moderate exercise — up to as much as an hour a day — the appetite may actually decrease.

Metabolism A measure of energy that is the sum of all the chemical processes that occur in the body.

The utilization of fat as a result of exercise is due to an increase in body metabolism. **Metabolism** is the amount and measure of energy needed for the body to function properly. It is the sum of all the chemical processes that occur in the body. It is interesting that this increased metabolic rate continues for as long as six hours after the exercise is stopped. One investigator noted as much as a 28 percent greater rate of metabolism four hours after exercising, as compared to the level of metabolism at the same time on days when there was no exercise.

To be effective, the exercise must be vigorous enough to raise a sweat. This means an increase of body heat and a utilization of calories. But if you are not accustomed to exercising regularly, start gradually and build up to this intensity over a period of time. Do not engage in vigorous exercise until you are fit enough to make the workouts enjoyable. What kinds of exercise should you engage in? Many types are excellent. Among them are tennis, handball, skiing, swimming, bicycling, running, dancing— almost any kind of exercise will help to trim off fat while at the same time adding zest and fun to one's life. These are recreational types of exercise, and they amount to acceptable "play" for people of all ages. You also spend calories doing chores, such as scrubbing floors, making beds, mowing grass, raking leaves, and building shelves. One very easy way to spend calories is by brisk walking. Do not, for example, park your automobile as close as you can to where you want to go. Instead, purposely park a good distance from your destination and then walk (see Chapter 12).

Fad Diets and Gimmicks

New diets claiming to reduce and control weight appear regularly. Be extremely cautious—many of these diets are dangerous. Often they depend on a rapid loss of water to cause a sudden drop in weight, which is not advisable.

Extravagant and erroneous claims are made by commercial diet programs because such advertising campaigns are designed to sell. The sales pitches and literature are enticing, some even suggesting that losses from specific areas of the body can be made to satisfy special needs. Some people, for example, want to lose pounds only from their hips or legs. This is really impossible to guarantee. Weight losses occur first from the largest fat deposits, wherever they are in the body.

Advertised programs rarely accomplish their claims unless they are craftily designed replicas of the simple calorie principle already described. In some cases, a person who is disturbed when the diet has not worked as advertised is then convinced by the diet hucksters that the program would have been effective if it were not for some personal peculiarity. If the diet is continued with perhaps a slight variation, the person is told, desired results will be achieved. A second sale is made, and usually the negative results are simply repeated.

Many diet clinics do not have medically approved programs and are not operated by trained technicians. The only real reduction you can be sure of is a slimmer wallet. Weight losses might be attained, but they are sometimes at the expense of good health. Avoid the fads, fraud, and quackery that characterize the advertised programs. If there are genuine weight problems of any sort, consult a physician or a qualified nutritionist to establish a proper program.

Gullible Americans may also purchase gadgets and gimmicks that are supposed to take away fat more easily and quickly than it was put on. These slimming belts, rollers, and similar devices may indeed flatten out rolls of fat and give a person an immediate, visual, and

YOUR HEALTH TODAY

Using Your Energy*

Activity	Calories per Hour
Moderate Activity	**200–350**
Bicycling (5½ mph)	210
Walking (2½ mph)	210
Gardening	220
Canoeing (2½ mph)	230
Golf	250
Lawn mowing (power mower)	250
Lawn mowing (hand mower)	270
Bowling	270
Fencing	300
Rowboating (2½ mph)	300
Swimming (¼ mph)	300
Walking (3¾ mph)	300
Badminton	350
Horseback riding (trotting)	350
Square dancing	350
Volleyball	350
Roller skating	350
Vigorous Activity	**over 350**
Table tennis	360
Ice skating (10 mph)	400
Tennis	420
Water skiing	480
Hill climbing (100 ft. per hr)	490
Skiing (10 mph)	600
Squash and handball	600
Cycling (13 mph)	660
Scull rowing (race)	840
Running (10 mph)	900

* The calorie expenditure noted here is approximately the same for a person weighing from 100–250 pounds.

Source: Adapted from material from the President's Council on Physical Fitness and Sports, Washington, D.C.

measurable reduction in the waistline or other part of the body on which they are used. But take the measurements fast! The fat is only squeezed in; ten minutes later, it will be back. Remember, there is no miracle method.

But What If You Are Underweight?

Relatively few people have the problem of being underweight, but it is indeed true that some people, particularly when they are young, may be below the average weight for their age and height. This might, of course, be normal for them and should not be a matter of great concern, but they may think they look too "twiggy." They feel uncomfortable in social situations, and therefore, primarily for cosmetic reasons, they want to "plump up." It is also true that underweight people—that is, those weighing more than 10 percent less than what the tables suggest as "ideal"—may become tired quickly. They may also be more susceptible to colds and other kinds of illnesses.

But being underweight is not necessarily the same as malnutrition. The typical underweight person simply spends more energy than is

Anorexia nervosa is an eating disorder that affects many adolescents. Anorexics virtually stop eating and may ultimately starve themselves to death. (Photo © 1982 Susan Rosenberg/Photo Researchers, Inc.)

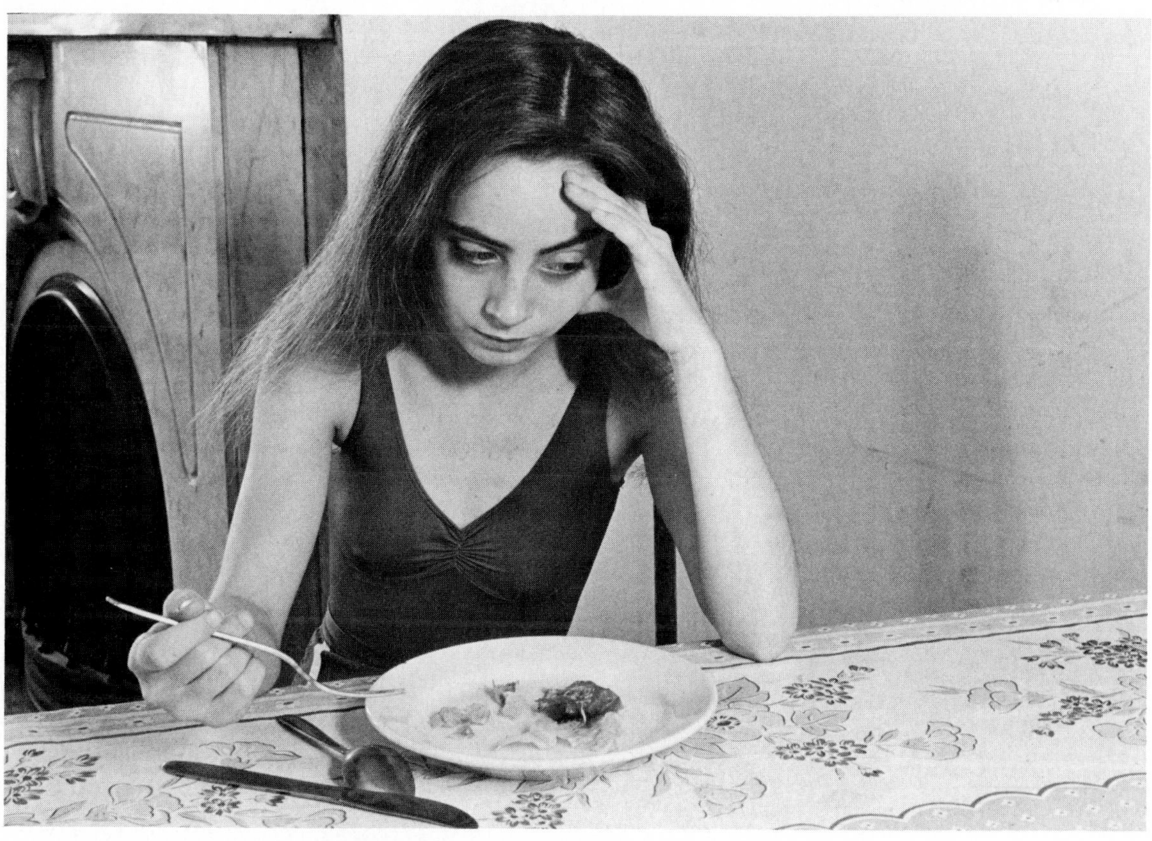

taken in and is thus undernourished as compared to the overweight person, who has an excess of nourishment. Malnutrition, however, is the result of poor or "bad" nutrition, a matter of eating the wrong kinds of foods. Even overweight people can suffer severely from malnutrition, which can become a serious physiological problem.

In most cases, however, being underweight can be corrected fairly easily. Weight is gained by taking in more calories. An addition of 3,500 calories above normal intake equals 1 pound in body weight. Gaining weight may require eating more than three meals a day, and the underweight person can generally enjoy the high-starch diet that is forbidden to one who is overweight. But be careful! Keep active, and do not let the gain be stored fat. Take in extra calories, making certain to get all of the nutritional essentials such as vitamins and minerals, but exercise as well. Build lean body weight—not fat!

Eating Disorders

In dieting to lose weight, some people become underweight from a purposeful and eventually psychological loss of appetite. If extreme and out of control, this leads to a clinically diagnosed disease called **anorexia nervosa,** a chronic, self-starvation that results from a personal feeling of being too fat. Anorexia nervosa's specific cause is unknown, but it generally strikes females during the teen years and peaks in the late teens, although cases have been identified in individuals over 30 years of age.

Anorexia nervosa A chronic, self-starvation disorder.

Often as a result of going on a fad diet to lose a few pounds, the adolescent female begins to feel a power over her eating habits but simultaneously begins to feel a preoccupation with the fact that she is fat. A revulsion syndrome sets in wherein any loose flesh is seen as fatness rather than a condition that exercise could help. This feeling of fatness becomes a severe emotional problem such that even with weight loss the feeling of fatness remains. As a result of the lack of eating, emaciation, skin discoloration, amenorrhea (loss of menstrua-

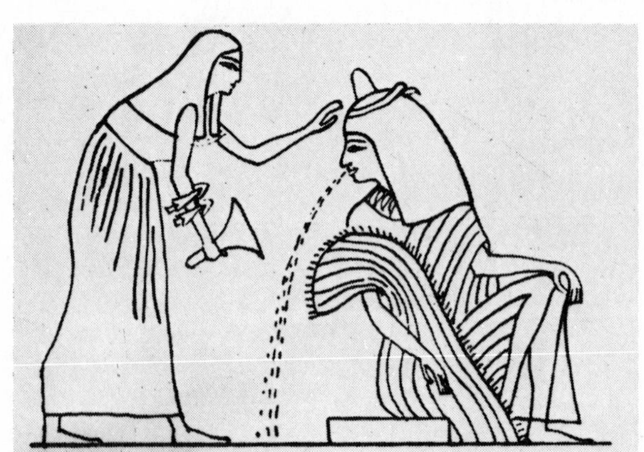

Ancient Egyptian drawing of a woman at a banquet vomiting—a drastic way of dealing with the age-old problem of overeating. This could also be an early depiction of what today is called bulimia. (Photo from the Bettman Archive)

tion), lowered blood pressure and body temperature, constipation, depression, and severe fatigue set in.

Another eating disorder is **bulimia,** also called the binge-purge syndrome. Bulimia involves a pattern of eating binges followed by self-induced vomiting and/or the consumption of a laxative in order to rid oneself of what was just consumed. Many bulimics are near normal weight but have an abnormal fear of becoming fat. The syndrome seems to be more prevalent in women than in men. If a person persists in this pattern of eating behavior, severe health problems, including kidney failure, infections, ulcers, and malnutrition can result.

Bulimia Binge-purge syndrome.

Both anorexia and bulimia require medical treatment combined with psychological counseling to restore the individual's sense of self-worth and good nutritional patterns. If you think that you may be a victim of either or both of these eating disorders, you can call the national helpline at 201-836-1800 or see your physician for advice.

Summary

Weight control is one of the most important aspects of preventive medicine today. Both the overweight and the underweight person are prone to fatigue and may feel uncomfortable in social situations as a result of low self-esteem. In addition, both the overweight and the underweight may be more susceptible to certain disorders. In the overweight, these include high blood pressure, heart disease, diabetes, digestive tract disorders, respiratory ailments, and gallbladder and kidney diseases.

Charts can be consulted to find out the ideal weight for people of different heights and body builds. For an accurate determination of the proportion of fat to lean tissue in the body, a physician, nutritionist, or technician can use either underwater weighing or skinfold measurements.

Obesity is defined as an excess amount of fatty, or adipose, tissue. Underweight people may be obese if they have an excess of fat but insufficient lean body tissue to be the desirable weight. Malnutrition is defined as eating the wrong kinds of foods and not supplying the body with the proper nutrients to satisfy its needs.

The body has two types of fat. Essential fats are temporary reserves that are stored in places like the liver, lungs, and spleen. The body draws upon these fats for the energy it needs to perform normal body functions. The other type of fat is storage fat, excesses beyond the body's requirements that collect as fatty tissue and contribute to obesity. In addition, there are two kinds of obesity. Hyperplasia is the result of an increased number of fat cells, and hypertrophy, which is easier to control, is the result of larger amounts of neutral fats contained in a normal number of cells.

One pound of weight is equal to 3,500 calories. Therefore, to lose one pound, a person must utilize 3,500 calories. A combination of calorie reduction and moderate exercise is generally the best way to achieve weight loss, which should be gradual—no more than 2 pounds a week. Anything more is not safe, and weakness, susceptibility to disease, and irritability may occur. Dieters who are reducing their calorie intake should make sure to eat nutritious, well-balanced meals, and those who are embarking on exercise programs should do so gradually. Crash programs should be avoided for both diet and exercise, and medical supervision should be sought for those who are more than moderately overweight.

Consumers should be wary of the extravagant claims and predictions that accompany advertisements for miracle diets. Many of these fad diets are dangerous, and weight-loss clinics are often not operated by trained personnel and do not have medically approved programs.

In some cases, purposeful dieting can go to extremes and lead to the psychological conditions called anorexia nervosa and bulimia, which can cause malnutrition, heart problems, and other disorders. In most cases, however, people are underweight because they spend more energy than they take in. They can correct the condition by obtaining medical and psychological help and by taking in more calories.

Review and Discussion

1. Describe some of the social reasons for losing weight.
2. What are some diseases associated with obesity? How does obesity affect longevity?
3. What is your ideal body weight?
4. Explain the skinfold technique for determining the amount of body fat.
5. What are hyperplasia and hypertrophy? How are they related to obesity?
6. Describe the environmental and medical causes of obesity.
7. Explain the set-point theory of obesity.
8. What is the relationship between calories and fat? How many calories are equivalent to a pound of fat?
9. When should a person decide to lose weight?
10. What is the most effective weight-loss program for most people?
11. Find two examples of claims made by commercial diet programs. Are these claims supported by scientific evidence?

Further Reading

Bailey, Covert. *Fit or Fat?* Boston: Houghton Mifflin Company, 1978.
A frank discussion of various ways to improve fitness, lose body fat, and feel good while doing both. Concepts of nutrition and aerobic exercise as they relate to weight control are presented. (Paperback)

Berland, Theodore. *Rating the Diets.* New York: New American Library, 1980.
An evaluation of a wide variety of diet programs in terms of medical safety and effectiveness. (Paperback)

Katch, Frank, and William McArdle. *Nutrition, Weight Control, and Exercise.* 2nd ed. Philadelphia: Lea and Febiger, 1983.
A basic discussion of how nutrition and exercise are directly related to and affect one's weight. Good tips for sensible weight control and loss or gain are presented. Explains nutrition and metabolism and also examines the caloric cost of foods and exercise. (Paperback)

Heyward, V. H. *Designs for Fitness.* Minneapolis, Minn.: Burgess Publishing Company, 1984.
Although the text concentrates on general fitness, Chapter 8, about weight reduction and control, is particularly appropriate and well written.

Mayer, Jean. *Overweight: Causes, Costs and Control.* Englewood Cliffs, N.J.: Prentice-Hall, Inc., 1968.
The classic book on the causes and control of obesity. (Paperback)

Part V
Disease

"The beginning of health is to know the disease."
Cervantes

Until a century ago infectious, or communicable, disease ranked first as the cause of death throughout the world. Slowly at first, and then with increasing momentum, scientists learned more about these diseases and their causes and effects and found weapons to prevent and conquer many of them. Today chronic diseases have replaced infectious diseases as the country's number one health problem. The prevention of such diseases is of special concern to young people. In Chapter 15, "Communicable Diseases," the pathogenic invaders that cause disorders from the irritating common cold to the deadly African sleeping sickness are discussed. Chapter 16, "Cancer," and Chapter 17, "Cardiovascular Diseases," concentrate on these two leading killers. "Other Noncommunicable Diseases," Chapter 18, describes risk factors, preventive measures, symptoms, and treatment of such familiar afflictions as allergies, diabetes, arthritis, epilepsy, and genetic diseases.

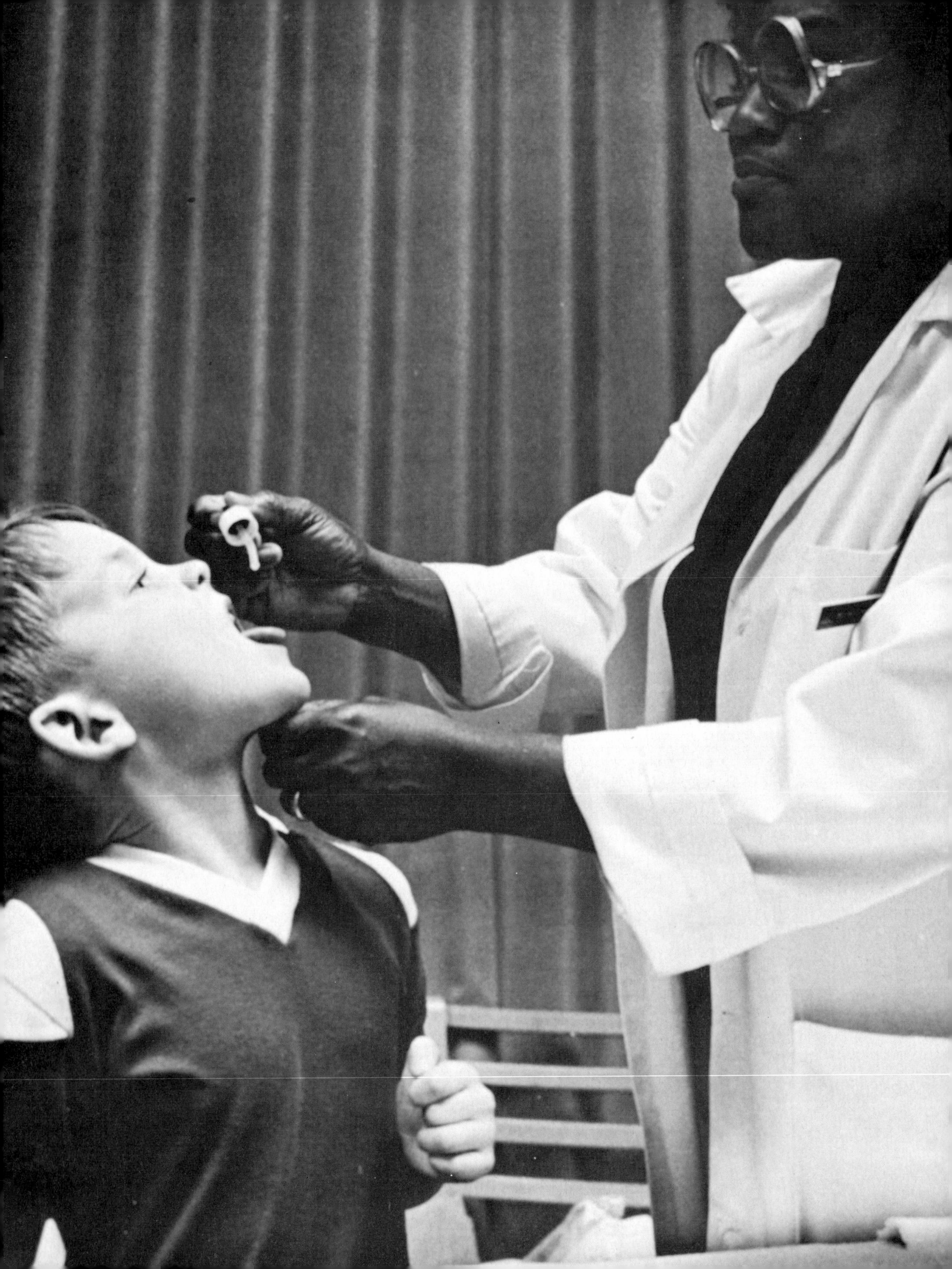

Chapter 15 Communicable Diseases

KEY POINTS

- ☐ Communicable diseases are diseases that can be transmitted from person to person, either directly or indirectly.
- ☐ Communicable diseases are caused by pathogens, or disease-causing organisms.
- ☐ The six basic types of pathogens are bacteria, viruses, rickettsias, protozoa, fungi, and parasitic worms.
- ☐ An infection is the invasion of body tissue that produces damage caused directly by the pathogen or by the toxins (poisonous substances) it produces.
- ☐ The human body has several lines of defense against pathogens, including the skin and mucous membranes, inflammation, the immune system, and interferon.
- ☐ Medical defenses against infection include public health measures, vaccination, and drug therapy.
- ☐ Communicable diseases vary widely in their cause, symptoms, and treatment.
- ☐ Although great progress has been made in the prevention and control of communicable diseases, further efforts need to be made.
- ☐ Acquired Immune Deficiency Syndrome (AIDS) is quickly becoming a public health problem of devastating magnitude.

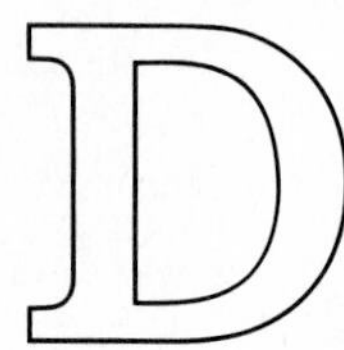

ISEASES that can be transmitted from person to person, either directly or indirectly, are called **communicable diseases.** The organisms that cause these diseases are termed **pathogens.**

Communicable disease Diseases that can be transmitted from person to person.

Pathogens Organisms that cause communicable disease.

Pathogenic, or disease-causing, agents such as bacteria and viruses can actually be transmitted not only from one human being to another, but also from an animal or insect to a human being or through the air we breathe, the water we drink, or the food we eat. Once inside the body, pathogens cause disorders, the effects of which range from merely irritating (the common cold) to deadly (African sleeping sickness).

The ease with which most pathogens can spread explains the numerous epidemic outbreaks of communicable disease that have plagued humanity since earliest times. Fortunately, the human body is well equipped to repel or render harmless many pathogenic invaders, and medical strategies such as vaccination, quarantine, and the use of antibiotics and other drugs are effective against many others. Medical advances over the past 100 years have controlled or contained such once-deadly diseases as smallpox and poliomyelitis, but many others remain serious problems.

Pathogens and Infections

A *microorganism* can be simply defined as any microscopic entity capable of carrying on living processes. A microorganism that is capable of causing a disease state is termed a *pathogenic organism.* The disease state caused by an invasion of body tissue by a pathogen is termed an **infection.** The vast majority of microorganisms are not pathogenic and pose no threat to human beings. However, there are still a significant number of pathogens which can cause disease states.

Infection Invasion of body tissue by a pathogen.

Pathogenic organisms range in size and complexity from submicroscopic viruses to animal-like varieties, such as protozoa and parasitic worms. The virulence, or disease-producing ability, of these pathogens varies greatly. There are six basic types of pathogens: (1) bacteria, (2) viruses, (3) rickettsias, (4) protozoa, (5) fungi, and (6) parasitic worms. An illustration and brief description of each type of pathogen can be found in Figure 15–1. In addition, each of the pathogens will be discussed later in the chapter.

The Infectious Disease Process

Infections may be either acute or chronic in development and local, focal, or systemic in impact. *Acute infections* develop rapidly and usually result in high fever and severe sickness. *Chronic infections,*

Illustrative plate	Group and size scale	Description	Examples of diseases caused	Mode of action
	Viruses (10 to 250 nanometers*)	Minute, submicroscopic particles composed of nucleic acids and protein; intracellular parasites	Rabies, polio, yellow fever, colds, influenza	Disrupt protein synthesis of cells, sometimes kill cells
	Rickettsia (less than 1 micrometer*)	Small bacteria always associated with insects and other arthropods	Typhus fever; Rocky Mountain spotted fever; Q-fever	Interfere with metabolism of host cells; all are intracellular parasites
	Bacteria (1 to 10 micrometers)	Single-celled, plantlike; abundant in the biosphere; secrete disease-causing toxins; are commonly found in a rod, spiral or spherical shape	Tuberculosis, syphilis, pneumonia, scarlet fever, boils, meningitis	Produce toxins and enzymes that destroy cells or interfere with their function
	Fungi (a few micrometers to several inches)	Single-celled or multicelled plantlike organisms; consist of threadlike fibers and reproductive spores, molds	Athlete's foot; most commonly diseases of the skin, hair, nails, and lungs	Release enzymes that digest cells
	Protozoa (a few to 250 micrometers)	Microscopic animals; each is single-celled	Malaria, amebic dysentery, and African sleeping sickness	Release enzymes and toxins that destroy cells or interfere with their functions
	Parasitic worms (1/32 inch to 20 or 30 feet)	Multicellular animals; common types are round or flat	Pinworm, trichinosis, tapeworms	Release toxins; compete for foods; block digestive tract and blood and lymph vessels

A nanometer is one billionth of a meter; a micrometer is one millionth of a meter; a meter is 39.37 inches.

Figure 15-1. Major Pathogen Groups. **(Source: Jones, Shainberg, and Byer, *Dimensions*, 4th ed. Copyright © 1979 by Kenneth L. Jones, Louis W. Shainberg, and Curtis O. Byer.) (Reprinted by permission of Harper & Row, Publishers, Inc.)**

on the other hand, develop slowly and exhibit symptoms that generally are milder but longer lasting. In a *local infection*, such as a boil, the infectious agent is restricted to one area of the body. Usually more serious in impact are *focal infections*, such as abcesses, in the course of which the pathogens themselves move from the initial site of the infection to other parts of the body. In *systemic infections*, such as typhoid fever, the pathogens are transported throughout the body via the circulatory system.

All infections develop in a process that can be broken down into three phases: (1) transmission of the pathogen from a source to a host, and invasion of the host's body by the pathogen; (2) the life cycle of the pathogen inside the host's body, and the body's reaction to it; and (3) the pathogen's exit from the body.

Transmission and Invasion

Humans and animals are the ultimate source, or *reservoir*, of almost all pathogens. Human sources usually exhibit symptoms of the infection caused by the pathogen they harbor. Less frequently, human sources will be *carriers*—individuals who harbor a pathogen without exhibiting any symptoms. There are three types of carriers: (1) healthy carriers, who have never contracted the disease caused by the pathogen they carry; (2) incubatory carriers, who have the disease in its early stage, before any symptoms are apparent; and (3) chronic carriers, who have recovered from the disease but still carry the pathogen. Because they seem to be uninfected, carriers pose a difficult health-control problem.

Pathogens spread from sources to new hosts in a variety of ways. Direct transmission from reservoir to host can occur through body contact or through droplets released from the mouth or nose of an infected person. Each of these routes of transmission is termed a "portal of exit."

Indirect transmission takes many forms. Pathogens may be ingested with food or water, or breathed in with air. Inanimate objects provide another vehicle for the spread of pathogens: a glass used by a person with a cold, for instance, may harbor viruses. Finally, other organisms, usually animals or insects, may carry a pathogen from reservoir to host. These are called **vectors.**

Vector Organisms that transmit pathogens from reservoir to host.

Once transmitted from a reservoir, the pathogen must be "caught" by the host: in order to infect body tissue, the pathogen must find or create a way of entering the host's body. Obvious candidates for these invasion routes are the body orifices: nose, mouth, urogenital tract, eyes, and ears. Other openings are provided by breaks in the skin (cuts and abrasions, for example). A few pathogens, such as ringworms, create their own openings by directly attacking the skin. All of the points can be thought of as links in a chain. Thus in order for transmission and invasion to occur these links must be in place (see Figure 15–2).

The Course of the Disease

Upon gaining access to the body tissue, a pathogen leads a parasitic existence, feeding off—or, in the case of viruses, manipulating—tissue cells in order to live and reproduce. As the pathogens multiply,

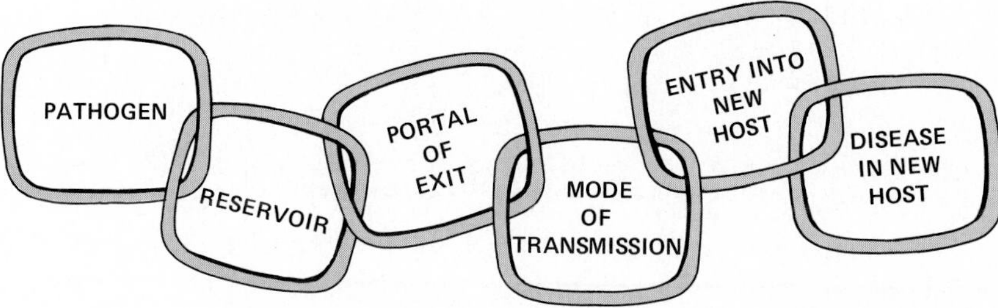

Figure 15-2. The Chain of Infection.
All of the links in the chain of infection must be in place before a disease is established. In order to control disease spread, a link in the chain must be broken.

sometimes producing toxins, they damage cells or pervert normal cell functions, thus producing disease. Typically, these disease have four stages:

1. *Incubation,* the time between the host's exposure to the pathogen and the onset of observable symptoms. The incubatory period can range from hours (for a cold) to months (for hepatitis).
2. *Prodromal stage,* the period during which early signs of the disease (a runny nose, for instance) appear. Since these symptoms typically are minor, the infected person often does not ascribe them to illness of any significance.
3. *Acute stage,* the stage when the disease is fully manifest and the body defenses have swung into action. With the host-agent reaction at its peak, symptoms are worst during this period.
4. *Convalescence,* the time when the body's defenses have successfully fought off the invader and the individual is recovering from the disease. Of course, particularly serious infections or secondary infections that strike an already weakened person can result in death rather than convalescence.

In most cases, this cycle ends with the expulsion of the pathogen. A few infectious diseases, such as malaria, are marked by recurrent cycles.

Exit of the Pathogen

During the acute and convalescent stages of an infection, the body often tries to flush out the invader, much as eyes flush out dust particles by producing tears. Pus, mucus, vomit, blood, or other fluids discharged either from superficial wounds and abscesses or from the nose, mouth, and urogenital tract serve to transport many infectious agents out of the body. Other invaders are expelled in coughs and sneezes, and pathogens that settle in the intestinal tract usually are excreted in feces or urine.

Body Defenses Against Infection

The human body has several lines of defense against pathogenic invasion. Unless weakened by injury, illness, or congenital defects, these defenses can cope with almost all infections.

Epithelial Defenses

Before a pathogen can attack body tissue, it must breach or bypass the barrier posed by the body's *epithelial defenses*—the layers of skin and mucous membrane that sheath the vulnerable inner parts of the body. A few pathogens can penetrate unbroken skin, but most can gain access to body tissue only through natural or injury-caused openings in the skin layer. Natural openings such as the nose and mouth are further protected by the mucous membranes that line the passageways leading from them. Other supplementary defenses include tearing, by which the eye cavities are flushed of foreign matter, and cilia, the hairlike fibers that protect the lungs from inhaled dust and microorganisms.

Inflammation

An infectious agent that succeeds in penetrating the epithelial barrier and establishing itself in body tissue triggers the body's second line of defense, the *inflammatory process.* The inflammation we see at the site of an infection actually stems from the body's attack on a pathogen, not vice versa. As the body automatically attempts to isolate and destroy the invader, fibrous tissue seals off the invasion site. A chemical compound called histamine is released by the damaged tissue, causing the local capillaries to dilate, and the flow of blood to the area is stepped up. With the increased blood flow (which produces the redness and swelling characteristic of inflammation) comes an increased supply of pathogen-destroying white blood cells. The dead tissue, pathogens, and white blood cells sometimes are flushed from the infection site in the form of pus.

Immunity

Inflammation provides an effective defense against most local infections but is too limited a mechanism to deal with particularly virulent and fast-spreading pathogens. Against these more serious threats, the body's most important defense mechanism is the immune system. Since immunity basically means "resistance to infection," both inflammation and the epithelial barrier can be viewed as part of the body's immune system. Specifically, however, **immunity** refers to a complex and variegated system by which the body defends itself

Immunity Body's ability to distinguish and neutralize foreign matter.

against particular types of infectious agents. Unlike the epithelial barrier and the inflammatory process, which defend body tissue against *all* foreign invaders, the immune system sets up specific defenses against specific pathogens, however they enter the body and wherever they spread within it.

Natural and Acquired Immunity. Immunity to an infectious disease can be either natural or acquired. *Natural immunity* means an inherent lack of susceptibility to a disease. Some pathogens simply cannot survive in the bodies of certain individuals.

Acquired immunity is a much more complex phenomenon, based on the body's ability to recognize the presence of a particular pathogen and produce agents that will destroy or neutralize it. Among the white blood cells that rush to an infection site during inflammation are *lymphocytes*. Once exposed to any antigen (foreign agent), lymphocytes retain the ability to recognize that antigen if and when it reappears in the body. Upon its reappearance, a type of lymphocyte called the T-cell lymphocyte directly attacks the antigen; another type, the B-cell lymphocyte, produces antibodies—chemical agents, the sole function of which is to destroy the specific antigen recognized by the sensitized lymphocytes.

This cycle of exposure-sensitization-reexposure-recognition-reaction is called active acquired immunity. It is acquired because it comes about only after exposure to a pathogen; it is active because the body manufactures its own antibodies and sensitized T-cells. Active immunity can be acquired either naturally (from an actual case of the disease) or artificially (from vaccines). Vaccines can be composed of four types of substances: (1) killed pathogens; (2) live but attenuated (weakened) pathogens; (3) pathogens of a disease closely related to but less severe than that for which immunity is desired; and (4) toxoids—nonpoisonous duplicates of the toxins produced by pathogenic bacteria.

Whatever its composition, a vaccine is designed to provoke the body's immune system into producing antibodies against a specific pathogen without actually causing the disease associated with that pathogen.

Interferon

The body's final line of defense against infection by viruses is *interferon*, a still-mysterious chemical substance released by cells that have been invaded by viruses. The principal effect of interferon is to protect nearby cells from viral invasion. It also helps the cell that releases it to resist the virus, but this resistance soon is lost. How interferon is produced and exactly how it aids immunity are not known. What does seem clear is that, unlike antibodies, interferon is effective against all viruses, not just the one that triggers its release.

Research into interferon is hampered by the fact that there are many different types of the substance, all of which are exceedingly

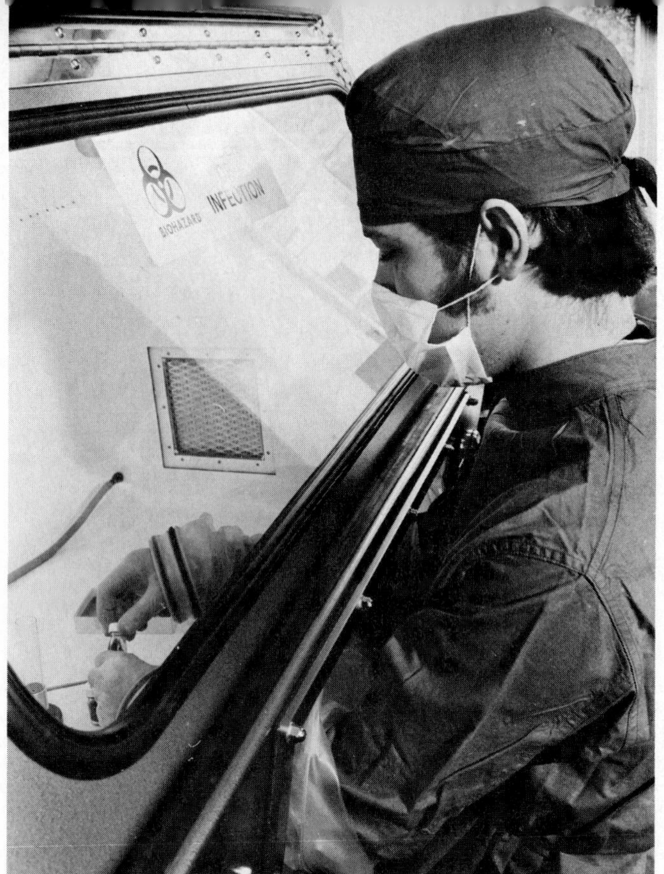

Limited quantities of human interferon can be processed from large amounts of human blood. Recently, however, researchers have developed techniques for producing human interferon synthetically in the laboratory. (Photo © Biophoto Association/ Photo Researchers, Inc.)

difficult to isolate and purify. Very limited quantities of human interferon (every living species apparently has its own interferons) can be processed, at fantastic expense, from large amounts of human blood. Recently, researchers have developed techniques for producing human interferon synthetically in the laboratory; through these techniques it may be possible to produce an effective form of interferon in greater quantity at lower cost. Administration of small doses of manufactured interferon to victims of viral infection and some types of cancer has provided encouraging, but still controversial, results.

Medical Defenses Against Infection

Communicable diseases present health professionals with the twofold problem of preventing the spread of infection and of curing infected individuals.

Public Health Measures

Public health measures are designed to stop communicable diseases before they get started, usually by preventing the pathogen from reaching a new host. Perhaps the classic example of this occurred during the building of the Panama Canal, when a team of doctors identified the *Aedes aegypti* mosquito as the vector of the yellow fever virus. The disease was virtually eradicated by eliminating or covering stagnant pools of water, the mosquito's prime breeding grounds. Today, insect-borne communicable diseases such as malaria are also combatted by spraying breeding grounds with insecticide and by providing individuals living in the areas with insect repellent.

Sanitation Laws and Public Health Codes. Communicable diseases spread via contaminated water and food supplies—typhoid fever, cholera, and dysentery, for example—present a different kind of health-control problem. Pathogens harbored in the excrement of infected persons can reach water supplies directly via sewage and food supplies indirectly via the hands of infected food handlers. To guard against these routes of infection, municipalities enforce sanitation laws aimed at insulating water used for drinking and bathing from the sewage system and ensuring that all persons who handle food in markets and restaurants follow sanitary procedures.

Quarantines. Still other sections of public health laws deal with *quarantine,* the enforced isolation of persons known to be infected by or suspected of carrying a pathogen. Quarantine has long been used to inhibit the spread of communicable diseases. During the late Middle Ages, when bubonic and pneumonic plagues killed off between one third and one half of the European population, unaffected towns and regions attempted forcibly to keep out refugees from plague-stricken areas. Modern health codes provide medical authorities with sweeping powers to quarantine any person liable to spread a communicable disease and to isolate, impound, or destroy property suspected of being contaminated. Quarantine laws are particularly useful in fighting outbreaks of diseases that spread rapidly in crowded environments.

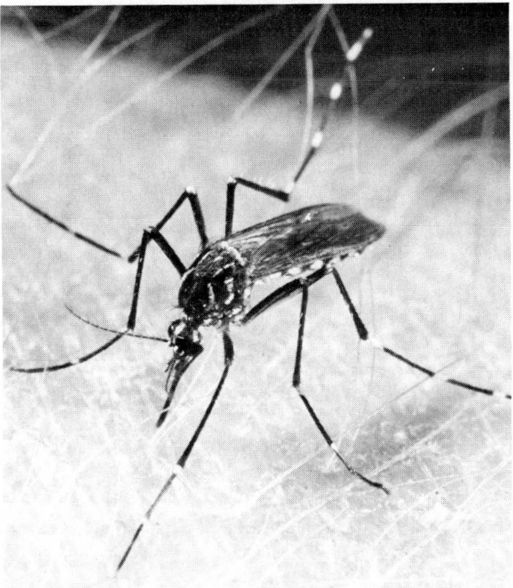

The *Aedes Aegypti* mosquito was responsible for the deaths of thousands of people during the construction of the Panama Canal, infecting its victims with the virus causing yellow fever. (Photo from Oxford Scientific Films/Photo Trends)

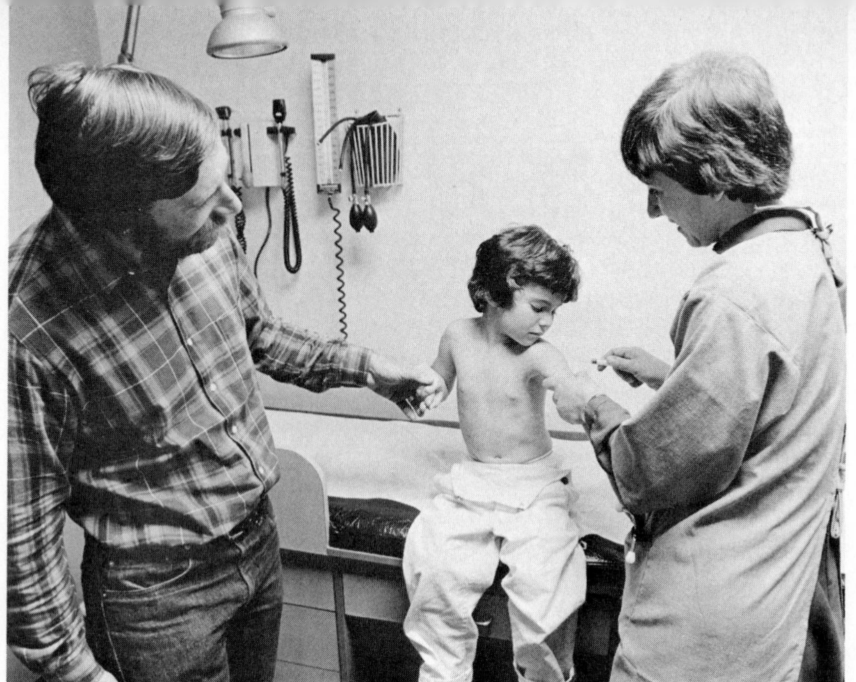

Vaccinations are one way of preventing or curing disease. (Photo © Donald Dietz 1981/Stock, Boston)

Mandatory Vaccinations. Aside from such public health measures, the principal medical weapon in the fight to prevent outbreaks of communicable diseases is vaccination. Mandatory vaccination programs in schools during the 1950s and 1960s all but wiped out poliomyelitis in the United States, where previously it had been a major threat to children. Often, vaccination is the only effective medical defense against virus-caused diseases, few of which can be treated with drugs.

Drug Therapy

For centuries it was known that certain naturally occurring substances could alleviate the symptoms of, or even cure, certain diseases. The Indians of South America, for instance, knew that a substance called quinine, obtained from the bark of cinchona trees, helped victims of malaria. How and why this occurred was not clear, however, until the late nineteenth and early twentieth centuries, when a series of scientific advances led to the isolation and identification of substances that destroy or inhibit the growth of pathogens. In 1928 the Scottish bacteriologist Sir Alexander Fleming discovered that a certain mold, *Penicillium notatum,* attacked and destroyed bacteria. The identification of penicillin led to the isolation and manufacture of a wide range of **antibiotics**—chemical substances produced by microorganisms that either destroy outright or interfere with the growth cycles of other microorganisms. A few years after Fleming's discovery, other researchers found that a synthetic substance called sulfanilamide inhibits the growth of a wide range of bacteria. Particularly during World War II, the so-called sulfa drugs derived from sulfanilamide played a major role in the treatment of bacterial infections. Now they have largely been supplanted by antibiotics, which generally are less toxic and more effective.

Antibiotics Chemical substances that destroy or interfere with microorganisms.

Drawbacks. With the development of antibiotic drugs, doctors for the first time could provide specific treatment to victims of many communicable diseases, including such feared killers as tuberculosis and pneumonia. Antibiotics have several shortcomings, however. In the first place, they are totally ineffective against all viral and many protozoal infections. Secondly, they often have harmful side effects on patients. Finally, the widespread use of antibiotics in the past 40 years has led to the emergence of drug-resistant strains of many pathogens.

Specific Pathogen-related Diseases

Bacteria

Bacteria are single-celled, plantlike organisms that reproduce by a process called fission, in which one cell divides itself into two cells. They come in three basic forms, differentiated by shape (see Figure 15–3). Some bacteria are aerobic (able to function only in the presence of oxygen), whereas others are anaerobic (unable to function in the presence of oxygen).

Bacteria Single-celled, asexual planklike organisms.

Bacteria live on, around, and between human cells. Within the body their effects are usually harmless and sometimes beneficial: some bacteria, for instance, produce enzymes vital to the digestive process. Only about a hundred species of bacteria are pathogenic to humans, but these hundred constitute the greatest single cause of human infection. All pathogenic bacteria (and all other pathogens, for that matter) are parasites that invade and live off body tissue, which they usually attack either directly or through the production of *toxins,* or poisonous substances.

Major bacteria-caused disorders include staphylococcus and streptococcus infections, most sexually transmitted diseases, the childhood diseases, diphtheria, tuberculosis, legionnaires' disease, and toxic shock syndrome.

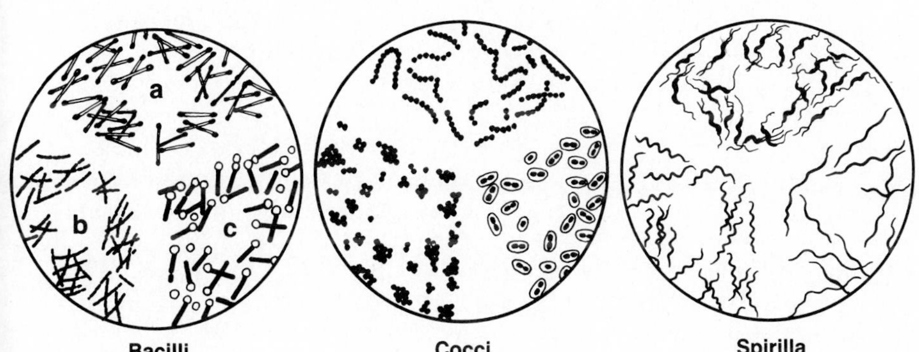

Figure 15–3. Bacteria Types.
Bacteria in the three major groups: bacilli (rod-shaped), cocci (spherical), and spirilla (spiral). Shown among the bacilli are those that cause diphtheria *(a)*, tuberculosis *(b)*, and tetanus *(c)*.

Major Bacterial Diseases

Staphylococcus bacteria Pathogenic bacteria occurring in irregular clusters.

Staphylococcal Infections. Among the many common bacterial diseases and disorders are those caused by **staphylococcus bacteria.** These are spherical microorganisms that usually appear in irregularly shaped clusters (*staphe* is Greek for "bunch of grapes"). Various strains of staph, as it is commonly called, cause such apparently disparate disorders as boils, food poisoning, and certain types of pneumonia. Both the skin and the internal organs are vulnerable to staph infection.

Humans comprise the principal reservoir of staphylococci, which are transmitted from reservoir to host either through direct contact or, less commonly, through infected objects. An estimated 30 to 40 percent of all human beings harbor staphylococci in their nostrils, and these carriers often infect the individuals themselves, as well as spreading the pathogen to others. The principal symptom of a staph infection is the appearance of a pus-filled skin infection, which may take the form of impetigo, a boil, a carbuncle, an abscess, or an infected cut or laceration. Pus draining from the infected area is a prime source of contagion; once the pus is gone, there is no danger of the infection spreading unless the individual affected is a carrier. More serious situations arise when staph pathogens infect the lungs, causing **staphylococcal pneumonia,** or are carried by the bloodstream from a surface infection to body organs or bone tissue, where they can produce life-threatening infections.

Staphylococcal pneumonia Serious infection caused by staph pathogens in the lungs.

Streptococcus bacteria Spherical, chain-forming pathogenic bacteria.

Streptococcal Infections. **Streptococcus bacteria** are spherical-shaped organisms that form chains rather than clusters. Some strains of streptococci are pathogens. Among the strep pathogens, the most important in human disease are the hemolytic streptococci, which produce a substance that destroys red blood cells. These pathogenic agents are responsible for streptococcal sore throat, scarlet fever, rheumatic fever, streptococcal pneumonia, and erysipelas (a severe and recurrent infection that spreads rapidly from a skin infection). They usually are transmitted through direct contact.

Streptococcal sore throat Infection that involves fever and swollen tonsils.

Scarlet fever Infection from strep pathogen causing vomiting and fever.

Streptococcal sore throat (strep throat), which reaches the acute stage after an incubation period of one to three days, is characterized by fever, soreness and redness in the throat, and, often, swollen tonsils. In some cases, the strep pathogen will produce a toxin that causes the telltale rash of scarlet fever. Severe cases of **scarlet fever,** accompanied by nausea, vomiting, and high fever, were once a significant cause of death in children aged five to eight. Today, death from scarlet fever is rare in the United States and other developed countries because of the availability of effective antibiotic drugs. Normally, the fever subsides within two weeks and no complications follow. Occasionally, however, the onset of strep throat or scarlet fever triggers an immune reaction that also attacks the heart and the joints. Although the inflammation and chest pain symptomatic of this reaction,

HARPER'S MAGAZINE ADVERTISER.

THE SANATORIUM, DANSVILLE, NEW YORK.

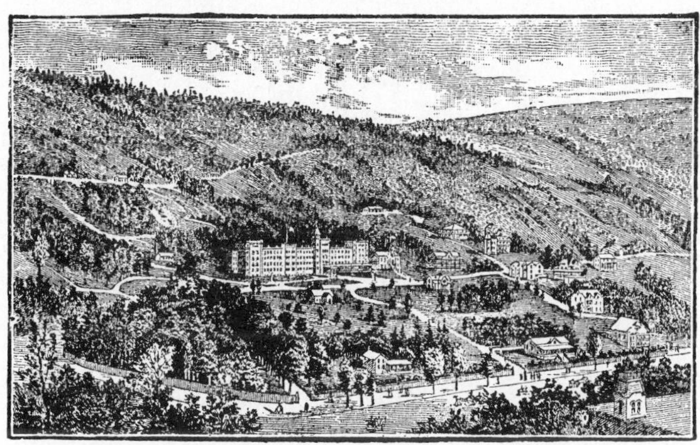

The largest Health Institute in America.

Built of Brick and Iron, and absolutely Fireproof. Heated throughout by Steam.

Fall and Winter most favorable for treatment.

Winters exceptionally mild. Pure water from Alkaline Calcic Spring. Perfect Sanitary Condition. Plentiful table. Special attention given to Diet. No Institution is so well equipped for giving baths of every kind, especially the famous Molière Bath, so effective in treatment of Malaria, Rheumatism, and Bright's Disease. Electricity, Massage, and Swedish Movements are specialties.

For illustrated circular and testimonials address

Drs. JACKSON and LEFFINGWELL,
DANSVILLE, NEW YORK.

Improved methods of detecting tuberculosis, such as chest x-rays and skin tests, and the development of antituberculosis drugs have made wards like this one obsolete. (Photo from EKM-Nepenthe)

commonly known as **rheumatic fever,** almost always subside, permanent heart damage may result.

Rheumatic fever Immune reaction from strep pathogen attacking heart, joints, and chest.

Tuberculosis. Once a worldwide scourge known as consumption, or the "white plague," **tuberculosis** is less feared today because of modern drug therapies. Between approximately 1900 and 1950, the tuberculosis death rate was cut by some 95 percent in the United States, where at one time it was a leading cause of death in adults. Although almost all developed countries have recorded a similar decrease in fatalities, in poorer parts of the world tuberculosis remains a formidable killer.

Tuberculosis Chronic disease infecting lung tissue.

Legionnaires' Disease. First identified after a fatal outbreak at a 1976 American Legion convention in Philadelphia, **legionnaires' disease** is actually a family of infections caused by the *Legionella pneumophilia* bacterium and related species. Researchers have yet to establish exactly how the pathogen is transmitted. The available evidence indicates that *L. pneumophilia* can live a long time in water (air-conditioning condensates provided the reservoir in the Philadelphia outbreak), that it enters a new host through the respiratory system, and that it most seriously affects individuals who have deficient immunity or an underlying chronic disease. An estimated 2 to 12 percent of all pneumonias in the United States result from *L. pneumophilia* infections.

Legionnaires' disease Infection that strikes mainly individuals with an immune deficiency.

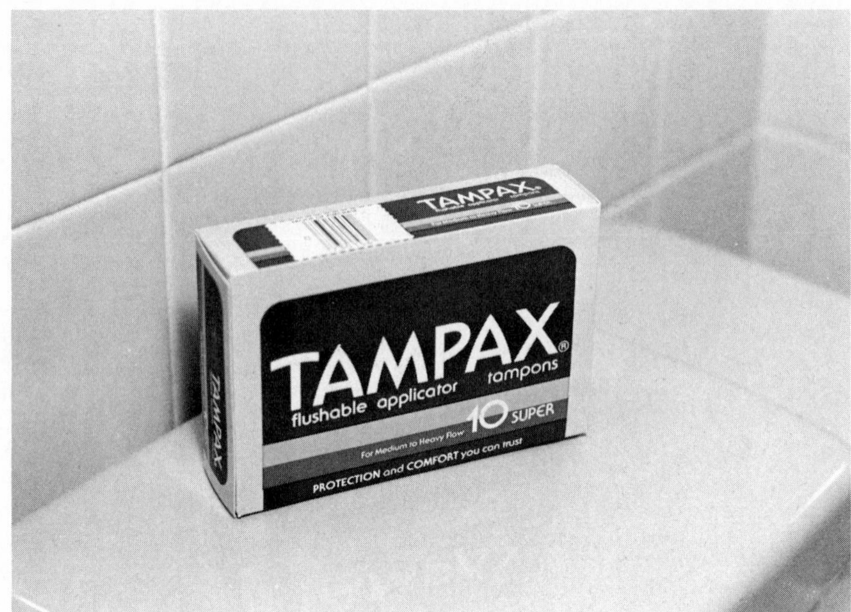

Toxic shock syndrome, a bacterial infection associated with the continuous use of superabsorbent tampons during menstruation, affects mainly women under age 30. (Photo by Paul Waldman)

Toxic Shock Syndrome Acute bacterial infection associated with continuous use of tampons.

Toxic Shock Syndrome. **Toxic shock syndrome** is an acute bacterial infection caused by staphylococcus and generally associated with the continuous use of tampons during the menstrual period. The condition usually affects menstruating women under age 30.

Tampons are clearly implicated in toxic shock syndrome, but their exact role is uncertain. Research has suggested that the tampons may contribute to the development of the syndrome by one or more of the following methods:

1. Introducing the bacteria *(S. aureus)* into the vagina during insertion.
2. Absorbing toxin from the vagina.
3. Traumatizing the vaginal mucosa during tampon insertion leading to infection.
4. Providing a favorable environment for the growth of the bacteria.

When toxic shock syndrome is not associated with menstruation, the bacteria seem to originate in bone, skin lesions, or lungs.

Toxic shock syndrome produces a sudden onset of high fever. Other symptoms include vomiting, diarrhea, and sudden low blood pressure, which sometimes leads to shock, and possibly death.

Treatment for toxic shock syndrome includes use of antibiotics other than penicillin. In addition, patients treated for toxic shock syndrome should use tampons intermittently, change them frequently, and discontinue use and notify their physician if they develop nausea, vomiting, diarrhea, or fever. Women who use tampons should choose tampons made entirely of cotton and avoid the super-absorbent type that holds a great deal of fluid and encourages prolonged use. Hands should be washed thoroughly before insertion, because the *S. aureus* bacteria are commonly found on the hands. Preventive measures are extremely important since about 9 percent of the cases of toxic shock syndrome prove fatal.

Viruses

Variously regarded as either very simple organisms or very complex molecules, **viruses** are submicroscopic particles made up of a nucleic-acid (DNA or RNA) core coated with protein. Free viruses exhibit none of the characteristics of living matter. In order to grow and multiply, they must invade a living host cell and utilize its genetic material. How they do this is not entirely clear. Apparently, they have the ability to commandeer a cell's genetic material and manipulate it to ensure their own survival and reproduction. As parasites inside cells, they usually damage or destroy the normal functioning of host cells and hence cause some of humanity's most widespread and serious diseases.

Viruses Pathogens composed of a protein coating and a DNA or RNA core.

Viruses are the most mysterious of all pathogens. They are too small to be seen with a light microscope and can only be identified under an electron microscope. Many researchers believe that some forms of cancer are caused by viruses that genetically "command" host cells to reproduce uncontrollably. Among the disorders definitely traced to viruses are influenza, the common cold, herpes I and II, viral hepatitis, smallpox, and poliomyelitis.

Major Viral Infections

The Common Cold. The viral infection of the upper respiratory tract known as the **common cold** is almost certainly the most widespread ailment afflicting humanity. It is also among the least preventable of infections: regardless of precautions, the average person will suffer at least one cold per year. One reason the common cold is so common is that the pathogen involved can be any one of more than 100 different types of viruses. These viruses are easily spread through direct contact or via droplets expelled from the nose or mouth by coughing, sneezing, or a so-called runny nose. Susceptibility to viral infection of the respiratory system varies greatly among people. In order to see how susceptible you might be to respiratory infections, complete Self-Assessment Exercise 15.1.

Common cold Viral infection of the upper respiratory tract.

The infection may be confined to the mucous membranes of the nose, or it may affect the throat and larynx, too. Coughing, sneezing, itchy or sore throat, tearing, a runny or stopped-up nose, and general malaise are common symptoms that normally persist no longer than

SELF-ASSESSMENT EXERCISE 15.1

Susceptibility to Respiratory Diseases

Directions Circle the number in the vertical column that best describes your behavior or habit.

	Frequency of Occurrence			
	Usually	**Often**	**Seldom**	**Never**
A. Symptoms				
1. Shortness of breath, as after climbing stairs	10	7	3	0
2. Coughing up sputum	15	12	4	0
3. Sore throat irritation	10	8	3	0
4. Glands swell in neck	5	3	1	0
5. Running nose (sniffles)	5	3	1	0
6. Fever	10	7	3	0
7. Feeling tired at end of day	5	3	1	0
8. Poor physical endurance	5	3	1	0
B. Behavior				
9. Smoking 10 or more cigarettes a day	20	15	5	0
10. Live in an air-polluted community	5	3	1	0
11. Work with chemicals, grain, dusts, or metallic vapors	5	3	1	0
12. Use aerosol hair sprays or deodorants	10	8	3	0
13. Use or work with pesticide sprays	5	3	1	0
14. Have dog or cat as pet	5	3	1	0
15. Have carpet on the floor	5	3	1	0
16. Have children under 5 years of age or come in contact with them	10	7	4	0
17. Work with children ages 6–12	10	7	3	0
18. Come in contact with people all the time	10	7	3	0
19. Eat an unbalanced diet	10	7	3	0
20. Do not get enough rest	5	3	1	0

	Frequency of Occurrence			
	Usually	**Often**	**Seldom**	**Never**
21. Get less than 8 hours sleep per day	5	3	1	0
22. Become overfatigued	5	3	1	0
23. Drink alcoholic beverages	5	3	1	0
24. Get feelings of depression	10	8	3	0
25. Feel life is not worth lifting	5	4	1	0
26. Life a sedentary life-style	10	8	4	0
27. Use hand when sneezing	5	3	1	0
28. Inhale air full of cigarette smoke	15	12	5	0
29. Become irritated at others	5	3	1	0
30. Have deadlines to meet	5	3	1	0
31. Have many crises or problems to solve	10	8	3	0
32. In company of friends or relatives suffering many colds or infections	5	3	1	0
33. Work or live in an air-conditioned office or house	5	3	1	0
34. Visit sick relatives	5	3	1	0
Total				

Scoring

1. Add the numbers you circled. This is your susceptibility score.

Interpretation

Classify your score in the appropriate score range

Score Range	Susceptibility to Respiratory Diseases
0–35	Exceptionally low
35–65	Some
66–90	Average
91–130	High
131+	Extremely high

(Continued)

Your susceptibility to respiratory diseases depends on many things, some of which are included in the behavioral variables. A few factors, like smoking cigarettes, being exposed to people, eating poorly, and feeling depressed collectively make one highly susceptible to respiratory infections. Some, like living in an air-polluted environment, having a pet, and not getting enough rest, are probably of lesser importance. There is an obvious vocational risk, for example, when working in a chemical or dust environment. Miners inhale fine dusts that irritate the lungs, causing miner's lung disease.

People differ in their ability to resist respiratory infections: Your behavior and life-style can help to protect your body against infection.

If you are susceptible to respiratory infections, you should identify those behavioral items you circled that have weighted values of 10 or more points. By eliminating these behaviors, you can lower your susceptibility to respiratory infections.

Source: Walter D. Sorochan. *Promoting Your Health,* New York, John S. Wiley, 1981. p. 300. Reprinted by permission of the author.

---

one week. Fever is rare, except in children (who are particularly susceptible). Although the symptoms usually are not serious, and death from the infection itself is unknown, the social impact of the common cold is great. Colds can occur in epidemic outbreaks that severely disrupt work, school, and home environments. There is no known cure.

Influenza Severe viral infection of the respiratory tract.

Influenza. Although various maladies are popularly ascribed to the "flu," **influenza** is properly defined as a viral infection of the respiratory tract. Sudden fever, coughing, headache, chills, and prostration characterize influenza, a highly contagious infection. Most victims recover unaided in about two to seven days. In the elderly or the chronically ill, however, influenza can be followed by such serious secondary complications as bronchitis and bacterial pneumonia. During flu epidemics, deaths from these secondary infections often number in the thousands.

The great public health danger posed by influenza stems from the characteristic swift spread of the infection, the nearly universal susceptibility to it, and the variety and number of the viral pathogens that cause it. Easily transmitted via droplets or direct contact, and even in airborne particles, influenza viruses move through a population with astounding speed. Since exposure to a particular strain confers (sometimes temporary) immunity to it, vaccination is an effective way of safeguarding those most likely to suffer from the deadly secondary complications. Periodically, however, entirely new strains appear, against which vaccination is useless. These new strains cause the great pandemics of influenza, such as the Hong Kong flu outbreak of 1968–1969. One such newcomer was responsible for the worldwide epidemic that killed approximately 20 million people in 1918 and 1919.

Infectious Mononucleosis. Another common viral disease, **infectious mononucleosis,** is caused by the so-called Epstein-Barr virus. It usually strikes children and young adults, sometimes in epidemic outbreaks. Along with such common symptoms of viral infection as sore throat and fever, mononucleosis is characterized by general fatigue, swollen lymph glands, and a high count of abnormal lymphocytes. In children, especially, the symptoms can be so mild as to pass unnoticed. The principal immediate danger for young adults is the possibility of rupturing the swollen spleen, so treatment centers around keeping the victim as inactive as possible during convalescence. There is no known cure for the disease, which normally runs its course in a period of one to several weeks.

Infectious mononucleosis Viral disease characterized by fatigue and swollen lymph nodes.

Exactly how the mononucleosis pathogen is transmitted is not known with certainty, although the evidence points to person-to-person spread via oral discharges (hence its reputation as the "kissing disease").

Viral Hepatitis. There are three distinct forms of **hepatitis** (infection of the liver). *Type-A hepatitis,* commonly called infectious hepatitis, is an acute infection whose symptoms appear suddenly and usually subside within a few weeks, although in serious cases they may persist for months. Most often the viral pathogen involved moves from person to person in food or water contaminated by the urine or feces of infected individuals. Crowded or substandard living conditions aid the spread of the disease.

Hepatitis An infection of the liver.

In contrast, *type-B hepatitis,* commonly called serum hepatitis, is a chronic disease that occurs endemically (as natural to a particular region or climate) rather than epidemically. Since it may be present in blood and other body fluids, it can be transmitted through transfusions of contaminated blood or blood products or through contaminated syringes and needles. Outbreaks often arise in hospitals and among drug users. It can also be transmitted by oral ingestion of contaminated material. Carriers are a major problem, because many people exposed to the virus show very mild symptoms and can communicate the disease for months or even years. Unlike infectious hepatitis, which ordinarily runs its course without serious consequences, some types of serum hepatitis can lead eventually to fatal complications, such as cirrhosis of the liver. A third form, very similar to type-B hepatitis, has been identified only recently and is known as non-A, non-B hepatitis.

All three types of viral hepatitis display early symptoms of nausea, loss of appetite, and fever (although fever is more common in victims of type-B hepatitis). These warning signals often are followed by jaundice, a yellowing of the skin that results from the damaged liver's progressive inability to remove bile pigment from the blood. Recently, a vaccine against type-B hepatitis has been developed.

Herpes Simplex. There are two kinds of **herpes simplex** *virus,* labeled *herpes I* and *herpes II.* Most humans harbor the herpes I virus,

Herpes simplex Virus that may recur with injury or stress.

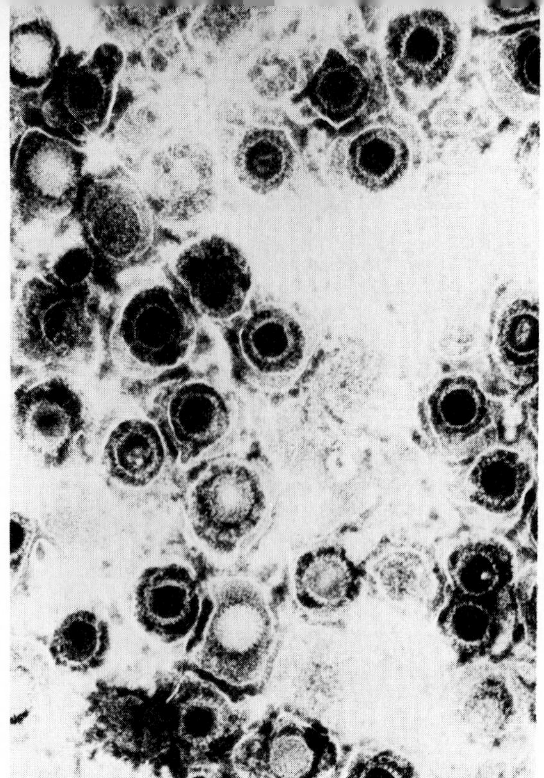

Microphotograph of herpes simplex viruses. (Photo courtesy of U.S. Center for Disease Control)

which lies dormant in the body after an initial childhood infection. Periodically, physiological injuries (other infections, sunburn) and changes (menstruation, pregnancy) or emotional stress will trigger a recurrence of the infection. Most recurrences take the form of cold sores on the lips or canker sores in the mouth, which usually disappear within ten days or so. Occasionally, the recurrence will involve encephalitis (inflammation of the brain), which is sometimes fatal.

Herpes II is a more serious infection that has become increasingly common. Whereas herpes I is acquired through direct contact with the saliva of an infected individual, herpes II normally is transmitted venereally, during genital-genital or oral-genital contact. Genital herpes is discussed under the section on sexually transmitted diseases in this chapter.

The Childhood Disease. Viral agents are responsible for most of the communicable diseases that commonly afflict children, including *varicella* (chickenpox), *rubeola* (ten-day measles), *parotitis* (mumps), and *poliomyelitis* (polio). The exceptions are *pertussis* (whooping cough) and *diphtheria,* which are caused by bacteria. Except for poliomyelitis, which can lead to permanent partial paralysis (and death, if the lungs are involved), ordinarily the only serious danger faced by the victims of these diseases today is the threat of secondary bacterial infections.

All of these disease are transmitted via infected droplets (see Table 15–1 for specific characteristics). They cannot be cured, but the widespread use of vaccines has greatly reduced the incidence of all except varicella. Parents are advised to see that their children are vaccinated for different diseases at the proper time (see Table 15–2).

Table 15-1 Childhood Diseases

Disease	Pathogen	Incubation Period	Common Symptoms
Poliomyelitis (polio)	Poliovirus types 1, 2, and 3	Usually about 7-12 days	Fever, headache, stiff back and neck, gastrointestinal disorder, often followed by paralysis
Infectious parotitis (mumps)	Paramyxovirus	12-26 days	Fever, swelling and tenderness of the parotid glands (near the ears) and other salivary glands
Rubella (3-day or German measles)	Rubella virus	14-21 days	Fever, malaise, swelling of lymph nodes, blotchy rash spreading from face to trunk[1]
Rubeola (10-day measles)	Measles virus	8-13 days	Fever, conjunctivitis, cold-type symptoms, bronchitis, blotchy rash that spreads from face all over skin
Varicella (chickenpox)	Varicella-zoster virus	2-3 weeks	Fever, malaise, widespread eruptions of the skin and mucous membranes, appearing first on the face and trunk
Pertussis (whooping cough)	*Hemophilus pertussis* bacterium	7-14 days	Early, mild nighttime cough; late, severe spasmodic cough, followed by loud whoop and expulsion of a thick, clear mucus
Diphtheria	*Corynebacterium diphtheriae*	2-5 days	Fever, sore throat, headache, nausea; toxin may damage cardiovascular and nervous systems

[1] If acquired by a woman in the early months of pregnancy, rubella may be passed on to the fetus, who may suffer retardation, deafness, cardiac defects, and other serious complications.

Table 15-2 Recommended Immunization Schedule for Children

At this age:*		A child should receive:	At this age:*	A child should receive:
2 months		DTP (first) TOPV (first)	18 months	DTP (fourth) TOPV (third)
4 months		DTP (second) TOPV (second)	about 4 years	DTP (fifth) TOPV (fourth)
6 months		DTP (third)	14-16 years and every 10 years thereafter	Td
15 months or later	Measles Mumps Rubella	Singly or combined		

DTP: Diphtheria and tetanus toxoids, with pertussis (whooping cough) vaccine

TOPV: Trivalent oral polio vaccine

Td: Combined tetanus and diphtheria toxoids (adult type)

* Some immunizations may properly be given sooner than indicated here.

Sources: American Academy of Pediatrics; U.S. Public Health Service

Table 15-3 Major Rickettsial Infections

Disease	Pathogen	Mode of Transmission	Common Symptoms
Typhus	*Rickettsia prowazekii*	Body lice or fleas	Headache, high fever, prostration followed by skin rash. Can be fatal without treatment.
Rocky Mountain spotted fever	*Rickettsia rickettsii*	Ticks	Fever, chills, headaches, and rose-colored rash on palms and soles that spreads over body. Can be fatal without treatment.
Q Fever	*Coxiella burnetii*	Dust particles	Typical rickettsial symptoms but without rash. Nonfatal.

Rickettsias

Rickettsias Bacteria-like organisms that cannot live without a host.

Rickettsias—organisms once classified somewhere between viruses and bacteria—are now known to be bacteria that have lost the ability to live as free agents in the environment. Since they can survive only within a living host cell, almost all rickettsial pathogens must be transmitted from infected animals or humans via bloodsucking insects. The insect that carries the rickettsial pathogen remains unaffected, but once the pathogen is injected into the bloodstream of an uninfected animal or human, it causes widespread inflammation. The diseases attributed to rickettsias are few in number but serious in their effects and include typhus, Rocky Mountain spotted fever, and Q fever. Most rickettsial infections can be treated with antibiotics if diagnosed in time. Several of the major rickettsial infections are listed in Table 15-3.

Protozoa

Protozoa Single-celled organisms that may be parasitic or pathogenic.

Often classified as animals, **protozoa** are single-celled microbes much larger than bacteria but usually too small to be seen with the naked eye. Some of the diseases caused by protozoa are malaria, African sleeping sickness, and amebic dysentery. Most protozoal diseases are a concern in underdeveloped nations but not in countries such as the United States.

Fungi

Fungi Simple plants lacking chlorophyll.

Fungi are very simple plants lacking chlorophyll. Without chlorophyll, they must live as parasites or as saprophytes (organisms that obtain nourishment from decaying matter). Only a small minority of fungi are pathogenic. The few that do cause human diseases are types of yeasts and molds. True yeasts (as opposed to the commercial product known by that name) are unicellular microorganisms, typically round or ovular in form, that reproduce by budding. Multicellular molds, on the other hand, reproduce by forming special spores, either sexually (by fusing nuclear material from separate cells) or asexually (by differentiation of the cytoplasm). The disorders caused by yeasts and molds are known collectively as **mycoses.**

Mycoses Infection caused by yeasts and molds.

Major Fungal Infections

Athlete's Foot. One of the best-known fungus infections is **athlete's foot,** the common name for ringworm of the foot. The infectious agents are various kinds of fungi that reproduce by forming spores and that can also infect the scalp, the skin in general, and the toenails. Athlete's foot is marked by scaled or cracked skin between the toes or by blisters. Skin infections occasionally spread to other parts of the body. Victims pick up the pathogens from contact with the infected skin of other persons or with contaminated surfaces or clothing. Fungicides applied to the affected areas usually eradicate the infection.

Athlete's foot Ringworm of the foot.

Valley Fever. Unlike athlete's foot and vaginal yeast infection (a sexually transmitted disease), **valley fever,** or coccidioidomycosis, is an internal infection that can affect the whole body. The pathogen, *Coccidioides immitis,* lives in the soil and releases spores that cause infection in humans when breathed in. In most cases the infection is characterized by an acute attack of influenzalike symptoms (fever, chills, and so forth) that occur after an incubatory period of from 1–4 weeks. More rarely, the infection will spread progressively through the body. This progressive, systemic form of the disease is highly fatal.

Valley fever A major fungal disease characterized by influenza-like symptoms that can affect the whole body.

Parasitic Worms

Parasitic worms enter the human body through ingestion or through contact with infected animals. The largest of all pathogens, all the parasitic worms are visible to the naked eye, and some (tapeworms) can grow several feet in length. *Nematodes* (roundworms) have long, slender, unsegmented bodies. *Cestapodes* (tapeworms) are segmented in form and appear as flat, tapelike bands. *Trematodes,* the third category of parasitic worm, are elongated, leaf-shaped flukes that usually possess one or more suckers, with which they can attach themselves to the walls of blood vessels or organs. A type of nematode known as *Trichinella spiralis* causes trichinosis. Trematodes feeding on organs or blood vessels can cause such disorders as cirrhosis and hepatitis.

Parasitic worms Visible pathogens that enter body through ingestion or animal contact.

Table 15–4 **Parasitic Worm Infections**

Worms and Infection	Specific Agents	Incubation Period	Common Symptoms
Nematodes (roundworms) Trichinosis	*Trichinella spiralis*	9 days after ingestion	Fever, swelling of upper eyelids, sore muscles, sweating, chills, prostration
Enterobiasis	*Enterobius vermicularis*	3–6 weeks	Generally mild and nonspecific; if severe, anal itching, irritability
Ascariasis	*Ascaris lumbricoides*	2 months after ingestion	Variable; if infection is pulmonary, coughing & fever; sometimes, abdominal pain, vomiting, and bowel obstruction
Cestapodes (tapeworms) Tapeworm disease	*Taenia saginata* (in beef) and *Taenia solium* (in pork)	8–14 weeks	Insomnia, weight loss, abdominal pain, digestive problems; if larval *T. solium* is ingested, infection may become systemic and chronic
Trematodes (flukes) Clonorchiasis	*Clonorchis sinensis*	Unknown	Early: loss of appetite, diarrhea; late: cirrhosis, hepatitis

Major Parasitic Worm Infections

Table 15–4 lists the major parasitic worm pathogens and the infections associated with them. Almost all of these infections begin with ingestion of adult or larval worms, often in cyst form, with contaminated or improperly cooked meat or fish. Less often, the worm travels the anal-oral route via the hands of an infected individual. After being incubated for a variable length of time in the intestinal tract, the pathogens often migrate to other parts of the body.

Parasitic worm infections are rarely fatal. The primary control measure is hygienic processing and proper cooking of food. Most victims can be treated successfully with drugs.

Sexually Transmitted Diseases

Sexually transmitted disease Infections transmitted principally by sexual contact.

The term **sexually transmitted diseases (STDs)** refers to all infections transmitted principally by sexual contact. They are also known as venereal diseases. Some infections of this kind, such as herpes, are virus-caused but most are produced by bacteria.

The people who are keeping the gonorrhea epidemic going are people who often don't know they have it.

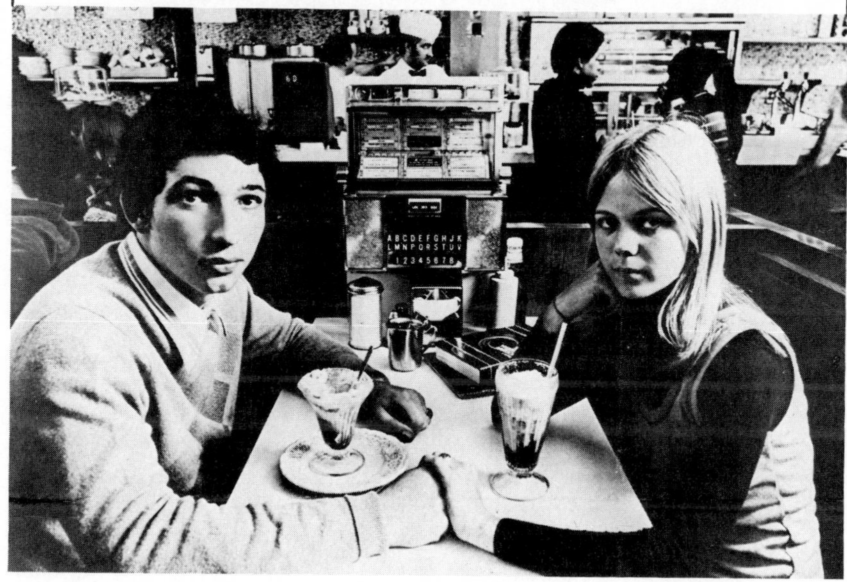

Sexually transmitted diseases infect more people than any other disease category except the common cold. It is important for everyone to become knowledgeable about the various sexually transmitted diseases and their symptoms. (Photo courtesy of Metropolitan Life Insurance Company)

Bacterial

Gonorrhea and syphilis are two of the most serious STDs and are both caused by bacteria.

Gonorrhea

Gonorrhea is caused by the *gonococcus bacteria,* which infect the mucous membranes of the urogenital tract. In males, a pus-filled discharge from the penis within 2–9 days after infection is characteristic of the disease. Painful urination is also a frequently early symptom. Although female victims often receive no warming signals they may experience painful urination and vaginal discharge. Inflammation of the genitalia and the urethra is a common symptom, and if the disease is not treated, the inflammation may spread throughout the urogenital system. It may eventually cause arthritis and also sterility in both men and women.

Gonorrhea Venereal disease that infects membrane of the urogenital tract.

Gonorrhea occurs worldwide in all age groups and both sexes. Perhaps because of relaxed sexual mores, incidence of the disease has reached near-epidemic proportions among adolescents and young adults in the United States. What makes outbreaks of gonorrhea especially difficult to control, despite the fact that antibiotic drugs are effective against most strains, is the fact that many female victims do not have observable symptoms. These unknowing victims can remain carriers of the infection for months or even years. Also, victims who promptly seek treatment sometimes are reluctant to identify their sexual partners.

Syphilis

Syphilis A common and serious venereal disease that if left untreated can result in death.

Undoubtedly the most serious sexually transmitted disease is **syphilis,** which in its late stages can result in blindness, heart failure, brain damage, and even death. The pathogenic agent is a spiral-shaped bacterium, *Treponema pallidum,* that is transmitted during sexual intercourse by exuded matter from skin or membrane infections or by fluids and secretions. Mother-to-fetus transmission often occurs; the result may be deformities in the bones, skin, eyes, and other parts of the infant's body. More rarely, the pathogen may enter a host via a transfusion of infected blood.

If left untreated, syphilis develops in three stages over the course of several years. In the first stage, beginning about 3 weeks after infection, a small, firm sore appears at the infection site. Perhaps 4–6 weeks later, the initial sore begins to disappear, and there are secondary eruptions of the skin and mucous membranes. These secondary symptoms subside after several weeks or months, and the disease apparently vanishes. Actually, however, it has passed into a latent phase that may last for a period as short as a few weeks or as long as 20 years. When the disease reemerges in its third and final stage, the victim may suffer chronic skin sores, tumors, serious heart damage, and progressive deterioration of the central nervous system. The longer the latency, the more severe the third-stage symptoms, which often directly or indirectly contribute to death.

There is no natural immunity to syphilis, and acquired immunity is tenuous at best. Untreated victims can communicate the infection to sexual partners for a period of up to four years. Penicillin usually can cure the disease in its first and second stages and end communicability within 24 hours of administration. As with gonorrhea, however, the relaxation of sexual mores and the problem of underreporting have frustrated attempts to control syphilis, and its incidence has risen noticeably in recent years. The emergence of drug-resistant strains of the disease has occurred in recent years.

Chlamydia

Chlamydia A recently recognized venereal disease that is similar to gonorrhea but twice as prevalent.

A sexually transmitted disease that has reached nearly epidemic proportions in the United States, affecting 3–10 million Americans, is **chlamydia.** *Chlamydia trachomatis* is the major cause of *nongonococcal urethritis (NGU),* a disease similar to gonorrhea but not caused by gonococcal bacteria. Not too long ago, chlamydia (or NGU, as it was then called) was considered a minor disease affecting a small number of men; but now it is thought to occur at least twice as frequently as gonorrhea and to affect women as well. In men, the symptoms are usually similar to a mild case of gonorrhea. Women often do not have immediate symptoms but the infection can lead to pelvic inflammatory disease, damaging the reproductive organs and causing sterility. Recently a faster, more accurate, and less costly test for chlamydia has been devised, and it is hoped that the test will be used routinely to screen out cases of the disease. Chlamydia is generally treated with the antibiotics erethromycin or tetracycline; penicillin is not effective.

Other STDs

Several other forms of sexually transmitted diseases are less common in the United States, including *chancroid, lymphogranuloma venereum,* and *granuloma inguinale.*

The prevalence of the major sexually transmitted diseases is a cause of concern for health authorities. They emphasize a few simple rules to keep these diseases under better control (see the box entitled "How to Prevent Spread of Sexually Transmitted Diseases").

Viral

Genital Herpes

The most common sexually transmitted disease is a herpes type II infection called **genital herpes:** over 20,000,000 people have genital herpes. The initial symptoms of genital herpes generally appear two to ten days after sexual contact. The symptoms include an itching and burning sensation during urination. After the initial symptoms and within a week, women usually develop small, painful blisters in the vagina, cervic, and urethra. Men usually develop similar painful sores on the shaft of the penis. Both men and women may exhibit an elevation of temperature and swollen lymph glands.

Genital herpes The most common sexually transmitted disease which causes painful, small sores.

The symptoms of genital herpes are usually most severe during the first infection. The acute illness may last from 3 to 6 weeks. Afterward, the infection appears to subside, but the virus remains in the body in what is termed a dormant phase. The individual can break out into a new infection at any time.

Some people never get recurrences. Some do occasionally; some, frequently. Many people have a recurrence 3 to 4 months after the first infection and then again every 2 months or so. Before the painful blisters come back, there may be early warning symptoms such as burning, itching, and tingling at the same place the earlier sores occurred.

Medical researchers do not know exactly what makes the virus recur, but many factors are thought to be "triggering" mechanisms. These factors include emotional stress, lack of sleep, poor diet, too much sun or wind, or even friction from wearing tight clothing. In general, recurrences tend to be less severe than the initial infection.

There is no cure for genital herpes or any herpes infection. Some relief can be obtained from a medication called acyclovir, prescribed by a physician. Formerly available only in ointment form, acyclovir is now on the market in oral form. This medication does not "cure" the disease but it reduces the severity of the symptoms.

Acquired Immune Deficiency Syndrome (AIDS)

AIDS Acquired Immune Deficiency Syndrome, characterized by body's inability to fight disease.

AIDS is a disease which has recently come into public view. Since the disease affects primarily male homosexuals (71 percent of cases), it has been coined the "gay plague."

AIDS was first diagnosed in 1979. The first victims were male homosexuals, and medical professionals felt that the disease was confined only to that population. Since 1979, AIDS cases have also appeared among heterosexuals who use drugs intravenously, Haitian immigrants, hemophiliacs, and a small miscellaneous group. Recent cases have suggested that the disease might even be transmitted during pregnancy, routine blood transfusions, and heterosexual contact with AIDS victims.

A victim of AIDS has a suppressed immune system, unattributable to any known cause. Because of the suppressed immune system the body loses its ability to fight off disease. As a result the victim becomes susceptible to a wide variety of rare diseases including:

- *Pneumocystis carinii pneumonia:* a parasitic pneumonia seen in 51 percent of AIDS victims. This form of pneumonia was previously associated with transplant patients and patients with blood disorders such as leukemia.
- *Kaposi's sarcoma:* a malignant angiosarcoma that causes distinctive penny-sized purplish lesions to appear on the skin, mucous membranes, and lymph nodes. This form of cancer is rare and was previously confined to older men of Italian and Jewish ancestry. Kaposi's sarcoma is seen in 30 percent of AIDS victims.
- *cryptosporidiosis:* a parasitic infection that causes chronic, diffuse, and watery diarrhea.
- *toxoplasmosis:* a parasitic infection that causes encephalitis.

Generally these diseases are not fatal to the patient with a normal immune-response system; however, these infections have proven fatal to AIDS victims.

AIDS has an extremely high fatality rate (75 percent for those cases

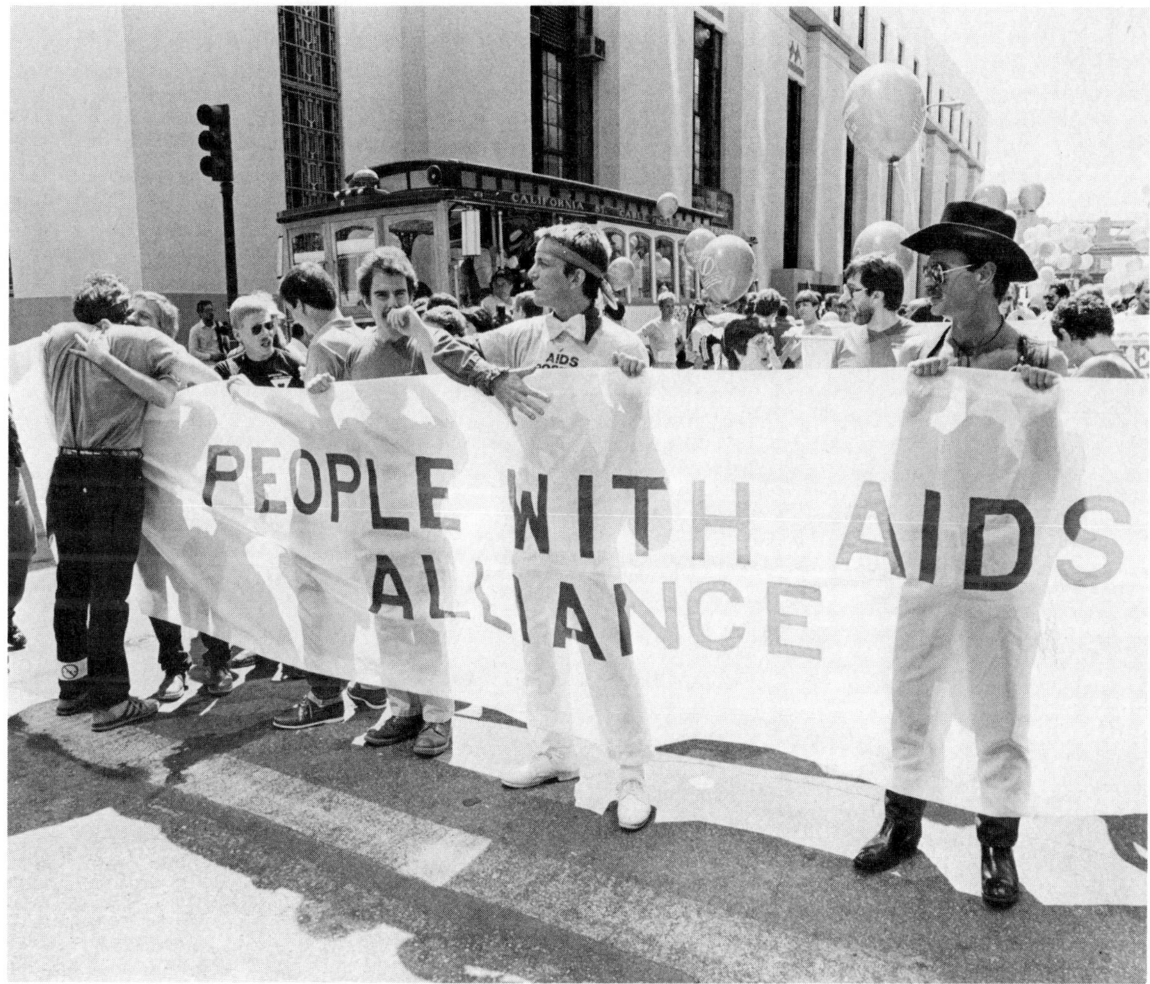

AIDS, by breaking down the body's immune system, causes its victims to become highly susceptible to a range of other potentially fatal diseases. (Photo © Robert V. Eckert, Jr./ EKM–Neptune)

diagnosed before June 1981). Some researchers and epidemiologists feel that unless a cure is found, anyone diagnosed with AIDS will eventually succumb to one of the related disorders common to patients with suppressed immune response systems.

The cause of AIDS remains unknown. Researchers have found evidence of the human T-cell leukemia lymphoma virus in 25 percent of AIDS patients. Most researchers suspect that AIDS results from an infectious agent, probably a new virus.

No laboratory test can detect whether or not a person has AIDS. In most cases there is an inverse ratio of helper T-cells, which activate the immune system, to suppressor T-cells, which prevent the immune system from overreacting to disease. A healthy person has twice as many helper T-cells as suppressor T-cells.

YOUR HEALTH TODAY

How to Prevent Spread of Sexually Transmitted Diseases

Except for common cold and flu infections, sexually transmitted diseases (STDs) are the most common infectious diseases in the United States today. Here are a few measures widely recommended by health authorities for persons who are sexually active:

- Familiarize yourself with the symptoms of each major type of STD and be alert for their appearance.
- Avoid any form of sexual activity with a person you know to be infected. This includes such activities as kissing and oral-genital sex, both of which can be means of spreading STDs.
- Consider using, or insisting on the use of, a condom during intercourse. When used properly, the condom can help to prevent the transmission of STDs; it must, however, be unbroken and be in place at any time the penis is in contact with the female body.
- If you know or fear that you have been infected, seek medical help promptly. Don't wait for serious symptoms to appear; prompt treatment is a major factor in controlling STDs, and delay can lead to serious complications.
- If you know or suspect that you have an STD, avoid all sexual activity until the condition is diagnosed and successfully treated.

One of the most puzzling questions regarding AIDS is, Why are the majority of AIDS victims male homosexuals? Researchers feel that possibly an infectious agent is in the semen of the infected person and is transmitted during homosexual activity through breaks in the anal mucosa during anal sex. The immuno-suppressive effect of semen is a contributing factor and helps to validate this popular theory.

It is interesting to note that the initial symptoms of AIDS make the syndrome difficult to diagnose; the initial symptoms often mimic those of less serious illness. Some of these symptoms include persistent fatigue, fever, diarrhea, night sweats, and swollen lymph nodes in the neck, armpits, and groin as well as a string of recurring viral infections such as colds, flu, and herpes simplex.

The incubation period for AIDS can vary from a few months to a few years. The period of communicability has not been established; thus, the person who feels healthy could be infecting many other people.

During the past six years AIDS has struck over 12,000 Americans. Of the total number of patients, approximately 50 percent have died already. That makes AIDS more lethal in terms of mortality rate than smallpox or toxic shock syndrome. Most of the surviving AIDS patients are expected to die from one of the associated disorders described earlier.

AIDS has become the number one public health problem in the United States. Given the extremely high fatality rate it is easy to see why public health professionals are anxiously trying to find a cure.

Protozoal

Trichomoniasis

Trichomoniasis is a protozoal infection of the lower genitourinary tract. Trichomoniasis affects about 15 percent of sexually active females and 10 percent of sexually active males. The mode of transmission of the protozoa *(Trichomonas vaginalis)* is through sexual contact. The organism grows best when the vaginal mucosa is more alkaline. Thus, the use of oral contraceptives is considered a predisposing factor to this infection.

Trichomoniasis Infection of the lower genitourinary tract.

The signs and symptoms of trichmoniasis are primarily confined to the female, since the male is usually asymptomatic. The signs and symptoms in the female include: gray or green-yellow discharge from the vagina and severe itching plus redness and swelling in the vaginal area. These symptoms may persist for a week to several months. If the symptoms are not treated, they may subside even though the infection actually persists.

The treatment for trichomoniasis is through use of a drug called Metronidazole. This drug is administered in small doses for 7 days or in a single large dose.

Fungal

Vaginal Yeast Infection

Another fungus, the yeast known as *Candida,* is responsible for **vaginal yeast infection,** or candidiasis. *Candida* used to be considered among the organisms normally found on the body, but many experts now see it as a purely pathogenic invader transmitted during sexual intercourse. The yeast infects the mucous membranes of the vagina, causing inflammation and watery discharges. Drugs taken in tablet or suppository form generally alleviate the symptoms, although recurrences are common unless the male partner is also treated.

Vaginal yeast infection A pathogenic fungus that causes watery discharges in women.

In general, STDs can be easily prevented—or at least the spread minimized—if people will take certain key actions. For a list of important STD prevention points, see the box entitled "How to Prevent Spread of Sexually Transmitted Diseases."

Problems in Prevention and Control

The prevention and control of many communicable diseases has been one of the great medical successes of the twentieth century. However, many are concerned that the successes of the past will lead to complacency, a feeling that the war against communicable diseases has been won and final victory achieved. They are concerned that this complacency will lead to deaths and disabling diseases that could have been prevented. Despite the successes, many problems remain.

The conditions of modern life often favor the spread of communicable diseases. The population explosion and the increasing numbers of people concentrated in cities have led to greater danger. More people living closer together means easier transmission of disease. The density of population creates problems with the disposal of human wastes and refuse. Untreated sewage is an ideal reservoir for many pathogens, and refuse serves as a breeding ground for rats and flies, two of the most important vectors spreading communicable diseases. Although these problems are more acute in the less-developed areas of the world, they remain a potential problem in developed areas and require continued attention.

With a growing number of people traveling more frequently, diseases can be spread much more rapidly than at any time in the past. Pathogens can be carried to new areas, where people have not been exposed previously and therefore have not acquired immunity. Many types of influenza have been spread in this way.

There is also concern about declining levels of acquired immunity. With the improvements in public health, many people have not been exposed to any forms of the pathogens during their early years and are therefore particularly susceptible when exposed, with a resultant epidemic outburst.

Another problem is that many pathogens have acquired a resistance to antibiotics. Bacteria multiply at incredible rates, and occasionally mutations occur that produce an organism more resistant to an antibiotic. This has occurred with strains of bacteria that cause meningitis, gonorrhea, and pneumonia, among others. The widespread use of antibiotics—some experts have maintained that it is overuse—seems certain to produce more of these strains. So far a good deal of success has been achieved by developing new forms of antibiotics, so that when a new strain becomes resistant to one type of antibiotic, another treatment can be used. However, many scientists are concerned that eventually we will run out of these back-up methods.

Finally, there is what is probably the major problem—a lack of concern among the public. Too often there is an overconfidence that leads people to neglect to take the necessary precautions. For example, children receive—on the whole—more careful medical attention than other groups, but declining immunization rates have led to legislation requiring immunization for school attendance. Several immunization procedures require booster shots after childhood—diphtheria, for example—and many people fail to receive them. Too often there is the mistaken belief that the diseases can be easily cured and that the preventive measures are therefore not worth the bother. Continued progress in the control and prevention of communicable diseases will depend on increased public awareness of the dangers that indifference can cause.

Summary

Communicable diseases are diseases that can be transmitted from person to person, either directly or indirectly. The disease-causing organisms are called pathogens.

The six basic types of pathogens are bacteria, viruses, rickettsias, protozoa, fungi, and parasitic worms. Bacteria are single-celled organisms that occur in three basic forms: cocci, bacilli, and spirilla. Only about 100 species are pathogenic to humans, but these are the greatest single cause of human infection. Viruses are submicroscopic particles that must invade a living host cell to grow and multiply. Rickettsias are bacteria that have lost the ability to live as free agents. They are transmitted by bloodsucking insects. Fungi are very simple plants lacking chlorophyll. The diseases they cause are called mycoses. Protozoa are single-celled organisms much larger than bacteria but usually too small to be seen with the naked eye. The largest pathogens are the parasitic worms, which are divided into the nematodes (roundworms), cestapodes (tapeworms), and trematodes (flukes).

Infection is the invasion of body tissue by pathogens that produce damage either directly or by the toxins they produce. The infectious disease process includes the transmission of the pathogen and invasion of the host organism, the life cycle of the pathogen in the host's body, and the pathogen's exit from the body. The disease passes through four stages: incubation, the prodromal stage, the acute stage, and convalescence.

The body has several types of defense against infection: epithelial defenses, inflammation, the immune system, and interferon. These defenses help both to prevent an infection and to limit the bad effects of an infection.

Outbreaks of communicable diseases can be sporadic, endemic, or epidemic. Public health measures, vaccination, and drug therapy are all important in prevention and control.

Bacterial diseases include staphylococcal and streptococcal infections. In some cases, a strep throat can lead to scarlet fever and rheumatic fever. Tuberculosis, legionnaires' disease, and toxic shock syndrome are also caused by bacteria.

Viruses are responsible for a large number of diseases, of which the common cold and influenza are the most widespread. Other viral diseases are infectious mononucleosis, viral hepatitis, herpes simplex, and various childhood diseases.

Rickettsial diseases are less well known but include several dangerous types: typhus, Rocky Mountain spotted fever, and Q fever. The major protozoal infections are malaria, African sleeping sickness, and amebic dysentery. Examples of fungal diseases are athlete's foot and valley fever. Parasitic worm diseases include trichinosis, roundworms, tapeworms, and flukes.

STDs can be caused by a variety of pathogens. One of the most serious STDs and a disease which could be the major public health problem of the century is AIDS.

Although great progress has been made in the prevention and control of communicable diseases, increased attention will be needed if further progress is to be made.

Review and Discussion

1. List the six basic types of pathogens and mention a major disease caused by each.
2. What are the major body defenses against infection?
3. Distinguish between the various types of immunity.
4. What is interferon and how is it thought to help the individual overcome infection?
5. Describe the major medical defenses against infection.
6. List and describe the most important public health measures used in disease control.
7. Distinguish between the major STDs.
8. Distinguish between staphylococcal and streptococcal infections.
9. Discuss what precautions can be taken to reduce the chances of contracting or spreading a sexually transmitted disease.
10. List the major childhood diseases and explain their symptoms.
11. Describe some of the major rickettsial diseases.
12. What are some of the factors causing concern about future progress in the prevention and control of communicable diseases?
13. Discuss why AIDS could potentially be the worst public health problem of the century.

Further Reading

Benenson, Abram S., ed. *Control of Communicable Diseases in Man.* 14th ed. Washington, D.C.: The American Public Health Association, 1985.
An official report of the American Public Health Association, containing detailed descriptions of all major communicable diseases. (Paperback.)

Corsaro, Maria, and Carole Korzeniowsky. *STD.* New York: St. Martin's Press, 1980.
A guide to the prevention and treatment of the sexually transmitted diseases.

Dowling, Harry F. *Fighting Infection.* Cambridge, Mass.: Harvard University Press, 1977.
A history of medical advances in the prevention and control of communicable diseases, written for the layman.

Purtilo, David T. *A Survey of Human Diseases.* Reading, Mass.: Addison-Wesley Publishing Company, Inc., 1978.
A good overview of both communicable and chronic diseases.

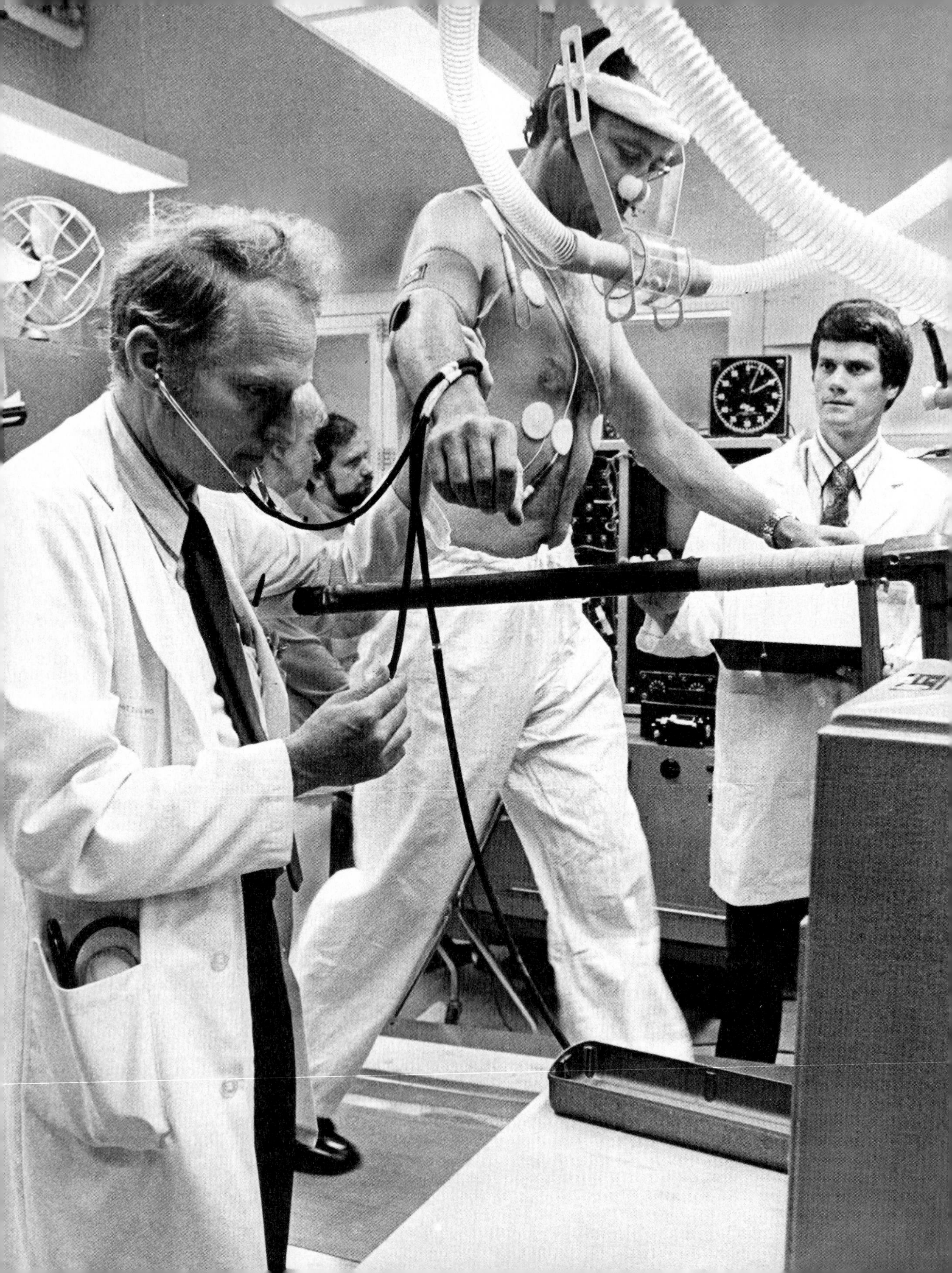

Chapter 16
Cardiovascular Diseases

KEY POINTS

- □ Cardiovascular diseases are the leading cause of death in the United States today.
- □ The principal risk factors associated with cardiovascular disease are cigarette smoking, a high intake of cholesterol, insufficient exercise, hypertension, obesity, and a family history of cardiovascular disorders.
- □ The cardiovascular system consists of the heart and a network of blood vessels.
- □ Arteriosclerosis, commonly called ''hardening of the arteries,'' is the single most significant factor in most cases of cardiovascular disease.
- □ Hypertension can cause severe and widespread damage to the cardiovascular system.
- □ A heart attack, or myocardial infarction, is the death from oxygen deprivation of a portion of the heart muscle.
- □ Other cardiovascular diseases include cerebrovascular accidents (or strokes), rheumatic heart disease, and congenital heart defects.
- □ Changes in life-style can decrease the risk of cardiovascular disease.

TODAY, the terms *heart attack, stroke, hardening of the arteries,* and *high blood pressure* are unpleasantly familiar to most Americans. Somewhat fewer people realize that these conditions are all manifestations of cardiovascular disease—disorders of the heart and the circulatory system. Even fewer are aware that since approximately 1940 more Americans have died from cardiovascular diseases than from all other causes combined. But the very familiarity of these terms represents a major victory for the medical community's vigorous campaign to awaken Americans to the dangers posed by cardiovascular diseases.

The origins of this campaign lay, paradoxically, in modern medicine's single greatest triumph: the conquest of acute communicable diseases. As recently as the 1920s, the country's top-ranking causes of death was influenza and pneumonia, with tuberculosis as the second-ranking cause. Beginning in the 1930s, however, the discovery of antibiotics and new vaccines, the implementation of effective public health control measures, and the establishment of proper nutritional standards helped bring about a dramatic decline in deaths from these and other communicable diseases. During the same period, the number of fatalities associated with cardiovascular diseases rose rapidly. By 1940 cardiovascular diseases were the leading cause of death in the United States; they remain first today, while major infectious diseases rank far behind.

Cardiovascular diseases are chronic, degenerative disorders that commonly take years, or even decades, to develop. It was inevitable, then, that as people lived longer, because of better nutrition and advances in the control of communicable diseases, more of them would suffer from heart and circulatory problems. But lengthened life span alone could not account for the increase in cardiovascular-related fatalities. A more subtle but equally important factor emerged during

Figure 16–1. Leading Causes of Death in the United States, 1981 Estimate.
(Source: National Center for Health Statistics, U.S. Public Health Service, DHHS)

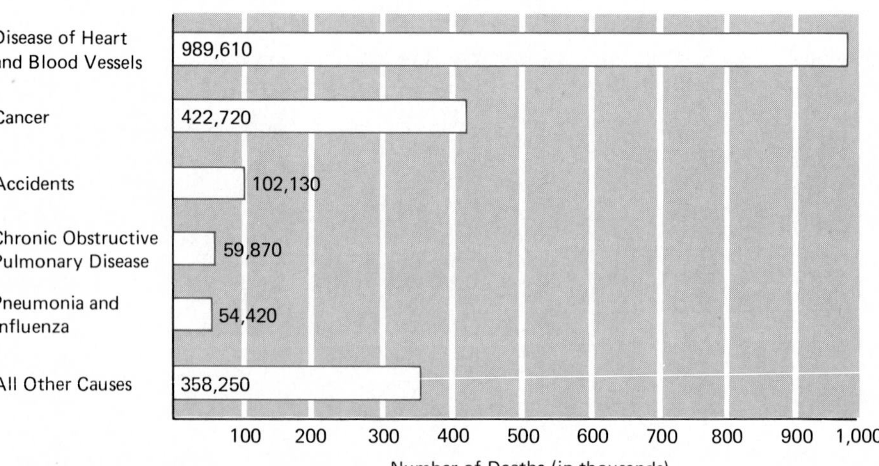

Perform a death-defying act.
Eat less saturated fat.
The American Heart Association

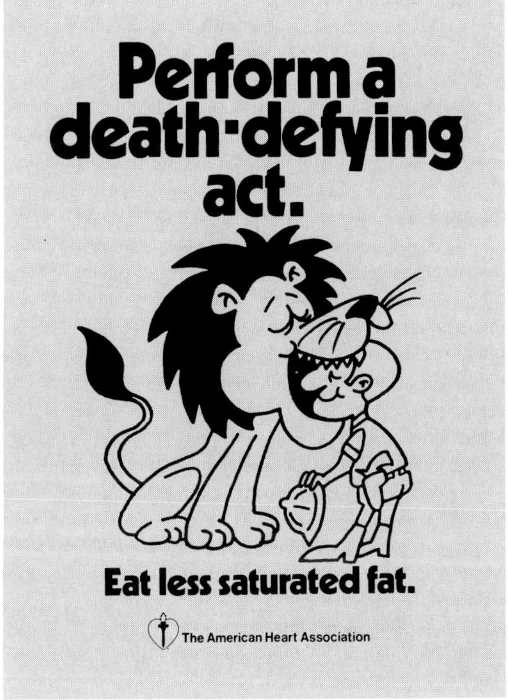

There is evidence that a diet rich in saturated fats (those from animal sources) can lead to cardiovascular disease. (Photo courtesy of American Heart Association)

the early 1950s, when autopsies were performed on the bodies of young soldiers killed in the Korean War. The autopsies revealed that a high percentage of these apparently healthy young men had discernible signs of cardiovascular disease. The implications were inescapable: obviously, degeneration of the cardiovascular system began much earlier than had been thought, and the problem was far more widespread than had been supposed.

Increasingly, doctors and researchers came to realize that the life-style, as well as the life span, of the average American contributed to the development of cardiovascular disease. In a landmark 1959 brochure entitled *A Statement on Arteriosclerosis, Main Cause of "Heart Attacks" and "Strokes,"* eight leading cardiologists and researchers identified the principal risk factors associated with this potent killer as cigarette smoking, a high intake of cholesterol, insufficient exercise, hypertension (persistently high blood pressure), obesity, and a family history of cardiovascular disorders. Except for the last named, all these factors could be related to the modern American life-style. In comparison with their forebears, Americans in the mid-twentieth century typically weighed more and got less exercise, smoked more and ate more saturated fats (a leading source of cholesterol), and were subject to more stress of all kinds. The result, according to the authors, was a sharp rise in cardiovascular disease.

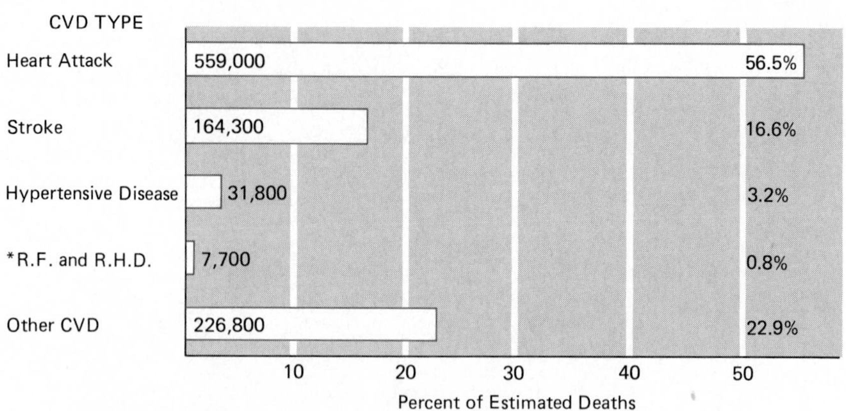

Figure 16–2. Estimated Deaths Due to Cardiovascular Diseases by Major Type of Disorder in the United States, 1981 Estimate. (Source: National Center for Health Statistics, U.S. Public Health Service, DHHS)

In subsequent years, medical and governmental bodies issued a series of pronouncements and warnings about the life-style risk factors associated with heart attacks and strokes. Having largely won the fight against infectious diseases, the medical community, in league with the federal government, now began to concentrate on the hidden side effects of the "good life" that had been made possible by widespread prosperity and medical advances. Results were not long in coming. By the early 1970s, deaths from cardiovascular diseases were declining at an appreciable rate (see Figure 16–2). There were many factors involved in this trend: a significant drop in the number of adult male smokers, a nationwide interest in physical fitness, a measurable decrease in the consumption of saturated fats, and a determined and successful campaign to detect and treat hypertension.

Despite the ongoing decrease in cardiovascular-disease fatalities, there is still a long way to go before this modern-day epidemic is brought under control. Cardiovascular problems are still by far the leading cause of death in the United States, as well as in Canada and northern Europe, and many thousands die prematurely from these problems.

The Cardiovascular System

Cardiovascular system The heart and the network of blood vessels leading to and from it.

The **cardiovascular system** consists of the heart and the intricate network of blood vessels leading to and from it. Blood circulates continuously through this network, delivering oxygen and other vital substances to and carrying waste products from every cell in the body. Blood flow is maintained by the pumping action of the heart.

The Circulatory System

The circulatory system formed by the blood vessels has two major components: the **pulmonary circulation,** which carries blood between the heart and the lungs; and the **systemic circulation,** which links the heart with the rest of the body. In the systemic circulation, blood moves from the heart through (sequentially and in order of decreasing size) the aorta, the arteries, the arterioles, and the capillaries. At the capillaries, the blood surrenders its oxygen and picks up waste material—principally carbon dioxide. Once the transfer is effected, the capillaries become venioles, which eventually combine into veins. Veins from the lower body converge into the inferior vena cava, those from the upper body form the superior vena cava, and the two venae cavae empty into the heart. Deoxygenated blood then enters the pulmonary circulation, moving from heart to lungs by way of the pulmonary arteries, cycling through the lungs to deposit waste and pick up oxygen, and returning to the heart via the pulmonary veins.

Pulmonary circulation Circulation of blood between the heart and lungs.

Systemic circulation Circulation of blood between the heart and the body (excluding lungs).

The Heart

The heart is a fist-sized, cone-shaped muscle located between the lungs, just to the left of the body's midline. Its exterior wall consists of a thick layer of muscle (the myocardium) sheathed by thin interior

Figure 16-3. The Heart (Left Front View).

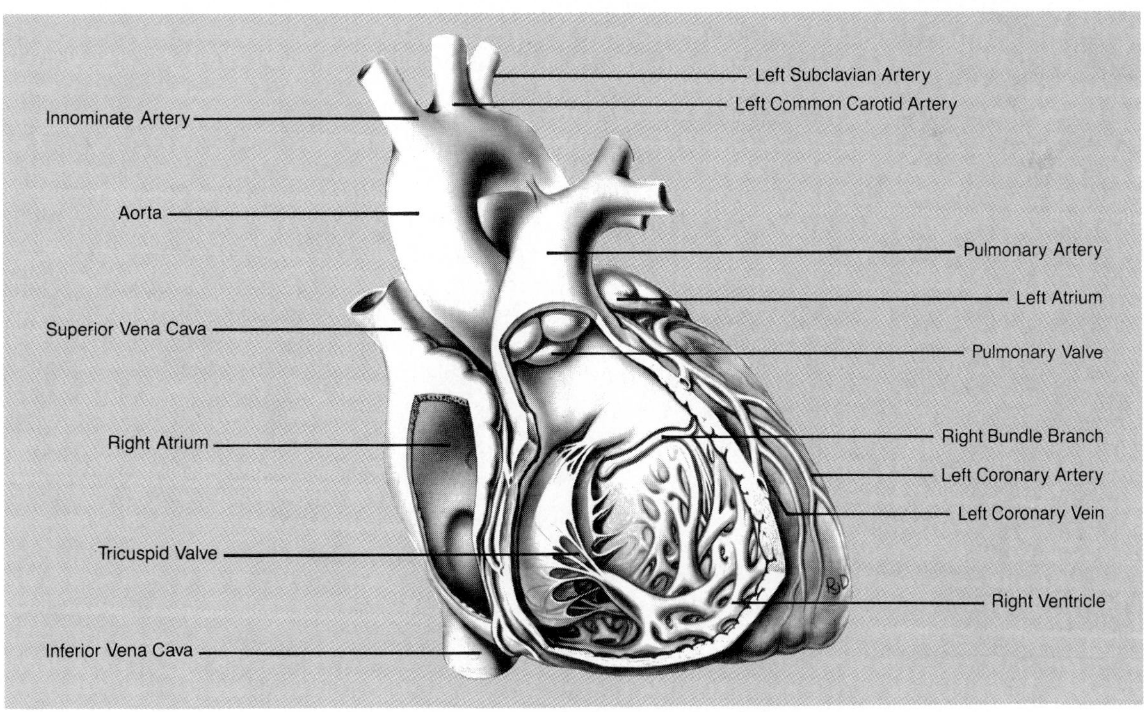

and exterior membranes (the endocardium and the epicardium, respectively). An interior wall of muscle (the septum) divides the heart vertically into right and left sides, each of which contains an upper chamber *(atrium)* and a lower chamber *(ventricle)*.

This four-part structure enables the heart to pump two incompatible flows of blood simultaneously and continuously. On the one hand, deoxygenated blood flows from the venae cavae into the right atrium, then through the tricuspid valve into the right ventricle, and finally through the pulmonary valve into the pulmonary artery. At the same time, oxygenated blood flows from the pulmonary veins into the left atrium, then through the mitral valve into the left ventricle, and finally through the aortic valve into the aorta. Because of the double sets of valves, which open and close in sequence, blood cannot back up when the heart contracts.

Systole The first phase of the heartbeat in which the heart pumps blood.

Diastole The second phase of the heartbeat in which the heart fills with blood.

Both sides of the heart contract simultaneously, generating a two-phase heartbeat. During the first phase, or **systole,** the ventricles contract, the mitral and tricuspid valves close (producing the characteristic *lub* sound heard through a stethoscope), the pulmonary and aortic valves open, and blood is ejected from the ventricles. In the longer second phase, or **diastole,** the ventricles relax and the atria contract, the lower set of valves closes (producing the *dub* sound) and the upper set opens, and blood pours into the ventricles from the atria.

Principal Cardiovascular Diseases

Arteriosclerosis and Atherosclerosis

Arteriosclerosis Hardening of the arteries.

Most forms of acquired cardiovascular disease originate with impairment of the blood flow through the blood vessels, a condition known generally as **arteriosclerosis** (commonly called "hardening of the arteries"). The root causes of arteriosclerosis are difficult to identify. Once thought to be an inevitable by-product of the aging process, it is now known to begin much earlier in life—even in childhood or adolescence. As arteriosclerosis progresses, the walls of the affected blood vessels thicken, harden, and become increasingly inelastic.

Atherosclerosis Accumulation of fatty deposits on the arterial walls.

Commonly, this process is exacerbated by the buildup of deposits of cholesterol and other fatty substances in the inner layers of the arterial walls. When such a deposit, or atheroma, hardens and expands, it can severely restrict the flow of blood. **Atherosclerosis,** the scientific name for this condition, is the most common form of arteriosclerosis; it is also regarded as the single most significant factor in most cases of cardiovascular disease.

High levels of cholesterol in the blood appear to play a major role in the development of atherosclerosis. In this condition, the arteries lose their resilience and become clogged by fatty deposits. A low-cholesterol diet and physical exercise, both of which apparently also help to control and possibly aid in reversing the condition, are recommended as preventive measures. Exercise apparently increases the level of **HDL (high-density lipoprotein),** one of the substances in the blood that carries cholesterol and other fat molecules. In some way, possibly by picking up cholesterol from arterial walls and carrying it away, HDL inhibits the accumulation of cholesterol in the arteries, so that the risk of coronary artery disease decreases. Depending on the doctor and on the patient's condition, various treatments are recommended for treating atherosclerosis when it has developed.

HDL (High density lipoproteins) Substances in the blood that carry various fat molecules.

Hypertension

Approximately one in ten Americans suffers from hypertension, the "silent killer." Hypertension is silent because it presents no obvious symptoms; it is a killer because it plays a direct role in thousands of deaths each year.

Hypertension is persistent elevation in blood pressure, the force exerted by the bloodstream on the walls of the arteries. In times of exertion or stress, when the body needs more oxygen, the blood pressure in normal individuals will rise as the heart pumps faster. Such temporary fluctuations in pressure can easily be accommodated by a healthy cardiovascular system. What arterial walls cannot tolerate indefinitely is a sustained onslaught of abnormally high pressure.

Hypertension Persistent elevation in blood pressure.

Measuring Blood Pressure

The only way to diagnose hypertension is through blood pressure readings, which are expressed as a composite of the systolic pressure and the diastolic pressure. During the heart's systole (contraction

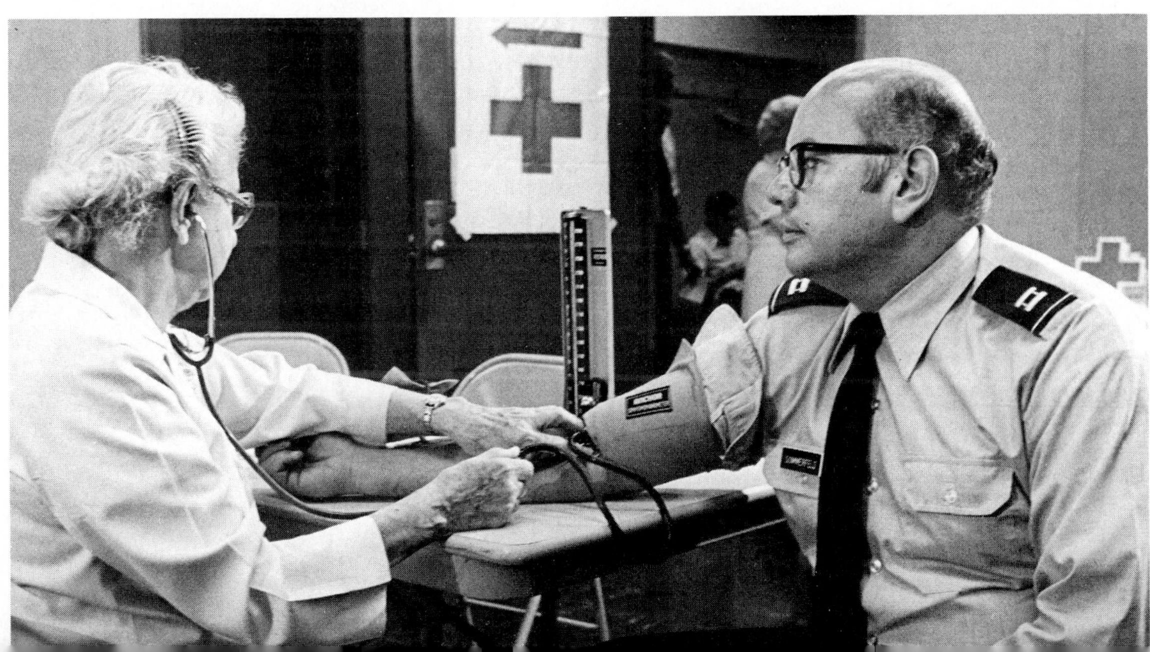

Hypertension is one of the principal risk factors in cardiovascular disease, and blood pressure screenings (often given free by health organizations) are among the most important preventive measures. (Photo courtesy of American Red Cross)

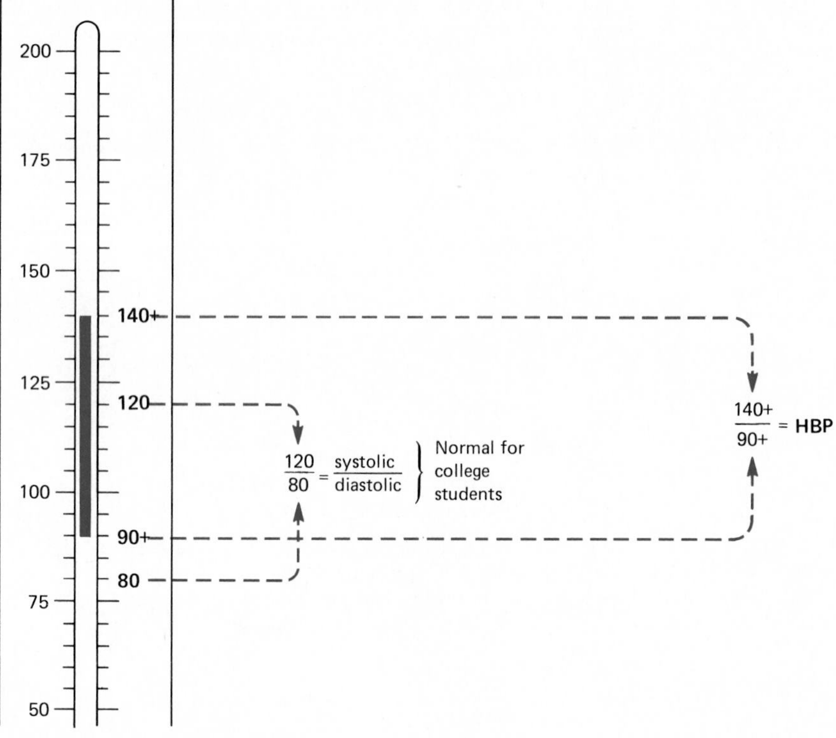

Figure 16–4. Blood Pressure Readings Depicting Normal Blood Pressure and High Blood Pressure for Adults. (Source: Walter D. Sorochan, *Promoting Your Health* [New York: John Wiley & Sons, Inc. 1981], 312)

phase), blood pressure is highest; during its diastole (relaxation phase), pressure on the arterial walls eases. The two pressures are measured in millimeters of mercury recorded on a *sphygmomanometer* (from the Greek words for "pulse" and "measure"), an inflatable cuff connected by a hose to a column of mercury. When the cuff is wrapped around a patient's left arm and inflated, the air pressure cuts off the flow of blood through the artery and pushes the mercury column to its highest point. As the cuff is deflated, the pressure drops until the blood flow resumes, and a characteristic sound can be heard through a stethoscope held over the artery. The height of the mercury column at this point represents the systolic pressure. A second reading of the mercury column, taken when the sound disappears, provides the diastolic pressure. The composite reading is given as, for example, 110/70—meaning 110 mm systolic pressure over 70 mm diastolic pressure.

Normal blood pressures range from about 120/80 for young adults to about 140/90 for persons over age 50. At any age, consistent readings higher than 140/90 can be said to signify hypertension. In some cases, hypertension arises from identifiable physiological causes: most commonly, from kidney diseases that lead to the overproduction of renin, an enzyme associated with constriction of the arteries.

Table 16-1 Guide to Interpretation of Diastolic Blood Pressure

140	
135	
130	**Severe Hypertension**
125	Organ damage is accelerated. Drugs can reverse some effects and may
120	prevent further damage.
115	
110	**Moderate Hypertension**
105	At 105 or above, drug treatment should begin.
100	**Mild Hypertension**
95	Drug treatment may begin. Have pressure checked at least three times
90	yearly.
85	
80	**Normal Blood Pressure**
75	Keep a record of them.
70	
65	

Source: With permission from *Consumer's Report,* October 1974, p. 735. Copyright © 1974 by Consumer's Union of the United States, Inc., Mount Vernon, N.Y.

Note: When the heart is relaxed, between beats, the pressure in the arteries is known as the diastolic blood pressure. In the numerical fraction that expresses blood pressure—e.g., 120/80—the diastolic pressure is the bottom figure.

Table 16-2 Guide to Interpretation of Systolic Blood Pressure

CVD Risk Level	Systolic (Upper) Blood Pressure	Category
1	100 or less	Very low risk
2	101-120	Below-average risk
3	121-140	Average risk
4	141-160	Above-average risk
5	161-180	High risk
6	181-200	Very-high risk

Source: P. Kuhne, "High Blood Pressure," in *Home Medical Encyclopedia* (London: Faber & Faber, 1960), pp. 57-58.

Essential Hypertension

When no such organic disorder exists, the individual is said to have **essential hypertension,** which accounts for over 90 percent of all cases of the disease. No one knows what causes essential hypertension, although heredity and diet have been strongly implicated. There is no doubt, however, that hypertension can cause severe and widespread damage to the cardiovascular system. Hypertension and atherosclerosis often go hand in hand, the one making the other worse until a cardiovascular crisis is provoked. In addition, hypertension in

Essential hypertension Consistent elevation of blood pressure with no apparent cause.

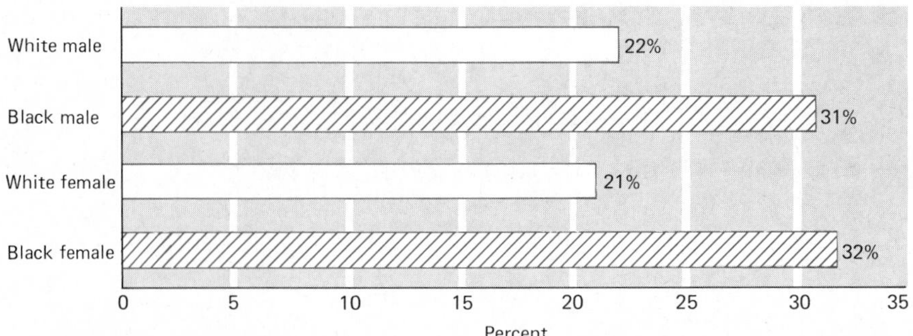

Figure 16-5. Hypertension Prevalence by Sex and Race, U.S. Adults Age 18 and Over: 1977 Estimate.
Black males and females have a higher incidence of hypertension than white males and females. (Source: Reprinted with permission from *Heart Facts: 1980,* American Heart Association, p. 20.)

and of itself can seriously damage the smaller arteries that supply the brain, kidneys, and eyes, leading to cerebrovascular accidents (strokes), kidney failure, and partial loss of sight.

Fortunately, hypertension can be controlled in most individuals, mainly through use of drugs. Three types of antihypertensive drugs are used, either singly or in combination: (1) *diuretics,* which increase urine flow and thus rid the bloodstream of excess salt and fluid; (2) *sympatholytic* drugs, which act on the sympathetic nervous system to lower blood pressure directly; and (3) *vasodilators,* which dilate the arterioles. Especially when combined with a low-salt diet, exercise regimens, and measures to reduce stress, drug therapy will lower blood pressure—but only for as long as therapy is continued. Hypertension cannot be cured, only controlled.

Coronary Heart Disease

Atherosclerosis is particularly dangerous when it occurs in the coronary arteries, which supply the heart with oxygenated blood. Obstruction of one or more of these arteries is by far the leading cause of myocardial ischemia—an insufficient flow of blood (ischemia) to the heart muscle (myocardium).

Angina pectoris Severe chest pain due to heart's sudden demand for more oxygen.

Myocardial ischemia often announces its presence in attacks of **angina pectoris** (literally, "chest pain"), sudden onslaughts of gripping pain that begin beneath the breastbone and may spread to the left shoulder, arm, and jaw. Most angina attacks occur after bouts of overeating or spells of physical exertion (particularly in cold weather), or in times of abnormal stress or excitement. During such episodes, the heart requires an increased supply of oxygen, which the obstructed arteries cannot deliver. As the victim's activity or stress level returns to normal, the angina pains disappear, only to return

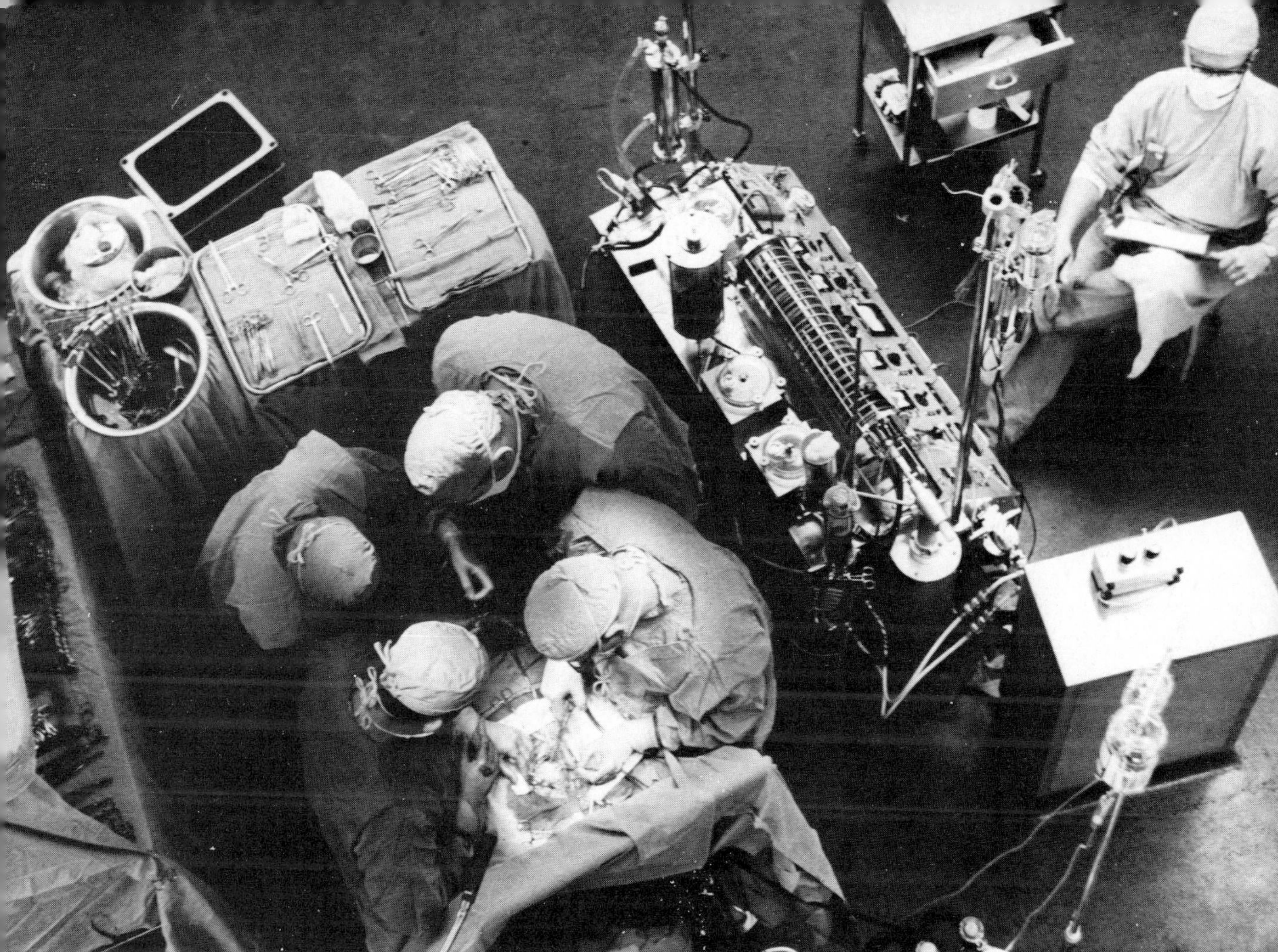

Overhead view of an operating room during open-heart surgery. (Photo courtesy of U.S. Department of Health and Human Services)

when the heart again must cope with more-than-usual demands. (Occasionally, angina strikes while the victim is pursuing normal activities, or even while the individual is at rest.)

Angina pectoris is rarely fatal, and quick relief of pain can be provided by tablets of nitroglycerin placed under the tongue. (Nitroglycerin dilates the coronary arteries, thereby easing blood flow.) Many persons ascribe mild attacks to indigestion or "heartburn" and do not seek further treatment. This is a serious mistake, because angina is a symptom of a deeper, underlying problem that can have fatal consequences. Specifically, the arterial obstruction announced by angina pains can lead to what is commonly called a heart attack.

Myocardial Infarction

A heart attack is in reality a **mycardial infarction,** the death from oxygen deprivation (infarction) of a portion of the heart muscle. Among the several possible causes of a myocardial infarction, the most common is the formation of a blood clot, or thrombus, in a coronary artery that is already obstructed partially by atheromas. Some-

Myocardial infarction Heart attack due to oxygen deprivation in part of the heart muscle.

times, atherosclerosis of the coronary arteries alone is responsible for an infarction. More rarely, a spasm in a coronary artery results in oxygen deprivation.

In any case, the effects of a myocardial infarction can be severe. Victims typically experienced crushing pain under the breastbone that may radiate down the left arm or up the left side of the face; this pain resembles that of angina pectoris, except that it is more intense and lasts longer. If the infarcted area is large enough, heart function can decrease so drastically that the victim will die within minutes. Death can also result from **arrhythmia,** a radical disruption of the rhythm of the heartbeat, caused by *fibrillation* (rapid, uncoordinated contraction of the ventricles).

Arrhythmia Radical irregularity of the heartbeat.

Treatment of heart attacks centers on alleviating the symptoms and stopping fibrillation. Victims admitted to hospitals are immediately given pain-killing drugs, to reduce the fear and stress that accompany heart-attack pain and place an added burden on the heart. They then are placed in coronary-care units (if such units are available), where their heart functions are monitored constantly by electronic devices. The emphasis here is on watching for fibrillation, which can be detected by electrocardiograph and controlled by drugs or the administration of electric shocks. If the damage to the heart muscle itself is not severe and incidents of arrhythmia do not persist, the patient will be discharged from the hospital after a few weeks. Convalescence, abetted by a program of physical therapy, may last for several weeks, or even for months after discharge. In most cases, scar tissue covers the infarcted area and victims return to normal life. However, the psychological trauma of undergoing a heart attack may inhibit their activities for some time, and they must face a heightened risk of suffering subsequent attacks.

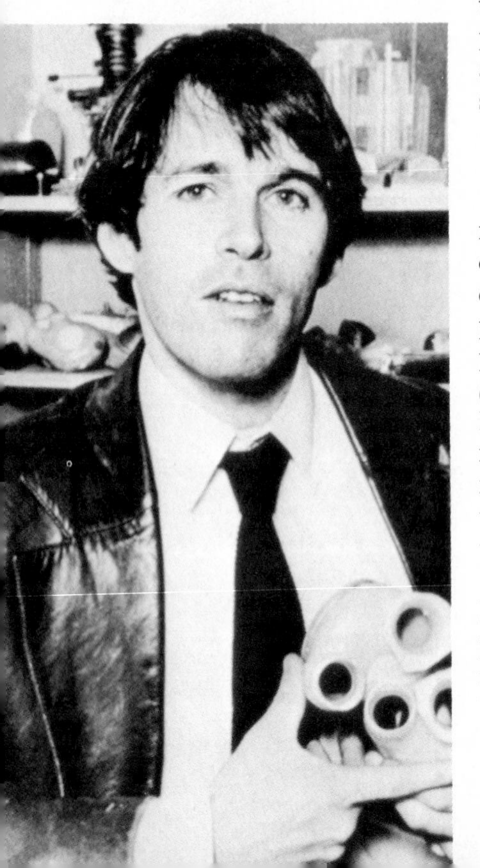

Dr. Robert Jarvik showing a polyurethane and Dacron mesh heart he designed. (Photo from United Press International)

Life-saving Procedures

Sudden death during a myocardial infarction, whether from arrhythmia or from massive damage to the heart, is far more likely to occur outside the hospital, particularly in communities that lack an emergency medical service (EMS). The value of an EMS is that medical personnel can reach most heart-attack victims within minutes of a phone call. If persons trained in *cardiopulmonary resuscitation (CPR)* arrive on the scene up to three or four minutes after a victim's heart has stopped beating, they often can restore circulation by means of this technique; it involves mouth-to-mouth breathing alternated with chest compression (see Chapter 19). Resuscitated individuals who reach coronary-care units have an excellent chance of survival.

Some individuals with advanced coronary heart disease can be helped by surgery. When coronary arteries are clogged by fatty deposits, the blockage sites can be pinpointed by an arteriogram (an X ray of an artery into which a special dye has been injected) and bypassed surgically in open-heart operations. *Bypass procedures,*

YOUR HEALTH TODAY

Living With Angina

Part of the success in controlling angina is attributable to various life-style changes made by the sufferer. The following life-style behaviors, if adhered to, will help keep angina under control:

- Follow the prescribed medication regimen suggested by your physician.
- Avoid excessive physical exertion or emotional stress.
- Avoid very cold weather.
- Stop smoking.
- Eat small meals and do so more often throughout the day.
- Rest briefly throughout the day.
- If you are overweight, shed some pounds.

which involve the rerouting of blood flow through surgically emplaced shunts in the coronary arteries, have proven helpful for persons with frequent and severe angina attacks, but whether or not they actually prolong life is a matter of dispute. Another controversial procedure is the use of *heart transplants,* that is, the replacement of a badly degenerated heart with a normal, functioning heart taken from a recently-deceased donor. Many heart-transplant patients now live for several years after the operation, but the problem of rejection (immune reactions to foreign proteins) remains formidable. More uniformly successful are pacemakers insertions, in which battery-powered pacemakers are implanted in hearts prone to arrhythmia.

Strokes (Cerebrovascular Accidents)

Strokes, also known as cerebrovascular accidents, the number-two killer among cardiovascular diseases, occur when one or more of the cerebral arteries becomes clogged or begins to hemorrhage (bleed profusely and uncontrollably), thus shutting off the flow of oxygenated blood to the brain. Once deprived of oxygen, brain cells die within minutes. The result may be death, paralysis, or impairment of one or more body functions.

The underlying causes of most strokes are atherosclerosis and hypertension. Many strokes are triggered by the formation of blood clots in atherosclerotic cerebral arteries, an event known as a **cerebral thrombosis.** (As noted above, clots are more likely to form in arteries already obstructed by fatty deposits.) In a **cerebral embolism,** another type of stroke, a mass detached from a clot or fatty deposit elsewhere in the circulatory system travels through the blood-stream

Stroke Cerebrovascular accident resulting from an obstruction of a vessel in the brain by a blood clot.

Cerebral thrombosis Formation of a blood clot in a cerebral artery.

Cerebral embolism Obstruction of a cerebral artery by a transported clot.

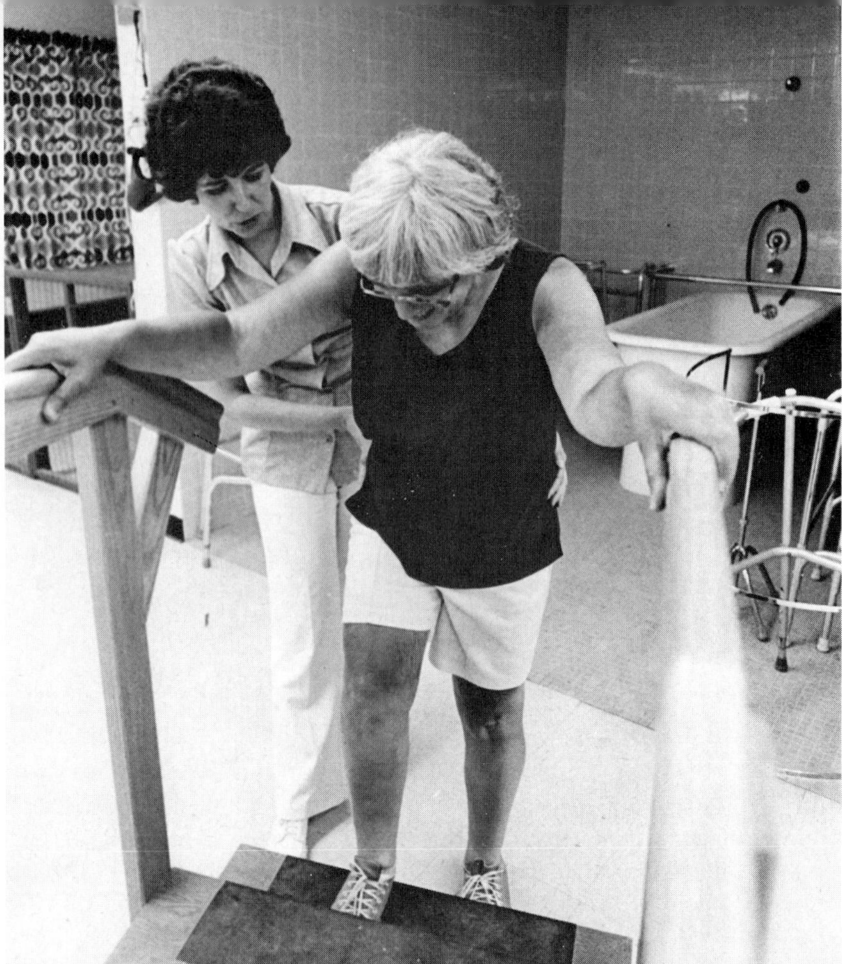

Often recovering stroke victims must relearn and practice basic skills, such as climbing stairs. Many need rehabilitative therapy to enable them to resume active lives. (Photo © Anne McQueen/ Stock, Boston)

Cerebral hemorrhage Seepage of blood into the brain due to a ruptured cerebral artery.

and clogs a cerebral artery. The third type of stroke, a **cerebral hemorrhage,** takes place when a cerebral artery bursts because of a head injury, the weakening of the arterial walls by arteriosclerosis, or the bursting of an aneurysm (a bulge in an arterial wall).

Whatever the cause, a stroke poses a grave threat to health and life, both because the brain is such a vital organ and because brain cells, unlike other body cells, cannot regenerate themselves. When brain cells die, the body functions they control degenerate or cease altogether. Depending on the affected area of the brain, the victim of a stroke may suffer partial paralysis, impairment of speech or sight, loss of memory, or any of a host of other disabilities. These effects may be permanent or temporary, depending on the extent of the damage. If the injury is massive enough and affects the vital functions of the body, death can occur almost instantaneously.

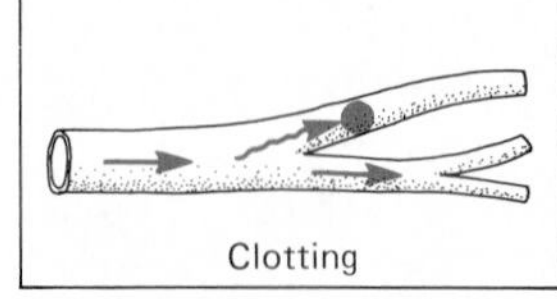

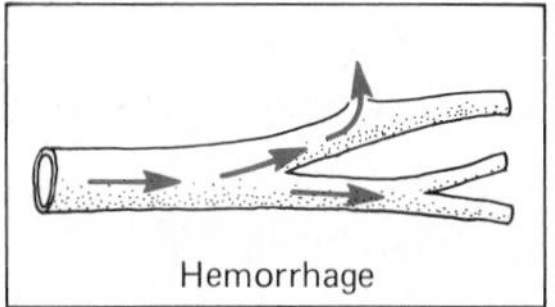

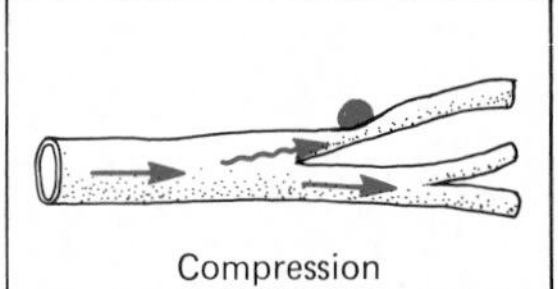

Figure 16–6. How Strokes Occur. (Source: With permission from *Facts About Strokes,* 1968, by the American Heart Association)

Potential victims of a major stroke often receive warning signals in the form of minor strokes; like angina pains, these symptoms of underlying arterial disease should be heeded as quickly as possible. In some cases, anticoagulants can be administered in an effort to prevent the formation of clots. An operation to open up obstructed arteries is another possibility. Both potential and actual victims should embark on a program of diet and exercise designed to reduce hypertension and should take antihypertensive drugs if prescribed. Survivors of major strokes face special difficulties in that, unlike most heart-attack victims, they must cope with one or several forms of physical or mental impairment. If paralysis is not permanent, patients who follow rigorous programs of physical therapy, usually under the guidance of a professional therapist, can recover partial or full function of speech, organs, limbs, or whatever other areas of the body were affected by the stroke.

Rheumatic Heart Disease

The most common cause of cardiovascular problems in children and young adults is **rheumatic fever,** a subsequent complication of a streptococcal infection (see Chapter 15) of the respiratory tract. In many cases, rheumatic fever leads to inflammation of and damage to the muscle layers, the lining, or the valves of the heart. Narrowing or impaired functioning of the mitral and aortic valves is a frequent occurrence. Rheumatic fever can also lead to inflammation of the sac surrounding the heart. Later in life, these conditions can contribute significantly to cardiovascular problems.

Rheumatic fever Damaging inflammation of the heart due to streptococcal infection of the respiratory tract.

Although rheumatic fever is preventable, because of the availability of antibiotics effective against streptococcal bacteria, the disease is still a leading cause of death from cardiovascular disease in the 5–15 age group. Primarily, this is because the symptoms of the original infection can be mild or even nonexistent, and because subsequent infections can accelerate damage to the heart. Rheumatic fever victims usually are given maintenance doses of penicillin, to prevent reinfections, for several years after the condition is diagnosed. If the valves are damaged, they sometimes can be repaired surgically or replaced altogether with artificial valves.

Betsy Sneith, 23, had a heart transplant in 1980 and gave birth to little Sierra on September 16, 1984. This was the first time in medical history that a woman with a transplanted heart had given birth. (Photo by Bill Nation/Sygma)

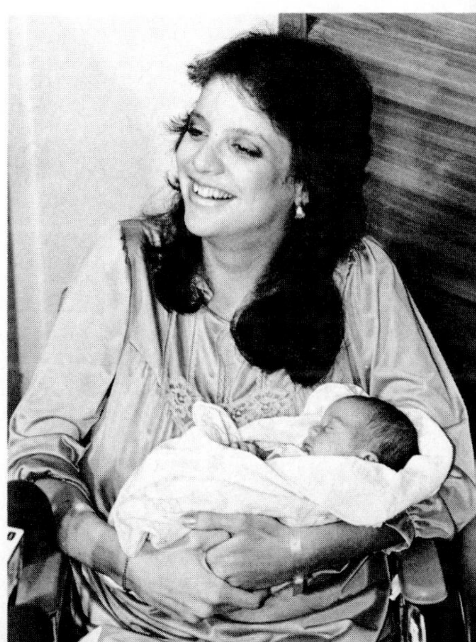

Congenital Heart Defects

Defects in the heart and the major blood vessels leading to and from it can appear during the time in which the heart develops in the embryo. Although the origin of most such congenital problems is unknown, studies have shown that mothers who contract German measles in the first three months of pregnancy give birth to a relatively high proportion of heart-damaged babies.

Any part of the heart can be damaged before birth, but the most common defects involve narrowing or insufficiency of the heart valves. Other frequently encountered defects include openings in the septum that allow the intermingling of oxygenated and unoxygenated blood, narrowing of the aorta, and the presence of an opening between the aorta and the pulmonary artery. Perhaps the best-known congenital heart condition is tetralogy of Fallot, or "blue-baby" disease, a combination of four defects: narrowing of the pulmonary valve, abnormal opening of the aorta, incomplete closing of the ventricular part of the septum, and enlargement of the right septum. The most obvious symptom of tetralogy of Fallot is a blue cast to the skin, caused by the presence of deoxygenated blood in the arterial circulation. Fortunately, open-heart surgery can correct these defects.

Risk Factors in Cardiovascular Diseases

Cardiovascular diseases are complex phenomena whose exact causes and mechanisms have thus far eluded scientific definition. No one knows precisely why one person with certain indicators will suffer a heart attack or a stroke whereas another person with the same indicators will not. It has become clear, however, that certain factors are associated with the development of cardiovascular disease. Some of these so-called risk factors, such as heredity and age, cannot be controlled by the individual. Others lie within our power to control or to avoid altogether. The controllable risk factors include improper diet, obesity, smoking, lack of exercise, and stress.

Controllable Risk Factors

People who eat properly, keep their weight within normal bounds, do not smoke, exercise regularly, and cope well with stress suffer fewer heart attacks and strokes. There is no doubt about this correlation, which has been demonstrated repeatedly in a wide range of studies. By altering your life-style to control these risk factors, you can significantly reduce your chances of dying from cardiovascular disease. Hence, it is worthwhile concentrating on these factors.

Diet

A major contributor to the development of atherosclerosis is cholesterol, a fatty substance manufactured by the liver. A certain level of cholesterol in the blood (serum cholesterol) is necessary for good health. Serum cholesterol levels above 200 mg/dl (milligrams per decaliter), however, have been implicated in the growth of fatty deposits in the blood vessels, and hence in the development of cardiovascular crises. High serum-cholesterol levels frequently are found in individuals whose diets contain a large percentage of saturated fats (those solid at room temperature), usually in the form of lard, dairy products, and animal fats. Several studies have shown that the incidence of heart attacks is much higher in areas with traditionally high-cholesterol diets (such as the United States, Canada, and northern Europe) than in those with traditionally low-cholesterol diets (such as Japan and the Middle East). To explore the possibility that ethnic or racial characteristics were the determining factors, researchers also studied emigrants from one type of culture to another and found that, for instance, ethnic Japanese who settled in the United States and adoped an American diet were more prone to develop cardiovascular disease than were their relatives in Japan.

Researchers have yet to uncover a direct causal link between high-cholesterol diets and cardiovascular disease, but the circumstantial evidence is overwhelming. Equally persuasive is the evidence that salt intake plays a role in high blood pressure; most doctors now recognize that a low-salt diet is a potent tool in treating hypertension, and thus in reducing the likelihood of heart attacks and strokes in hypertensive individuals. Another possible dietary culprit is sugar, although this is still a matter of debate.

Figure 16-7. Life-style Factors Contributing to the Risk of Cardiovascular Disorders.

This illustration summarizes the multi-factorial causes of cardiovascular diseases (CVD). Many health habits, initiated in early childhood by parents, are precursors to CVD. CVD may remain asymptomatic but build up in youth, and then erupt in middle age (symptomatic). (Source: Adapted from Walter D. Sorochan, *Promoting Your Health* [New York: John Wiley & Sons, Inc., 1981], 314.)

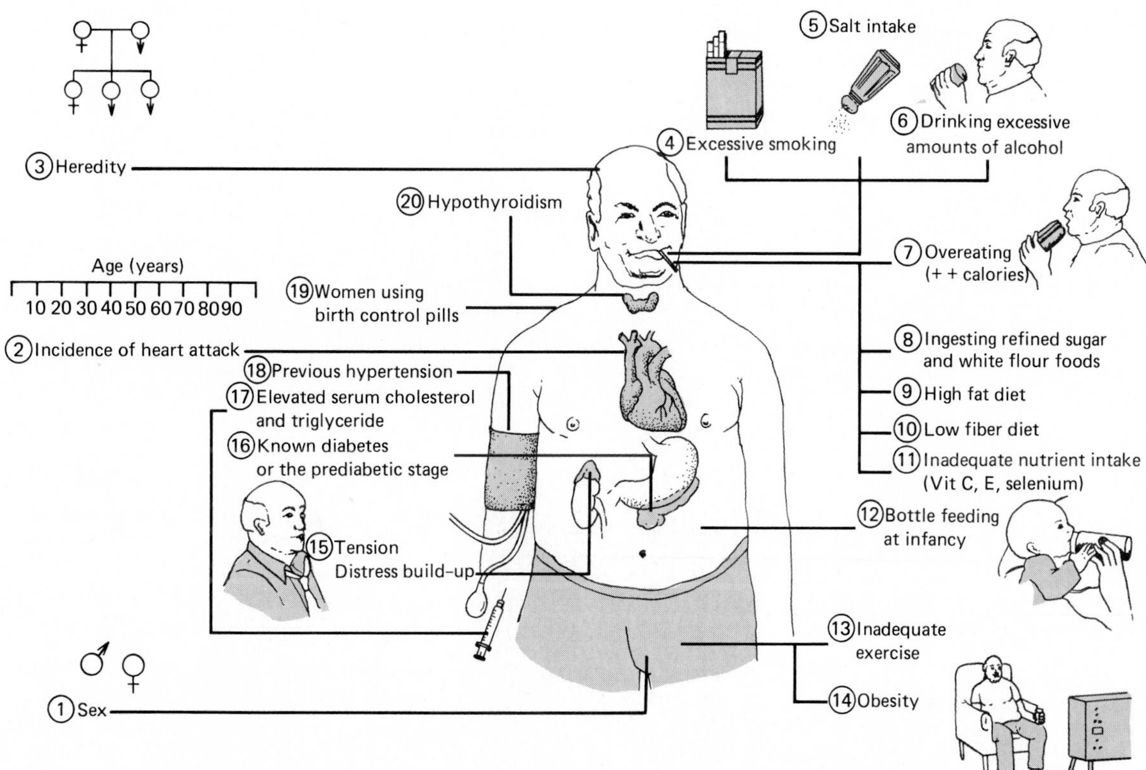

Obesity

Diets high in saturated fats, red meat, and refined sugar lead directly to obesity, another risk factor. Individuals with higher-than-normal weight for their height and age are more likely to suffer from hypertension and diabetes (in itself a risk factor). Particularly at risk are individuals whose body weight exceeds the norm by 30 percent or more.

In addition to sugar and fats, a significant (and often overlooked) contributor to obesity is alcohol, which adds an enormous number of empty calories to the diets of many Americans. By reducing alcohol intake to no more than two ounces a day, cutting down moderately on high-calorie foods, and engaging in regular exercise, most Americans could avoid this risk factor entirely.

Smoking

A number of studies have linked smoking with significantly greater risk of heart attacks and other circulatory diseases. One ten-year survey, conducted by the American Heart Association, found that middle-aged men who smoke a pack of cigarettes a day are twice as likely to have a heart attack as those who do not smoke. When cigarette consumption rises above a pack a day, the danger of heart attack is three times higher than the risk for nonsmokers.

Cigarette smoking apparently contributes to cardiovascular disease in several ways. The carbon monoxide inhaled in cigarette smoke reduces the amount of oxygen in the blood, thereby forcing the heart to work harder. Nicotine, another constitutent of cigarette smoke, increases the heartbeat, causes the arterioles to constrict (a prime cause of hypertension), and destroys vitamin C (which breaks down serum cholesterol). Finally, there is some evidence that smokers are more prone than others to suffer *fatal* heart attacks, probably because nicotine affects the heartbeat.

Fortunately, all of these deleterious effects are reversible. Within months or, at most, a few years after quitting, ex-smokers are no more likely to suffer heart attacks than anyone else. Even cutting down the number of cigarettes smoked daily will substantially reduce the risk of cardiovascular trouble. For those who refuse to quit or to cut down, the best advice is to avoid inhaling cigarette smoke, or to inhale as little and as shallowly as possible.

Lack of Exercise

In highly industrialized societies, the prevalence of labor-saving devices and sedentary occupations has led to a marked decline in the amount of physical exercise engaged in by the average person. This modern trend has undoubtedly affected the overall level of physical fitness in the United States. Lack of exercise increases the ratio of body fat to muscle, and thereby encourages obesity and degrades the functioning body systems. Perhaps more important than the bad effects of a failure to exercise are the positive effects of regular physical exertion. Physical activity strengthens the cardiovascular system by, among other things, increasing the oxygen-carrying capacity of the system, lowering the heart rate, and, by burning off excess calories, aiding weight control.

The assertions of some jogging enthusiasts to the contrary, regular and strenuous physical exercise alone will not confer immunity to heart attacks. (One of the highest rates of cardiovascular disease in the world, for example, can be found among the rural population of Finland — farmers and lumberjacks who work strenuously but who have an extremely high-cholesterol diet.) The available evidence indicates strongly, however, that the more sedentary your life-style, the higher are your chances of developing cardiovascular problems. For people in nonactive occupations, the most healthful form of exercise is a regular program of jogging, vigorous walking, swimming, or well-rounded exercises.

Stress and Personality

The amount of stress inherent in modern life — and the individual's reaction to it — has emerged as one of the most intriguing and controversial topics in present-day studies of cardiovascular disease. Indisputably, emotional stress temporarily stimulates the heart to beat faster and raises both blood pressure and serum-cholesterol levels. Whether sustained exposure to stressful situations leads to permanent damage to the cardiovascular system is still uncertain, however.

In the 1950s and 1960s, Dr. Meyer Friedman and Dr. Ray Rosenman developed a model of coronary-prone behavior they labeled the Type A pattern. Type A persons are aggressive, hard-working, achievement-oriented individuals who tend to be time-conscious, intolerant of interruptions, impatient, and irritable. They also are unable to shift easily into the more relaxed (Type B) life-style that would be better for their health.

Several studies have borne out the two doctor's hypothesis that Type A persons are more likely to suffer heart attacks, irrespective of other risk factors, than persons with a different pattern of behavior. Other studies have failed to support this conclusion, however. One of the most difficult problems facing researchers in this area is how to test for Type A behavior. The written tests normally employed are subject to a wide range of interpretations, and the criteria behind the tests are controversial.

Unavoidable Risk Factors

People cannot choose their physiological inheritance, stop the aging process, or (except to a limited extent) prevent the occurrence of diabetes. These unavoidable risk factors are associated with the incidence of cardiovascular disease.

Perhaps the most important of these factors is heredity. In a relatively few families, early developing and severe cardiovascular disease appears in generation after generation, for unknown reasons. More often, individuals seemingly inherit a greater or lesser tolerance for high blood pressure, high serum-cholesterol levels, and atherosclerosis. Among other hereditary factors, race and sex are linked statistically, if not causally, to the incidence of heart and circulatory disorders. Blacks, for instance, are statistically more likely than whites to have hypertension, and men in general are statistically more prone than women to have heart attacks. These statistical patterns may denote inherent characteristics of blacks and men, or they may merely reflect the impact of other risk factors associated with black culture or male roles.

The once widely held belief that cardiovascular disease was an inevitable by-product of the aging process has long since been disproved. Although aging does weaken the cardiovascular system to some extent, and although blood pressure normally rises after the age of 50, all the available evidence suggests that atherosclerosis and hypertension are not age-related disorders.

Diabetes, the final risk factor, may or may not be unavoidable. Obesity and diet almost certainly contribute to the onset of diabetes,

YOUR HEALTH TODAY

Ways to Maintain a Healthy Cardiovascular System

1. Stop smoking cigarettes or decrease the number of cigarettes you now smoke and try not to inhale the smoke.
2. Start a program of regular endurance exercise (especially if you are a smoker). Become more physically active—take the stairs instead of the elevator, walk or bicycle to the store instead of driving, and so on. "You are as old as your arteries."
3. If you are overweight, undertake a weight reduction program that will help you adjust your caloric intake to appropriate levels.
4. Lower your fat intake, particularly the saturated fats, such as fried foods, fatty meats, cold cuts, and dairy products rich in fats.
5. Eat a diet high in fresh fruits and vegetables and low in refined sugar products (cakes, cookies, candy, and so on).
6. Cut down on your salt intake. Americans eat much more salt than their bodies need, and salt is involved in high blood pressure.
7. Reduce your intake of alcoholic beverages. Many studies have indicated that alcohol consumption aggravates the cardiovascular system and multiplies other risk factors.

Source: Walter D. Sorochan, *Promoting Your Health.* (New York: John Wiley & Sons, Inc., 1981), 316.

but it is unclear how significant these factors are. At any rate, diabetic individuals should do everything in their power to control the disease, which is a principal factor in cardiovascular problems among older people.

What Can Be Done

Unlike the infectious diseases that plagued humanity until well into the twentieth century, cardiovascular diseases, the great scourge of modern industrial society, are to a large degree preventable. The steady if unspectacular decrease in the cardiovascular-disease death rate in recent years clearly indicates that by changing our life-style in certain ways, we can prevent tens of thousands of premature deaths annually. (For further information on how to maintain a healthy cardiovascular system see the box on "Ways to Maintain a Healthy Cardiovascular System.")

Whatever the impact of unavoidable risk factors, there is much we can do to lessen the effects of those risk factors that we can control. Taking the following self-assessment test, "RISKO: A Heart Hazard Appraisal," will give you a clearer picture of the interplay of risk factors in cardiovascular disease. Every risk factor that you avoid or bring under control represents a vital step on the road to good health.

Some words of caution. The American Heart Association, which developed the RISKO test, emphasizes the following points for people who take it:

- If you have diabetes, gout, or a family history of heart disease, your real risk of developing heart disease will be greater than indicated by your RISKO score. If your score is high and you have one or more of these additional problems, you should give particular attention to reducing your risk.
- If you are a woman under 45 years or a man under 35 years of age, your RISKO score represents an upper limit on your real risk of developing heart disease. In this case your real risk is probably lower than indicated by your score.
- If you are a woman whose use of estrogen has contributed to a high RISKO score, you may want to consult your physician. Do not automaticaly discontinue your prescription.
- Using your weight category to estimate your systolic blood pressure or your blood cholesterol level makes your RISKO score less accurate. Your score will tend to overestimate your risk if your actual values on these two important factors are average for someone of your height and weight. Your score will underestimate your risk if your actual blood pressure or cholesterol level is above average for someone of your height or weight.

SELF-ASSESSMENT EXERCISE 16.1

RISKO: A Heart Hazard Appraisal

Introduction:

In the United States it is estimated that close to 550,000 people die each year from coronary heart disease. Scientists have identified a number of factors which are linked with an increased likelihood or risk of developing coronary heart disease. Some of these risk factors, like aging, being male, or having a family history of heart disease, are unavoidable. However, many other significant risk factors can be modified.

RISKO scores are based upon four of the most important modifiable factors which contribute to the development of heart disease. These factors include your weight, blood pressure, blood cholesterol level, and use of tobacco. If you are a woman, your score will also take into account your use of estrogen.

The RISKO score you obtain measures your risk of developing heart disease in the next several years, provided that you currently show no evidence of such disease. It is not a substitute for a thorough physical examination and assessment by your physician. Rather, it will help you learn more about your risk of developing heart disease and will indicate ways in which you can reduce this risk.

Men

Find the column for your age group. Everyone starts with a score of 10 points. Work down the page *adding* points to or *subtracting* points from your score.

1. Weight

Locate your weight category in the table on the facing page. If you are in . . .

	54 or Younger		55 or Older	
	Starting Score	10	Starting Score	10
weight category A	Subtract 2	______	Subtract 2	______
weight category B	Subtract 1	______	Add 0	______
weight category C	Add 1	______	Add 1	______
weight category D	Add 2	______	Add 3	______
	Equals	☐	Equals	☐

2. Systolic Blood Pressure

Use the "first" or "higher" number from your most recent blood pressure measurement. If you do not know your blood pressure, estimate it by using the letter for your weight category. If your blood pressure is . . .

		54 or Younger	55 or Older
		Score ☐	Score ☐
A	119 or less	Subtract 1 ___	Subtract 5 ___
B	between 120 and 139	Add 0 ___	Subtract 2 ___
C	between 140 and 159	Add 0 ___	Add 1 ___
D	160 or greater	Add 1 ___	Add 4 ___
		Equals ☐	Equals ☐

3. Blood Cholesterol Level

Use the number from your most recent blood cholesterol test. If you do not know your blood cholesterol, estimate it by using the letter for your weight category. If your blood cholesterol is . . .

		54 or Younger	55 or Older
A	199 or less	Subtract 2 ___	Subtract 1 ___
B	between 200 and 224	Subtract 1 ___	Subtract 1 ___
C	between 225 and 249	Add 0 ___	Add 0 ___
D	250 or higher	Add 1 ___	Add 0 ___
		Equals ☐	Equals ☐

4. Cigarette Smoking

If you . . . .

(If you smoke a pipe, but not cigarettes, use the same score adjustment as those cigarette smokers who smoke less than a pack a day.)

	54 or Younger	55 or Older
do not smoke	Subtract 1 ___	Subtract 2 ___
smoke less than a pack a day	Add 0 ___	Subtract 1 ___
smoke a pack a day	Add 1 ___	Add 0 ___
smoke more than a pack a day	Add 2 ___	Add 3 ___
	Final Score Equals ☐	Final Score Equals ☐

Weight Table for Men
Look for your height (without shoes) in the far left column and then read across to find the category into which your weight (in indoor clothing) would fall.

Weight Category (lbs.)

Your Height FT	IN	A	B	C	D
5	1	up to 123	124–148	149–173	174 plus
5	2	up to 126	127–152	153–178	179 plus
5	3	up to 129	130–156	157–182	183 plus
5	4	up to 132	133–160	161–186	187 plus
5	5	up to 135	136–163	164–190	191 plus
5	6	up to 139	140–168	169–196	197 plus
5	7	up to 144	145–174	175–203	204 plus
5	8	up to 148	149–179	180–209	210 plus
5	9	up to 152	153–184	185–214	215 plus
5	10	up to 157	158–190	191–221	222 plus
5	11	up to 161	162–194	195–227	228 plus
6	0	up to 165	166–199	200–232	233 plus
6	1	up to 170	171–205	206–239	240 plus
6	2	up to 175	176–211	212–246	247 plus
6	3	up to 180	181–217	218–253	254 plus
6	4	up to 185	186–223	224–260	261 plus
6	5	up to 190	191–229	230–267	268 plus
6	6	up to 195	196–235	236–274	275 plus
Estimate of Systolic Blood Pressure		119 or less	120 to 139	140 to 159	160 or more
Estimate of Blood Cholesterol		199 or less	200 to 224	225 to 249	250 or more

Because both blood pressure and blood cholesterol are related to weight, an estimate of these risk factors for each weight category is printed at the bottom of the table.

(Continued)

Women

Find the column for your age group. Everyone starts with a score of 10 points. Work down the page *adding* points to or *subtracting* points from your score.

1. Weight

		54 or Younger		55 or Older	
		Starting Score	**10**	**Starting Score**	**10**
Locate your weight category in the table on the facing page. If you are in . . .	weight category A	Subtract 2	____	Subtract 2	____
	weight category B	Subtract 1	____	Subtract 1	____
	weight category C	Add 1	____	Add 0	____
	weight category D	Add 2	____	Add 1	____
		Equals	☐	**Equals**	☐

2. Systolic Blood Pressure

		54 or Younger		55 or Older	
Use the "first" or "higher" number from your most recent blood pressure measurement. If you do not know your blood pressure, estimate it by using the letter for your weight category. If your blood pressure is . . .	A 119 or less	Subtract 2	____	Subtract 3	____
	B between 120 and 139	Subtract 1	____	Add 0	____
	C between 140 and 159	Add 0	____	Add 3	____
	D 160 or greater	Add 1	____	Add 6	____
		Equals	☐	**Equals**	☐

3. Blood Cholesterol Level

		54 or Younger		55 or Older	
Use the number from your most recent blood cholesterol test. If you do not know your blood cholesterol, estimate it by using the letter for your weight category. If your blood cholesterol is . . .	A 199 or less	Subtract 1	____	Subtract 3	____
	B between 200 and 224	Add 0	____	Subtract 1	____
	C between 225 and 249	Add 0	____	Add 1	____
	D 250 or higher	Add 1	____	Add 3	____
		Equals	☐	**Equals**	☐

4. Cigarette Smoking

		54 or Younger		55 or Older	
If you	do not smoke	Subtract 1	____	Subtract 2	____
	smoke less than a pack a day	Add 0	____	Subtract 1	____
	smoke a pack a day	Add 1	____	Add 1	____
	smoke more than a pack a day	Add 2	____	Add 4	____
		Equals	☐	**Equals**	☐

5. Estrogen Use

Birth control pills and hormone drugs contain estrogen. A few examples are: *Premarin *Ogan *Menstranol *Provera *Evex *Menest *Estinyl *Meurium.

*Have you ever taken estrogen for five or more years in a row?

*Are you age 35 years or older and now taking estrogen?

	54 or Younger	55 or Older
	Score ☐	Score ☐
No to both questions	Add 0 ____	Add 0 ____
Yes to one or both questions	Add 1 ____	Add 3 ____
	Final Score Equals ☐	Final Score Equals ☐

Weight Table for Women
Look for your height (without shoes) in the far left column and then read across to find the category into which your weight (in indoor clothing) would fall.

Your Height FT IN	Weight Category (lbs.) A	B	C	D
*4 8	up to 101	102–122	123–143	144 plus
4 9	up to 103	104–125	126–146	147 plus
4 10	up to 106	107–128	129–150	151 plus
4 11	up to 109	110–132	133–154	155 plus
5 0	up to 112	113–136	137–158	159 plus
5 1	up to 115	116–139	140–162	163 plus
5 2	up to 119	120–144	145–168	169 plus
5 3	up to 122	123–148	149–172	173 plus
5 4	up to 127	128–154	155–179	180 plus
5 5	up to 131	132–158	159–185	186 plus
5 6	up to 135	136–163	164–190	191 plus
5 7	up to 139	140–168	169–196	197 plus
5 8	up to 143	144–173	174–202	203 plus
5 9	up to 147	148–178	179–207	208 plus
5 10	up to 151	152–182	183–213	214 plus
5 11	up to 155	156–187	188–218	219 plus
6 0	up to 159	160–191	192–224	225 plus
6 1	up to 163	164–196	197–229	230 plus
Estimate of Systolic Blood Pressure	119 or less	120 to 139	140 to 159	160 or more
Estimate of Blood Cholesterol	199 or less	200 to 224	225 to 249	250 or more

Because both blood pressure and blood cholesterol are related to weight, an estimate of these risk factors for each weight category is printed at the bottom of the table.

What Your Score Means

0–4 You have one of the lowest risks of Heart Disease for your age and sex.

5–9 You have a low to moderate risk of Heart Disease for your age and sex, but there is room for improvement.

10–14 You have a moderate to high risk of Heart Disease for your age and sex, with considerable room for improvement on some factors.

15–19 You have a high risk of developing Heart Disease for your age and sex, with a great deal of room for improvement on all factors.

20 & over You have a very high risk of developing Heart Disease for your age and sex and should take immediate action on all risk factors.

Warning

- If you have diabetes, gout, or a family history of heart disease, your actual risk will be greater than indicated by this appraisal.
- If you do not know your blood pressure or blood cholesterol level, visit your physician or health center to have them measured. Then figure your score again for a more accurate determination of your risk.
- If you are overweight, have high blood pressure or high blood cholesterol, or smoke cigarettes, your long-term risk of heart disease is increased even if your short-term risk is low.

Source: Reprinted with permission, American Heart Association.

Summary

More Americans die from diseases of the heart and the circulatory system than from all other causes combined. This modern preeminence of cardiovascular causes of death coincided with the lengthening of the average life span, made possible by the control of communicable diseases. It also coincided with the significant changes in diet and life-style in modern industrial societies. Only in the past 20 years or so, as both medical professionals and laypersons have come to understand the relevance of life-style factors, has the death rate from cardiovascular diseases declined.

The cardiovascular system consists of the circulatory system (the blood vessels) and the heart. Most disorders in this system arise from damage to or blockage of arteries, which carry oxygenated blood throughout the body. Atherosclerosis (clogging of the arteries by fatty deposits) and hypertension (persistently high blood pressure) are the underlying causes of most cardiovascular crises. Myocardial infarctions (heart attacks) and angina pectoris are crises precipitated by coronary heart diseases (blockage of the arteries that supply the heart). Clogging of the arteries of the brain can lead to strokes (cerebrovascular accidents). Two other major forms of cardiovascular disease are rheumatic heart disease, caused by a streptococcal infection, and congenital heart defects.

The ultimate causes of cardiovascular disease are unclear, but there is strong evidence that certain life-style factors play an important role in its development. These so-called risk factors, which can be controlled or avoided by the individual, include dietary intake of saturated fats and salt, cigarette smoking, obesity, lack of exercise, and stress and personality. Unavoidable risk factors include heredity, age, and diabetes. By dealing with the controllable risk factors, most people could significantly reduce the chances of dying from cardiovascular disease.

Review and Discussion

1. Why have cardiovascular diseases become the major cause of death in industrial countries?

2. Describe the circulation of blood through the cardiovascular system, paying particular attention to the heart's role as pump.

3. What are arteriosclerosis and atherosclerosis? How do they contribute to coronary heart disease?

4. What is hypertension? How does it affect the cardiovascular system?

5. What is the difference between systolic and diastolic pressure? What is the range of normal blood pressure for a young adult?

6. What is angina pectoris? What life-style changes are necessary to control it?

7. What are the signs and symptoms of a myocardial infarction?

8. What is a stroke, or cerebrovascular accident? How does it occur? What are its consequences?

9. What are the effects of rheumatic heart disease on the heart?

10. What are the most common congenital heart defects? How do they occur?

11. What are some of the risk factors in cardiovascular disease? Which are controllable?

Further Reading

American Heart Association. *The Heart Book.* New York: Elsevier-Dutton Publishing Company, 1980.
A detailed discussion of cardiovascular diseases with a strong emphasis on the medical explanations and on methods of treatment.

American Heart Association. *Heart Facts 1985.* New York: American Heart Association, 1984.
An annual report containing the latest information on cardiovascular diseases. (Pamphlet)

DeBakey, Michael. *The Living Heart.* New York: Charter Books, 1978.
A prominent physician's explanation of the cardiovascular system.(Paperback)

Friedman, Meyer, and Ray H. Rosenman. *Type A Behavior and Your Heart.* New York: Fawcett Books, 1978.
A discussion of the relationship between psychological traits and cardiovascular disease. (Paperback)

Roth, Oscar, and Lawrence Galton. Heart Attack. Chicago: Contemporary Books, 1980.
A question and answer guide to heart attacks, for the general public. (Paperback)

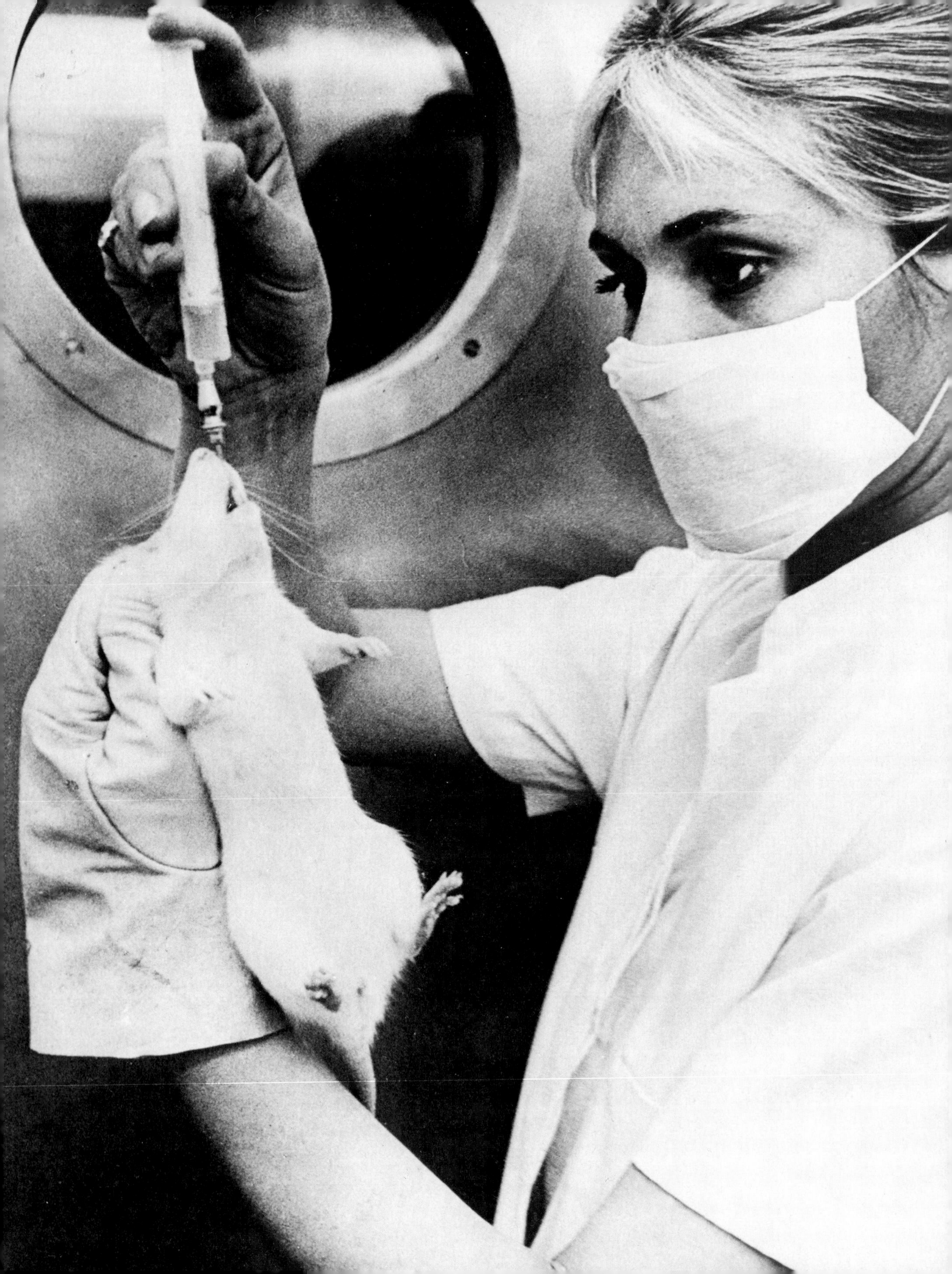

Chapter 17
Cancer

KEY POINTS

- ☐ Cancer refers to a group of diseases characterized primarily by the uncontrolled growth of abnormal cells.
- ☐ Cancer cells can spread, or metastasize, from the original tumor throughout the body.
- ☐ The most common types of cancer are malignancies of the skin, the lungs, the breast, the colon and rectum, the uterus, the blood-forming tissues, and the lymphatic system.
- ☐ More Americans die from lung cancer than any other form of cancer.
- ☐ Cancers have several known or suspected causes, the most prominent of which are radiation, carcinogens (cancer-causing substances), and viruses.
- ☐ Avoidance of risk factors offers the best chance of preventing cancer.
- ☐ Early detection is the most crucial factor in successfully treating cancer.
- ☐ Aids to early detection include self-monitoring for the warning signals of cancer, annual physical examinations, and a variety of early-detection tests.
- ☐ Currently, approximately 45 percent of all cancer patients survive at least five years—the accepted criterion for cure.

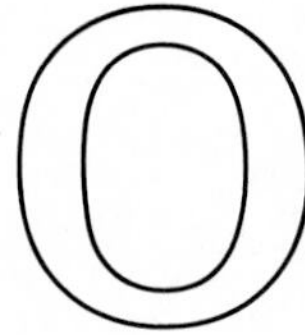

F ALL the major diseases that afflict us today, perhaps the most feared—and in many ways the most mysterious—is cancer. Cancer is actually a group of diseases characterized primarily by the uncontrolled growth of abnormal cells. As they multiply, these cells often spread from their original site (which may be in any type of body tissue) to other areas of the body, destroying normal tissue and impairing body functions. If left unchecked, this process can be fatal.

In modern times, cancer has become an increasingly prominent and feared cause of death. Although facets of modern life—in particular, cigarette smoking and chemicals in the environment—undoubtedly have contributed to the increased incidence of cancer, the lengthened life span of twentieth-century humans is probably the dominant factor behind the rise of this killer. The longer an individual lives, the greater the chance of developing cancer. It is now the second-leading cause of death (behind cardiovascular disease) in the United States, Canada, and Europe.

These statistics are frightening enough, but they alone cannot account for the deep-seated dread of cancer that pervades modern industrial societies. Fear represents the single most frustrating aspect of cancer treatment. Cancer specialists agree that the present cure rate of about 45 percent could be significantly increased simply by earlier detection of the disease. And the best way to achieve early detection is to consult a doctor as soon as any of the warning signals indicated in Figure 17–1 appears.

Several of these signals seem common enough to shrug off, and those that are unmistakably serious, such as the sudden appearance of a lump or unusual bleeding, often engender such fear of cancer that the victim will postpone seeing a doctor, hoping that the symptom will just go away. Both of these responses must be avoided. Most persons who promptly seek a diagnosis find out that they don't have cancer after all. If cancer is diagnosed, their chances of remission or cure will be greatly enhanced by early detection.

Origins and Pathology

With a few exceptions, such as brain cells, all body cells have the ability to duplicate themselves by cell division. This reproductive capacity is vital to life and health; without it, any damage to the body would be permanent. When enough new cells have been produced to fulfill the body's requirements, normal cells stop reproducing.

Cancer cells, on the other hand, do not stop reproducing. Exactly why this is so remains a mystery. At first, cancer cells may look like normal cells of the tissue in which they appear. As they multiply, however, they tend to become more and more abnormal in appear-

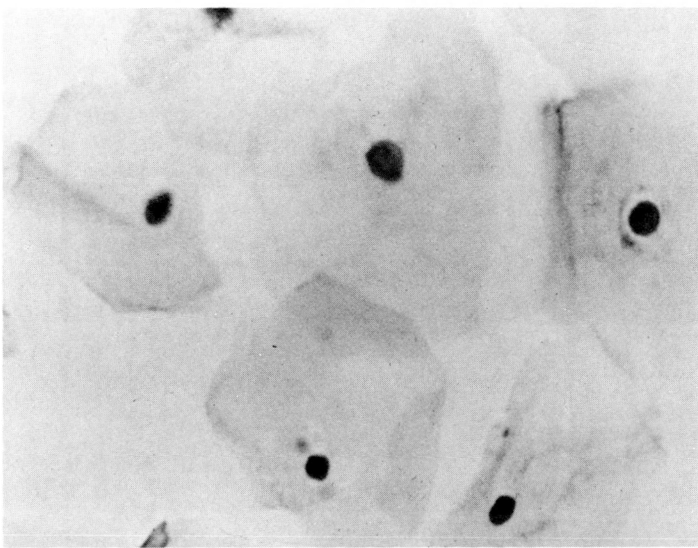

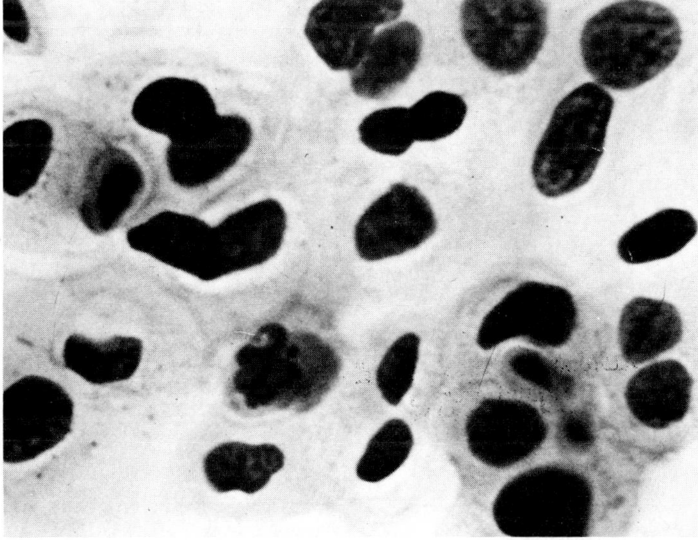

Normal cells from the cervix *(top)* and cancer cells from the cervix *(bottom).* Several characteristic features of cancer cells can be seen: The nuclei (the dark spots in the center of the cells) are much enlarged, and the cells vary greatly in size. (Photo courtesy of American Cancer Society)

Figure 17-1. Key Warning Signs of Cancer. (Source: American Cancer Society; used with permission.)

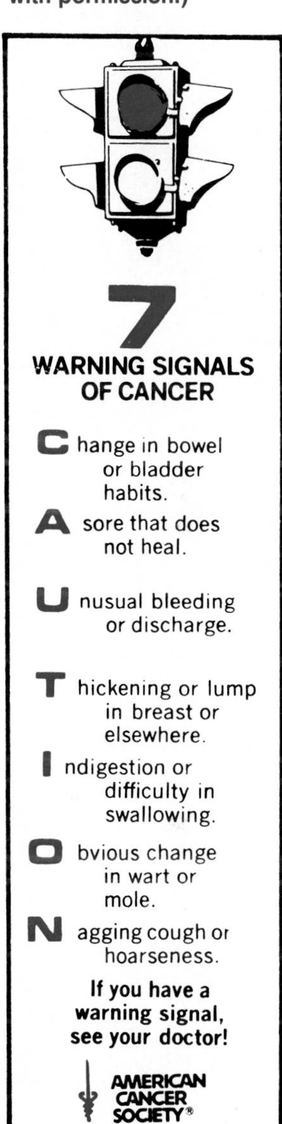

ance, as well as in behavior. Unlike normal cells, cancer cells vary greatly in size. The nuclei usually are much enlarged, and budding and fragmentation are common. There is great variation in the number of chromosomes, and sometimes they, too, fragment. The nucleus may divide in a normal manner, whereas the cell may not, and there may be many more granules than usual in the cytoplasm.

Tumors

Neoplasms New growths; tumors resulting from uncontrolled reproduction of abnormal cells.

Tumor Masses of new tissue.

Benign tumor Tumor restricted to growth within a capsule of connective tissue.

Malignant tumor Dangerous tumor that multiplies unhindered, supplanting normal cells.

The uncontrolled reproduction of abnormal cells leads to the formation of **neoplasms** (“new growths”), or **tumors**—masses of new tissue that serve no useful purpose. Tumors can be either benign or malignant in nature. All cancers stem from malignant tumors.

Benign tumors grow within capsules of connective tissue that restrict them to a local area. Further, the cells in benign tumors ordinarily reflect to some degree the structure and function of the normal cells of their tissue of origin; and since they remain somewhat specialized, they tend not to invade other types of tissue. Benign tumors, therefore, are stable and localized growths that are not inherently life-threatening. They can pose problems, however, if by virtue of their size or positioning they block crucial blood vessels or hinder the functioning of body systems. Once removed surgically, benign tumors usually will not recur.

Malignant tumors are fundamentally different and far more dangerous. Unhindered or only partially enclosed by connective-tissue capsules, malignant cells multiply rapidly, feeding off and ultimately supplanting normal cells. As entirely unspecialized units, malignant cells are capable of radical mutations; and because they adhere only loosely to one another, they easily can break away from the original tumor. These characteristics make malignant cells ideal invaders and colonizers of other tissues.

Metastasis

Metastasis Internal disease transmission through infiltration of malignant cells.

Cancer would not be such a deadly disease if malignancies spread only by direct extension into adjacent areas. Such localized growth, while potentially serious, at least confines the initial, or primary, tumor to a specific area on which treatment can be focused. Unfortunately, malignant cells not only can infiltrate neighboring tissues, but also are capable of breaking off from the primary tumor and traveling to distant parts of the body. This process of disease transmission, called **metastasis,** can take place via body cavities, the circulatory system, or the lymphatic system. Once established in a new area, often far away from the primary tumor, malignant cells grow into new tumors, which in turn can establish additional colonies in yet other areas of the body. In this way, a single malignant tumor can be responsible for the spread of the cancer throughout the body.

Because of metastasis, early detection is *the* crucial factor in cancer survival rates. Unless a malignancy is detected before it metastasizes extensively, the prognosis usually is poor. Each and every colony must be eradicted in order to rid the body of cancer—frequently an impossible task if the colonies are numerous and widely distributed.

Types of Cancer

Although cancers are popularly known by site names (lung cancer, breast cancer, etc.), oncologists (physicians who specialize in the treatment of cancer) prefer to classify them by tissue type. **Carcinomas,** the most common type of cancer, arise in the epithelium, the tissue layers that cover the exterior surfaces of the body and sheathe its internal organs and glands. Most cancers of the skin, lung, breast, stomach, intestines, prostate, and uterus are carcinomas, which tend to metastasize via the lymphatic system or by infiltrating body cavities. Considerably less common are **sarcomas,** cancers of the connective tissue (muscle, cartilage, bone) that frequently travel through the circulatory system. **Leukemias** and **lymphomas** are systemic cancers that arise, respectively, in the blood-forming tissues (primarily bone marrow) and in the lymphatic system. More specialized cancers include **gliomas** (nerve-tissue tumors) and **melanomas** (cancer of the melanin cells, which impart darkish coloring to the skin and hair).

Carcinoma Most common cancer, occurring in body's surface tissue.

Sarcoma Cancer of the connective tissues (muscle, cartilage, and bone).

Leukemia Cancer of the blood-forming tissue.

Lymphoma Cancer of the lymphatic system.

Glioma Nerve-tissue tumors.

Melanoma Cancer of the skin cells containing melanin.

A specific cancer's degree of malignancy and pattern of metastasis depends more on the type of tissue in which it originates than on the site of the primary tumor. Carcinomas of the skin, for example, have more in common with carcinomas of the lung than with melanomas. But since site names are universally used to classify cancers, we will discuss individual types by site of origin. Figure 17–2 indicates the different types of cancer, by site, and the proportion of cancer deaths associated with each of these types of cancer.

Skin Cancer

Of the more than 400,000 new cases of skin cancer diagnosed in the United States each year, all but a small percentage are localized growths that are easily detected and cured. Most commonly, skin cancers involve surface lesions that, although cancerous, rarely metastasize. But even though these disorders are usually minor, no cancer should be taken lightly. Any cankerlike sore that does not heal should prompt an immediate visit to the doctor.

A far more deadly form of skin cancer is melanoma, whose principal danger signal is a mole that for no apparent reason enlarges and begins to itch. If left untreated, the primary tumor (composed of cancerous melanin cells) will metastasize through the blood vessels, spreading cancer throughout the body. Every year, some 14,000 Americans are diagnosed as having melanoma, and about 5,000 die from it.

Excessive exposure to the ultraviolet rays of the sun has been implicated in the development of skin cancer, and fair-skinned individ-

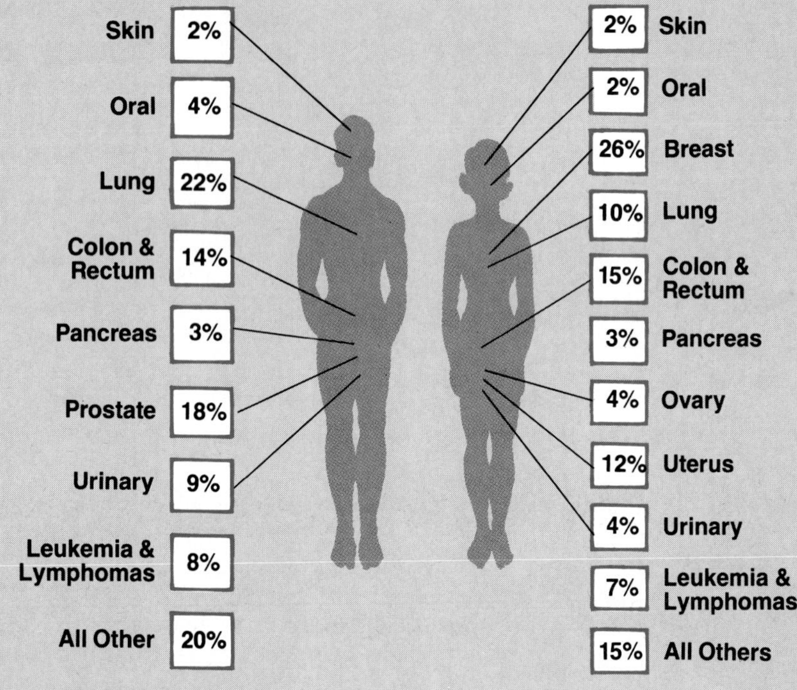

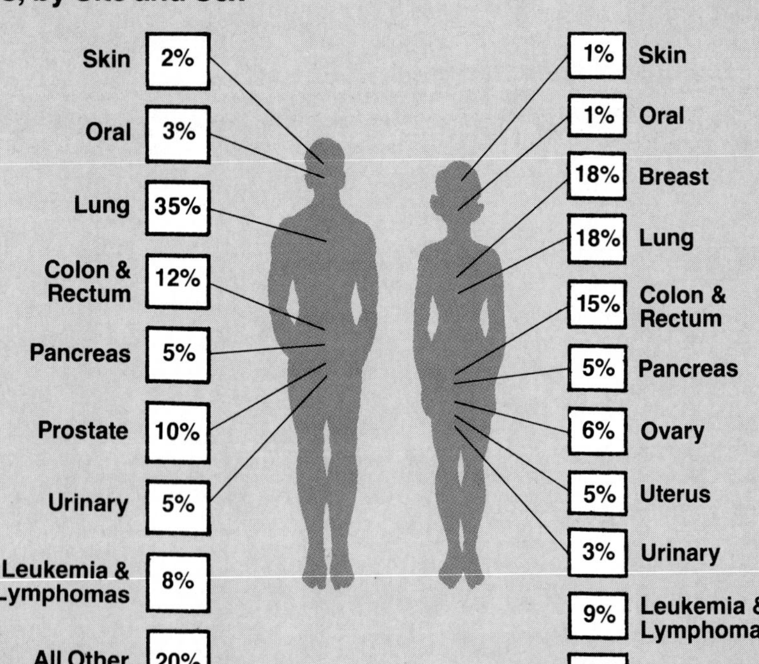

Figure 17–2. Percent of Cancer Cases and Deaths, by Site and Sex.
Estimates for 1984 show that lung cancer in men and breast cancer in women are still the most common forms, and the leading killers. (Nonmelanoma skin cancer and localized carcinomas are not included in the figures for cancer cases.) (Source: American Cancer Society; used with permission.)

uals apparently are more prone to suffer from it than are dark-skinned people. An effective filtering agent will block out most of the sun's ultraviolet radiation.

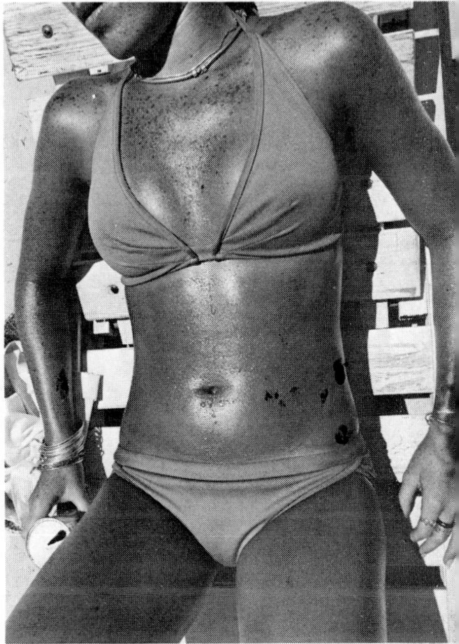

Suntanning has been seen as a sign of leisurely pleasure. However, doctors assert that it can cause skin cancer. (Photo © Antonio Mendoza/The Picture Cube)

Lung Cancer

More Americans die from lung cancer than from any other type of malignancy, and yet lung cancer is one of the most preventable forms of the disease. The reason for this paradox is cigarette smoking, which has been associated with approximately 75 percent of all incidences of lung cancer.

Typically, lung cancer begins as a carcinoma in the bronchial tree, the complex of passageways leading from the throat to the lungs themselves. From the bronchi, cancerous cells infiltrate one or (more rarely) both lungs, then metastasize via the lymphatic system throughout the upper body. Metastasis is rapid and lethal; untreated victims seldom survive longer than six to nine months after the onset of the disease. Most lung-cancer patients die from degeneration of the respiratory system or from secondary infections, usually after much suffering. Even with the most radical treatments, including radiation therapy and surgical removal of a cancerous lung, fewer than one in ten patients survives for five years (the accepted criterion of cancer cure).

The lung cancer death rate among women is rising at an alarming rate (16 percent in 1982 to 18 percent in 1984). In the near future lung cancer will be the leading cause of cancer deaths among women. If you are concerned about your risk of lung cancer, complete Self-Assessment Exercise 17.1, "What Is Your Risk of Lung Cancer?"

Colon-Rectum Cancer

In number of cases and number of deaths it causes, cancer of the colon and rectum ranks second only to lung cancer, and like that deadly disease it is becoming more common in the United States and Europe. Dietary habits may be responsible for this increase: fat-rich, fiber-poor diets have been correlated statistically to high rates of colon-rectum cancer. There also is evidence that the precancerous polyps from which the malignancy often arises may be inheritable.

Colon-rectum cancer tends to spread slowly from the primary tumor, involving first the lower digestive tract and then neighboring organs. If detected early, it can often be cured by surgical removal of the cancerous area. Once the disease becomes widespread, however, cure becomes difficult. Noticeable changes in bowel habits and non-hemorrhoidal bleeding from the rectum are the usual danger signals. An annual rectal examination provides the best chance for early detection.

Breast Cancer

Breast cancer is historically the number-one killer of women among cancers, although it is now being challenged for that position by lung

SELF-ASSESSMENT EXERCISE 17.1

What Is Your Risk of Lung Cancer

	A	B	C	D
	50–60	61+ or 40–49	25–40	Under 25
1. Age (at present)	10	5	0	0
	10+ Years	5–9 Years	1–4 Years	Few Months or Do Not Smoke
2. Number of years smoking cigarettes (or as ex-smokers)	40	30	15	0
	30–40	11–29	5–10	Do Not Smoke or Ex-smoker
3. Number of cigarettes you now smoke per day	20	15	5	0
	10–14	15–19	20–24	25+ or Do Not Smoke or Ex-smoker
4. Age you started smoking	10	7	3	0
	20 Years	10–19 Years	1–9 Years	Few Months or Never
5. Number of years working in coal mine or rock quarry	10	7	4	0
	20 Years	10–19 Years	1–9 Years	Few Months or Never
6. Number of years working in asbestos factory	20	15	5	0
	20 Years	10–19 Years	1–9 Years	Few Months or Never
7. Number of years working in other jobs such as sandblasting, tunneling, fiberglass, or grain elevator	5	3	1	0
	20 Years	10–19 Years	1–9 Years	Few Months or Never
8. Number of years working in chromium plating factory	5	3	1	0

	A	B	C	D
	Yes	—	—	No
9. Unexplained chronic coughing	5	—	—	0
	5+	3–4	1–2	None
10. Repeated episodes of respiratory infections (flu, pneumonia, or bronchitis) in past year	5	3	1	0
	Always	Often	Sometimes	Never
11. Feeling shortness of breath	5	3	1	0
12. Feeling tired or exhausted	5	3	1	0
13. Wheezing (chest) while breathing	5	3	1	0
Total				

Scoring: First, add up the total number of points under columns A, B, C, and D. Second, add up all row totals and once a total score has been calculated find the range your score is in from the chart below.

1. Lung Cancer

(a) For nonsmokers:

Score Range	Degree of Susceptibility
0–5	Low
6–17	Moderate
18–50	High
51+	Extremely high

(b) For smokers and (ex-smokers):

Score Range	Degree of Susceptibility
23–25	Moderate
26–35	Above moderate
36–54	High
55–90	Very high
90+	Extremely high

Source: Walter D. Sorochan. *Promoting Your Health,* New York, John S. Wiley. 1981, p. 322. Reprinted by permission of the author.

cancer. It is a sex-specific disease, striking more than 110,000 American women, but fewer than 1,000 men, a year. Most malignancies of the breast originate in the lining of the mammary ducts, grow slowly and remain localized for long periods of time, then metastasize via the lymphatic system. Treatment consisting of radical or modified mastectomy followed up by chemotherapy has proven quite effective, especially when the lymph nodes are not extensively involved. Currently, about 87 percent of all victims survive at least five years. Where the cancer has spread, however, the survival rate is under 50 percent.

Early detection is vital to successful treatment. Every woman over 20 should examine her breasts for unusual lumps at least once a month, and annual examinations by a physician are recommended after age 40.

Uterine Cancer

The uterus, the pear-shaped organ in which fetuses develop, is also a common site for cancer in women. Most uterine cancers are carcinomas of the cervix (the passageway from the vagina to the uterus) or of the endometrium (the lining of the uterus). In either case, unusual bleeding or discharge is a warning signal. Sexual intercourse at an early age and a history of many sexual partners are risk factors associated with cervical cancer. Endometrial cancer victims often show a history of infertility, high blood pressure, obesity, and late menopause. In recent years, cure rates for both kinds of uterine cancer have risen dramatically, to about 81 percent for cervical cancer when detected early and 88 percent for the endometrial variety when detected early—principally because of widespread use of the early-detection Pap test.

Prostate Cancer

The prostate is a small gland located below the neck of the bladder in men; its sole function is to produce the milky fluid released during sperm emission. Among men over 60, cancer of the prostate is a leading cause of death. If the malignancy is confined to the prostate itself, surgical removal of the gland can produce complete cure. Unfortunately, the disease often is diagnosed only after the primary tumor has metastasized into adjacent tissues, in which case the survival rate decreases radically. Difficulty in urinating usually accompanies the onset of the disease.

Oral Cancer

The term *oral cancer* is used to describe all malignancies of the lips, tongue, mouth, or throat. Twice as many men as women are afflicted with this type of cancer, the risk factors of which include the smoking or chewing of tobacco and heavy alcohol intake. Sores that bleed easily and difficulty in chewing or swallowing are among the normal danger signals. Dentists and dental hygenists trained in oral-cancer detection can spot its manifestations at an early stage, but such training is by no means universal. The survival rate varies substantially, depending on the site; the overall average is about 40 percent.

Leukemia

Cancer of the blood-forming tissues, such as bone marrow, is known generally as leukemia. The name is derived from the disease's outstanding symptom, an abnormally high count of immature leukocytes (white blood cells) in the bloodstream. Fully developed leukocytes comprise one of the body's principal defenses against infection. Immature ones cannot perform this vital task, and when present in large numbers they crowd out normal white blood cells, red blood cells (which carry oxygen to body tissues), and platelets (which control hemorrhaging). The consequent degeneration of the blood system leads to death from a variety of causes, of which secondary infections are the most common. Early signs of the disease may include fatigue, paleness, frequent infection, easy bruising, and nosebleeds or other hemorrhaging.

Leukemia's progression can be either acute or chronic. Acute leukemia, which accounts for a large proportion of the cancer deaths among children, is a particularly deadly form of cancer that until recently killed almost all its victims within a year's time. Newly developed chemotherapies have produced longer and longer remissions, and the overall survival rate for acute lymphocytic leukemia (a common type) is now about 30 percent. However, acute granulocytic leukemia (which is more common among adults) has a much lower survival rate.

Chronic leukemia is chiefly a disease of adulthood. Its slower progression boosts its five-year survival rate to around 35 percent, but most of its victims eventually succumb to secondary infections.

Lymphomas

The lymphatic system is a network of vessels that parallels and supplements the main circulatory system. Lymph, the colorless fluid carried in the lymphatic vessels, resembles blood but has no platelets or red blood cells. Its principal function is to carry away from the circulatory system bacteria and other harmful agents, which are collected in the lymph nodes scattered throughout the system from the neck to the groin. Of the various types of malignancies that can arise in this system, including lymphosarcomas and Hodgkin's disease, most begin in the lymph nodes, remain within the system through their early and middle stages, and spread to neighboring tissue only when the disease is far advanced. The principal symptom of almost all lymphomas is enlargement of the involved nodes and, in many cases, of the spleen.

When detected in the early, localized stage, lymphomas can often be eradicated with radiation therapy. Within the past decade, highly effective chemotherapy programs have dramatically raised the five-year survival rate for persons with more advanced lymphomas. Hodgkin's disease, in particular, has become a heartening success story. A lymphoma that tends to strike young adults (especially males), Hodgkin's disease once was almost uniformly fatal unless diagnosed at a very early stage. Today, up to three-fourths of all victims survive at least five years, and apparently are cured.

Known and Suspected Causes

Carcinogen Cancer-causing substance.

The identification of the causes of cancer remains complicated. Most studies establishing links between a potential risk-increasing factor and cancer take many years to conduct and are very expensive. Since the biochemical mechanisms of cancer cells are not fully understood, the studies are open to interpretation, leading to controversy (particularly when economic interests are at stake). However, in some cases, such as smoking and lung cancer, the evidence of a causal connection is overwhelming. Known or suspected factors in the development of cancer include radiation, **carcinogens** of various kinds (including those in tobacco), viruses, heredity, and diet.

Radiation

Electromagnetic radiation, the energy released in waves by the motion of electric charges, can take the form of radio waves, microwaves, infrared or ultraviolet radiation, X rays, or gamma rays. Normal cells bombarded with an abnormal amount of electromagnetic radiation of any kind often undergo changes, or mutations, some of which apparently produce malignancy. Prolonged and excessive exposure to the ultraviolet rays of the sun, for example, has long been associated with an increased incidence of skin cancer. More dangerous are large doses of X rays. Until the 1950s, knowledge of the dangers posed by X rays was limited, and patients, radiologists, dentists, and technicians alike were insufficiently protected during X-ray examinations. The result was a high incidence of leukemia and other cancers among these groups. Today, only relatively small doses of X rays are given at any one time, and patients, as well as hospital and dental personnel, are carefully shielded. Patients undergoing X-ray examinations or radiation therapy should request a gonadal shield if they are not given one, because the reproductive organs are particularly sensitive to radiation.

Some elements, such as radium and uranium, spontaneously release radiation and so pose an extreme hazard to individuals exposed to them. Before the dangers of their jobs were properly understood, uranium miners were exposed to large amounts of that dangerous element, and factory workers who applied luminous paint to watch and clock dials regularly ingested radium by using their mouths to moisten paint brushes. These practices led to high rates of lung cancer among uranium miners and of bone cancer among radium workers (because ingested radium salts are deposited in bone tissue). Also prone to develop cancer are all individuals exposed to the enormous amounts of radiation released by nuclear weapons. Survivors of the atomic bombs dropped on Hiroshima and Nagasaki, as well as unshielded observers of open-air nuclear weapons tests of the 1940s and 1950s, are at greater risk of developing leukemia, because blood-forming tissues are highly susceptible to damage from nuclear radiation.

Carcinogens

A wide range of chemicals and drugs are classified as known or suspected carcinogens (cancer-promoting substances) or cocarcinogens (substances that when combined with other chemicals promote cancer). Carcinogens are identified in two ways: (1) by statistical correlation in studies matching the incidence of cancer with individuals exposed to suspected carcinogens; (2) by laboratory experiments in which animals whose physiological processes resemble those of humans are administered doses of suspected carcinogens and monitored for cancer.

Research on carcinogens has sparked much criticism, especially from industries in which profits depend upon manufacturing or using allegedly cancer-causing substances. Usually, critics point out that no researcher has ever discovered an exact mechanism linking a carcinogen to the development of cancer and that no laboratory experiment has ever shown that carcinogens produce cancer in human beings. The statistical and experimental evidence associating some substances with cancer is so overwhelming, however, that the lack of an identifiable mechanism (a difficult phenomenon to isolate in even the simplest of disease processes) seems a weak objection at best. The predictive value of laboratory tests on certain animals has been demonstrated many times in the past.

Tobacco

Many studies, carried out in different countries, have demonstrated that individuals who smoke cigarettes are anywhere from six to twenty times more likely (depending on the number and kind of cigarettes smoked) than nonsmokers to suffer from lung cancer. Laboratory experiments support this conclusion: for instance, dogs taught to smoke cigarettes (through tubes) will often develop lung cancer.

Tobacco smoke apparently precipitates cancer in several ways. So-

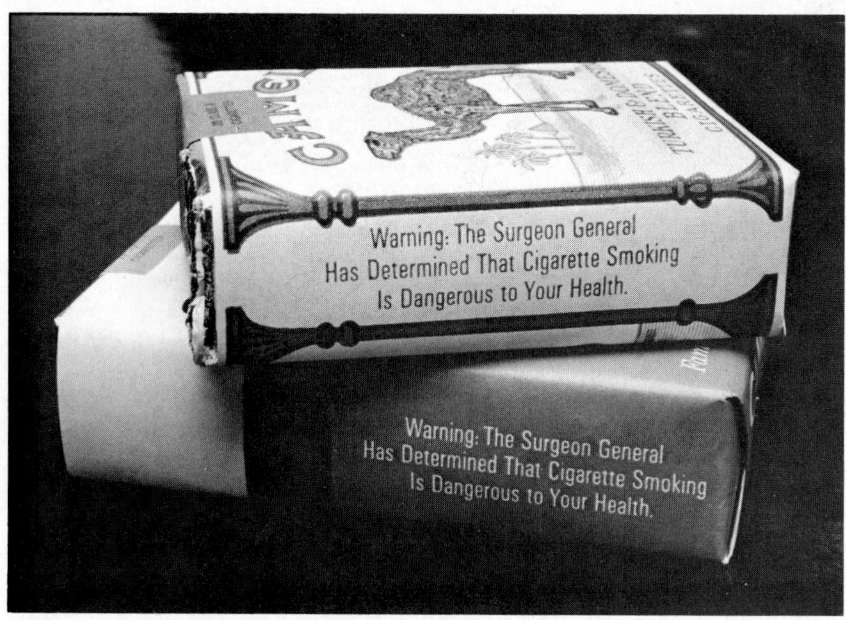

The federal government continues to alert the public to the health hazards of cigarette smoking. (Photo © Joel Gordon 1979/Joel Gordon Photography)

called tar, a major constitutent of cigarette smoke, contains several known carcinogens and cocarcinogens. Equally important is the destructive effect of inhaled cigarette smoke on the inner surfaces of the bronchial passages, where most malignancies of the lung originate. The bronchi of long-term smokers often display a precancerous condition in which the cilia (threadlike hairs, the constant sweeping motion of which clears the passages of foreign substances) are immobilized or destroyed and the passages themselves are clogged with mucus. This condition may be reversible once the irritation is removed.

The use of cigarettes low in tar and nicotine, as well as those equipped with a filter, does reduce the risk of lung cancer — but only if the person who switches to a safer cigarette does not increase the number of cigarettes smoked nor inhale more deeply. And whether or not the cigarette of choice is low in carcinogens, the irritating effect of constant smoking imperils the smoker. Fortunately, the available evidence indicates that smokers who quit the habit radically reduce their chances of dying from lung cancer.

Carcinogens in the Workplace

Carcinogens are often found in industry. Occupation-related cancer is especially prevalent wherever coal tar or its numerous derivatives (benzene, napthalene, creosote, pitch) is an integral part of the industrial process. The carcinogenic properties of asbestos were much publicized a few years ago, although less because of that substance's widespread use in industry than because of its presence in home appliances, such as hair dryers, and in insulation.

Such substances were not widely recognized as carcinogens until an unusually high number of workers in the industries involved were diagnosed as having cancer. Since such diagnoses typically occur 20 or 30 years after the initial exposure, what might be called a cancer time bomb is ticking away among hundreds of thousands of industrial workers exposed to carcinogens before the dangers were recognized and safety rules implemented. Today, employers are required by law to inform employees of possible carcinogens in the workplace and to take all measures necessary to minimize exposure to dangerous substances.

Carcinogens in the Environment

Pollution of the air, water, and soil by industrial wastes, automobile emissions, improperly dumped chemicals, and insecticides represents a significant, if largely unquantified, source of carcinogens breathed in or ingested by the general public. Many carcinogens are present in the enviroment around the factories in which they are used or produced. In addition, the hydrocarbons released in automobile exhausts have been shown to act as carcinogens, although this problem has eased somewhat as tougher emission-control standards have been implemented. In general, it is thought that city dwellers run a slightly higher risk (perhaps 10 percent) of developing lung cancer than rural inhabitants, because of the higher levels of air pollution found in cities. Those who live in the vicinity of carcinogen-emitting factories are even more at risk, as are those who, usually unknowingly, live on land where the soil or groundwater has been contaminated by carcinogenic chemicals dumped by industrial users.

Carcinogens in Food

Much controversy surrounds the subject of carcinogens ingested in food and drink. In the past 50 years, an increasing number of preservatives and additives have appeared in foods, and several of these very widely used substances have been associated with malignancies.

A particularly complex debate centers around **nitrates** and **nitrites,** which are added to many luncheon meats and to hot dogs, ham, and bacon, among other foods. These substances are used both to retard the growth of bacteria, and thus prevent food poisoning, and to impart a pinkish color that supposedly adds to the products' attractiveness. Some scientists have argued that ingested nitrates and nitrites combine in the body with amines to produce nitrosamines, which are known carcinogens. This claim is backed up with experiments on animals and with studies of populations whose diet is high in nitrates. Critics of these studies argue that nitrates and nitrites are destroyed in the cooking process. Although the issue is still controversial, the Food and Drug Administration has been attempting to limit the amount of nitrates and nitrites in cured meats. Similar controversies involve such additives and preservatives as BHT and MSG.

Nitrates Controversial substances used in foods to retard bacterial growth.

Nitrites Like nitrates, used as a meat preservative despite evidence of carcinogenic potential.

Perhaps the most notorious example of a carcinogenic prescription drug is that of diethylstilbesterol (DES), a synthetic estrogen (female

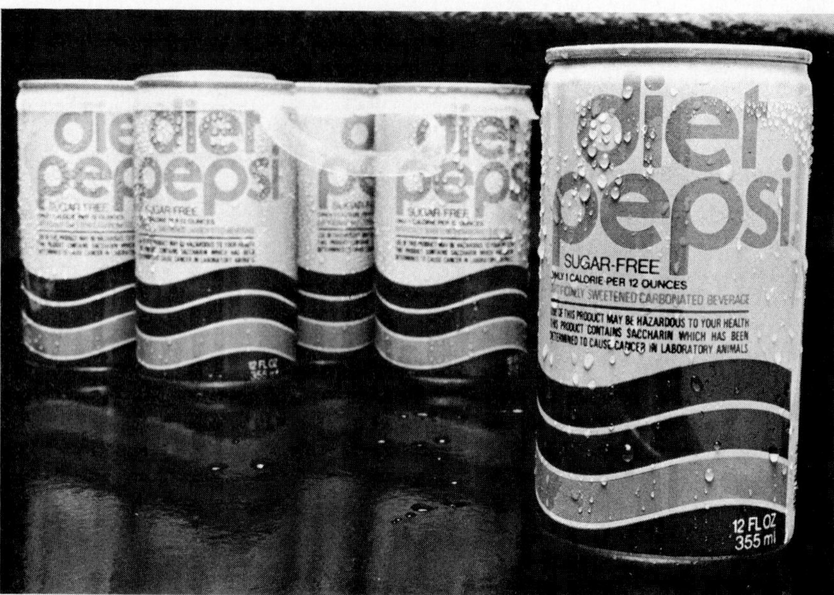

Recently it was determined that saccharin, often found in diet soda drinks, is a cancer-causing ingredient. The Department of Health is trying to alert the public to this fact, and many soda manufacturers are now using NutraSweet. (Photo © Joel Gordon 1978/Joel Gordon Photography)

sex hormone). DES was hailed as a miracle drug in the 1950s, when it was used to aid women prone to miscarriages. Then in the late 1960s, doctors began reporting an alarmingly high incidence of vaginal cancer among the daughters of mothers who had used DES. Subsequent research identified DES as a carcinogen, and it was taken off the market. Synthetic estrogens are still used, however, to ease the discomforts of female menopause and male prostate disease. In both cases, careful monitoring by a physician is essential to minimize the risk of cancer.

Viruses

Although it is known that viruses, the submicroscopic agents responsible for many communicable diseases, can cause cancer in animals, no human-cancer virus has ever been isolated. Viruses interest cancer researchers because they can survive and multiply only by infiltrating normal cells and subverting their hosts' functions—for example, causing them to multiply abnormally or using their resources to produce more viruses. This process seems so cancerlike that some scientists believe it will turn out to be the key to the mystery of why cells turn malignant.

Most closely linked to cancer is the herpes virus, which causes cold sores, fever blisters, and the sexually transmitted disease of the same name. A herpes variant known as the Epstein-Barr virus is almost always present in tissues affected by Burkitt's lymphoma, a rare cancer found only in certain parts of Africa. Herpes simplex virus regularly turns up in tissue samples revealing the precancerous stage of cervical cancer, and herpes-like particles have been associated with leukemia.

Other types of cancer linked to viruses include a sarcoma of the nose and pharynx and Hodgkin's disease. In one noteworthy study, conducted at Harvard's School of Public Health, investigators found a high correlation between the incidence of Hodgkin's disease and an earlier bout of infectious mononucleosis, a viral infection.[1]

Heredity

Very few cancers are directly inheritable. (An exception is retinoblastoma, a very rare tumor of the eye.) The incidence of breast, uterine, and lung cancer among blood relatives does exceed statistical probability, but any argument in favor of a genetic factor in cancers must take into account the fact that family members share a similar environment. Hereditary influences seem most likely in the case of breast cancer, whose victims tend to be related by blood to at least one other victim, and least probable in the case of lung cancer, because the family's predisposition here may often be toward smoking rather than toward developing cancer.

Diet

Researchers have noted that colon-rectum cancer is more prevalent in societies, the traditional diet of which is high in fats and low in fiber. One possible explanation for this phenomenon hinges on the length of time it takes different types of food to pass through the intestines. Fats are difficult to digest and remain in the intestines for a longer period of time than do fibrous foods. According to the theory, the constant irritation of prolonged digestion caused by fat-rich diets predisposes the intestinal tissues to malignancies, much as the constant irritation of smoking predisposes the lung tissues to cancer.

Another possible dietary link to cancer is cholesterol, which, some scientists believe, overstimulates the metabolism of breast tissue and thus promotes the development of breast cancer. Buttressing this theory is the fact that a statistically significant percentage of breast-cancer victims have high-cholesterol diets.

Prevention and Early Detection

Assessing Your Risk

The American Cancer Society has published a simple, basic test to help you assess some important risk factors for common types of cancer (see Self-Assessment Exercise 17.2). The test also describes a few safeguards that can help to protect you against some of the most basic risks.

SELF-ASSESSMENT EXERCISE 17.2

Your Cancer Risk

Your risk of developing cancer increases with age and depends on life style and your personal/family medical history. This short test covers some important aspects of cancer risks or warnings as determined by the American Cancer Society. Circle Yes or No to answer each question, then look at the Safeguards that follow.

For Men and Women

1. Do you smoke cigarettes? . . . . Yes No
2. Do you work with any of these substances—arsenic, vinyl chloride, asbestos, nickel, chromates, uranium? . . . . Yes No
3. Do you have a light complexion and spend much time in the sun? . . . . Yes No
4. Have any of your close relatives had colon or rectum cancer? . . . . Yes No

For Women Only

1. Have you noticed vaginal bleeding after the occurrence of menopause? . . . . Yes No
2. Do you have vaginal bleeding between menstrual periods? . . . . Yes No
3. Do you take hormones for menopausal symptoms? . . . . Yes No
4. Have you or any of your close relatives had breast cancer? . . . . Yes No
5. Was your first child born after you were 30 years old? . . Yes No

Even if you have answered No to all of these questions, you should still talk with your physician about how often you need cancer-related checkups.

Explanations and Safeguards

Men and Women

1. **Smoking:** Your risk of developing lung cancer and other cancers, heart disease, and emphysema increases, depending on how many cigarettes you smoke per day. If you do smoke and stop smoking now, your risk factors will decrease. *Safeguard:* Don't smoke.

2. **Workplace Hazards:** Your risk of developing certain cancers increases with the number of years of exposure to the substances listed, but with uranium and asbestos, it further increases if you also smoke cigarettes. *Safeguard:* Wear protective clothing and masks, and don't smoke.

3. **Skin Cancer:** Avoid overexposure to sunlight, but if you have a light complexion you need extra protection. *Safeguard:* Ask your pharmacist for a good sunscreen cream or lotion.

4. **Colon/Rectum Cancers:** Your risk increases if polyps of the colon "run in the family" or if close relatives have had colorectal cancer. Blood in the stool can be a sign of cancer. *Safeguard:* See your physician once a year after age 40. Find out how often you need a rectal examination, proctoscopy, and test for hidden blood in the stool.

Women Only

1, 2, & 3. Uterine Cancer: Bleeding between menstrual periods may be a sign of cancer of the endometrium or cervix. *Safeguard:* See your physician for a pelvic examination, Pap test, and other diagnostic tests as needed.

1, 2, & 3. Endometrial Cancer: Your risk increases after age 50. Women taking hormones after menopause have a higher risk of developing endometrial cancer. *Safeguard:* Report abnormal vaginal bleeding to your physician.

4, 5. Breast Cancer: Your risk increases after age 50. A personal or family history of breast cancer places you at increased risk of developing breast cancer. Women who have never had children or had their first child after age 30 are also at higher risk. *Safeguard:* Ask your physician how often you need a physical examination of the breast and mammography (x-ray examination). Do breast self-examination once a month.

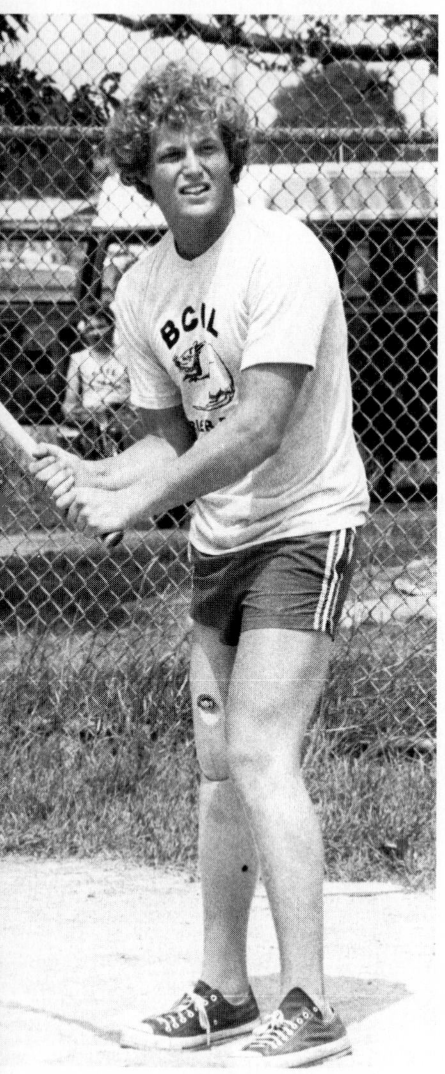

Edward Kennedy Jr., the son of Senator Edward Kennedy, lost a leg to cancer, but still pursues an active life. (Photo from United Press International)

Lung and skin cancer are the most prominent, but not the only, examples of largely preventable malignancies. You can reduce your chances of developing other types of cancer as well by knowing and avoiding their possible causes or risk factors. Many risk factors are harmful to overall health anyway, so it makes sense to avoid them whether or not you fear cancer. A high-fat, low-fiber diet, for example, may promote colon-rectum cancer, and it certainly *does* increase your risk of developing cardiovascular disease. And cigarette smoking, the single most dangerous cancer risk factor, is a definite contributor to heart and circulatory problems.

But even the healthiest life-style will not ensure a cancer-free life. After avoidance of risk factors, the most important weapon available in the fight against cancer is early detection of the disease. The common types of malignancy can be treated successfully if diagnosed before extensive metastasis takes place. To maximize your chances of survival if cancer does strike, you must be aware of and act promptly upon noticing the seven CAUTION signals noted by the American Cancer Society and listed earlier in this chapter. In addition, you should consult with your physician — especially if you appear to be at high risk — about regular cancer checkups. You should take advantage of the numerous early-detection tests and procedures available, most of which must be administered by a physician or a specially qualified technician.

Procedures for Early Detection

A guide to prevention and early detection of the six most common cancers is provided in Table 17–1, which lists risk factors, warning signals, and early-detection tests associated with each type of malignancy. The risk factors and warning signals are largely self-explanatory, but some of the early-detection tests may be unfamiliar to most laypeople. Of the tests for lung cancer, the chest X ray is the most widely used, but it will not always detect a malignancy in time to permit successful treatment. Newer techniques such as sputum cytology (analysis of sputum samples for indications of cell changes) and the use of a fiberoptic bronchoscope (a device that permits direct examination of the bronchi) are designed to detect lung cancer in its earliest stages; although their value is debated, they are recommended for high-risk individuals.

Several of the other tests mentioned in Table 17–1 are simple procedures that can be performed quickly and easily in the course of a physical examination. Every woman over a certain age (40, according to the American Cancer Society) should have her breasts examined by a physician at least once a year. Persons of both sexes over age 40 should make sure that their annual checkups include a digital rectal examination, and some people should have a more extended examina-

Table 17–1 **Watching Out for Cancer**

Site	Risk Factors	Warning Signals	Early Detection
Lung	Heavy cigarette smoking or smoking for 20 or more years; exposure to certain industrial substances	Persistent cough, sputum streaked with blood, recurrent attacks of pneumonia or bronchitis	Difficult to detect early; X ray, sputum cytology, and fiberoptic bronchoscope may be used to diagnose
Breast	Over age 50: no children, or first child after age 30	Lumps or thickening in the breast; other breast changes such as swelling, puckering, dimpling, skin irritation; distortion or scaliness of nipples; nipple discharge, pain, or tenderness	Breast self-examination, physical exam, mammography
Uterus	Early age at first intercourse, multiple sex partners, history of infertility, failure of ovulation, estrogen therapy, late menopause, combination of diabetes, hypertension, and obesity	Unusual bleeding or discharge	Pap test
Colon/ rectum	Family history of colon/rectum cancer; personal or family history of polyps in colon or rectum; ulcerative colitis; (possibly) dietary factors	Unusual bleeding, change in bowel habits	Digital rectal examination, proctoscopy, other tests
Skin	Excessive exposure to the sun, fair complexion, occupational exposure to certain carcinogens	Unusual skin condition, change in size or color of mole or other darkly pigmented spot	Self-examination
Oral cavity	Heavy smoking and drinking, use of chewing tobacco	A sore that bleeds easily and does not heal; lump or thickening; reddish or whitish patch that persists; difficulty in chewing, swallowing, or moving tongue or jaws	Dental examination

Source: American Cancer Society

tion, such as a **proctoscopy,** with the use of a hollow, lighted tube. The **Pap test,** named after its inventor, Dr. George Papanicolaou, is perhaps the single most effective early-detection method currently available and should be part of a woman's regular physical exam. This painless procedure, which involves the analysis of vaginal fluid and

Proctoscopy Inspection of the rectum with a special instrument.

Pap smear Detection method for cervical cancer.

tissue taken from the wall of the cervix, is almost uniformly successful in detecting cervical cancer before it spreads.

A far more controversial procedure is mammography, the use of X rays to detect abnormal lumps or lesions in the breasts. Some physicians feel that such tests are both unnecessary and dangerous for most women. Experts generally agree, however, that mammography can be a valuable diagnostic aid for high-risk women.

The only early-detection test that can be administered without the aid of a doctor or technician is the breast self-examination. From her early 20s on, every woman should examine her breasts at least once a month, preferably right after menstruation. The recommended procedure for breast self-examination is given in Figure 17–3; following this procedure is a valuable means of detecting breast cancer at an early stage.

A form of cancer which affects young men is cancer of the testes, although its incidence is not high. Figure 17–4 explains the facts about testicular cancer—a form of cancer that can be detected early—and the methods of self-examination.

Treatment

Surgery is the preferred form of treatment for cancer when the primary tumor is not in a vital organ and has not begun to invade the tissue around it. In the past, a surgeon usually removed healthy tissue along with the tumor, trying to make sure that no cancer cells remained. Today many surgeons feel that such radical procedures are unnecessary; they believe that the body's defense mechanisms will destroy any stray cancerous cells left over after the primary tumor is removed. In cases such as a mole that has become cancerous, however, it seems safer to take much more of the skin around than appears necessary.

If the cancer has invaded nearby lymph nodes, the surgeon can remove these as well. But if the malignancy has metastasized to distant parts of the body or sent cells into the bloodstream, surgery is useless. Chemotherapy and radiation, the treatments of choice for metastasized cancer, often are used today in conjunction with surgery in an effort to eliminate new colonies that might have passed unnoticed.

Cancers of the skin, colon and rectum, uterus, and breast can, as a rule, be successfully treated by surgery. In the case of breast surgery, a difference of opinion has arisen over how much tissue to remove. Radical breast removal, including the lymph nodes of the armpit, has in many cases been supplanted by "lumpectomy," the removal of the lump only, with equally good survival rates.

Figure 17–3. How to Examine Your Breasts. (Source: © 1977, American Cancer Society)

FOR WOMEN ONLY

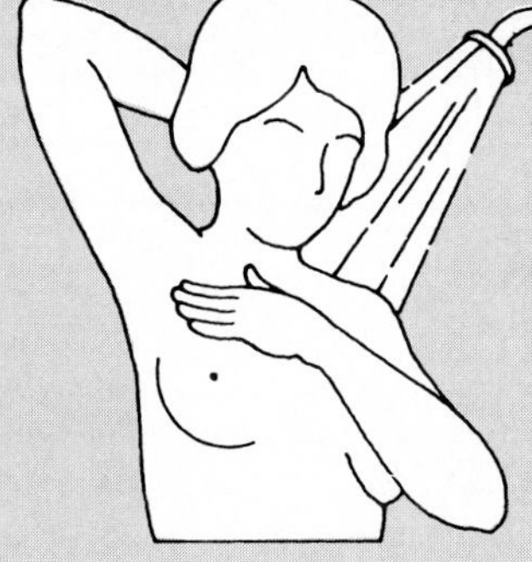

1 **In the Shower:**

Examine your breasts during bath or shower; hands glide easier over wet skin. Fingers flat, move gently over part of each breast. Use right hand to examine left breast, left hand for right breast. Check for any lump, hard knot, or thickening.

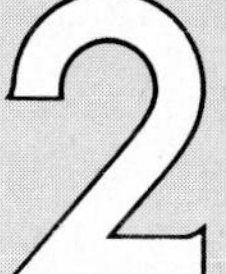

2 **Before a Mirror:**

Inspect your breasts with arms at your sides. Next, raise your arms high overhead. Look for any changes in contour of each breast, a swelling, dimpling of skin, or changes in the nipple.

Then, rest palms on hips and press down firmly to flex your chest muscles. Left and right breast will not exactly match—few women's breasts do.

Regular inspection shows what is normal for you and will give you confidence in your examination.

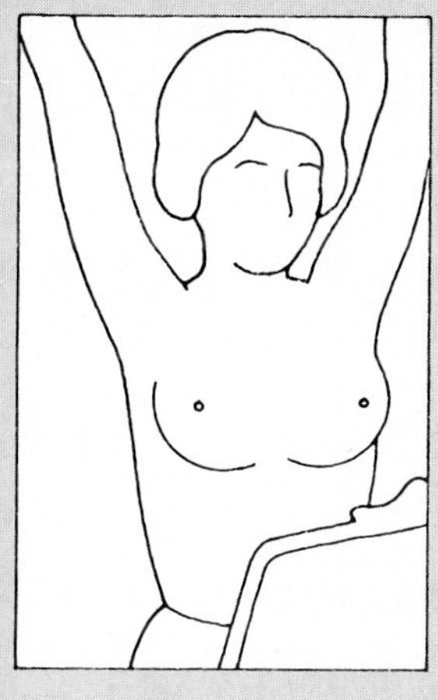

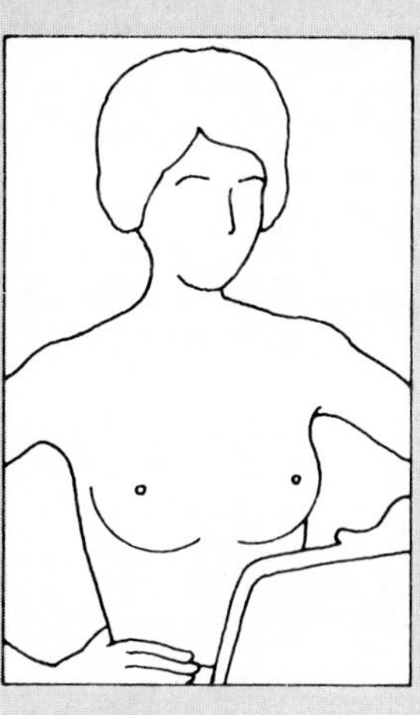

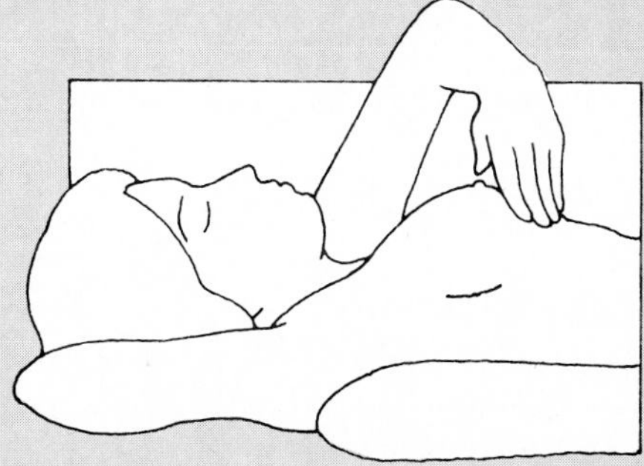

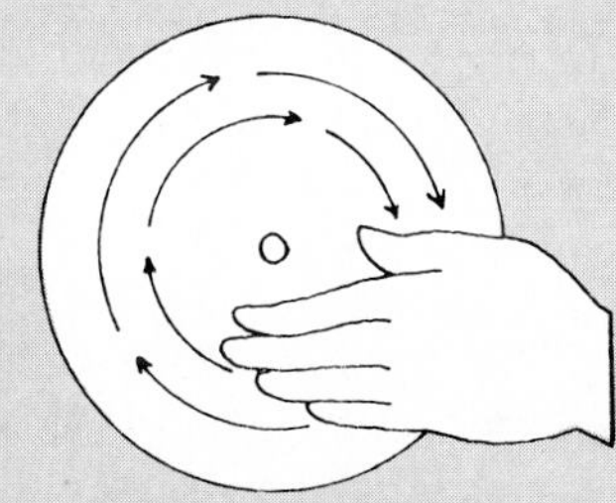

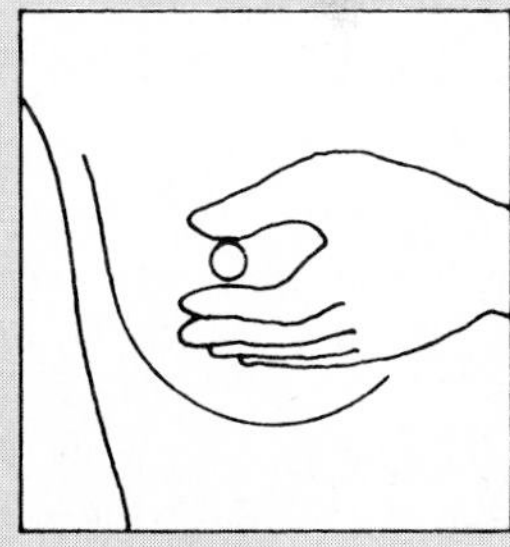

3 **Lying Down:**

To examine your right breast, put a pillow or folded towel under your right shoulder. Place right hand behind your head—this distributes breast tissue more evenly on the chest. With left hand, fingers flat, press gently in small circular motions around an imaginary clock face. Begin at outermost top of your right breast for 12 o'clock, then move to 1 o'clock, and so on around the circle back to 12. A ridge of firm tissue in the lower curve of each breast is normal. Then move in an inch, toward the nipple. Keep circling to examine *every part of your breast,* including nipple. This requires at least three more circles. Now slowly repeat procedure on your left breast with a pillow under your left shoulder and left hand behind head. Notice how your breast structure feels.

Finally, squeeze the nipple of each breast gently between thumb and index finger. Report any discharge, clear or bloody, to your doctor promptly.

Figure 17-4. How to Examine Your Testes.

FOR MEN ONLY

Cancer of the testes—the male reproductive glands—is one of the most common cancers in men 15 to 34 years of age. It accounts for 12 percent of all cancer deaths in this group.

If discovered in the early stages, testicular cancer can be treated promptly and effectively. It's important for you to take time to learn the basic facts about this type of cancer—its symptoms, treatment, and what you can do to get the help you need when it counts.

A MAJOR RISK FACTOR

Men who have an undescended or partially descended testicle are at a much higher risk of developing testicular cancer than others.

However, it is a simple procedure to correct the undescended testicle condition. See your doctor if this applies to you.

WHAT ARE THE SYMPTOMS?

The first sign of testicular cancer is usually a slight enlargement of one of the testes, and a change in its consistency.

Pain may be absent, but often there is a dull ache in the lower abdomen and groin, together with a sensation of dragging and heaviness.

WHAT CAN I DO?

Your best hope for early detection of testicular cancer is a simple three-minute monthly self-examination. The best time is after a warm bath or shower, when the scrotal skin is most relaxed.

Roll each testicle gently between the thumb and fingers of both hands. If you find any hard lumps or nodules, you should see your doctor promptly. They may not be malignant, but only your doctor can make the diagnosis.

Following a thorough physical examination, your doctor may perform certain x-ray studies to make the most accurate diagnosis possible.

TREATMENT

Surgery is usually the preferred treatment, and in certain cases it may be used together with radiation therapy or chemotherapy.

A GOOD CHANCE OF CURE

Although the five-year survival rate for all cases of testicular cancer is 68 percent, the most common type of testicular cancer—seminoma—has a survival rate approaching 100 percent in cases detected and treated early.

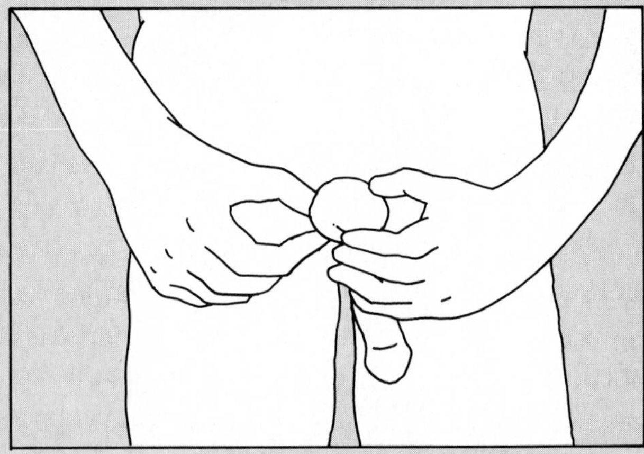

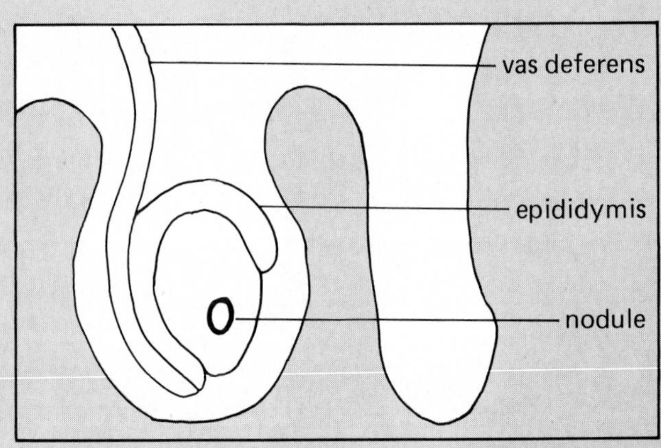

Source: American Cancer Society.

Radiation Therapy

Because malignant cells are more sensitive than normal cells to damage by radiation, X rays can selectively kill cancer cells without killing healthy tissue. In addition, X-ray machines can produce radiation of different wavelengths, allowing the therapist to select the degree of penetration desired. The radiotherapist also can focus the stream of radiation precisely on the malignant area. The growing use of particle accelerators, which provide simultaneous streams of different kinds of particles that penetrate to different depths, further adds to the value of **radiation therapy** in treating many cancers.

Radiation therapy Use of X-ray machines to treat cancer.

Sometimes the radiotherapist will choose to implant rods of irradiated cobalt at the site of the cancer. The cobalt in these rods stays radioactive for some time, emitting cell-destroying gamma rays without requiring the patient to make regular visits to the hospital. When the radioactivity is lost, the cobalt package must then be replaced.

Chemotherapy

Chemotherapy, the use of drugs or other chemicals to fight disease, is the newest and most promising avenue of cancer treatment. Almost unknown 25 years ago, chemotherapy has become the most effective form of treatment available against several types of cancer, including leukemia, lymphomas, and metastasized breast cancer. Most chemotherapy programs employ batteries of various drugs, administered both orally and intravenously. The scores of anticancer drugs currently in use can be divided into three general categories:

Chemotherapy Use of drugs or chemicals to treat cancer.

1. Drugs that upset normal metabolism of the cell.
2. Hormones that inhibit tumor growth.
3. Drugs that increase the body's resistance to the tumor cells (immunological agents).

Drugs That Upset Normal Cell Metabolism

Drugs that upset normal cell metabolism make it impossible for the cell to use the materials it ordinarily uses. The difficulty in employing such agents is that normal cells are affected along with cancerous cells, though at a slower rate.

An interesting example of this type of drug is so-called nitrogen mustard, a derivative of mustard gas. During World War I, both sides used mustard gas, which burned away exposed areas of skin and destroyed the lungs. Decades later, researchers noted that mustard gas also destroys white blood cells and conjectured that it may destroy abnormal white cells faster than normal ones. If so, it might work wonders in treating leukemia victims, who have an enormous supply of abnormal white cells. Nitrogen mustard turned out to have

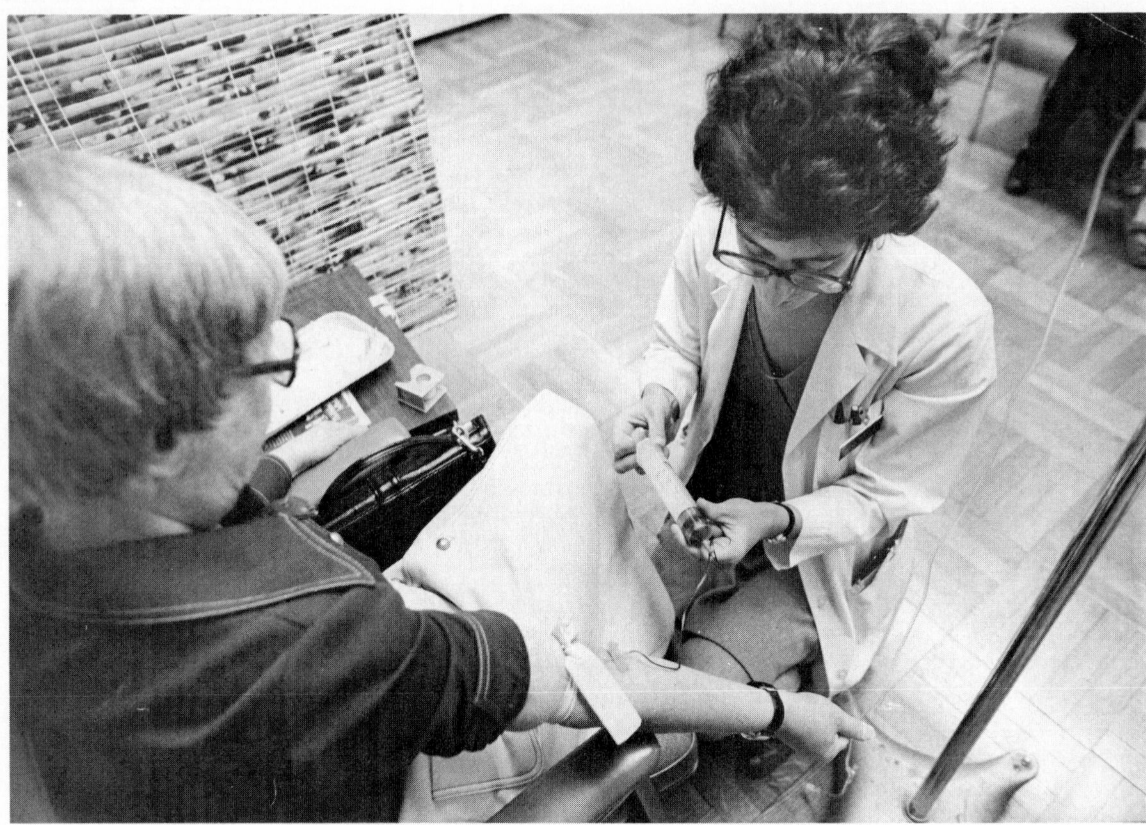

Chemotherapy is a method of cancer treatment involving the use of drugs to fight the disease. It has been relatively successful in the fight to overcome some forms of cancer. (Photo © Sepp Seitz 1982/Woodfin Camp & Associates)

exactly this beneficial effect, not only against leukemias, but also against lymphomas and Hodgkin's disease.

Hormones That Inhibit Tumor Growth

Hormones that inhibit tumor growth are especially effective against tumors of the endocrine glands and other organs that normally depend on hormones. This kind of therapy makes the patient much more comfortable, although it doesn't cure. It has been used against thyroid cancer and against cancer of the breast, uterus, prostate, and kidney.

Immunological Agents

Among drugs that increase immune capability, 5-fluorouracil is a prime example. When this agent is used on skin lesions, tissue at the site of the cancer becomes hypersensitive to cancer cells, and in some cases lesions heal without any scar. Even premalignant cells can be eradicated. The potential ability to destroy precancerous and cancerous cells by an immunological reaction is very important, since as many as 10 million living Americans now are estimated to have precancerous or cancerous skin lesions.

The basic problem with all forms of chemotherapy is that the substances used are powerful systemic agents, some of which are extremely toxic and most of which have undesirable side effects (nausea, hair loss, weakening of the body's defenses against infection). In the ongoing search for less toxic and more selective chemical agents, the most promising and widely publicized discovery has been **interferon,** a protein manufactured naturally in the body. When viruses invade a cell, the cell sometimes reacts by producing interferon, which acts to prevent the multiplication of the virus. Researchers hope that interferon can be targeted against cancerous cells, shutting down their ability to multiply and thus neutralizing them without any side effects on normal cells. Recently, genetically engineered bacteria have been used to produce interferon, increasing the supply and lowering the cost. However, experimental results have been inconclusive.

Interferon A protein released by body cells to combat viruses.

Summary

Cancer refers to a group of diseases characterized primarily by the uncontrolled growth of abnormal cells, which often spread from their original site to other areas of the body. Early detection is the most important factor in successfully treating cancer, and a doctor should be consulted as soon as any of the warning signals appear.

Cancer arises when cells fail to stop dividing and form tumors. Tumors may be benign, when they are restricted to a local area, or malignant, when they spread rapidly. When cancer cells break away from the original tumor and travel to other parts of the body, they are said to metastasize.

Cancers can be classified by tissue type. Carcinomas arise in the epithelium; sarcomas in connective tissue (muscle, cartilage, bone); leukemias in the blood-forming tissue; lymphomas in the lymphatic system; gliomas in nerve tissue; and melanomas in the melanin cells in the skin.

Most skin cancers are localized and easily detected and treated but should not be taken lightly. Melanoma is a far more deadly form, the principal danger signal of which is a mole that enlarges and begins to itch. If left untreated, it will metastasize.

More Americans die from lung cancer than from any other form of malignancy. Cigarette smoking is associated with it in about 75 percent of all cases. It typically begins as a carcinoma in the bronchial tree and rapidly metastasizes.

Colon-rectum cancer has been associated with dietary habits. It spreads slowly and if detected early can often be cured by surgery. Breast cancer is the number-one killer of women among cancers, but lung cancer will soon assume this position. Most malignancies begin in the lining of the mammary ducts, grow slowly, but then metastasize via the lymphatic system. Other forms of cancer include uterine cancers, cancer of the prostate, oral cancer, leukemia, and lymphomas.

Known and suspected causes of cancer include radiation; carcinogens, including tobacco, chemicals in the workplace and environment, food additives, and drugs; viruses, heredity; and diet.

Prevention and early detection are essential in reducing the number of deaths from cancer. Prevention is based on a healthy life-style and the avoidance of specific risk factors. Early detection techniques include self-monitoring, annual physical examinations, and a variety of early-detection tests.

The treatment of cancer takes three forms: surgery, radiation therapy, and chemotherapy. Surgery is effective when the primary tumor has not begun to invade the tissue around it. Radiation therapy is based on the fact that malignant cells are more sensitive than normal cells to radiation; X rays and radioactive materials are used. Chemotherapy makes use of drugs that increase the body's resistance to the tumor cells. These drugs achieve success in many cases, but often produce undesirable effects.

Review and Discussion

1. What are the seven warning signs of cancer in the acronym CAUTION devised by the American Cancer Society?

2. Define benign tumor, malignant tumor, and metastasis.

3. Name and describe the six tissue types of cancer.

4. Name and describe the major types of cancer by body site.

5. What is the relationship between radiation and cancer?

6. Describe the major types of carcinogens.

7. Discuss viruses, heredity, and diet as risk factors in cancer.

8. What preventive measures can reduce the risk of cancer?

9. Discuss the major self-monitoring and early detection tests.

10. Describe the procedures for breast self-examination and for testicular self-examination.

11. What are the three main forms of treatment of cancer? In what cases are they used?

Further Reading

Cancer Facts and Figures 1985. New York: American Cancer Society, 1984.
The latest information on cancer—one of the many useful pamphlets available from the American Cancer Society. (Paperback.)

Pelletier, Kenneth R. *Mind as Healer, Mind as Slayer.* New York: Delacorte Press, 1977.
Includes a discussion of the relationship between psychological factors and cancer.

Prescott, David, and Abraham S. Flexer. *Cancer.* Sunderland, Mass.: Sinauer Associates, 1981.
A description of the causes of cancer and its treatment and prevention. (Paperback.)

Rosenbaum, Ernest H., and Isadora Rosenbaum. *A Comprehensive Guide for Cancer Patients and Their Families.* Palo Alto, Calif.: Bull Publishing Company, 1980.
A guide for the cancer patient, family, and friends. (Paperback.)

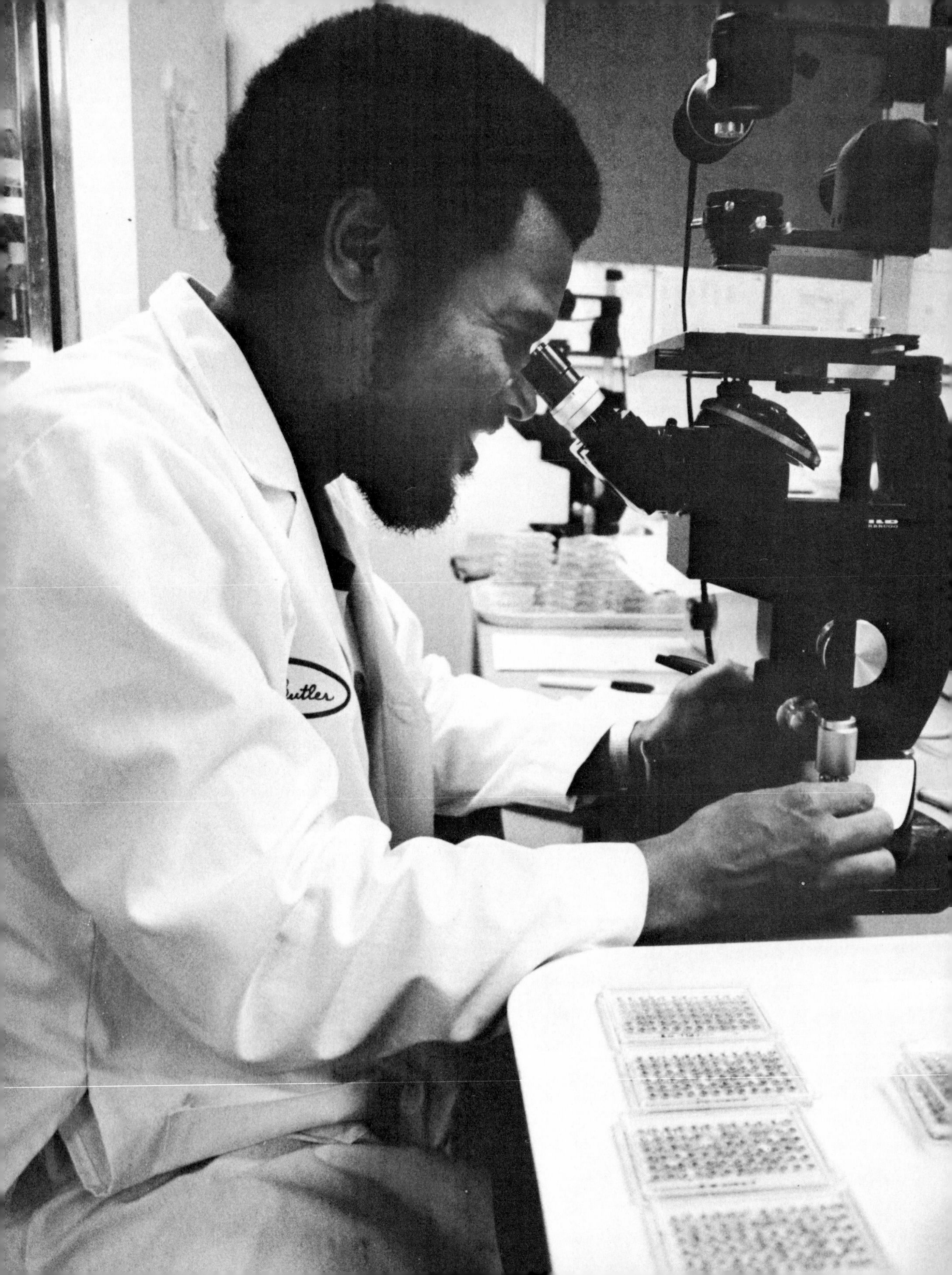

Chapter 18

Other Noncommunicable Diseases

KEY POINTS

- ☐ Unlike communicable diseases, which are spread by pathogens, noncommunicable diseases result when body systems, for a variety of reasons, malfunction or break down altogether.
- ☐ Immune-system disorders include allergies, autoimmune disorders, and immune deficiencies.
- ☐ Diabetes is a chronic disease of the pancreas that interferes with the body's ability to utilize sugar and starches to produce energy.
- ☐ Arthritis refers to a group of diseases that attack the body's joints or connective tissue.
- ☐ Chronic respiratory disorders, such as asthma, chronic bronchitis, and emphysema, interfere with the body's ability to take in oxygen and expel carbon dioxide.
- ☐ Some common genetic-related disorders include Down's syndrome, phenylketonuria (PKU), sickle-cell anemia, muscular dystrophy, and cystic fibrosis.
- ☐ Epilepsy and multiple sclerosis are neurological disorders that usually begin in younger years.

CARDIOVASCULAR diseases and cancer, covered in Chapters 16 and 17, are two of the most serious and widespread types of noncommunicable diseases — disorders that cannot spread from one person to another. In this chapter we will discuss other major noncommunicable diseases.

Unlike communicable diseases, which are caused and spread by pathogens, noncommunicable diseases develop when environmental conditions, genetic defects, negative life-styles, or as-yet inexplicable factors cause body systems to malfunction or break down altogether. A relatively minor flaw in the fine tuning of the body's immune system, for example, causes the immune-response disorders — notably, allergies — that plague millions of people. Most chronic respiratory diseases, on the other hand, are caused by negative life-styles or environmental conditions (smoking, air pollution, and so forth).

Generally, noncommunicable diseases are chronic disorders that develop slowly and recede slowly (if at all). Even the deadliest of noncommunicable diseases, such as emphysema and muscular dystrophy, take years to develop. Less serious noncommunicable disorders (asthma, arthritis, allergies) can plague a victim over decades. Except for disorders caused wholly or primarily by negative life-styles and environmental conditions (chronic bronchitis, emphysema, some cases of osteoarthritis), few noncommunicable diseases can be prevented from developing. Even fewer can be cured completely.

The very nature of noncommunicable diseases makes them difficult

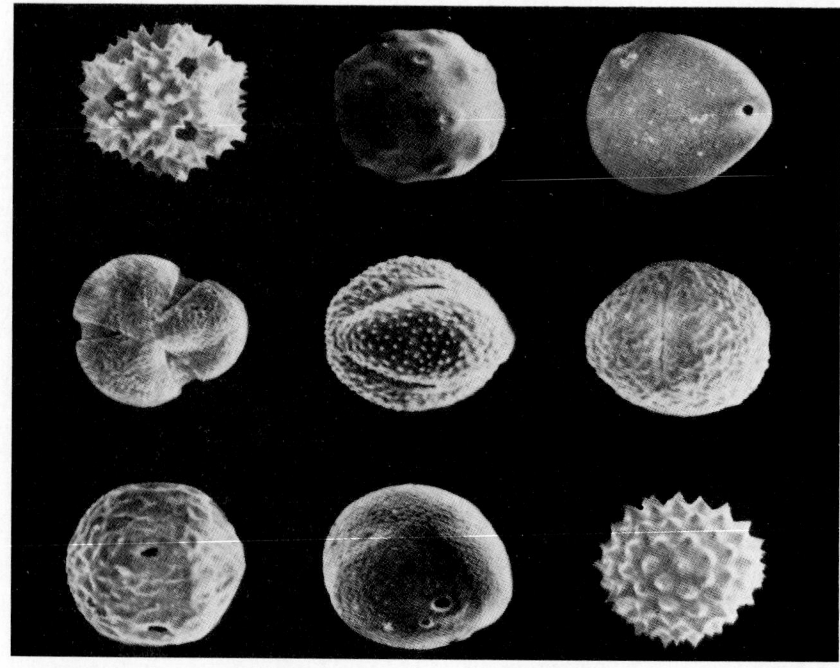

Electron-microscope photographs of pollen grains, all of which are common causes of allergies. From top to bottom in each row, starting at top left: dandelion, box elder, American elm, black walnut, sagebrush, Johnson grass, pecan, white oak, giant ragweed. (Photo from Wide World)

to deal with effectively. To find the cause of an infection, one needs only isolate the pathogen. Public-health measures can then be developed to help limit the spread of an infectious disease, and it will often be possible to immunize the body against the pathogen involved. When cases of the disease develop, antibiotics and other drugs can be used to kill or neutralize the pathogen that caused it. On the other hand, discovering the exact mechanism of a noncommunicable disorder entails the much more formidable task of isolating the underlying, often well-hidden, factor or factors that cause the body to malfunction. Little wonder, then, that research has failed to identify the mechanisms that lead to the development of such diseases as diabetes and arthritis.

Given the complexity of the human body, the possibilities for malfunction are almost endless. The number of noncommunicable diseases is staggering, since practically any organ or organ system may break down. In this chapter we will focus on some of the more common types: immune disorders, diabetes, arthritis, emphysema, chronic bronchitis, asthma, and genetic-related diseases.

Immune Disorders

The workings of the immune system were described in Chapter 15. Basically, *immunity* is the mechanism whereby the body produces specific antibodies and sensitized T-cells to fight off infection caused by specific **antigens** (foreign proteins such as foods, pollens, and chemicals that are capable of producing an allergic reaction). Without this marvelously complex and effective defense system, our bodies would be helpless before the onslaught of innumerable pathogens. Sometimes, however, the body's immune response can be *too* sensitive to invasion by foreign bodies, triggering body defense mechanisms, the effects of which are far more severe than called for by the antigen involved. This hypersensitivity to a particular antigen is known as an **allergy.** Another type of immune disorder occurs when, occasionally, a person's immune system, for some unknown reason, attacks the body tissue it is supposed to defend; this is called an autoimmune disorder. Finally, some immune systems respond inadequately or not at all to invasion by certain antigens; this type of immune-system malfunction is known as immune deficiency.

Antigens Foreign proteins capable of producing an allergic reaction.

Allergy Hypersensitivity to a particular antigen.

Allergies

Over 35 million Americans suffer from allergies, which collectively comprise one of the most widespread maladies known to humanity. Among all diseases, communicable and noncommunicable alike, perhaps only the common cold claims as many victims, year in and year out.

Allergens		Reactions
Substances Inhaled	Household and industrial dust, lint, kapok, tobacco, feathers, glue, insecticide, cottonseed, wool, pollen, flaxseed, dander, face powders, smog	Asthma, hay fever, eczema, allergic bronchitis, migraine headaches, angioneurotic edema
Substances Swallowed	Meat, fish, eggs, cereals, chocolate, tomatoes, aspirin, codeine, morphine, barbiturates, quinine, alcohol	Intestinal complaints, serum sickness, asthma, eczema, migraine headache, hives
Substances Injected	Venom from insect bites, serum, drugs, antibiotics	Hives, giant hives, eczema, serum sickness, respiratory allergies
Substances Contacted	Plant oils (poison ivy, oak, sumac), plant products (waxes, gums, resins, adhesive plaster), cosmetics, chemicals, hair lacquer, dusts, textiles, soaps	Contact dermatitis, rashes, angioneurotic edema, eczema, giant hives, asthma
Infectants	Bacteria, fungi, worms, protozoa	Asthma, nonseasonal hay fever, hives, rashes, intestinal disorders
Physical Agents	Heat, cold, ultraviolet light, irritation	Intestinal disorders, hives, asthma, respiratory allergies

Figure 18-1. Some Common Allergic Reactions.

Essentially, an *allergy* is an overreaction by the body's immune system. For whatever reason—inherited predisposition is the most likely suspect—the immune systems of certain individuals react strongly to antigens that basically are harmless and normally have no effect on other persons. An ordinarily harmless antigen that triggers

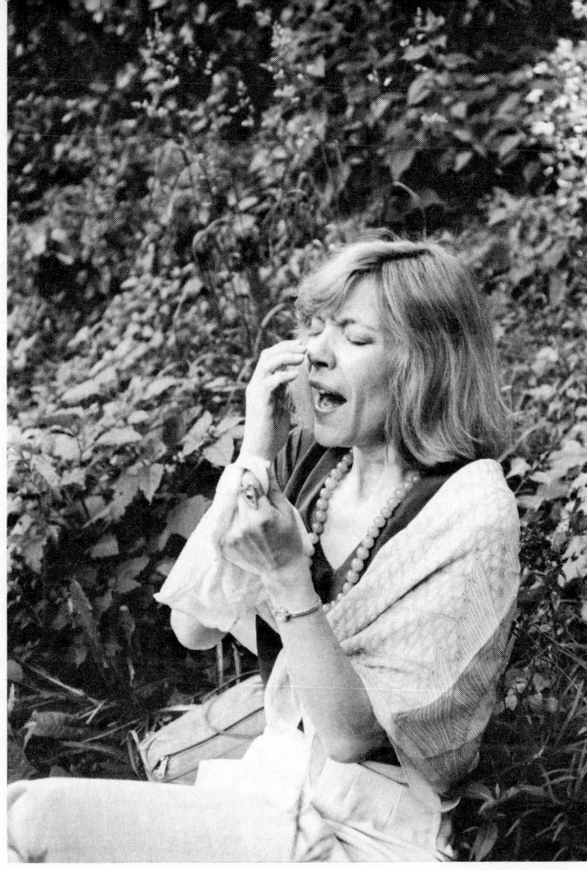

Hay fever is a seasonal allergy that irritates the respiratory system. (Photo © Jim Anderson 1982/Woodfin Camp Associates)

an allergic reaction is called an **allergen.** Allergens take several forms. Many, such as pollens, dust, and animal hair, are airborne particles breathed in by the victim; others are ingested (many types of food and drugs) or acquired through direct contact (poison ivy, certain types of chemicals). Even such common physical agents as light and heat can produce an allergic response (see Figure 18–1).

Allergen An antigen that triggers allergic reaction.

Although any foreign substance entering the body can produce an allergic reaction, some substances are more apt than others to do so. Perhaps the most well-known allergens are pollens, which are responsible for the seasonal allergy known as hay fever. A respiratory-system allergy, hay fever is characterized by watery eyes, runny nose, and frequent sneezing. It usually strikes in the spring and in late summer and fall, when the pollen count in the atmosphere reaches its highest levels.

Treatment

Allergies usually cannot be cured, but they frequently can be controlled by **desensitizing** the individual. Desensitization is a two-step process. First of all, an allergist (a doctor specializing in the treatment of allergies) tests the individual for the degree of sensitivity to various allergens. This is accomplished by introducing allergens into the body, via scratches or injections, and then monitoring the skin reaction to each allergen. After gauging the patient's sensitivity to spe-

Desensitize To alleviate allergic reaction by building the body's tolerance to allergens.

cific allergens, the allergist periodically injects into the body a serum made up of allergens to which the patient is sensitive. The strength of the allergens in the serum is increased with each injection until the patient is receiving the maintenance dose, regular injections of which often lead to desensitization. If the patient does become desensitized, the reaction to the allergens gradually decreases in severity, and sometimes disappears altogether.

While undergoing desensitization, the patient also is given doses of antihistamine drugs, which often help alleviate the symptoms of allergic reactions. Antihistamines, unlike antibiotics, do not treat the disease itself, merely its manifestations; thus, they are of only limited value in fighting allergies.

Autoimmune Disorders

Autoimmune disorder Production of antibodies by the body's immune system against its own tissues.

Little is known about the causes of **autoimmune disorders,** which arise when the immune system produces antibodies that attack the body's own tissues. All body tissue is subject to autoimmune attack, but connective tissue (bone, muscle, cartilage, ligaments, etc.) seems particularly vulnerable. There is some evidence, for example, that the inflammation of the joints characteristic of rheumatoid arthritis, as well as the damage to muscles and joints that often accompanies lupus erythematosus and rheumatic fever, stem from autoimmune attacks. Other diseases of possible autoimmune origin include Hashimoto's thyroiditis (an inflammation of the thyroid gland) and myasthenia gravis (a muscle-weakening disease).

Treatments

Immunosuppressive drugs Drugs that block the production of antibodies.

At present, there is no satisfactory treatment for autoimmune disorders. Most patients are treated with **immunosuppressive drugs,** which block the production of antibodies, but these substances have serious drawbacks. Some are too toxic for use in non–life-threatening situations, and all of them weaken the body's best defense against infection.

Immune Deficiency

Some persons, either congenitally or because of a later immune disorder, are unable to produce the antibodies needed to fight antigens. In its most extreme form, congenital immune deficiency, this disorder leaves an individual defenseless against nearly all antigens; such persons must live in a constantly sterile environment, or risk the near certainty of death from even the most minor of infections. One of the most recently discovered immune disorders is AIDS, discussed in Chapter 15. More commonly, immune-deficient individuals are prone to frequent but nonfatal infections and bear an increased risk of developing certain types of cancer. There is no known cure for this condition.

Diabetes

Diabetes, or diabetes mellitus, is a chronic disease of the pancreas that prevents the body from utilizing sugars and starches to produce energy. Normally, the sugars and starches we eat are converted into **glucose,** a type of sugar, and then stored in the liver; there, the glucose is acted upon by **insulin,** a hormone secreted by the pancreas. Insulin-treated glucose then is carried through the bloodstream to body tissues, which use it as fuel for energy production. In a person afflicted with diabetes, either not enough insulin is manufactured or the insulin that is produced does not properly act upon the glucose. In either case, body tissues cannot utilize the glucose, which accumulates in the bloodstream and is expelled from the body in urine. Lacking glucose, body tissues must burn fats to produce energy — a situation that if left untreated eventually results in **acidosis** (abnormal acidity in body fluids), coma, and death. Fortunately, diabetes usually can be controlled (although not actually cured) through insulin injections, proper diet and exercise regimens, and oral drugs.

Diabetes Pancreas disease that prevents body from utilizing sugars and starches to produce energy.

Glucose Form in which sugar is converted by the body to be stored in the liver.

Insulin Pancreatic hormone that enables glucose to be used for energy production.

Acidosis Abnormal acidity in blood and body fluids.

The cause of this noncommunicable disorder is unknown. Hereditary predisposition seems to play a role, as do excess weight and the aging process. Overweight persons more than 35 years of age whose families have a history of diabetes are particularly at risk. Females are twice as likely as males to develop diabetes, especially if they are taking oral contraceptives or have given birth to an unusually large baby. In all, over 10 million Americans suffer from some form of diabetes, and the number and proportion of known diabetics is rising at a rate of about 6 percent a year. The early symptoms of diabetes are often hidden, that is, without noticeable symptoms. Completing Self-Assessment Exercise 18.1 will give you some idea of whether or not you might be a "hidden diabetic."

Approximately 10 percent of diabetics suffer from juvenile-onset diabetes, which, as the name implies, usually strikes children and young adults. Less severe in impact, but far more frequent in occurrence, is maturity-onset diabetes. Both forms of the disease can lead, over a period of years, to the widespread breakdown of blood vessels and hence to such grave complications as blindness, arteriosclerosis, kidney failure, and frequent infections. Diabetes currently is the fifth leading cause of death by disease, ranking even higher if deaths from diabetic complications are included.

Type I Diabetes

The form of the disease known as Type I or juvenile-onset diabetes is characterized by sudden onset; excessive urination, thirst, and hunger; fatigue, general weakness, and weight loss; an increased

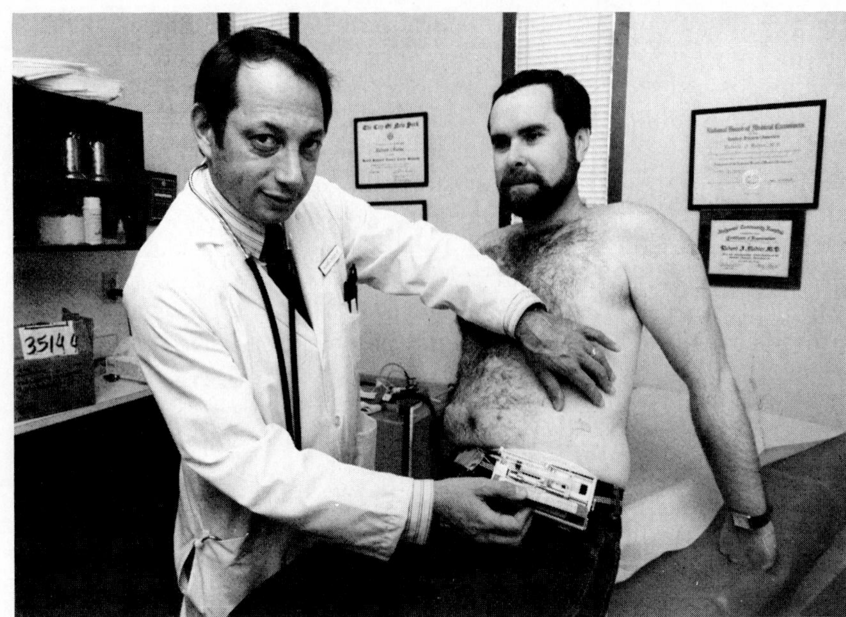

A doctor with a patient wearing an insulin pump. Still in the experimental stage, the pump offers hope to diabetics who do not respond well to insulin injections. (Photo by Tony Korody/Sygma)

number of slow-healing infections, particularly of the foot; blurred vision; and itching of the skin. Victims of juvenile-onset diabetes almost invariably are **insulin-dependent;** that is, their pancreases fail to produce any or sufficient insulin, which must be received through daily injections. (It cannot be taken orally, because stomach acids would destroy it.)

Insulin dependence Diabetic condition that requires victim to obtain insulin through injections.

Before Sir Frederick Banting and Charles Best isolated insulin in 1921, individuals who developed juvenile-onset diabetes usually died within a few weeks, from diabetic coma. Today, daily injections of insulin processed from animal pancreases almost ensure a longer life span, although the life-threatening complications noted previously pose serious dangers later in life.

It is important to remember that insulin does not cure diabetes: it merely provides an artificial means of enabling the diabetic's body to process sugar. Since it is an artificial process, insulin therapy must be carefully and constantly monitored to prevent the development of potentially fatal problems.

There are two opposite dangers. On the one hand, diabetics must guard against **insulin shock,** which develops when the blood-sugar level falls too low because of an excess of insulin injected, too-strenuous exercise, or too little food digested. Insulin shock occurs suddenly, and some form of sugar must be ingested shortly after the symptoms manifest themselves. For this reason, insulin-dependent diabetics should carry with them a candy bar or some other source of sugar. On the other hand, if the insulin level in the blood falls too low, acidosis and coma can result. The only remedy is an insulin injection.

Insulin shock Serious bodily reaction to excessively low level of blood sugar.

SELF-ASSESSMENT EXERCISE 18.1

Are You a Diabetic? Checklist

	Yes	No
Are you over 40?		
Any diabetics in your family?		
Are you overweight?		
Any sudden weight loss?		
Are you constantly thirsty?		
Do you eat excessively?		
Do you urinate frequently?		
Do you tire easily?		
Do wounds heal slowly?		
Any pain in fingers or toes?		
Any changes in vision?		
Does skin itch frequently?		
Are you often drowsy?		
Have you had any babies weighing over 9 pounds at birth?		
Do you have a craving for sweets?		
Total		

Interpretation:

Every "yes" you checked on the quiz raises the possibility that you could be a "hidden diabetic."

Read the section on diabetes for more information.

Source: Walter D. Sorochan, *Prompting Your Health,* (New York: John S. Wiley, 1981) p. 349. Reprinted by permission of the author.

Type II Diabetes

In contrast to Type I diabetes, Type II or maturity-onset diabetes develops more slowly and presents fewer and milder symptoms. Many victims are unaware that they have the disease until a laboratory test reveals its presence. In most cases, proper diet and exercise suffice to control this form of diabetes. Until very late stages of the disorder, victims ordinarily are not insulin-dependent, since their pancreases retain some insulin-secretion capability. Although juvenile-onset sufferers are more prone to develop complications, maturity-onset victims also must face the distinct possibility of blood-vessel degeneration and its often fatal results. Weight control is vital to slowing the disease: for some reason, the insulin process is hindered far more in overweight diabetics.

Hypoglycemia

Hypoglycemia Condition that occurs when blood sugar falls very low due to too much insulin in bloodstream.

If the pancreas produces too much insulin, rather than too little, the blood-sugar level will fall unacceptably low. This condition, known in general as **hypoglycemia,** appears in insulin-dependent diabetics in the form of insulin shock. Hypoglycemia often arises from other causes, however. A prolonged high-carbohydrate diet will induce this condition: a heavy intake of carbohydrates sets off an increased production of insulin, which in turn leads to a too-rapid conversion of blood sugar into fats and thus a drop in the blood-sugar level. Symptoms include fatigue, restlessness, weakness, and irritability. If left unchecked, hypoglycemia can lead to coma and death. A proper low-carbohydrate diet usually will control the problem.

Strictly speaking, diabetes and hypoglycemia are opposite conditions, yet there is a close relationship between the two. In adults hypoglycemia frequently progresses into maturity-onset diabetes, so it is important to bring hypoglycemia under control as soon as possible. Perhaps because of a recent spate of publicity, however, hypoglycemia has become an overused diagnosis. The body's reaction in this area is as yet not fully understood, and many conditions diagnosed too quickly as hypoglycemia have turned out to be something else entirely. Such misdiagnosis can have serious consequences.

Arthritis

Arthritis Inflammation of the joints.

The term **arthritis,** which literally means "inflammation of the joints," is used to signify more than 80 forms of rheumatic disease that attack the body's joints and/or connective tissue. There is no single cause of this chronic condition and no cure. Apart from cardiovascular disease, arthritis is the most widespread chronic illness in

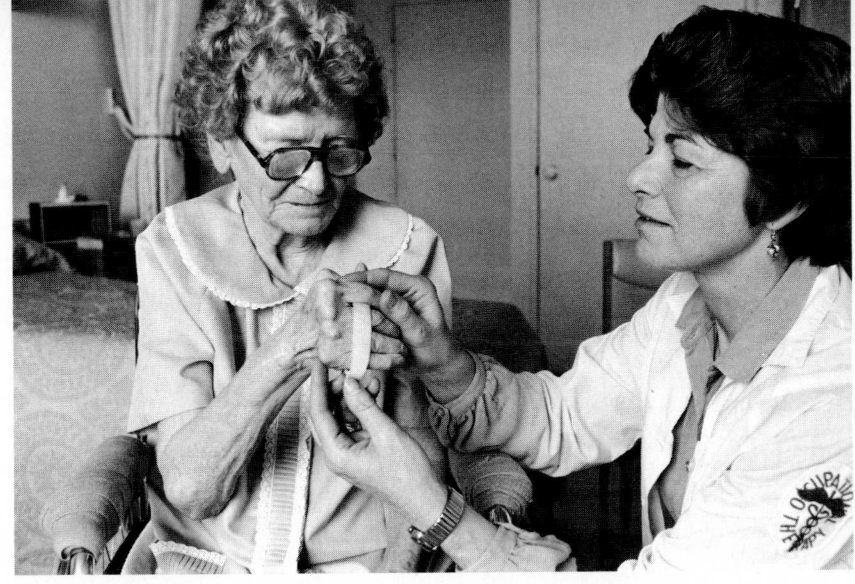

An arthritic patient being fitted with a special device to help with manual dexterity. (Photo © Joel Gordon 1982/Joel Gordon Photography)

the United States. At any one time, an estimated 35 million Americans are disabled to some extent by the painful inflammation it causes; of these victims, approximately 20 million are afflicted with arthritis severe enough to require medical treatment. Although it is popularly thought of as an affliction exclusively of old age, arthritis can develop even in children, and more than 300,000 of its victims are under 45 years of age. The three most common forms of arthritis are rheumatoid arthritis, osteoarthritis, and gout. In order to see if you are susceptible to arthritis, complete Self-Assessment Exercise 18.2, entitled "Susceptibility to Arthritis Inventory."

Rheumatoid Arthritis

This is the most common form of the disease and the most severe in effect. Over 5 million Americans suffer from **rheumatoid arthritis,** which manifests itself as swelling and inflammation in a joint or joints. The condition is chronic and often progressive: prolonged inflammation can lead to permanent deformation of joints. To a much greater extent than other types of arthritis, the rheumatoid variety can afflict persons at a young age—even children. (Juvenile arthritis, one type of rheumatoid arthritis, is particularly crippling.) Most victims are between 25 and 50 years of age, and about 75 percent are women.

Rheumatoid arthritis Prolonged inflammation of the joints, leading to their deformation.

The cause of rheumatoid arthritis is unknown. Because the presence of an abnormal antibody, called the rheumatoid factor, usually accompanies manifestation of the disease, many researchers believe that it arises from an autoimmune disorder. During the periodic flare-ups of inflammation, which sometimes are accompanied by fever and fatigue, the pain can be excruciating, and much or all function in the affected joints can be lost temporarily. These periods of exacerbation are followed by spells of remission. In many cases, chronic inflammation eventually results in **ankylosis,** or fusing, of the joints, which thereafter are permanently unable to function. Ankylosed joints are

Ankylosis Permanent fusing of the joints.

SELF-ASSESSMENT EXERCISE 18.2

Susceptibility to Arthritis Inventory

Instruction: Circle the category beside each item that you feel best describes your situation.

	Mother Father	**Sisters Brothers**	**Aunts Uncles Grandparents**	**None**
1. Heredity—relatives who had, or were treated for, arthritis, rheumatism, or gout	50	40	20	0
	40+ years	**40–30 years**	**30–20 years**	**20–0 years**
2. Age—female	60	40	20	5
male	20	10	5	1
	Never	**1–2 Times per Week**	**3–4 Times per Week**	**Daily**
3. Amount of physical activity—frequency of exercise	25	20	5	0
	0–30 minutes	**30–45 minutes**	**45–60 minutes**	**1–2+ hours**
Length of exercise or activity per frequency	15	10	3	0
	5+ times	**3–4 times**	**1–2 times**	**Never**
4. Number of times bones have been broken in your lifteime	10	7	3	0
	10+ years	**5–9 years**	**2–4 years**	**1–0 year**
Playing (body-contact) sports	10	7	1	0
	50+ pounds	**25–49 pounds**	**10–24 pounds**	**0 pounds**
5. Overweight	30	20	10	0

	None	**½–1 Hour**	**1–2 Hours**	**2+ Hours**
6. Amount of rest per day from all activity	10	7	2	0
	4–5 hours	**5–6 hours**	**6–7 hours**	**8+ hours**
7. Amount (hours) of sleep per day	10	7	3	0
	10+ drinks per week	**6–9 drinks per week**	**1–5 drinks per week**	**0 drinks per week**
8. Drinking alcoholic beverages	25	20	10	0
	Never	**Once a Week**	**3 Times per Week**	**1–2 Times per Day**
9. Diet—eat fresh fruits and vegetables (minerals, vitamins C and A)	30	10	3	0
	Never	**1–2 Times per Week**	**3 Times per Week**	**1–2 Times per Day**
Drink whole or skim milk; eat cheese (minerals and vitamins)	10	7	3	0
B vitamins	20	15	5	0
	Always	**Often**	**Sometimes**	**Never**
10. Emotional stress				
Work stress or crises	25	20	5	0
Home or family stress	10	7	3	0
Crises of living	15	10	5	0
11. Rash—skin or face	30	20	5	0

(Continued)

12. Pain or stiffness in joints	75	50	25	0
13. Climate (live in cold)	10	7	3	0
14. Dampness (live in damp weather)	10	7	3	0

Scoring: Add up all numbers circled.

Interpretation:

	Degree of Risk
250+	High
250–100	Average
99–0	Low

Read the section on arthritis for more information.

Source: Walter D. Sorochan, *Promoting Your Health,* New York, John S. Wiley, 1981, p. 347. Reprinted by permission of the author.

responsible for the deformities characteristic of severe and progressive rheumatoid arthritis. The course of the disease, however, varies with the individual.

Treatment

Although there is no cure for rheumatoid arthritis, in recent years major progress has been made in controlling the symptoms of the disease, alleviating the pain suffered by its victims, and preserving or restoring function in arthritic joints. The first stage of treatment combines physical therapy (exercises during periods of remission, hot baths, bed rest) with the administration of salicylates, or aspirin—the single most effective drug used in treating arthritis. Aspirin is so effective because it both reduces inflammation and relieves pain and because its side effects are mild. Throughout the course of the disease, patients usually are urged to take aspirin several times a day. If pain and inflammation worsen despite physical therapy and aspirin, a wide range of powerful medications can be administered including corticosteroids, which are injected directly into the affected joints in order to reduce inflammation.

Osteoarthritis

Osteoarthritis Mild form of arthritis related to aging process.

Osteoarthritis, also called degenerative arthritis, develops much more slowly than rheumatoid arthritis and usually is milder in effect. Its onset apparently is related to the aging process and/or to severe stress on and damage to joints. Victims, therefore, tend to be either persons over 50 or individuals whose joints have been badly damaged by trauma or by continual abuse. (Many football players, for instance, develop osteoarthritis in one or both knees.) The condition first becomes evident in the wearing down of articular cartilage, which cushions the bones hinged in a joint. As the cartilage is destroyed, the bones become deformed and abnormal growths, called lips, appear along their edges. The combination of worn-down cartilage and bone growths restricts the functioning of the joint, causing stiffness and pain. Eventually the joint becomes enlarged or otherwise deformed.

Unlike rheumatoid arthritis, osteoarthritis develops unilaterally: that is, it appears in one knee but not the other, one hip but not the other, and so forth. More women than men are afflicted with osteoarthritis, and overweight people tend to suffer more severely from it because of the added stress on the joints. Treatment is similar to that for rheumatoid arthritis. Since only one joint is involved in most cases, joint-replacement surgery provides a particularly effective course of treatment in individuals whose joints have degenerated severely.

Chronic Respiratory Disorders

Through the complicated process of breathing, or respiration, life-giving oxygen is supplied to all body tissues and poisonous carbon dioxide is expelled from the body. Respiratory diseases degrade or obstruct this process by damaging the lungs. All such diseases are serious, since good health depends on the adequate functioning of the oxygen–carbon dioxide exchange.

Just as respiratory infections like pneumonia and tuberculosis are among the most feared of communicable diseases, so asthma, chronic bronchitis, and emphysema are among the most crippling of noncommunicable diseases. The real tragedy of these chronic obstructive pulmonary diseases (COPDs), as they have come to be called, is that, with the exception of one form of asthma, they are highly preventable disorders. As long as people continue to smoke cigarettes, work and live in hazardous or polluted environments, and fail to treat promptly and completely all respiratory infections, COPDs will continue to cripple and kill thousands of victims each year.

Asthma

Asthma is a chronic narrowing, or hyperreactiveness, of the bronchioles—the passageways in the lungs that carry air to the alveoli, or air sacs. Hyperreactive bronchioles respond much too drastically to any of various stimuli, spasmodically opening and closing and

Asthma Chronic narrowing of the bronchioles.

thus obstructing the flow of air through the lungs. The classic symptom is wheezing, which often is accompanied by paroxysms of coughing and tightness in the chest. In particularly severe cases, the victim will wake up several times a night, wheezing and fighting for breath.

An estimated 10 million Americans suffer from asthma of one sort or another, although considerably fewer seek medical attention for this condition. Of those who are treated, about 75 percent have *extrinsic asthma,* which is caused by an allergic reaction. The other 25 percent of asthmatics suffer from *intrinsic asthma,* which is brought on by a respiratory infection. In some cases, emotional or mental stress will trigger or exacerbate asthma attacks. All forms of the disease are characterized by sudden and periodic attacks that can be severe enough to impair the breathing function and cause death. (About 4,000 – 5,000 Americans die during asthma attacks each year.)

Treatment

Bronchodilators Drugs that open air passages to the lungs.

There are three facets to the treatment of asthma: (1) providing immediate relief to victims during attacks; (2) attempting to lessen the incidence and severity of future attacks; (3) discovering and dealing with the causes of the disease. Immediate relief can be obtained from injections of epinephrine (or adrenaline, as it is more commonly known) or from **bronchodilators** (drugs that open up the bronchioles) given in tablet or aerosol form. Chronic, harsh attacks that do not yield to other treatment can be lessened with cortisone injections, although potentially serious side effects rule out this course of treatment in most cases. Finally, the root cause of the disorder must be identified and attacked. If the asthma is extrinsic in origin, the allergen involved can either be avoided (by eliminating it from the diet, for instance) or treated (with allergy shots). In particularly serious cases in which the allergen is airborne, the victim is urged to move to an allergen-free climate. Intrinsic asthma often can be cleared up by eliminating the infection that causes it. Where stress is found to be the culprit, a program is started to reduce the patient's mental and emotional tension.

Chronic Bronchitis

Whereas most cases of asthma cannot be prevented from developing, because they stem from allergic reactions, almost all forms of *chronic bronchitis* are preventable. Smoking, continual exposure to airborne pollutants (usually in the workplace), and chronic, untreated infections are the principal causes of this disease, which involves inflammation of the bronchioles. In normally functioning bronchioles, foreign particles breathed into the lungs are trapped by the mucous membranes. They are then swept out of the lungs and into the throat in mucus propelled by the undulating action of tiny, hairlike fibers known as cilia. Constant and prolonged irritation of the

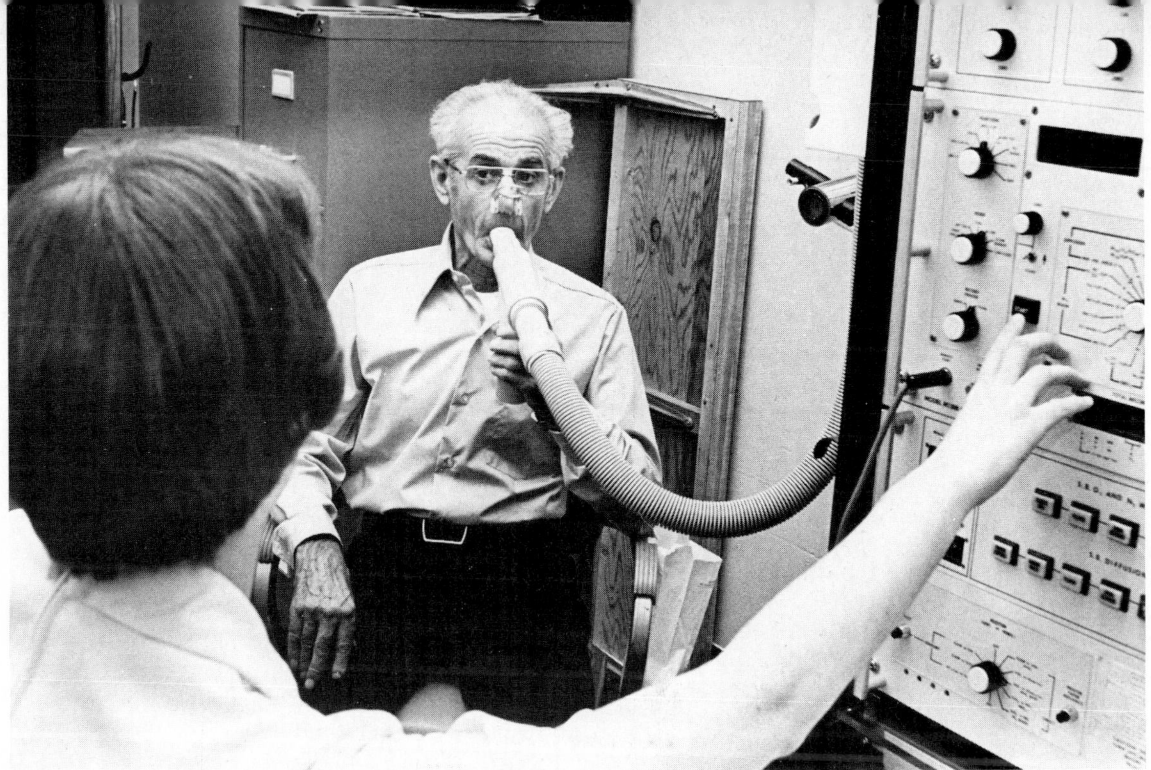

A coal miner taking a breathing test to determine the existence of black lung disease. New regulations on clean air in mines may lessen the danger of this and other chronic lung diseases of miners. (Photo from United Press International)

membranes eventually leads to inflammation of the bronchiole lining and destruction of the cilia. As the cilia cease to function, mucus builds up in the bronchiole to the point that it blocks the airway and thereby triggers the reaction known commonly as coughing, which is the body's attempt to clear the bronchioles. The fits of coughing that characterize chronic bronchitis, as opposed to those symptomatic of asthma, are productive: that is, they expel large amounts of mucus. Other symptoms of the disease include wheezing (usually less pronounced than the asthma variety) and shortness of breath.

Chronic bronchitis can be alleviated or cured entirely be removing the cause of irritation, whether that cause is smoking, pollutants, or infection. Normally a nonfatal condition, bronchitis is most dangerous in children and in adults who have an underlying disease that also affects the respiratory system. If left untreated, it can develop into emphysema, a far more deadly condition. Drugs used in the treatment of chronic bronchitis include bronchodilators, antihistamines, and antibiotics.

Emphysema

The most serious of all chronic respiratory conditions is *emphysema*, a long-term deterioration of the air sacs, or alveoli. Some localized damage to the alveoli is common in older people and in most cases is not serious. When the deterioration affects large areas of the lungs, however, blood will not be properly provided with oxygen and cleansed of carbon dioxide. If the damage is widespread and irreversible, death is the eventual outcome. Men over 45 are the prime candidates for this condition. Heavy smokers are particularly at risk, as are those who work in particle-laden environments such as coal mines. A history of chronic bronchitis or asthma often precedes the onset of emphysema.

Treatment

Although emphysema cannot be cured, its progress can be slowed by a therapy program that combines instruction in beneficial breathing techniques with the administration of bronchodilators and other drugs that ease the passage of air through the lungs. In the later stages of the disease, antibiotics are used to combat the ever-present threat of secondary infection.

Genetic-Related Disorders

Chromosomal abnormalities Genetic disorders related to a defect in the structure or number of chromosomes.

Gene abnormalities Specific problems inherent in the genetic DNA.

The complex mechanisms of heredity are subject to a wide variety of disorders, most of which occur too infrequently or are too poorly understood to warrant mention here. The two major categories of genetic-related disorders are **chromosomal abnormalities** (defects in the structure of the chromosome or an abnormal number of chromosomes) and **gene abnormalities** (specific problems inherent in the DNA—the actual genetic code which makes up the gene).

Fortunately, chromosomal abnormalities are quite rare. Somewhat more common are gene abnormalities. The genetic information contained in genes dictates many characteristics. Mutant genes are almost always detrimental to the person who inherits them, because the human body is so closely adapted to its environment that a sudden change in its basic constituents is bound to cause problems. The only reason abnormal genes do not cause far more problems than they do is that every individual receives duplicate sets of genes, one from each parent. If one set contains a defective gene, the normal gene in the other set often will suffice to ensure normality. The most common genetic-related disorders include Down's syndrome, phenylketonuria, sickle-cell anemia, muscular dystrophy, and cystic fibrosis.

Down's Syndrome

Down's syndrome Chromosomal abnormality characterized by physical malformations and some degree of mental retardation.

Down's syndrome is a chromosomal abnormality that is characterized by physical malformations and some degree of mental retardation. The condition is present at birth (congenital). Down's syndrome is due to the presence of three 21st chromosomes instead of the two that normally would make up the 21st pair. The term *trisomy* refers to the presence of three chromosomes; hence, Down's syndrome has been called *trisomy 21*.

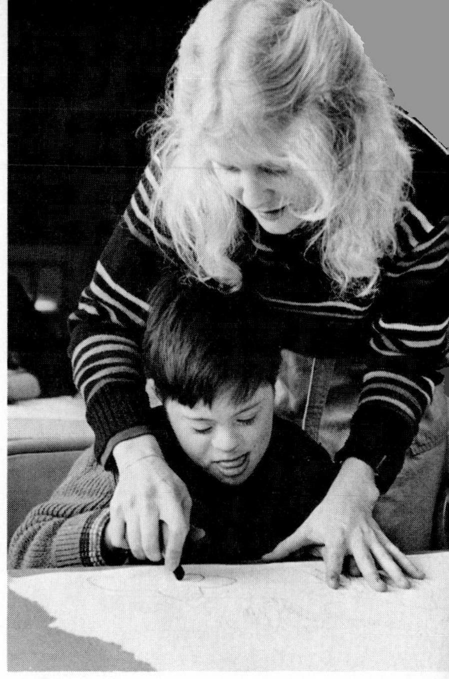

A teacher with a victim of Down's syndrome. (Photo © Susan Lapides 1981/ Design conceptions)

The physical malformations that result from the trisomy 21 condition include a small, flattened skull; a short, flat-bridged nose; wide-set eyes; a protruding tongue; and short, broad hands. This appearance was once called "mongolism" because the characteristics resembled those of persons of the Mongolian race; this term is not used anymore. As a child with Down's syndrome grows older, he or she remains below average in height and evidences some degree of mental retardation.

The mechanism by which three 21st chromosomes are formed is not clearly understood. The best explanation is that during the process of meiosis, when the chromosomes are reduced by half in the ovum, the 21st pair of chromosomes fails to separate. The result is an ovum with 24 chromosomes (two 21st chromosomes) instead of the normal 23 chromosomes. When the ovum is fertilized by a normal sperm carrying 23 chromosomes, the result will be a child born with three 21st chromosomes, or 47 total chromosomes instead of the normal 46.

Women at greatest risk of producing an ovum with an extra 21st chromosome are those over 35 years of age. As a woman gets older, the risk becomes greater. There is no cure for Down's syndrome. Depending upon the degree of physical malformations and mental retardation, the child can often be helped to live a productive life.

Phenylketonuria

The disorder known as **phenylketonuria (PKU)** is inherited as a recessive trait. Symptoms begin in early infancy and consist of vomiting, skin rash, irritability, an odor caused by abnormal urine, and abnormal movements. If not treated, it leads to mental retardation.

Phenylketonuria (PKU) Inherited absence of a certain enzyme which increases levels of phenylalanine in the blood.

The cause is the absence of an enzyme that metabolizes phenylalanine, an amino acid found in many proteins. Consequently, levels of phenylalanine in the blood are excessively high, and the body excretes a large amount of a chemical called phenylketone in the urine.

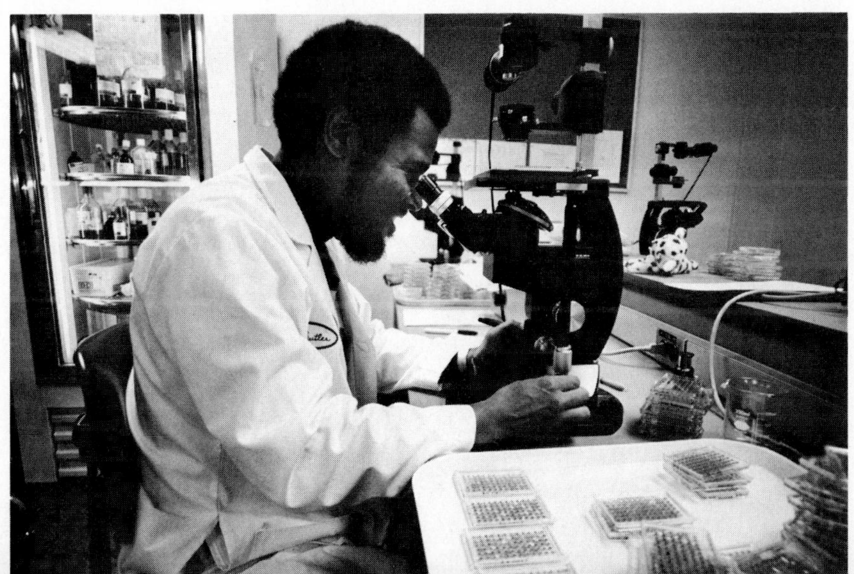

A lab technician performing tests for genetic disorders such as PKU. (Photo © Christopher Morrow/Stock, Boston)

The symptoms, especially mental retardation, may be prevented by a diet low in phenylalanine, and commercial foods are available for infants with the disease. However, since complications can arise if the level of phenylalanine falls too low, blood levels must be measured regularly.

PKU occurs in about one out of every 20,000 white persons, and most victims are blond and blue-eyed; PKU is rarely found in blacks. Many states require that a blood test for PKU be given to all babies shortly after birth.

Sickle-Cell Anemia

Sickle-cell anemia Genetic disorder whereby red blood cells have a reduced oxygen-carrying capacity.

Sickle-cell anemia is a genetic disorder in which the red blood cells, after releasing the oxygen they carry, change their shape from round to a thin, curved form resembling a sickle. As a result, the cells cannot circulate freely but clog blood vessels, especially the smaller ones. Since the red cells break down, the delivery of oxygen to the body is reduced, and the victim does not grow as rapidly as a normal individual.

The disease can occur in a very mild or a very severe form. In the mild form, the individual rarely suffers from the disease. In the severe form, pain is felt in the limbs, the abdomen, the lower back, and the head. The lungs, bones, spleen, kidney, heart, and brain may be affected. It should be emphasized that the complications are not present all the time. Even individuals with the most severe form have long periods during which they feel relatively well. The mild form generally occurs when individuals receive the trait from one parent. Even though they may not be ill, they are carriers and will pass the trait on to 50 percent of their offspring. The severe form occurs when the trait is received from both parents; the victim has a reduced life expectancy and will pass along the disease to any offspring.

The majority of affected families are black, although the disease is also found in southern India, Italy, Greece, and Turkey. It is estimated that in the United States roughly one in ten black people carries the trait and one in 400 has the disease in the severe form. Although no cure is available, adequate medical attention may prevent serious crises and prolong the lives of chronically ill patients.

Muscular Dystrophy

Muscular dystrophies Inherited diseases that cause degeneration of muscle tissue.

The **muscular dystrophies** are a group of chronic, inherited diseases that affect the body's muscle tissue. Most muscular dystrophies are sex-linked and appear only in young males; some, however, can strike either sex. The principal characteristic of this type of disease is the degeneration of the muscle tissue, whose cells swell and rupture.

The muscles become either overdeveloped or wasted, and eventually the nerves that serve the affected areas degenerate. Because its victims lose control over muscle movement, muscular dystrophy is popularly regarded as a disorder of the nervous system; it is actually a disorder of the muscle fiber itself, and the deterioration of the nervous sytem is secondary.

Authorities actually differ on whether the muscular dystrophies are separate diseases or merely different manifestations of the same disease. The symptoms, in any case, are similar. The muscles affected initially may be limited to those of the arms and legs, or they may include those of the face. By early adolescence, the victims usually have lost so much muscle function that they must be confined to a wheelchair. There is no known cure. Programs of physical therapy, similar to those designed for victims of poliomyelitis, may help muscular dystrophy patients retain some muscle function, but they cannot prevent the progression of the disease. Death is the common outcome of progressive muscular dystrophy, although many victims of milder forms of the disease may enjoy a normal life span.

Cystic Fibrosis

Cystic fibrosis is a genetic-related disorder involving the exocrine (externally secreting) glands, such as the sweat glands and the mucus-secreting glands. For unknown reasons, abnormally sticky secretions obstruct the ducts leading from mucus-secreting glands, which eventually swell to form cysts (liquid-filled cavities). These cysts impair the functioning of the organs with which they are associated—most commonly, the pancreas and the lungs. The sweat glands, meanwhile produce sweat that contains far more salt than is normally found—a key symptom in diagnosing the disease. As the disease progresses, the pancreas usually stops producing the enzymes and electrolytes needed for digestion, and the lungs degenerate, showing symptoms similar to those of emphysema and bronchitis. The earliest discernible symptoms usually appear before the victim is one year old. Most often, parents first notice the characteristics of intestinal obstruction, including an inability to gain weight, a swollen abdomen, and the frequent passage of bulky and foul-smelling stools. If the lungs become involved, serious difficulties in breathing follow; extensive lung damage or secondary infections can cause death in particularly severe cases.

Cystic fibrosis Genetic-related disorder involving exocrine glands.

Almost all cases of cystic fibrosis are diagnosed in infancy. Of the approximately 1 in 1,500 American babies who inherit some form of the disease, most are Caucasian and a high percentage are born in the northeastern part of the country. Treatment is concentrated on alleviating the effects of the disease on the major organs involved, since a complete cure is impossible at the present time. With early diagnosis and proper therapy most victims reach adulthood, unless the damage to the nervous system is especially severe.

Common Neurological Disorders

Neurological disorders involve one or more structures of the nervous sytem. Since the nervous system is the controller and coordinator of all body systems, any neurological problem can have profound implications. Two common disorders of the nervous system found in youthful populations include epilepsy and multiple sclerosis.

Epilepsy

Epilepsy Sudden discharge of electrical energy in the brain.

Epilepsy is a condition in which a sudden discharge of electrical energy in the brain takes place. The resulting physical response to this discharge of electrical energy is termed a *seizure*. It is estimated that epilepsy affects approximately 1 to 2 percent of the population. In addition, most cases of epilepsy (75 percent) are diagnosed before age 18.

Grand mal seizure Type of epileptic seizure characterized by violent muscle spasms.

Petit mal seizure Type of epileptic seizure characterized by a daydreaming appearance.

There are three major types of epileptic seizures: grand mal, petit mal, and psychomotor. In a **grand mal seizure** the individual loses consciousness, the body stiffens, and alternating episodes of muscular spasm and relaxation occur. The seizure usually stops in 2 to 5 minutes.

Petit mal seizures are generally characterized by a brief change in level of consciousness and are most commonly found in children. Symptoms of petit mal include blinking or rolling of the eyes, a blank stare, and slight mouth movements. The individual has a daydreamer's appearance. The seizure lasts from 1 – 10 seconds, and seizures can reoccur as often as 100 times a day.

Psychomotor seizure Type of epileptic seizure characterized by involuntary muscle movements.

Psychomotor seizures are characterized by brief involuntary muscular jerks of the body or extremities, which may occur in a rhythmic fashion, lip smacking, and incoherent speech. These seizures do not usually last long.

Anticonvulsant drug therapy Use of drugs that prevent convulsions

The clinical diagnosis of epilepsy is based on the occurrence of one or more seizures and proof that the condition which led to the seizures is still present. The cause of epilepsy is unknown, thus it is often difficult to identify the predisposing factors associated with observed seizures. **Anticonvulsant drug therapy** (drugs that prevent convulsions) has been very successful in treating epilepsy and the associated seizure and has allowed the individual suffering from epilepsy to live a normal life.

Multiple Sclerosis

Multiple sclerosis (MS) is a neurological disorder characterized by a progressive "stripping away" of the **myelin sheath** that covers the axon structure of the **neurons,** or nerve cells, in the brain and spinal cord. The degeneration, or demyelination, of the myelin sheath causes a variety of symptoms, which are related to the extent of the stripping away. In general, the greater the extent of demyelination, the more profound the physical symptoms.

Multiple sclerosis (MS) Neurological disorder characterized by the demyelination of neurons in brain and spinal cord.

Myelin sheath The axon covering of neurons.

Neuron Nerve cell.

The onset of MS occurs mostly between ages 20 and 40 with an average age of onset at 27. This is why MS has been termed a young person's disease. The exact cause of MS is unknown, but current theories suggest that there is some viral involvement.

When MS begins, the most common symptoms include visual problems and some sensory impairment marked by numbness and tingling sensations, especially in extremities. Symptoms can progress in magnitude to a point where there is almost complete muscle dysfunction, urinary disturbance, and emotional problems, including mood swings, euphoria, or depression. The symptoms may be so mild that a patient may be unaware of them or so intense that he or she may become completely disabled.

Diagnosis of MS is difficult, because years may go by between the onset of relatively minor symptoms and the diagnosis. There is no cure for MS, and the average survival time after the onset of symptoms is estimated at 27 years.

Summary

Noncommunicable diseases are chronic disorders that arise from breakdowns of or malfunctions in body systems. Typically, such disorders progress slowly, gradually crippling or impairing bodily functions. Most are not directly fatal, although several may contribute significantly to the ultimate cause of death. Since they are not caused by pathogens, these diseases cannot be spread from one victim to another. The absence of a pathogen also makes their causative agents difficult to isolate, however, and greatly hampers treatment. Except for those caused principally by harmful life-styles (most chronic respiratory disorders and some forms of arthritis), few noncommunicable diseases are preventable, and almost none can be cured. Treatment usually centers around alleviation of the symptoms or efforts to control or arrest the progress of the disease.

In addition to cancer and cardiovascular diseases (see Chapters 16 and 17), the major groups of noncommunicable diseases include immune disorders, diabetes, arthritis, chronic respiratory disorders, and genetic-related disorders. Malfunctions of the body's infection-fighting immune system include allergies, one of the most widespread of human disorders; autoimmune disorders, in which the immune system attacks the body's own tissues; and immune deficiencies. Diabetes mellitus, a pancreatic disorder that prevents or degrades the production of insulin and thereby impairs the body's ability to process sugars and starches, can take the acute form of juvenile-onset diabetes or the slower-developing form of maturity-onset diabetes. In either case, insulin therapy can help control the disease, although it cannot cure it. Equally incurable are the three principal forms of arthritis, a rheumatic disease that inflames and cripples the body's joints and/or connective tissue: rheumatoid arthritis, osteoarthritis, and gout. Contrary to popular conception, many types of arthritis can strike at any age.

Chronic respiratory disorders are lung diseases that impair the functioning of the respiratory system. Asthma, the most common of these disorders, involves a narrowing of the passageways to the lungs; its cause is unknown. Chronic bronchitis and emphysema, on the other hand, are largely preventable disorders caused in many cases by cigarette smoking or repeated exposure to airborne pollutants. Emphysema is one of the few noncommunicable diseases that is directly and almost invariably fatal. Another such exception to the rule is muscular dystrophy, a chronic degeneration of the muscle tissue caused by a breakdown in the mechanisms of heredity. Other genetic-related disorders include Down's syndrome, sickle-cell anemia, phenylketonuria (PKU), muscular dystrophy, and cystic fibrosis. Two of the common neurological disorders usually affecting a young population include epilepsy and multiple sclerosis. Both of these disorders vary in the intensity of symptoms and impact on a person's life.

Review and Discussion

1. Compare communicable and noncommunicable diseases. Why are noncommunicable ailments so resistant to treatment?

2. List and describe examples of the three types of immune disorders.

3. Explain in detail the process involved in an allergic reaction.

4. What is diabetes? What are the differences between juvenile-onset and maturity-onset diabetes?

5. Describe three common forms of arthritis and how each is commonly treated.

6. What are the symptoms of asthma? How can it be treated?

7. What are the causes and symptoms of chronic bronchitis and emphysema?

8. Distinguish between gene abnormalities and chromosome abnormalities.

9. Describe phenylketonuria (PKU) and the two forms of sickle-cell anemia.

10. Distinguish between muscular dystrophy and cystic fibrosis.

11. Explain the three types of seizures associated with epilepsy.

12. Describe the symptoms associated with multiple sclerosis.

Further Reading

Alexander, Dale. *Arthritis and Common Sense.* New York: Simon and Schuster, 1981.
A discussion of arthritis and its treatment for the layperson. (Paperback.)

Biermann, June, and Barbara Toohey. *The Diabetic's Total Health Book.* New York: Pocket Books, 1982.
A popular guide to the treatment of diabetes. (Paperback.)

Knight, Allan. *Asthma and Hay Fever.* New York: Arco Publishing, 1981.
A discussion of the causes, symptoms, and treatment of two common medical problems. (Paperback.)

Ropp, Doris J. *Allergies and Your Family.* New York: Sterling Publishing Company, 1981.
A practical approach to the problems of living with allergies. (Paperback.)

Part VI

Community Well-Being

Health care is a human right that concerns world organizations, our government from the federal to the local level, private industry, voluntary groups, and most importantly, each and every one of us. Conservationists have long concentrated on preventing the disappearance of any species that appears to be losing the battle with its environment. The dangers imposed by technology, overpopulation, and air, water, and noise pollution, as well as the effects of nuclear energy on health, now force us to think of ourselves as an endangered species. "Safety and Accident Prevention," Chapter 19, stresses how to circumvent and reduce accidents, the leading cause of death for young people between the ages of 15 and 24. "Consumer Health," Chapter 20, includes information on health standards, health insurance, selecting medical care, and ways of guarding against quackery and questionable advertising claims for some health products. The last chapter, "Environmental Health," reinforces the importance of safeguards that will prevent our hospitable environment from becoming one that is hostile.

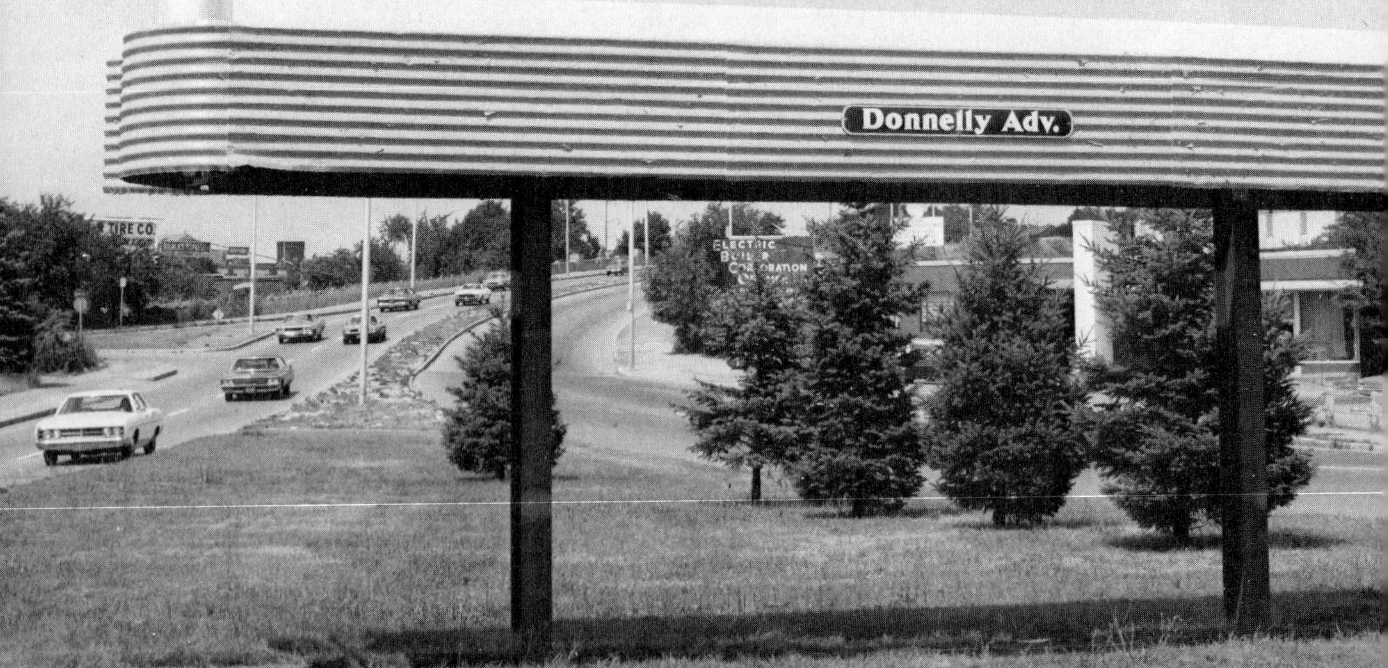
THERE'S A NAME FOR PEOPLE
WHO DON'T USE SEAT BELTS.
STUPID!
Donnelly Adv.

Chapter 19
Safety and Accident Prevention

KEY POINTS

- ☐ Accidents are the fourth leading cause of death in the United States, causing more than 100,000 deaths each year.
- ☐ About 85 percent of all accidents are the result of human error; other causes include environmental hazards and mechanically defective or poorly designed products.
- ☐ Appropriate preventive measures can significantly reduce the risks of accidents.
- ☐ Psychological, physiological, and cultural factors are often contributing elements in accidents stemming from human error.
- ☐ Traffic accidents are the leading cause of accidental death, and alcohol is implicated in at least half of all fatal collisions.
- ☐ Not wearing safety belts doubles your chance of being hurt seriously in a crash.
- ☐ Other types of accidents include falls, fire, poisoning, drownings, and sports injuries.
- ☐ Emergency first-aid care includes techniques to slow severe bleeding, to provide artificial respiration, and to help shock victims.

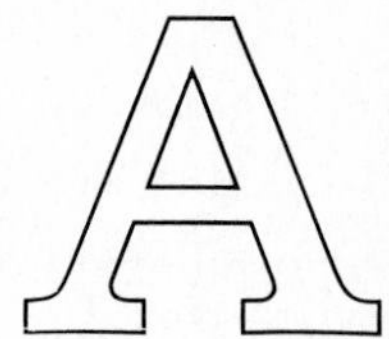

DRIVER falls asleep at the wheel. A small child drinks a bottle of cleaning fluid. An elderly person stumbles while emerging from the bathtub. Faulty electrical wiring bursts into flame. The list is endless. Accidents occur so frequently that they often elicit little surprise, save a sad shake of the head over the carelessness typically involved.

Clichés such as "Accidents will happen" make light of the fact that accidents are the fourth leading cause of death in the United States, and the first leading cause for people between the ages of 1 and 38. This age group includes the majority of college students. Accidents claim over 100,000 victims annually and result in more than 10 million disabling injuries. Also, accident-related suffering is not purely physical: the financial toll amounts to more than $40 billion annually in lost wages, medical and hospital costs, and property damage. For young people—those between the ages of 15 and 24—accidents account for more deaths than all other causes combined.

Accident Sequence of sudden, unplanned events resulting in injury or damage.

By definition, an **accident** is a sequence of sudden, unplanned events which may result in personal injury or property damage. There are usually several factors involved in each accident. For example, an overhead light burns out; a harried homemaker stands on a chair to change the bulb; the doorbell rings and she hastily jumps off the chair; she misjudges the distance between the chair and the floor and her foot slips; she lands awkwardly, painfully spraining her ankle. Clearly, had the light not broken, had the woman not been in a hurry, had she stood on a sturdy ladder instead of a chair, had the doorbell not rung, or had the woman stepped off the chair carefully, she might not have been injured.

Accidents and Accident Victims

More than half of all accidents are motor-vehicle related, and alcohol consumption is a factor in approximately 50 percent of these mishaps. Other accidents occur at home, on the job, and in public places.

Motor-vehicle crashes—the leading killer of individuals between the ages of 15 and 24—usually involve a car, motorcycle, or moped colliding with a fixed obstacle. Accidents that occur at home usually involve the very old or the very young (about one third of those killed are 75 or older). Most of these fatalities are attributable to falls, but death or serious injury may also result from fire, poison, suffocation, or use of firearms. There have even been accidents of children drowning in buckets of water.

On-the-job accidents often result from malfunctioning or inadequately shielded machinery or from the worker's failure to use protective equipment. Work-related environmental hazards also claim many victims, as in the case of coal miners with black lung disease and asbestos workers with cancer due to inhalation of toxic dust.

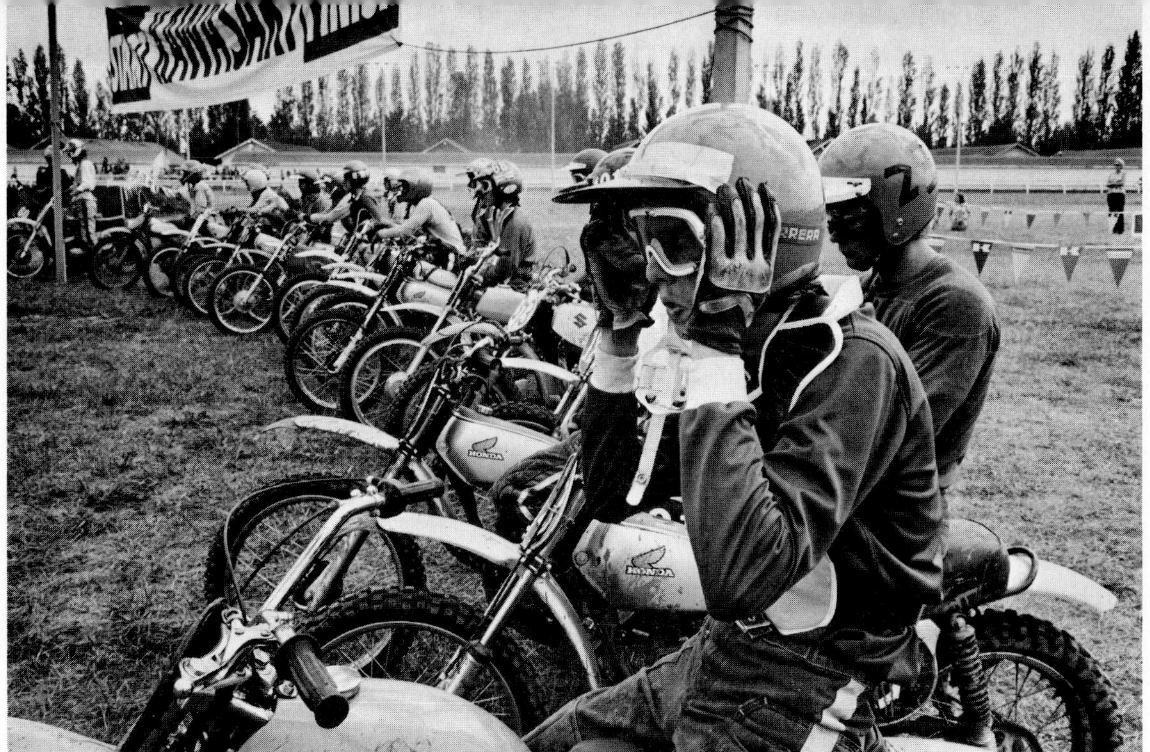

Accidents are the leading cause of injury and death among teenagers and young adults, partly because of their participation in high-risk activities such as motorcycling. (Photo by Charles Harbutt/Archive Pictures)

Many victims of other accidents in public places were participating in recreational activities, particularly water sports, such as boating, swimming, water skiing, or scuba diving. Others are killed or injured while riding on a public conveyance (bus, train, subway, or airplane), and fires in public buildings claim many lives. Children are vulnerable to accidents both in school and as they are transported to and from school.

Causes of Accidents

About 85 percent of all accidents are due to human error or unsafe behavior. Accidents caused by human failure are rarely the result of sheer chance or carelessness. Psychological, physiological, and cultural factors are usually involved. (To test your susceptibility to accidents, complete Self-Assessment Exercise 19.1 at the end of this chapter.) When our emotions are altered by *psychological conditions* — when we are very angry, very happy, very anxious — we may act unpredictably. We are "not ourselves," and thus we may perform tasks haphazardly, ignoring important details. On the other hand, people who are accident-prone may have deep-seated personality traits or attitudes that make them susceptible to mishaps. Some people respond to dares and similar challenges; others enjoy showing off; still others believe that they are powerless to control their destiny, and thus do not take steps to minimize risks.

Physiological factors that may contribute to accidents include sensory impairments (particularly defective sight or hearing); fatigue; handicaps such as epilepsy; and muscle or nerve disorders that impair coordination. Psychoactive drugs such as tranquilizers and amphetamines, and some medicines, such as cough syrups and antihistamines, may induce drowsiness, dizziness, and confusion.

Cultural factors are often contributing elements in accidents stemming from human error. In our fast-paced society, many of us neither have the patience nor take the time to perform tasks carefully. Also, the emphasis on competitiveness, aggressiveness, and rugged individualism may drive people to flaunt their physical prowess—leaping fences, climbing trees, playing tackle football, hockey, or basketball with almost brutal zeal. Firearms—the legacy of our frontier heritage—can be found in many American homes, where their misuse often results in tragedy.

Accidents also result from *environmental hazards* (rain, ice, lightening, floods, earthquakes), and a small percentage of accidents are caused by poorly designed or *defective devices or equipment* (such as cribs that allow a baby's head to become caught between the bars or a roof that caves in under the weight of too much snow).

Traffic Accidents

When consumer advocate Ralph Nader wrote *Unsafe at Any Speed* in 1965, automobiles rolled off the assembly line with few built-in safety guarantees. Nader's book presented evidence that automobile injuries and fatalities could be greatly reduced if safety standards and design changes were introduced. Its publication led to the passage of the National Traffic and Motor Vehicle Safety Act of 1966. Before 1966 lap seatbelts had become standard equipment in most cars, and

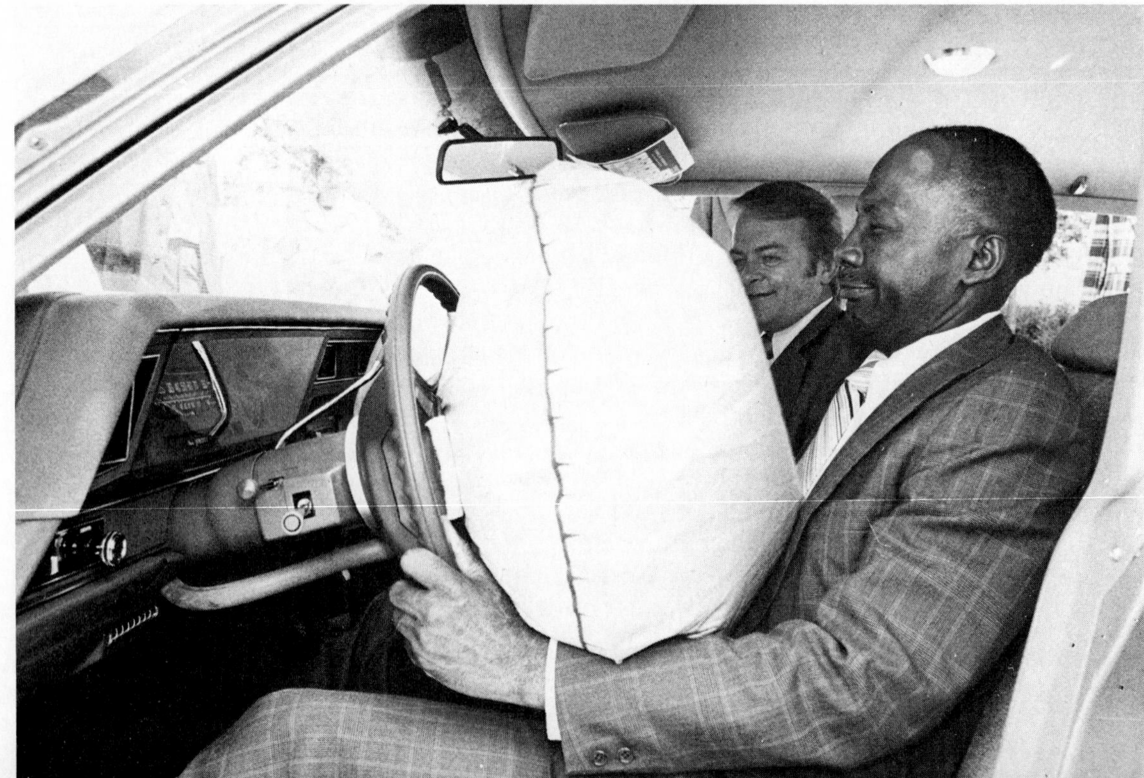

The use of air bags would substantially reduce the danger of injury or death in automobile collisions. (Photo from Wide World)

some vehicles contained energy-absorbing steering assemblies and penetration-resistant windshields. The 1966 act, however, mandated sweeping reforms: all automobiles manufactured in 1968 were required to include crash avoidance equipment such as redundant braking systems (emergency brakes) and side-view lights, and to provide for reduced light reflection in the driver's eyes. Since then, manufacturers have eliminated sharp parts on the dashboard, removed projecting ornaments from hubcaps, installed roll bars to prevent the roof from collapsing if the car rolls over, and added shoulder belts, outside rear-view mirrors, larger and sturdier tires, and padded interiors. Other design changes being tested include rupture-resistant gas tanks, air bags to cushion car occupants during a crash, energy-absorbing bumpers, and engines that will slant downward rather than into the driver in head-on collisions.

States vary in their inspection requirements. Most states require a 1⁄16-inch tread on tires, but this is inadequate for wet-weather driving. There is evidence, however, that federal safety regulations have had a significant impact. For a three-year period ending in 1978, some 37,000 fewer deaths were recorded than would have been expected without the introduction of safety standards. Still, in 1980 almost 50,000 people—three quarters of them male—died in accidents involving cars, light trucks, vans, motorcycles, or mopeds.

Many deaths result from people failing to wear safety belts. In fact, approximately 35,000 people die each year in cars, vans, or light trucks equipped with safety belts. It has been estimated that about 50 percent of these deaths could have been avoided had the people only worn their safety belts. According to the U.S. Department of Transportation, a common cause of death and injury to children in automobiles is being crushed by adults who are not wearing safety belts. The Department estimates that about one out of four serious injuries to passengers is caused by occupants being thrown into each other. When they wear safety belts, drivers have more control over their cars in emergency situations and are thus likely to avoid an accident.[1] (For more information on the effectiveness of safety belts see the box entitled "Safety Belt Fact Sheet.")

Drinking Drivers

Even a couple of drinks can turn a driver into a potential killer. Alcohol is not a stimulant but a depressant: it dulls mental capacities, slows reflexes, impairs judgment, and causes drowsiness. Significantly, people under the influence of alcohol often don't realize that they are not functioning at peak efficiency, so they may attempt to drive. It is very hard to set individual limits on how much liquor can be safely tolerated in drivers. Most people set their own standards: perhaps one drink per hour if they plan to drive. However, the fact remains that at least half (and possibly more than two-thirds) of all motor vehicle crashes are alcohol-related. Drunken drivers most

YOUR HEALTH TODAY

Safety Belt Fact Sheet: How Effective Are Safety Belts?

Most people accept the fact that wearing safety belts offers protection in a crash, but too few bother to find out exactly how much protection they can expect. If they asked, they would probably be surprised by the answer. While researchers may differ by a few percentage points either way, average figures coming out of safety belt studies look like this:

- Safety belts cut the number of serious injuries received by 50 percent.
- Safety belts cut fatalities by 60 to 70 percent.

To put these figures in other words, not wearing a safety belt doubles your chance of being hurt seriously in a crash. Serious injuries received in crashes often involve the head or spinal cord. In fact, in the U.S., auto accidents are the number one cause of epilepsy (from head injury) and paraplegia (from damage to the spinal cord). The restraining action of safety belts—especially shoulder belts—helps explain why they so drastically reduce the likelihood of being seriously hurt. Wearing just a lap belt gives you twice as good a chance of living through a crash as you'd have if you wore no belt at all. And using a lap/shoulder belt combination makes your chances of survival *three to four times better* than they are if you drive beltless. One important note: These improved chances of escaping injury or death thanks to safety belts hold true *regardless of speed.* Whether you're going 5 mph or 75 mph, you're a lot better off using belts.

Safety belts help occupants in five ways:

1. There is the *"ride down" benefit,* in which the belt begins to stop the wearer as the car is stopping.
2. The belt keeps the *head and face* of the wearer from striking objects like the wheel rim, windshield, interior post, or dashboard.
3. The belt *spreads the stopping force widely across the strong parts of the body.*
4. *Belts prevent vehicle occupants from colliding with each other.*
5. Belts help the driver to *maintain* vehicle control, thus decreasing the possibility of an additional collision.

Source: U.S. Department of Transportation, National Highway Traffic Safety Administration.

often injure themselves by hitting a fixed obstacle, such as a tree. When the crash involves another motorist, however, it is usually head-on, with the drunken driver veering over from the opposite lane. A driver who drinks is 20 times more likely to have an accident than is a sober driver.

Law enforcement officials have had difficulty applying rules governing drinking and driving. In the aftermath of an accident, it is hard

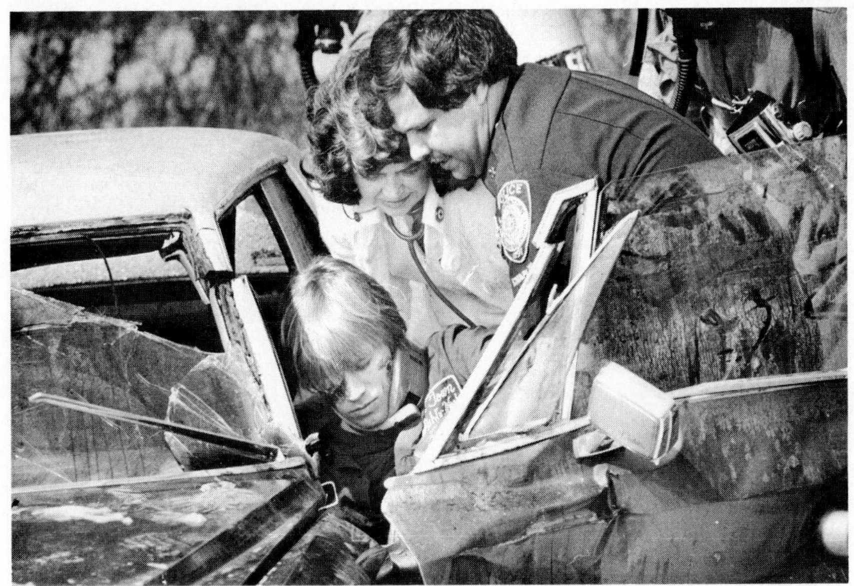

Traffic accidents can result from carelessness, drinking while driving, or a mechanical failure in the car. Statistics show that wearing safety belts can prevent death in a serious accident. (Photo by Michael Hayman/ Photo Researchers, Inc.)

to determine the concentration of alcohol in the blood of the driver and others involved, especially if they have been injured. Tests may be unavailable or inadequate, or time may reduce the accuracy of the tests. In some areas, the average age of victims in alcohol-related car crashes has been declining, a trend that has led many states to raise the minimum drinking age to 21. This movement to raise the minimum drinking age to 21 has begun to spread to many more states, stirring up a great deal of controversy along the way. The Federal Government has expressed its support of this movement, by threatening to remove federal highway funds from states not having a minimum drinking age of 21.

How To Handle Some Common Emergencies

Learning to be a good driver is an important skill that may save your life, or the lives of others, some time in the future. One aspect of good driving is to drive defensively, alert and ready to handle a possible sudden emergency, such as those that follow.

Someone Is Coming at You Head-on. If a car is coming directly at you, the best defensive step is to move over to the extreme right of your lane. A common mistake is to get into the lane the other driver should be in, which is exceedingly dangerous. Perhaps the other driver, overcoming a temporary drowsiness, may quickly swerve back to the correct lane only to find your car there. Often the other driver is passing someone and has misjudged the time it will take to do it. Blow your horn, brake, and veer to the right. Don't count on the other driver to size up the situation and drop back.

You Have Parked on a Hill and Your Car Starts Moving. Get into the car as quickly as possible and hit the brakes while turning the steering wheel toward the curb or toward another obstruction, being careful to direct the vehicle away from pedestrians. This type of mishap usually occurs when a driver turns off the ignition but does not put the car in neutral or park and neglects to use the emergency brake. On cars that have a manual shift, place the gearshift lever in reverse when parking on a hill and facing downhill. When parking on a hill and facing uphill, be sure that the gearshift lever is in forward gear. In addition, always turn your wheels toward the curb when parking on an incline.

Your Lights Fail. Brake to slow the car and get off the road. Using a flashlight (something every car should be equipped with, along with flares), try to locate and repair the trouble. Check the fuses first. If they are unimpaired, call for emergency road service and wait until help comes. Do not drive in the dark without lights.

A Tire Blows Out. Your car will be pulled abruptly to the side of the blown-out tire. The natural reaction is to slam on the brakes. Don't do it! Grip the steering wheel and concentrate on staying in your lane regardless of speed. Allow the care to slow by itself, then brake *gently* and get off the road.

The Road Is Wet or Icy and You're Skidding. Do not brake. That will often just pull the car faster to the side of the skid and possibly turn the vehicle over. Remove your foot from the accelerator and concentrate on steering. Turn the steering wheel in the direction of the skid, taking care not to skid to the other side.

The Car Ahead of You Stops Suddenly. Put on your brakes and steer straight if you are too close to swerve. Remember that there may be traffic in the adjacent lanes, too. Because drivers are sometimes forced to brake abruptly (if, for example, a child runs into the road), it is important to leave yourself sufficient space to stop. Do not tailgate. Allow at least one car length for every 10 miles of speed (three car lengths if you are going 30 miles per hour; five car lengths if you are going 50 miles per hour, and so forth).

Motorcycles, Mopeds, and Bicycles

Motorcycles have become increasingly popular. They get excellent mileage, and they are easy to maneuver and park. Mopeds, or motorized pedal bicycles, are light, flexible, and require relatively little fuel. Unfortunately, two-wheeled vehicles, especially motorized ones, are the most dangerous form of transportation. Not only do other drivers have trouble seeing them on the road, but cyclists are relatively unprotected should they become involved in an accident. Helmets, which are required for motorcyclists in some states, have substantially reduced the incidence of head injuries.

A person attempting to aid an injured cyclist should remove the helmet carefully, so as not to worsen injuries to the central nervous system. If the helmet provides full coverage to the face, the glasses should be removed first. Expand the helmet laterally to clear the ears;

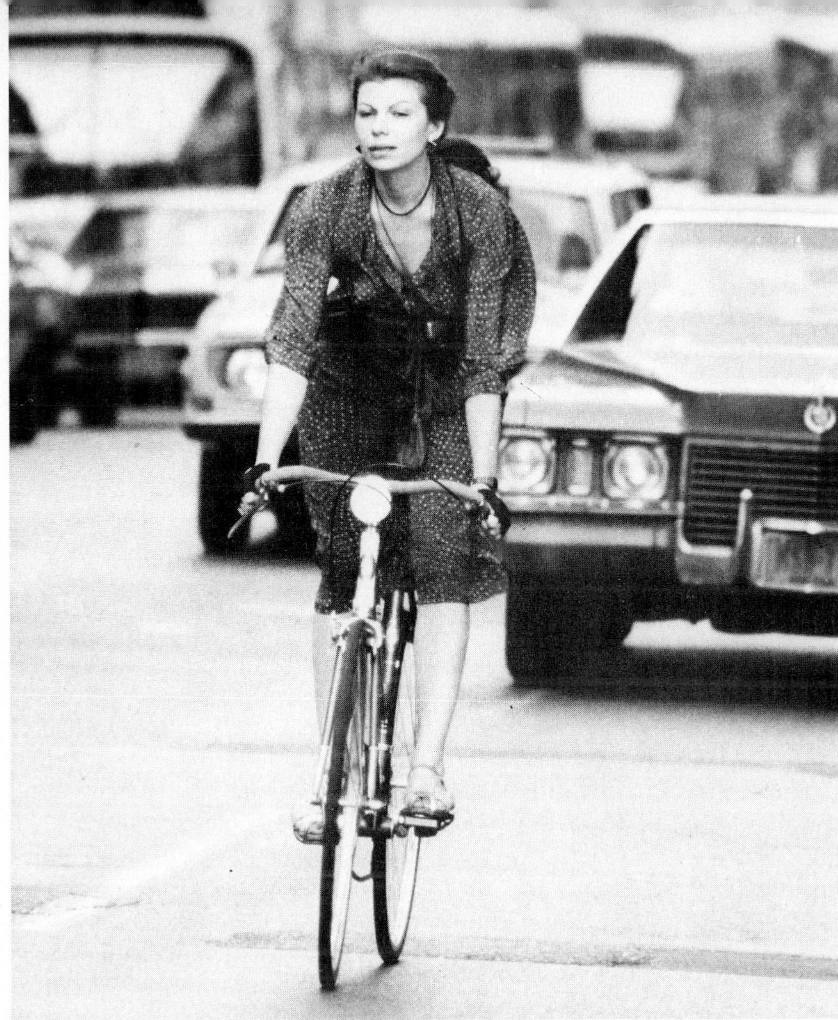

A bicycle rider during rush hour. Coping with city traffic demands extreme alertness and a thorough knowledge of bicycle safety and traffic laws. (Photo from Wide World)

the helmet must then be tipped backward and raised over the nose. *Keep the head and neck rigid:* any tilt may cause further damage to an already injured spine.

In recent years the growing concern about fuel supplies and the growing enthusiasm about physical fitness have sparked a particular interest in bicycle riding. Unfortunately, the sharp increase in the number of bicycles on the road has resulted in some alarming accident statistics. Between 1961 and 1971, deaths involving bicycles increased by 70 percent, compared to 44 percent for motor vehicles. (Most often, bike-related injuries do not involve cars.) Many injured cyclists are children, who are unaware that they are required to observe the same rules as those that prevail for motorists (for example, stopping for red lights and stop signs, signaling for turns, keeping to the right side of the road, giving the right of way to pedestrians). Other basic safety rules include:

- Keep both hands on the handlebars.
- Walk your bicycle through busy intersections and when making a left turn through heavy traffic.

- Make yourself visible. Retroreflective tape is helpful.
- If cars are parked along the curb, watch for drivers who may be about to open a door.
- Wear a helmet.
- Don't wear long coats, scarves, wide pants, or skirts that may catch in the spokes.
- Do not carry passengers.
- Avoid trick riding, racing, or snaking between two lanes of traffic.
- Watch carefully for pedestrians.

When choosing a bicycle, make sure that it's the proper size for your height and weight. Are there easy-to-operate hand or foot brakes? Are there protruding bolts, gear controls, or sharp fenders that could hurt you in the event of a fall? Are the lights and reflectors in good repair? Check that the posts for the seat and handlebars are thrust at least 2½ inches into the frame.

Pedestrians

The young, the old, and persons under the influence of alcohol are the most likely pedestrian victims of traffic accidents. A child is almost twice as likely to be hurt as a pedestrian than as a passenger in a car. Children may be unable to cope with complex traffic patterns, they may dash into the road in pursuit of a ball, or they may not be properly supervised by adults. Persons over 65 may have impaired hearing, lack agility, or have trouble seeing, especially at dusk or night, when most pedestrian-related accidents occur. Also, it may sometimes be difficult for senior citizens to finish crossing a street before the light changes.

The best rule for the pedestrian is: make sure that you can be seen. Wear light-colored clothes at night and don't jaywalk. Where there is no sidewalk, stay on the left side of the road. In an unlit rural area carry a flashlight. Some motorists have difficulty seeing at night, and few states are equipped to test night-driving ability in their examining centers.

Home Accidents

Although the number of crippling injuries suffered at home is slowly declining, some three million people in the United States are temporarily or permanently disabled on their own property each year. Only motor-vehicle-related mishaps account for more accidental deaths.

Home accidents are not a major factor in the 15- to 24-year-old group, but for the population as a whole, falls and fires claim many victims. To avoid falls, safety experts recommend that both indoor and outdoor steps be well lit and have sturdy handrails. Stairways should be free of obstructions at all times, and carpeting should be in good repair. Tubs and shower surfaces should be covered with non-skid mats, decals, or a textured surface. A bathroom night-light is a good investment. Wipe up spills immediately. Climb only with the aid of a sturdy, well-maintained ladder. Small rugs also represent a hazard; they should not be placed in heavy household-traffic areas.

Fire

About half the deaths from fire in the United States occur in private dwellings. Roughly 6,000 die each year in home fires, and another 100,000 are injured severely enough to require medical attention.

Because smoke always precedes flames, smoke detectors are vital safety devices: they can sound a warning alarm before escape routes are blocked. Nearly half the households in the United States now have smoke detectors, as compared to 28 percent in 1977, and in some instances the installation of these devices is required by law. As a result, according to the Federal Emergency Management Agency, although the number of residential fires has risen, death and injury rates have dropped. A smoke detector usually gives a warning within two minutes of a fire's start; the usual household fire takes about seven minutes to become so serious as to prevent escape.

Smoke detectors can be powered by the household electrical system or by battery. A battery-operated alarm is advisable, because an electric system may malfunction in case of fire. Some models are electric with a battery back-up system. Experts recommend installation of detectors in ground-floor hallways near the foot of stairs and in hallways outside of bedrooms.

To prevent fires, certain precautions should be taken:

- Be sure home wiring is in good condition. Don't put extension wires under carpets where they can't be seen. Walking or placing heavy furniture on the wires can damage the insulation. Avoid overloading electrical outlets.
- Don't smoke in bed and be sure the ashes of smoking products are cold when you empty ashtrays (never into wastebaskets).
- Don't allow rags or papers to collect, especially if the rags have been used to wipe up oil, paint, fuel, or other combustible material. They may ignite from spontaneous combustion.
- Use space heaters carefully. Keep them away from rugs, flammable material, and small children.

If a fire breaks out, here are some rules to follow:

- Get everybody out of the house. It's a good idea to keep a knotted heavy rope, or a rope ladder, in second-floor bedrooms so that you are not dependent on stairs. Stay close to the floor (at about crawling height) while making your way to a door or window.

Heated air and carbon monoxide, a colorless, odorless—and deadly—gas, tend to rise toward the ceiling. Test doors before opening them. If panels or knobs are warm, use a different escape route. (Practice your exit plan before you need it, especially in the dark, so every family member knows what to do.)

- Once everyone is out of the house, call for help.
- If you are trapped in a room, cover your nose and mouth with a pillow or wet cloth, put wet cloths around the crack in the door, position yourself near a slightly opened window, and wait for help to arrive.
- Don't waste time getting dressed or collecting things to save. Have a predetermined place to meet other family members once you are out of the house.
- If clothing catches fire, smother the flames with a blanket or coat, or roll on the ground. *Do not run.*
- Keep a fire extinguisher handy near the door or exit for small fire emergencies.

Poisoning

For young adults, poisoning by solids or liquids is the most common home-related accident. Most cases of poisoning involve overdoses of barbiturates, heroin, or tranquilizers. Many common household products, however, are highly toxic and constitute a threat to young children, who will eat almost anything, regardless of taste.

A major step toward the prevention of accidental childhood poisoning was taken in 1970, when Congress passed the Poison Prevention Packaging Act. Special safety caps requiring matching of arrows or applying pressure while turning have proved to be effective in reducing ease of opening for little children. Unfortunately, many adults, particularly the elderly, have experienced difficulty with safety caps.

What to Do. Symptoms of poisoning vary. In general, if a person has sudden abdominal pain, burns around the lips or mouth, contracted or dilated pupils, or a chemical odor on the breath, suspect poisoning. Try to find out what poison has been swallowed. If you can, locate the original container and label to give to medical personnel for identification. Other steps to be taken are as follows:

If the victim is conscious and not having convulsions, give a glass of water to dilute the poison. (A person who has taken an overdose of tranquilizers, barbiturates, opium, or alcohol should be given warm, but not hot, coffee or strong tea. The caffein acts as a stimulant.) Call for help immediately. (Keep numbers of the emergency rescue squad, the poison control center, and your doctor handy by your telephone.) Induce vomiting unless the substance swallowed is a strong acid (such as disinfectant), a strong alkali (such as ammonia), or a petroleum product (such as kerosene or gasoline). Lye and acid burn the mouth and food passages; petroleum products can be breathed into the lungs and cause pneumonia. Keep the person warm and quiet.

YOUR HEALTH TODAY

Basic Principles of First Aid

1. Call an ambulance or a physician immediately or instruct someone else to call.
2. Keep calm and try to keep other people calm. Often the best thing that can be done in an emergency is to protect the injured person from well-meaning but clumsy and possibly harmful attempts at helping.
3. Allow the best-trained person present to take over the responsibility of administering first aid.
4. Examine the victim carefully and determine what immediate help is needed. If there is more than one injury, attend to the most serious injury first.
5. Never give fluids to an unconscious person. The fluid may enter the air passages and block them.
6. Do not move victims unless it is necessary. They should lie quietly until a doctor or an ambulance arrives. The safest place is usually on the ground or the floor, so that they cannot fall and suffer further injury. Victims should be covered and kept warm.
7. Protect victims from injuring themselves further; do not allow them to move about restlessly. Keep bystanders away.

If the patient vomits, save some of the regurgitated material for analysis. Do not give counteragents to neutralize. Do not give oils.

If the victim is unconscious, or becomes unconscious, keep the airway open. Call the emergency rescue squad. When necessary, give mouth-to-mouth resuscitation or cardipulmonary resuscitation (CPR) if you know the technique. Do not give fluids. Do not induce vomiting. If the person is vomiting, position the person on the side so the vomitus drains from the mouth. As in the case of a conscious patient, save some of the regurgitated material for analysis.

If the victim has convulsions, try to protect the individual from these movements. Do not try to restrain the person, however. Do not force anything between the teeth. Do not induce vomiting. Do not give any fluids. Watch for obstruction of the airway and use CPR or mouth-to-mouth resuscitation where feasible and necessary. After a convulsion, turn the patient on the side so that fluid drains from the mouth. Again, keep the person warm and quiet.

Poison Prevention. To prevent accidental poisoning, various steps can be taken:

- Store all chemicals, medicines, alcoholic beverages, and drugs out of reach of children, preferably in a locked cabinet.
- Never store harmful products in food containers, such as soft drink or milk bottles.
- Keep medicines and cosmetics in their original, labeled containers. Do not take medicine in the dark.

- Avoid inhaling insecticide, weed killers, and spray paint.
- Never tell a child that medicine is candy.
- Keep syrup of ipecac (a formula that induces vomiting) on hand, especially if there are children in the home.

Job-related Accidents

For decades the scene of crippling injuries and accidental deaths, the workplace has become relatively safe in recent years. Between 1912 and 1976, accident fatality rates dropped by 71 percent, largely as a result of organized safety campaigns. Nevertheless, job-related accidents still kill more than 12,000 people each year; another 2.2 million are injured on the job, 80,000 of whom become permanently disabled.

The Occupational Safety and Health Act (OSHA), which became law in 1970, established minimum health and safety standards in most workplaces. The law is enforced by compliance officers, who focus most of their attention on construction sites and factories. The most hazardous occupations are roofing, stevedoring, mining, preparing meat and meat products, and working with sheet metal, lumber, and wood products.

Employers are required to tell their employees if they are being exposed to toxic fumes, gases, or chemicals, some of which have been linked to cancer, lung disorders, and other life-threatening illnesses. Efforts are also underway to limit worker exposure to extreme heat, dust, and deafening noise, which also represent job-related health hazards. Those interested in reducing workplace mishaps are con-

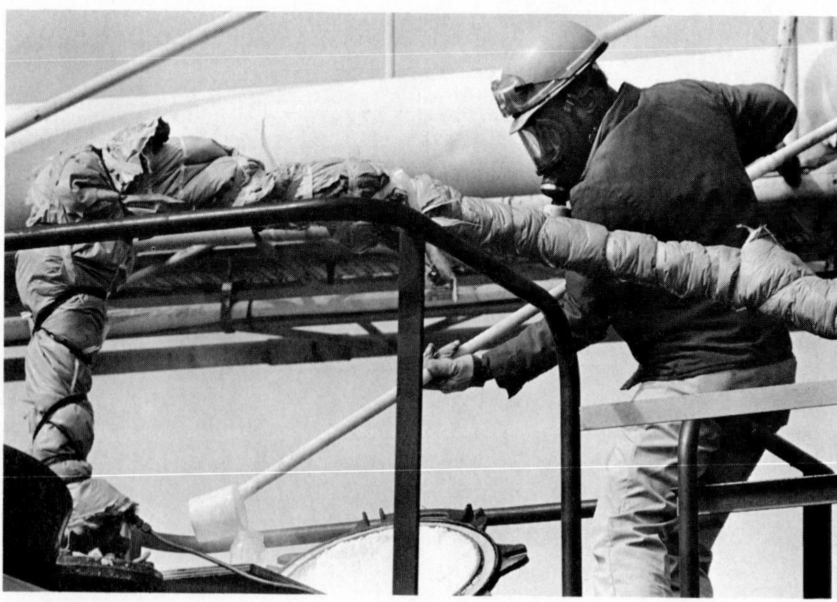

A worker testing chemicals. The Occupational Safety and Health Act (OSHA), passed in 1970, established minimum health and safety standards in the workplace. (Photo © John Coletti/Stock, Boston)

cerned about the sharp increase in the labor force of women over 35 and young people from 14 to 25, the most accident-prone group in the population.

Both unsafe environmental conditions and irresponsible behavior on the part of some workers contribute to accidents on the job. It is important that factories and other industrial plants be properly ventilated, well lit, carefully laid out, and kept free from clutter. Guards for machines are essential. Workers may be overconfident about using power tools and thus injure themselves with electric saws or drills, or they may fail to use protective gear, such as hard hats, ear plugs, goggles, and special gloves. Industries should employ a staff physician and/or nurse and provide a well-equipped first-aid center.

Public Accidents

Public accidents include falls, drownings, firearm-related injuries, and burns that occur on public property or in public buildings. Often large numbers of people are involved and complex rescue methods are required.

In the United States over 30,000 deaths and close to 3,000,000 injuries occur each year in accidents involving air, rail, and water transportation. As air travel becomes more and more extensive, accidents may increasingly occur because of a lack of well-trained pilots and ground staff or because air traffic regulations are not adequately adapted to the heavy volume of landings and takeoffs.

Fortunately, emergency-care systems have improved enormously in the United States. In addition, more than 500 areas now have 911 as a telephone number for reporting emergencies and getting help.

Swimming

Drownings are the fifth leading cause of accidental deaths in public places and the second overall cause of accidental death for young adults. Teenage boys are the most likely drowning victims. More than 50 percent of all drownings occur when people unexpectedly find themselves in the water, as when a boat overturns, a fisherman tumbles off a dock, or a child falls into an open well. Ironically, many drowning victims are excellent swimmers who overestimate their abilities and become exhausted while swimming in unguarded water, develop cramps, or ignore hazardous swimming conditions (sharp rocks, strong currents, or debris). As with many accidents, alcohol is often a factor: in more than half the drowning victims who are over 15, the blood alcohol level is high.

Here are a few common water safety tips:

- Never swim alone in unguarded water.
- Do not swim when overheated, overtired, or immediately after eating.

- Before diving, check to see that the water is deep enough, that nothing is hidden beneath the surface, and that there are no swimmers in close proximity.
- Lower yourself into cool water slowly; give your body time to adjust to the change in temperature.
- Teach children to swim at the earliest age possible. Most youngsters are ready by the time they are five.
- Never leave a small child unattended in a bathtub or near a pool, open well, fish pond, or other body of water—even for a few seconds.

School Sports

Despite helmets, shoulder pads, knee pads, and other protective devices, *football* is the most physically punishing of all sports, accounting for almost two-thirds of all elementary and secondary school athletic injuries. Furthermore, football casualties tend to be more serious and are more likely to be fatal than basketball, track and field, and baseball injuries. (However, deaths are relatively rare.)

The most frequent—and most dangerous—football injuries involve the head, which is sometimes used as a battering ram in blocking and tackling. Although it is true that the construction of helmets

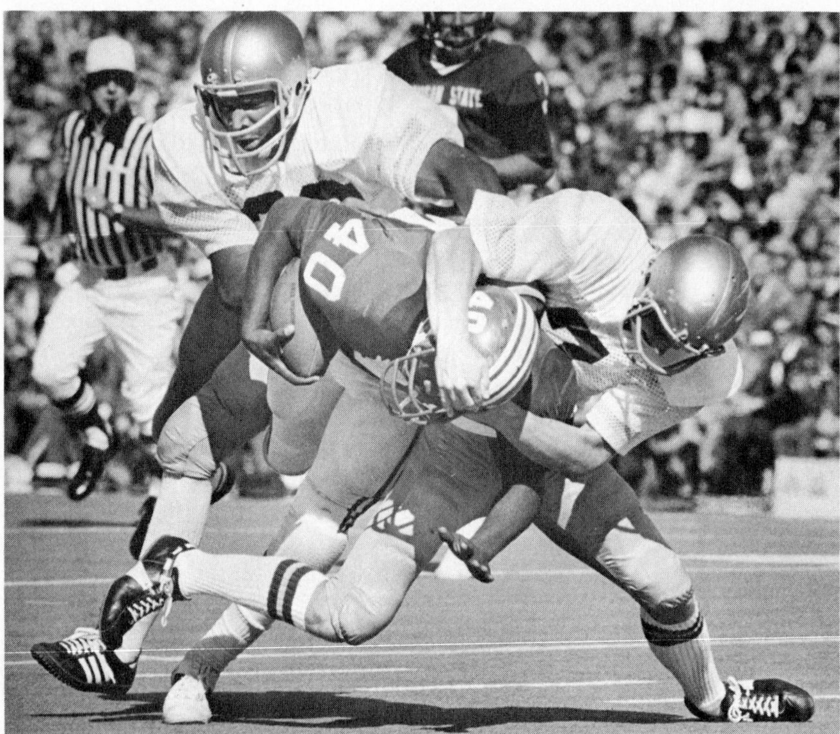

Football is a leading source of sports injuries. (Photo © Michael Hayman/Photo Researchers, Inc.

has improved, the American Medical Association's Committee on Sports Injuries says that shock-absorbing material encased in a firm plastic shell is essential. A face mask covered with rigid, cushioned material that does not protrude more than 1¼ inches from the nose is also advised. Dentists suggest the use of a mouthpiece that separates the biting surfaces and protects the lips from the teeth. There is evidence that the use of short, soccer-type cleats, or traditional football shoes but with heel cleats covered by a disk, rather than long cleats, cut down on knee and ankle injuries.

Two important innovations that have reduced Little League *baseball* injuries are flip-type sunglasses that will not shatter upon impact at 100 mph, and helmets that offer more protection to the temples and ears than the headgear worn by most major league baseball players.

Helmets for *wrestlers* became mandatory for competition in 1969. In gymnastics, the formula for safety involves well-conditioned and trained athletes, good supervision, proper maintenance of equipment, and careful placement of mats on hard surfaces. Track and field participants encounter relatively few hazards. Use of foam rubber and air-cushioned landing pits in the high jump and pole vault have proven valuable. Freed of the fear of a hard, bruising landing, some jumpers have attempted increasingly high leaps, setting new world records in the process.

Water Sports

Water skiing results in some 200 injuries and about 35 deaths in the United States each year. This count is not especially high, considering that many people water ski; still, there are some general rules to be observed by both the skier and the boat driver:

- Wear a good flotation device (a safety jacket or belt), preferably one recommended by the United States Coast Guard. A proper safety jacket should roll an unconscious person into an upright position by supporting the head and neck with the face out of water.
- Learn to ski from a knowledgeable instructor or from an accomplished skier.
- Keep a safe distance from docks, boats, debris, swimmers, and fishermen. Steer clear of shallow water and watch out for submerged objects just below the surface.
- Learn the basic hand signals to communicate with boat drivers and other water skiers.
- A person other than the driver should ride in the boat to observe the skier.
- When completing a tow, come in slowly parallel to the shore, not straight at it.
- Fall backward if you must fall. Falling forward cause the tips of the skis to dig into the water, resulting in knee and ankle injuries.

- Handle the tow rope carefully to avoid torn muscles and rope burns.
- Driver and observer should both remain seated. A driver who rides on the back of the seat or on the boat gunnel—presumably to get a better view of the skier—risks being tossed overboard.

The most significant difficulty associated with *scuba diving* is panic. If the air supply apparatus malfunctions or if the diver feels threatened by a marine animal, the diver may lose control and thrash about. This leads to carbon dioxide retention, oxygen deprivation, and, ultimately, exhaustion. Drowning or cardiac arrest can result.

Knowledge of emergency techniques (resting, floating to the surface, use of life vests), possession of proper equipment, and careful assessment of diving conditions before entering the water help to prevent the panic cycle.

The body's reaction to cold can also be very serious. A wet suit is a considerable help in a variety of water sports. In a wet suit an individual can tolerate water temperatures of 40 degrees Fahrenheit for up to six hours. However, a drop in body temperature even to 94°F (from the normal 98.6°F) results in confusion, disorientation, and loss of coordination. At 90°F one loses consciousness, and at 88°F the heart stops beating. This cooling of the body is referred to as **hypothermia.** Hypothermia can occur anytime an individual is engaged in an activity which exposes him to cold, wetness, wind, and exhaustion. To treat loss of body heat, the patient should be warmed to 104°F. Alcohol should never be given.

Hypothermia Abnormal lowering of the body temperature.

Emergency Care for Accident Victims

When a serious accident occurs, even under the best of circumstances it may be several minutes before medical help arrives at the scene. It is therefore essential that every person have at least a basic knowledge of emergency first-aid care. The following techniques are presented in order of priority: putting first things first may save a life.

Respiratory Failure

A person will die in about six minutes if the oxygen supply is cut off. Respiratory failure occurs if the air passage is blocked by a foreign object, or in cases of heart attack, inhalation of toxic gases, drowning, shock, chest wounds, or lung disorders. When breathing has stopped, mouth-to-mouth rescue breathing is the emergency measure of choice.

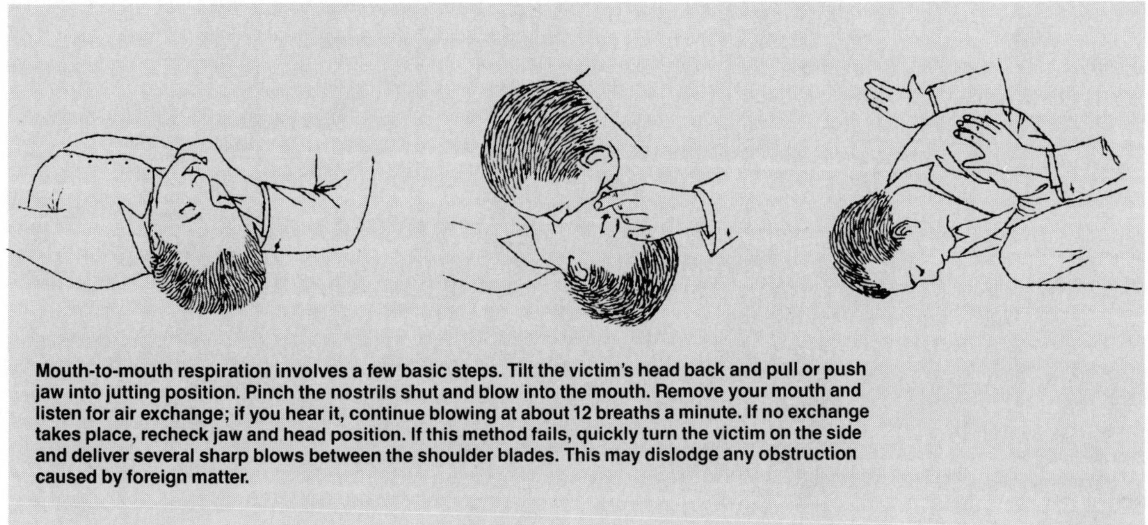

Mouth-to-mouth respiration involves a few basic steps. Tilt the victim's head back and pull or push jaw into jutting position. Pinch the nostrils shut and blow into the mouth. Remove your mouth and listen for air exchange; if you hear it, continue blowing at about 12 breaths a minute. If no exchange takes place, recheck jaw and head position. If this method fails, quickly turn the victim on the side and deliver several sharp blows between the shoulder blades. This may dislodge any obstruction caused by foreign matter.

Figure 19-1. Performing Artificial Respiration.

Mouth-to-Mouth Artificial Respiration

You begin this procedure by tilting the victim's head back, lifting it either with a hand under the neck or by pressing up and back on the chin. (If you choose the chin, be careful to put your hand on the bone, not on the soft tissue under the chin.) This will keep the tongue out of the airway. Take a few seconds—about five—to see if the victim's chest rises and you can hear air escaping from the mouth. Call for help. If the victim is not breathing, start mouth-to-mouth resuscitation by sealing your mouth tightly around the victim's and blowing in. Hold the nostrils shut so that no air leaks out.

Begin by quickly giving four full breaths without emptying your lungs between them. Look and listen again for exhalation of air and feel the victim's carotid (neck) pulse in the groove between the Adam's apple and the muscle at the side of the neck. If there is a pulse and no breathing, continue with the mouth-to-mouth resuscitation, giving at least one breath per five seconds for an adult. Take a deep breath yourself for each of these; it's important to keep enough volume going in to make the chest rise. You won't feel much resistance if the airway is clear.

When the victim's chest is expanded, raise your mouth, turn your head to the side, and listen for exhalation. Watch for the chest to fall, then repeat. Soon the patient's own breathing will start, and by that time the help you called for may have arrived (see Figure 19-1).

Cardiopulmonary Resuscitation

When the heart has stopped beating and the victim is unconscious and not breathing, **cardiopulmonary resuscitation (CPR)** is the necessary method. In this technique, bascially, the person administering

Cardiopulmonary resuscitation (CPR) Emergency technique used to revive heartbeat and breathing.

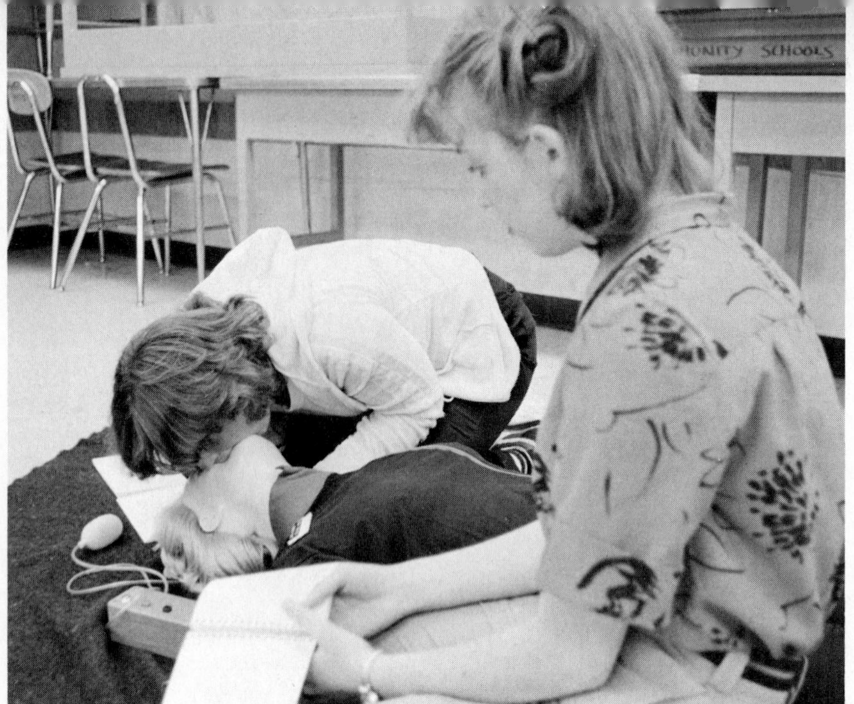

College students receive training in cardiopulmonary resuscitation. (Photo © Frank Siteman/Photography/The Picture Cube)

CPR places his or her mouth over the victim's and forces air into the lungs. The rescuer also presses down on the victim's chest to force the heart to pump blood.

The actual technique is rather complicated and requires special training in order to be carried out properly, but the use of CPR is not restricted to medical personnel. Any person can learn, and many should. It has been estimated that if one out of three Americans were trained in CPR, bystanders might be able to save between 100,000 and 200,000 lives each year by beginning treatment before the arrival of the rescue unit. Heart attacks cause about 550,000 deaths in the United States each year. More than 60 percent of these deaths occur before the patient reaches the hospital. Laypersons trained in CPR could prevent many such deaths.

Fortunately, CPR is being taught in classes to those who want to be able to help in emergencies. Programs are being developed in connection with, among other groups, the Boy Scouts, the American Red Cross, the Jaycees, and the General Foundation of Women's Clubs. The American Heart Association and the American Red Cross set guidelines for such instruction. Courses involve practice on mannequins designed to provide the kind of chest movement, airway obstruction, and resistance of the breastbone that are encountered in real life.

First Aid for Choking

If a person's air passage is completely blocked by food or a foreign object, stand behind the person and place your clenched fist against the belly just under the ribcage, with the thumb side inward. Then grasp your fist with your other hand, thrusting sharply upward and backward three or four times (see Figure 19–2). The pressure on the stomach forces air out of the lungs and the expelled air pushes the obstruction out of the airway. Repeat the procedure if necessary. This technique, known as the **Heimlich maneuver,** has saved many lives. It can also be performed with the victim lying on the back. Note: you should attempt the Heimlich maneuver only if the individual cannot breathe. If a person is able to cough or speak, there is sufficient time to seek medical help.

Heimlich maneuver Technique used to expel foreign matter lodged in a choking victim's windpipe.

If a baby is choking, hold the baby's face down on your arm, with your hand supporting the face. Spread your fingers so that air can reach the mouth and whatever is in the mouth can fall out. Give four sharp blows to the back between the shoulder blades.

Choking accidents among children can often be prevented by observing a few simple rules:

- Keep small objects such as marbles and coins out of the reach of infants and toddlers.
- Do not give small children nuts, popcorn, hard candy, unpeeled apples, or any other food that may lodge in the throat.
- Select sturdy toys that have no detachable or easily broken parts. Manufacturers are required to provide warnings when a toy is unsuitable for small children.

Stand behind the choking victim and wrap your arms around the person's waist.

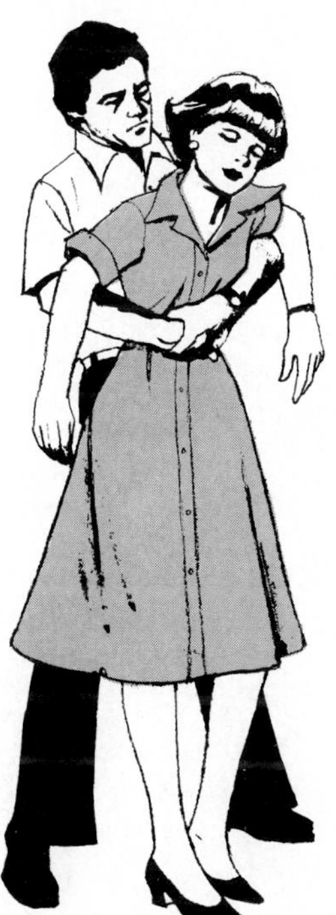

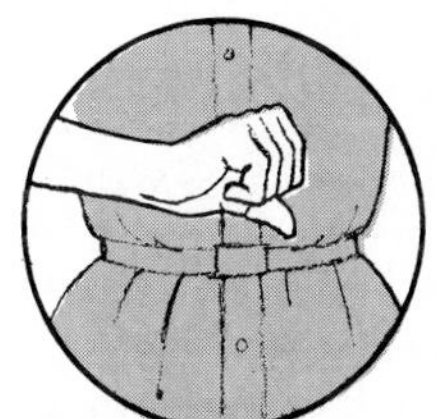

Place your fist against the victim's abdomen above the navel and below the rib cage.

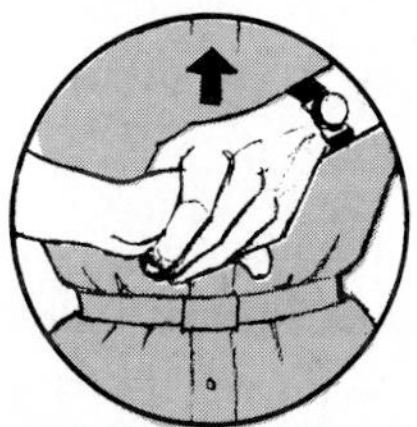

Grasp your fist with the other hand and press it into the abdomen with a sharp upward thrust. Repeat the maneuver if necessary.

Figure 19-2. Heimlich Maneuver for Adults.

Loss of Blood

If the victim is losing blood rapidly, death can follow in a few minutes. To control severe bleeding, apply direct pressure on the wound by firmly placing the palm of your hand on a dressing or clean cloth immediately over the whole area of the wound. If the pad or dressing is thick it will absorb blood and allow clotting. Wrap a pressure bandage around the wounded area, securing the pad or dressing in place. This will free your hands for other tasks. If there are no broken bones, raise the wounded arm, leg, or head. This reduces blood pressure on the injured area, slowing the flow of blood through the wound.

Brachial artery Main artery in the arm located on the inner side.

Femoral artery Main artery of the leg.

Pressure point technique Manual application of pressure to key arteries to stop the bleeding.

Tourniquet Apparatus used to stop blood flow from a life-threatening wound.

If bleeding still hasn't stopped, press the **brachial artery** if the victim has an arm wound. Grasp the victim's upper arm with your thumb on the outside and your other fingers on the inside. In this way you will squeeze the artery against the arm bone. (Use this technique *while* applying direct pressure and elevation, not as a substitute.) For an open leg wound, apply pressure to the **femoral artery.** With the victim lying flat on the back (if possible), place the heel of your hand on the artery and lean forward. Continue applying direct pressure and keep the limb raised (see Figure 19–3).

Techniques used to stop bleeding by manually applying pressure to key arteries are called **pressure-point techniques.** In a life-threatening emergency where these methods cannot be effectively employed, a **tourniquet** may be used. See Figure 19–3 for an illustration of some first-aid techniques to control bleeding.

Shock

In any accident the victim may go into shock, and the alert rescuer should learn what to look for and what to do. The kind of shock related to injury is not the same as electric shock or the shock that comes from getting too much insulin. The pulse is faint and probably cannot be felt at the wrist, but the carotid or femoral artery pulse will be noticeable. Blood pressure is very low or not perceptible at all, and the skin will be pale or bluish. If shock is untreated, at later stages the eyes will appear sunken and the pupils dilated.

The following steps should normally be taken to aid shock victims:

- If no obvious injuries make it unadvisable, you should place the patient in a lying-down position to ease blood circulation. (If you suspect an injury of the neck or spine, do not move the victim except to protect from further injury.) If the individual is unconscious, the best position is on the side, so that fluids or vomited material will drain from the mouth. Make sure there is an open airway.

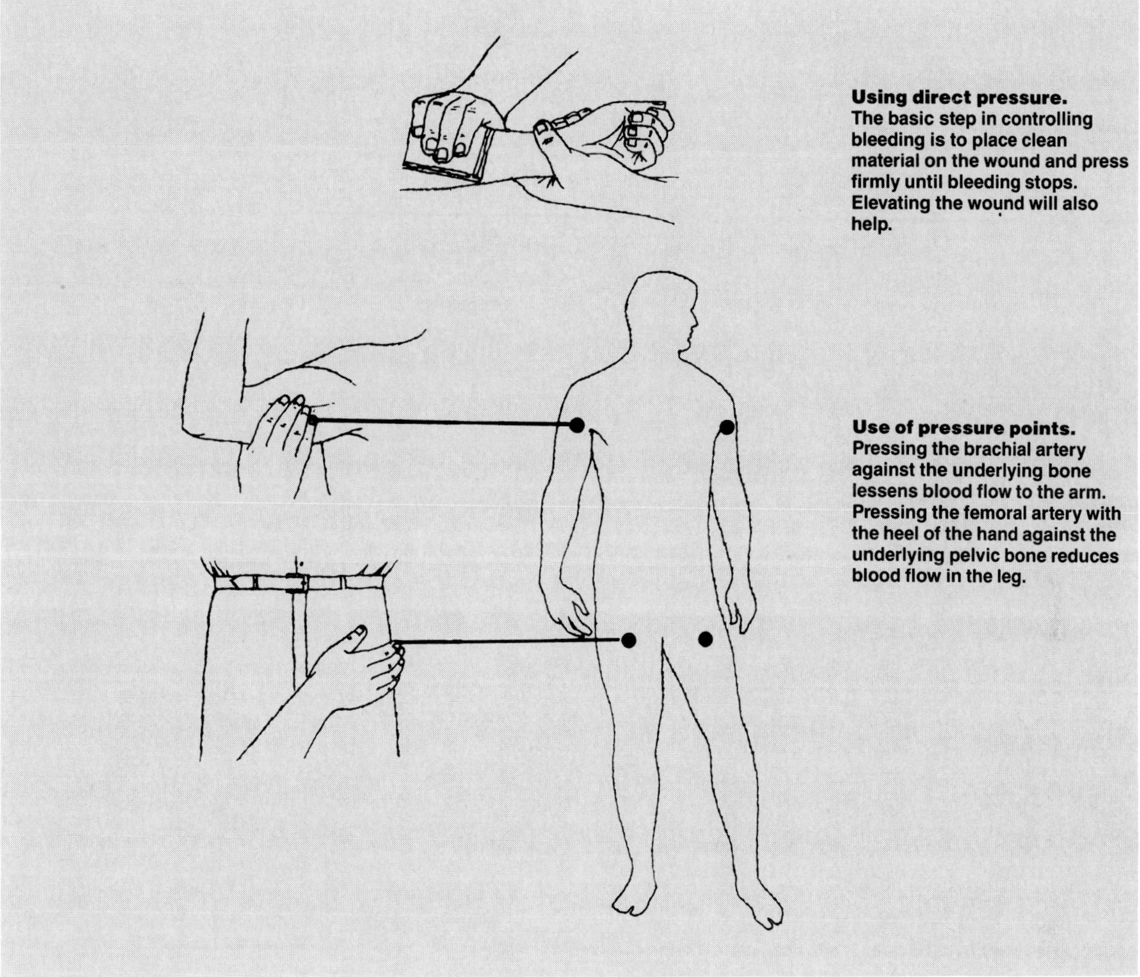

Figure 19-3. How to Stop Bleeding.

- Call for help. If nobody comes within a half hour or so and the patient is conscious, give a half glass of moderately warm water, with salt and baking soda if available. Measure one level teaspoon full of salt and a half teaspoonful of soda to a quart of water. Repeat the half-glass dose (four ounces) after 15 minutes. For a child in shock, give half the amount.
- If the person in shock has a head injury, keep the patient flat or prop up the head, but never have the head lower than the feet. You can place a blanket over and under the patient to prevent chilling until help comes.

As a general rule, it is more important to treat for severe bleeding or for an obstructed airway than for shock. Blood loss or inability to breathe normally can kill very quickly.

SELF-ASSESSMENT EXERCISE 19.1

Susceptibility to Accidents Inventory

Directions: Circle the number in the frequency column opposite the behavioral statement that best describes your behavior or best fits you.

Behaviors	Frequency			
	Usually or Always	Often	Sometimes/ Seldom	Never
A. Recreational Activities				
1. Fly a private plane or glider	5	3	1	0
2. Skydive	5	3	1	0
3. Drive a racing car or dune buggy	5	3	1	0
4. Drive a motorcycle, snowmobile, or power boat	5	3	1	0
5. Skin dive or scuba dive	5	3	1	0
6. Drive on weekends to go skiing or camping	5	3	1	0
7. Board or body surf	5	3	1	0
8. Hunt	5	3	1	0
9. Play body contact sports, like football, hockey etc.	5	3	1	0
10. Snow or water ski	5	3	1	0
11. Mountain climb or spelunk	5	3	1	0
12. Swim alone	5	3	1	0
Total	+	+	+	
B. Vocational				
13. Work with explosives or chemicals	5	3	1	0
14. Work as a lineman	5	3	1	0
15. Work in constructing bridges, high rise buildings, etc.	5	3	1	0
16. Smoke cigarettes in no-smoking areas	5	3	1	0
17. Drive 20,000 miles or more per year	5	3	1	0

Behaviors	Frequency			
	Usually or Always	Often	Sometimes/ Seldom	Never
18. Work in a noisy environment	5	3	1	0
19. Work with X-ray or ultraviolet equipment	5	3	1	0
20. Work with hot metals	5	3	1	0
21. Work with heavy construction materials or equipment	5	3	1	0
Total	+	+	+	
C. Home				
22. Store cleaning materials, insecticides, etc., in unlabeled or improperly labeled containers	5	3	1	0
23. Store old clothes, papers, paints, or solvents in garage or attic	5	3	1	0
24. Cut lawn when grass is wet	5	3	1	0
25. Have inadequate lighting in stairways	5	3	1	0
26. Use long light or TV electric cords	5	3	1	0
27. Smoke cigarettes in bed	5	3	1	0
28. Use underground electrical appliances or extension cords	5	3	1	0
29. Leave electrical appliances connected when not in use	5	3	1	0
30. Have slippery shower or bathtub floor	5	3	1	0
31. Smoke cigarettes while using aerosol cans (e.g., hairspray)	5	3	1	0
32. Have small rugs that skid on floor	5	3	1	0
33. Do own house repairs	5	3	1	0
34. Store guns and ammunition at home	5	3	1	0
35. Have windows nailed shut	5	3	1	0

(Continued)

Behaviors	Frequency			
	Usually or Always	Often	Sometimes/ Seldom	Never
36. Have stairs without adequate handrails	5	3	1	0
37. Use pot holders (towel) to handle hot pots and pans	5	3	1	0
38. Forget to replace burned-out lightbulbs	5	3	1	0
39. Wear high heel shoes	5	3	1	0
40. Cannot locate shutoff switch for electricity	5	3	1	0
41. Wear pants with wide cuffs	5	3	1	0
42. Cannot locate shutoff valve for water	5	3	1	0
43. Cannot locate shutoff valve for gas or oil	5	3	1	0
44. Cannot locate flashlight or do not have one	5	3	1	0
45. Postpone getting fire extinguisher (or do not have one)	5	3	1	0
Total	+	+	+	
D. Personality				
46. Tend to overlook "doing things"	5	3	1	0
47. Postpone making repairs to car, house, boat etc.	5	3	1	0
48. Postpone paying bills on time	5	3	1	0
49. Get a kick out of taking chances	5	3	1	0
50. Postpone getting sleep	5	3	1	0
51. Feel tired a lot	5	3	1	0
52. Drink beer or alcoholic beverages	5	3	1	0
53. Procrastinate, then rush to meet deadlines	5	3	1	0
54. Have difficulty in making decisions	5	3	1	0
55. Trip over obstacles	5	3	1	0

Behaviors	Frequency			
	Usually or Always	Often	Sometimes/ Seldom	Never
56. Experience failure more often than success	5	3	1	0
57. Worry over your clumsiness and lack of coordination	5	3	1	0
58. Have difficulty seeing faraway objects (without glasses)	5	3	1	0
59. Get mad or lose temper often	5	3	1	0
60. Get into trouble with others	5	3	1	0
61. Have difficulty hearing others speak	5	3	1	0
62. Feel you are more important than others	5	3	1	0
63. Have a sense of power when driving	5	3	1	0
64. Worry over what happened the day before	5	3	1	0
65. Carry a knife with a blade more than 6 in. long	5	3	1	0
66. Carry a gun or handle one	5	3	1	0
Total	+	+	+	
E. Pedestrian				
67. Wear dark clothes at night	5	3	1	0
68. Cross street wherever it is convenient	5	3	1	0
69. Step off curb when waiting for light to change	5	3	1	0
70. Cross intersection when light is red or amber	5	3	1	0
71. Expect cars to stop for you	5	3	1	0
72. Jaywalk to cross street	5	3	1	0
73. Walk in same direction as traffic	5	3	1	0
74. Walk frequently at night	5	3	1	0

(Continued)

Behaviors	Frequency			
	Usually or Always	Often	Sometimes/ Seldom	Never
75. Walk after drinking alcoholic beverages	5	3	1	0
Total	+	+	+	
F. Bicycling				
76. Ride with poor or no brakes	5	3	1	0
77. Ride with low or unchecked air pressure in tires	5	3	1	0
78. Ride on sidewalk	5	3	1	0
79. Ride at night without a headlight	5	3	1	0
80. Ride without light reflectors	5	3	1	0
81. Forget to give traffic signals	5	3	1	0
82. Ride two abreast on street	5	3	1	0
83. Like to show off	5	3	1	0
84. Ride with handlebars curled low	5	3	1	0
Total	+	+	+	
G. Driving (car/motorcycle)				
85. Park improperly or illegally	5	3	1	0
86. Drive when tired	5	3	1	0
87. Drive at excessive speeds for conditions	5	3	1	0
88. Cut in and out of traffic	5	3	1	0
89. Drive when ill or upset	5	3	1	0
90. Drive when under drug medication	5	3	1	0
91. Drive after having two or more beers or cocktails	5	3	1	0
92. Forget to buckle safety belt or harness	5	3	1	0

Behaviors	Frequency			
	Usually or Always	**Often**	**Sometimes/ Seldom**	**Never**
93. Driver over 20,000 miles a year	5	3	1	0
94. Carry gasoline in a can in trunk of car	5	3	1	0
95. Drive when signal lights and brakes do not work	5	3	1	0
96. Drive car or motorcycle with engine not tuned up	5	3	1	0
97. Drive with leaky exhaust	5	3	1	0
98. Drive with low air pressure in tires or with worn-out tires	5	3	1	0
99. Drive with mechanical problems	5	3	1	0
100. Drive in rain or icy conditions	5	3	1	0
101. Drive with poor car brakes	5	3	1	0
102. Have poor judgment of distance	5	3	1	0
103. Receive traffic citations or warnings	5	3	1	0
Total	+	+	+	

Scoring: Add the circled numbers in each section.

Interpretation:

Score Range	Degree of Susceptibility
151–520	Extreme
70–150	Average
0–69	Low

It is more important to pay attention to how you score in each section than to interpret your total score for this inventory. A total score for all sections is included although your scores in each separate section are more important.

Confer with your health science and safety instructor about your reactions to this inventory. Select alternative behaviors and habits that will make you less prone to accidents. Another alternative would be to modify some of your habits and behaviors that structure your present life=style.

You can avoid accidents and still experience exciting adventures.

Most of the topics covered in the inventory are discussed in this chapter.

Source: Walter D. Sorochan, *Promoting Your Health,* New York, John S. Wiley, 1981, p. 259–264. Reprinted by permission of the author.

Summary

Accidents are the fourth leading cause of death in the United States, claiming over 100,000 victims annually and resulting in more than 10 million disabling injuries. For young people—those between the ages of 15 and 24—accidents account for more deaths than from all other causes combined. More than three quarters of all accidents are mainly the result of human error, but accidents also result from environmental hazards, mechanical failures, and poorly designed products.

Psychological, physiological, and cultural factors are significant in increasing the risks of accidental injury or death, but appropriate preventive measure can decrease the risks.

At least half of all accidents are motor-vehicle-related, and alcohol is a factor in some 50 percent of these mishaps. Safety standards and design changes have helped to reduce the number of motor-vehicle-related fatalities. The growing popularity of motorcycles, mopeds, and bicycles has led to an increasing number of accidents involving two-wheeled vehicles.

The very young and the very old are the most likely victims of home accidents, which include falls, fires, and poisonings. On-the-job accidents may result from malfunctioning or inadequately shielded machinery or from a worker's failure to use protective equipment. Work-related environmental hazards also claim many victims. Accidents in public places include airplane crashes and other public-transportation mishaps, drownings, and sports injuries. Football is the most dangerous of all team sports, accounting for almost two-thirds of all elementary and secondary school athletic injuries. The number of injuries resulting from water sports—such as water skiing, scuba diving, and boating—could be reduced if more participants obtained proper instruction and observed safety rules.

Knowledge of how to treat severe bleeding, respiratory failure, cardiac arrest, choking, and shock may play a vital role in saving lives. In cases where the victim has stopped breathing, is unconscious, and has no pulse, cardiopulmonary resuscitation (CPR) is required; this technique can be properly learned by taking an approved course, and it has saved many victims on the verge of death.

Review and Discussion

1. Compare the roles of human error and the environment as the cause of accidents. What psychological and other factors contribute to human error related to accidents?

2. Explain the role of age, type of motor vehicle, and alcohol consumption as causative factors in accidental injury or death.

3. Why, in your opinion, are there fewer deaths among workers on the job than there are in the home environment?

4. How do drugs and medicines increase one's chances of being involved in an accident?

5. List several improvements and safety features of the modern automobile that have contributed to the marked reduction in auto accidents, injury, and death.

6. Describe some basic bicycle safety rules.

7. Name several precautions which may be taken to avoid becoming the victim of a fall in or around the home.

8. Describe safety precautions to be followed when attempting to escape from a home fire at night.

9. Explain the value of knowing how to perform cardiopulmonary resuscitation. Where can this lifesaving skill be learned in the community?

10. Explain the steps that should be taken to treat a victim of shock.

Further Reading

Aaron, James E., A. Frank Bridges, Dale O. Ritzel, and Larry B. Lindaver. *First Aid Emergency Care,* 2d ed. New York: Macmillan Publishing Co., Inc., 1979.
Very good first aid text with excellent chapters on safety philosophy and how to examine an injured person. (Paperback.)

American Red Cross (National Headquarters), 17th and D Streets, N.W., Washington, D.C. 20006.
Publishes books and pamphlets on many safety topics including CPR and first aid. Check local or state office for information.

Breyfogle, Newell D. *The Common Sense Medical Guide and Outdoor Reference.* New York: McGraw-Hill Book Company, 1981.
An excellent reference for hikers, backpackers, campers, recreation leaders, and others who spend a lot of time out-of-doors, containing sections on first aid, survival techniques, and reactions to adverse climate. (Paperback.)

Mroz, Joseph H. *Safety in Everyday Living.* Dubuque, Iowa: William C. Brown Company, 1978.
A very well-written, easy-to-understand book on all phases of accidents and safety.

National Safety Council, *Accident Facts,* 1984 ed., 444 North Michigan Avenue, Chicago, Illinois 60611.
One of the many magazines and pamphlets published by the NSC on all areas of safety and accident prevention. Most libraries will have several NSC publications in their collection. (OZ1.64, 1984)

Strasser, Marland K., James E. Aaron, and Ralph C. Bohn. *Fundamentals of Safety Education.* 2d ed. New York: Macmillan Publishing Company, Inc., 1973.
Very good overview of the accident problem and a philosophy of safe human behavior. The authors investigate psychological factors behind accidents.

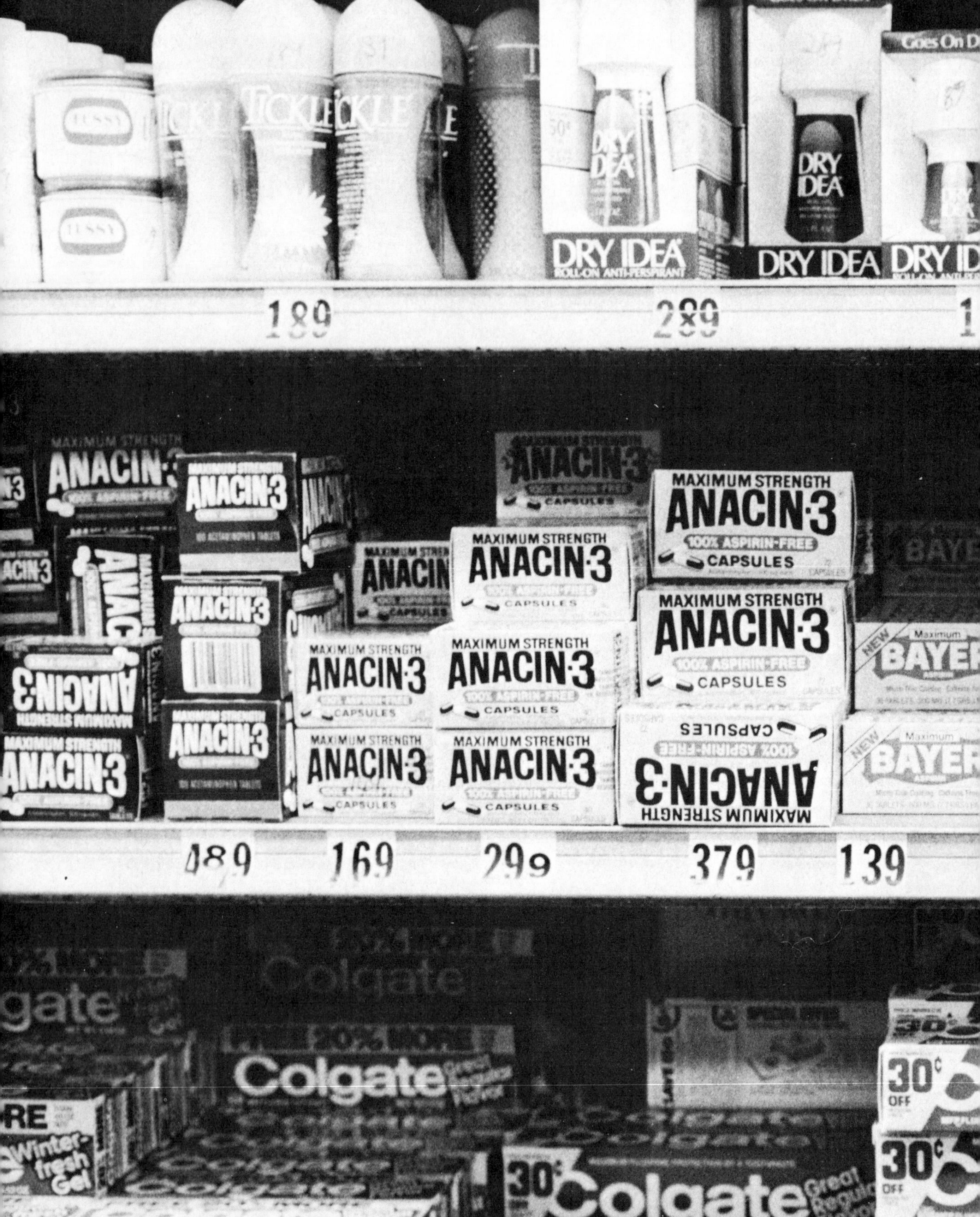

TUSSY
TICKLE
Goes On Drier!
DRY IDEA
DRY IDEA
ROLL-ON ANTI-PERSPIRANT
189
289
MAXIMUM STRENGTH
ANACIN-3
100% ASPIRIN-FREE
CAPSULES
489
169
299
379
139
NEW
Maximum
BAYER
Colgate
FREE 20% MORE
Winter-fresh Gel
30¢ OFF
Great Regular Flavor

Chapter 20
Consumer Health

KEY POINTS

- ☐ The physician you choose should have sound scientific training, treat you courteously, answer your questions, and not expose you to excessive treatments.
- ☐ Over-the-counter drugs, which usually relieve symptoms rather than treat illness, are generally safe but may be harmful when improperly used.
- ☐ You may ask your doctor to prescribe generic drugs, when possible, which are cheaper than their brand-name equivalents.
- ☐ The principal types of private health insurance are hospitalization, major medical, and disability; as an alternative to traditional insurance, health maintenance organizations provide comprehensive prepaid health care.
- ☐ Quackery is the purveying of misinformation about health, often in the form of "secret" remedies directed at the gullible.
- ☐ It is best to approach advertisements critically, examining their direct claims and looking for propaganda techniques or subliminal elements.
- ☐ Be aware of consumer protection laws and the agencies to which you may complain if you buy an unsafe product.
- ☐ Consumer protection agencies exist at the national, state, and local levels.

IN DAYS gone by, people were much more directly responsible for the quality of their foods and medicines than they are today. They butchered their own livestock, grew their own fruits and vegetables, preserved foods by salting, canning, and other methods, and made their concoctions for use as medicines. Those who made no mistakes survived and fared well. But in our modern society, very few people directly produce the goods that they need. Most of us, instead, are consumers, dependent on other people for the safe and sanitary processing of the products we use. In one sense, we are buying one product or another, but in another sense, we are buying good health or bad.

The wide variety of foods and drugs available means that today we must make choices that formerly we would not have had to make. We may choose a healthful diet, or we may rely excessively on junk foods. We may dose ourselves with various remedies at the slightest twinge of discomfort, or we may confine our use of painkillers and other drugs to times when they seem necessary. We may choose a product —whether tobacco, soft drink, cold remedy, or face cream—on the basis of an appealing advertisement, or we may try to examine such ads critically before making a purchase and consider what effect, if any, the product will have on our health.

Medical Care

In past centuries, the customary treatments for certain conditions were often useless, and sometimes even harmful. Today, a patient often has several alternatives to choose among, including the best conventional medical therapy, forms of treatment being studied experimentally, and treatments by less conventional systems.

Conventional Medical Treatments

A hundred years ago, many Americans still had no easy access to any kind of professional medical services, and many others lived in places where there was only one doctor, perhaps serving several communities. City dwellers may be surprised to hear that in many areas of the country there is still a shortage of skilled medical personnel and medical services; but even in cities, finding good medical care is not a simple matter. For one thing, because of the complexity of modern medicine, many physicians are specialists of one kind or another, and many of those who are in general practice have all the patients they can handle.

More and more doctors are now being trained, and according to estimates made by the Graduate Medical Education National Advisory Committee, by 1990 there will be 70,000 more physicians than required.[1] Nevertheless, because of uneven distribution by geographical area and specialty, there will still be some shortages.

Fear or the high cost of medical care discourages some people from finding doctors until an emergency arises. This is hardly the best time to choose one; you should know where you will go for medical help before you have an urgent need for it.

If you are relocating to a new area, the best way to find a new doctor may be to ask your current physician for a recommendation. Calling a county medical society is another way of locating a new doctor. The society will provide you with a list of qualified physicians, although they will not recommend a particular one.

Close friends can also be helpful in recommending physicians. However, regardless of whom a friend may recommend, you still should make sure that the individual is competent and uses sound diagnostic and therapeutic techniques. Therefore, you must see to it that your new physician has acceptable credentials, including an M.D. (medical doctor) or D.O. (doctor of osteopathy) degree. Affiliation with a good hospital, particularly a teaching hospital of a medical school, is an added advantage. If not a general practitioner, your family doctor may be an internist (specializing in internal medicine) or a **family practitioner** (specializing in the varied medical problems a family is likely to experience).

Family practitioner Physician who specializes in care of the entire family.

Medical Training and Specialties

A **medical doctor,** or M.D., first goes through undergraduate school with a premedical training program, typically in the sciences. The program lasts three to four years and generally culminates in a bachelor of arts or bachelor of science degree. This is usually followed by four years of medical school—two spent in comprehensive science courses and two in clinical work covering the full spectrum of the medical field. After medical school, the new doctor spends one or two years as an intern, practicing under the supervision of other doctors; then come one or more years of residency training if the doctor elects to specialize in a particular field rather than to become a general practitioner. The accompanying box lists some of the most common medical specialties and briefly describes the scope of each.

Medical doctor (M.D.) Physician who has completed premedical and medical training plus an internship and residency.

An **osteopathic physician** (D.O), or osteopath, gets the same basic premedical training as the M.D. and also usually goes through four years of medical school. In addition to standard medical practices, osteopathic training includes manipulation, a technique not required in most other medical schools. Manipulation is the manual application of pressure to stretch and relax muscles and ligaments and to realign spinal vertebrae. According to osteopathic theory, this technique helps increase the body's natural resistance to disease. More than 75 percent of the osteopathic physicians are family practitioners; others enter specialties comparable to those for M.D.'s.

Osteopathic physician (D.O.) Specialist in manual application of pressure, or manipulation.

YOUR HEALTH TODAY

A Glossary of Common Medical Specialties

- An **allergist** is concerned with the diagnosis and treatment of allergies.
- An **anesthesiologist** administers drugs that render a patient unconscious during an operation.
- A **cardiologist** specializes in the diagnosis and treatment of heart problems and diseases.
- A **dermatologist** treats diseases of the skin.
- A **gastroenterologist** deals with problems of the stomach and intestinal tract.
- A **gynecologist** is a specialist in the problems and diseases of the sexual and reproductive organs in women.
- A **hematologist** is a specialist in the study of the blood.
- An **internist** specializes in the diagnosis and nonsurgical treatment of diseases of adults, whatever system of the body may be involved.
- A **neurologist** treats disorders of the nervous system.
- An **obstetrician** is concerned with the care of women during pregnancy, labor, childbirth, and after childbirth.
- An **ophthalmologist** treats problems and diseases of the eyes.
- An **orthopedist** corrects deformities of the musculoskeletal system, mainly by means of surgery.
- An **otolaryngologist** is an ear, nose, and throat specialist.
- A **pathologist** deals with identification of diseases and their causative agents.
- A **pediatrician** specializes in the care and treatment of children.
- A **proctologist** treats diseases and problems of the anus, rectum, and colon.
- A **pulmonologist** deals with diseases of the lungs.
- A **psychiatrist** is concerned with the study, treatment, and prevention of mental illnesses.
- A **radiologist** is a specialist in the use of X rays in the diagnosis and treatment of disease.
- A **surgeon** treats diseases, injuries, and deformities by means of operative procedures.
- A **urologist** specializes in diseases of the urinary tract, whether male or female, and in disorders of the genital organs in males.

Doctor of podiatric medicine (D.P.M.) Specialist in diseases and disorders of the feet.

Doctor of dental surgery (D.D.S.) Dentist specializing in disorders of teeth and gums.

Doctor of medical dentistry (D.M.D.) Dentist.

A **doctor of podiatric medicine** (D.P.M) goes through the same premedical training as do M.D.'s and D.O.'s, then completes four years of podiatric medical college to become a specialist in the diseases and disorders of the feet.

A **doctor of dental surgery** (D.D.S.) or **doctor of medical dentistry** (D.M.D), each otherwise known as a dentist, follows a four-year premedical program with four years in dental college to learn to diagnose and treat diseases and disorders of the teeth and gums.

All of the doctors listed are entitled to the use of hospitals for care of patients and can also prescribe medications. Other medical care practitioners described here do not have these privileges.

A **clinical psychologist** usually has a doctor of philosophy degree (Ph.D.) in clinical psychology, which is ordinarily obtained by completing four years of preprofessional training and then an additional four to five years of professional training in psychology. A clinical psychologist diagnoses and treats behavior disorders but cannot prescribe drugs. For this reason, a clinical psychologist often works with a psychiatrist, who can prescribe drugs for a patient if they are needed.

Clinical psychologist Professional who diagnoses and treats behavior disorders.

Judging the Quality of Medical Care

In medicine, as in other fields, incompetence occasionally exists. You should be concerned about the quality of care you are receiving if you are required to take three or more medicines of different types daily, if you have to visit the doctor's office too regularly, or if you are given injections every time you visit the doctor. Be sure to ask your doctor any questions you have about your care. If the answers are not to your satisfaction, perhaps you should seriously consider changing doctors. Remember that you have a right to quality medical care. The physician is your employee. If you are not satisfied with the care you receive, you have the right to change employees. Of course, most competent physicians will do their best to provide you with quality care, but you also should expect to be treated courteously and with concern and to be given answers to your questions.

If you are given treatment you suspect to be incompetent, report it to the county medical society. Chances are that others have complained about this individual, and your complaint may be the one necessary to warrant a professional investigation. Be sure you document the precise reasons for your dissatisfaction.

No matter how healthy one may feel or seem to be, it is always a good idea to have a regular, full physical examination by a medical doctor every few years. (Photo by Paul Conklin)

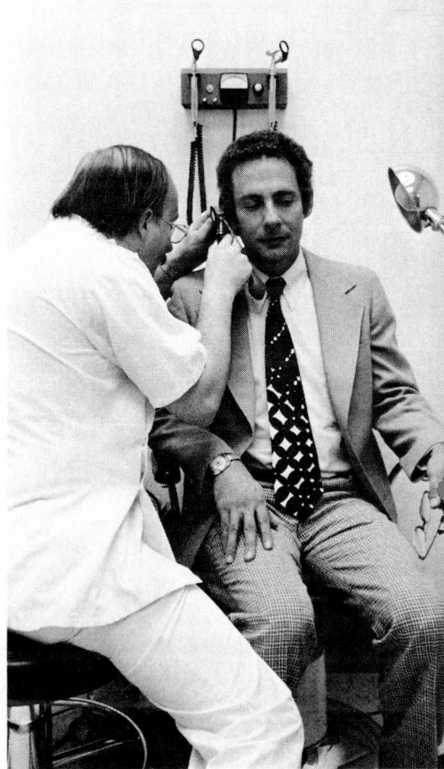

Physical Examinations and Screenings

It has been shown that the yearly physical examination is not very cost-effective, especially for those under the age of 40. However, when you find a new physician, it's a good idea to have a baseline physical so that the doctor will have an accurate record of your state of physical and mental health. A good physical examination would generally include an evaluation of the patient's general appearance and of the condition of the eyes, ears, nose, mouth and throat, neck, lungs, heart, breasts, lymph nodes, back, abdomen, sex organs, rectum and anus, legs, feet, bones and joints, and reflexes. In addition, certain laboratory tests would be ordered. For young adults a complete physical every five years is usually sufficient; after age 40, every three to five years; after 50, every two to three years; and after 60, yearly. Otherwise, you generally need to visit a doctor only when you have a specific problem.

However, various screenings for particular health problems should be done more often. For example, it's a good idea to have your blood pressure checked at least twice a year, but this need not be done by a physician. In addition, tests for heart problems and different types of cancer are important. For more information, see Chapters 16 and 17 of this book and check with the American Cancer Society or the American Heart Association in your area.

Second Opinions

Sometimes there is more than one acceptable way to treat an ailment, and there will be differences of opinion among doctors about which should be preferred. Surgeons, for example, may lean toward a surgical solution to a condition that could instead be treated with medication or physical therapy. However, any surgery, even though minor, carries some risk; and in general, surgery should be avoided unless it seems necessary. In order to help prevent unnecessary surgery, many insurers, including Blue Cross/Blue Shield and Medicare, will pay for a second opinion from another doctor whenever elective surgery has been recommended.

If any doctor or dentist recommends a treatment that seems risky or extreme to you, whether medical or surgical, you should get a second opinion. In some circumstances, if the two opinions differ, you might even consider getting a third opinion. Whenever you have doubts about a proposed treatment, you should get whatever information you need to resolve them before undertaking it.

Alternative Systems of Healing

The following systems of healing are not as well documented scientifically as those described previously, but each has enthusiastic supporters.

Chiropractor Doctor who treats partial dislocations of the vertabrae.

A doctor of chiropractic medicine (D.C.), or **chiropractor,** typically has at least two years of preprofessional college training or the equivalent and then attends a college of chiropractic medicine for four years—two years spent studying basic science plus two years of clinical practice. A chiropractor diagnoses and treats incomplete or partial dislocations of the spine and uses a variety of techniques, most commonly the X ray, to make the diagnosis. The true chiropractic philosophy states that all diseases are related to spinal dislocations and that a disease can be treated by a manipulation of the spine. As an example, you might take an aspirin to kill the pain when you have a headache, but a chiropractor would look for the cause of the tension that produced the headache—generally a tightening of muscles in the neck that in turn affects the blood vessels and nerves in the head. The chiropractor would try to relieve the tension to eliminate the headache. Chiropractors are not permitted to prescribe drugs.

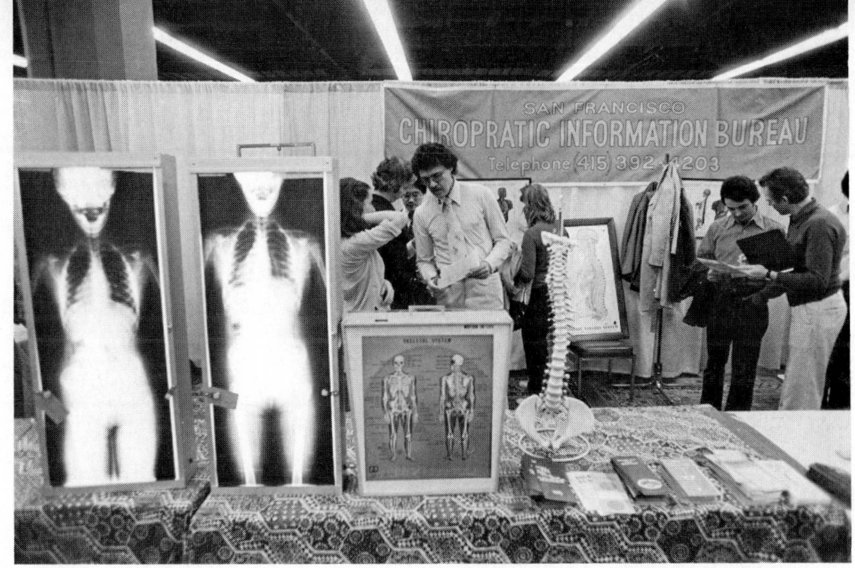

Chiropractors attribute illnesses to spinal dislocations, and their treatment involves manipulation of the spine. (Photo © Peter Menzel/ Stock, Boston)

Naturopathic doctor Practitioner who treats diseases with natural cures such as vitamins and spinal manipulations.

A **naturopathic doctor (N.D.),** or naturopath, completes at least two years of preprofessional college training or the equivalent and then attends a naturopathic medical college for four years, receiving two years of basic medical sciences and then two years of clinical practice. Naturopaths believe that all diseases and disorders can be cured by natural methods, such as diet, vitamins, and spinal manipulation. Most states do not permit naturopathic physicians to prescribe drugs.

No single accreditation agency for chiropractors and naturopaths is recognized by the federal government; thus, neither field of practice is an officially recognized profession. For the same reason, there are no standards of practice and accountability for weeding out incompetent practitioners. The states vary in their restrictions and regulations; some states allow chiropractors and naturopaths virtually free rein, while other states are much less liberal in their allowances.

Acupuncture Therapeutic technique whereby fine needles are inserted in specified parts of the body.

Acupuncture is a form of therapy that has been used in the Far East for thousands of years. The theory behind it is that there are fields (meridians) of energy that flow through the body and that if needles are inserted at the proper points, it is possible to balance these fields and restore a person's health. Inserting needles in the right spots is also thought to block pain impulses; hence, acupuncture has been extensively used as an anesthetic.

In 1971 an acupuncture boom was launched in the United States as a result of reports from people who had visited China and subsequent media promotion of this technique as a panacea. The American Medical Association, however, has stated that acupuncture is still not widely employed in American medical care, since it does not relieve pain totally. Many doctors and scientists feel that there is no medical basis for the use of acupuncture and that the effects some patients report stem strictly from psychological causes. Even in China, the limitations of the technique are realized: physicians there screen patients who appear nervous or whose operations may be complicated, and in such cases acupuncture is not used.

Over-the-counter and Prescription Drugs

OTC Drugs and Cosmetic Aids

Over-the-counter drug (OTC) Nonprescription drug.

Americans spend billions of dollars every year for **over-the-counter (OTC) drugs,** that is, those for which no prescription is necessary. Most of these drugs are effective if used for their intended purposes and according to the directions provided. Few OTC drugs are really cures for illnesses; rather, they give relief from annoying symptoms.

Just because a drug is sold over-the-counter doesn't mean that there is no danger in taking the drug. Some OTC drugs, especially those that treat the symptoms of colds and allergies, contain active ingredients that can affect such things as vision, motor coordination, and reasoning ability. It is important that consumers use OTC drugs as they would prescription drugs, that is, in a safe manner. Therefore, each consumer using an OTC drug should read and understand the caution and warnings for the user that appear on the label. In addition, the directions for use of the OTC drug should be closely followed. Finally, keep in mind that, in general, OTC drugs only treat symptoms—they should not be relied upon to cure a medical condition. Therefore, if symptoms continue to persist even after use of the proper OTC drug or if the frequency of symptoms increases, then the consumer should consult a physician immediately and not attempt to self-diagnose or prescribe. Before reading about the various OTC drug products, why not see how well you understand the effectiveness of these products. Self-Assessment Exercise 20.1 will help you see how well you understand the effectiveness of these drugs.

Aspirin

An effective pain reliever, aspirin is the most common of all the over-the-counter drugs. It is taken primarily to reduce fever or to relieve headaches and aches and pains, including those associated with colds and similar ailments. It is widely used to relieve symptoms of arthritis. For these purposes, its effectiveness is unquestionable. Some people are allergic to aspirin, however, and those who take aspirin regularly over a long period of time may develop iron-deficiency anemia; a minimal but constant loss of blood which results from irritation to the stomach lining. Some aspirin is buffered to reduce this irritation.

Advertisements to the contrary, all aspirin works essentially the same way. Some brands combine aspirin with decongestants, antacids (bufferins), or other drugs and thus contain varying amounts of pure

SELF-ASSESSMENT EXERCISE 20.1

How Well Do You Understand the Effectiveness of OTC Drug Products?

Directions: Check "True" or "False" for each of the following statements.

Statement	True	False
1. Aspirin can cure headaches.	____ True	____ False
2. Aspirin helps to cure colds and flu.	____ True	____ False
3. Time-released cold capsules are the best form of cold medications.	____ True	____ False
4. Sore throat medications, especially those containing antiseptics, are effective because the medications kill bacteria and viruses causing the sore throat.	____ True	____ False
5. All suntan lotions are effective in preventing skin problems caused by too much sun.	____ True	____ False
6. Sleep aid products contain medications that act on the sleep centers in the brain.	____ True	____ False
7. Cough medications are successful in curing a cough.	____ True	____ False
8. Acne OTC Products are effective in curing acne.	____ True	____ False
9. Detergent-type shampoos are the best shampoos to use on one's hair.	____ True	____ False
10. Laxatives cure constipation.	____ True	____ False

Scoring: All answers are false. OTC products, for the most part, do not cure anything. They are merely ways to treat symptoms. Reexamine the questions or statements you responded "true" to and evaluate your use of this particular OTC product.

aspirin; but by and large, the higher price charged for one brand compared to another represents sales and advertising costs rather than greater effectiveness. Always read the label to ascertain the amount of aspirin as opposed to other contents, and use only as directed. Children's doses, for example, are considerably less than doses for adults. Do not be hesitant about buying aspirin generically.

Cold Remedies

The term "common cold" is somewhat misleading, for there are many different types of colds; the causative agents of some are well recognized, while those of others are not. The characteristic common to nearly all colds is an effect on the membranes of the respiratory tract, typically causing stuffiness and such discomforts as coughing, a runny nose, and headache. A cold usually runs its course in about ten days, but afflicted Americans spend many hundreds of millions of dollars on hoped-for relief. In general, the over-the-counter cold medicines do not hurry the disappearance of the cold, but most do no harm. Some give relief by reducing congestion, helping to lower fever temperatures, or eliminating general aches and pains. Time-release remedies are no better than the others. When choosing medicines for colds, read the labels carefully. Avoid taking "shot-gun" remedies that include drugs to alleviate symptoms you don't have; thus, you can avoid exposing yourself to excessive side effects.

Laxatives

Constipation is another disorder that has spawned many would-be cures. The best laxatives are natural, but many kinds of over-the-counter drugs are sold to help relieve constipation, racking up sales in the hundreds of millions of dollars annually. Most are harmless if used as directed, but if used in excess they can be harmful. When constipation is a genuine problem, it may require a doctor's attention to determine the cause. Most commonly, constipation is the result of some transient tension. Some of the over-the-counter laxatives do indeed loosen the bowels, sometimes even causing the opposite effect—diarrhea. A disturbing fact is that many over-the-counter laxatives may in the long run promote constipation. So if constipation appears to be aggravated rather than alleviated, the person should stop using the product and should probably see a doctor—definitely so if the constipation persists.

Finally, it is important to note that if a person desires to use a laxative, it is better and safer to use a bulk-forming laxative (e.g., Metamucil) as opposed to a bowel-stimulant laxative (e.g., Feenamint, Ex-lax). Studies have shown that people who use bowel-stimulant laxatives on a regular basis can develop a physical dependence on the laxative. This finding has not been demonstrated for the bulk-forming type of laxative.

Sore Throat Medicines

Sore throats often accompany colds and can make even swallowing water painful. Sometimes they are the result of dry, overheated conditions indoors, particularly in winter, and the condition can be corrected by humidifying the house or room involved. But sore throats are often caused by infections, either viral or bacterial. If left untreated, such an infection can lead to damage to the kidneys or the heart. A sore throat, particularly if it lasts for 2 weeks or longer, should not be taken lightly and needs the attention of a physician. Mouthwashes and medicated lozenges do not eliminate an infection, but they may give temporary relief. For most sore throats, warm salt water may be just as effective.

Cough Aids

A cough is an action which is controlled by a cough center located in the brain. The most common cough stimulus is irritation in the respiratory tract. Coughs can be caused by colds or other infections that affect the respiratory tract or by any irritant, such as cigarette smoke. Most people tend to play down the potential severity of a cough; it is important to note that the typical coughs following a cold can also be associated with much more serious diseases, such as pneumonia or cancer.

Most OTC cough medications are shotgun remedies that contain from two to ten different drugs aimed at the various links in the cough mechanism. Some of these ingredients might help some people, but for the most part, OTC cough medications are expensive and ineffective. The best advice is that if a cough lasts more than one week, one should see his or her physician. If there is an identified source for the irritation to the respiratory tract, then staying away from the source should reduce the frequency of coughing.

Sleep Aids

There are many prescription medications which can deal with a condition called insomnia, or difficulty in sleeping. These prescription medications are effective but can lead to a dependence. Most OTC sleep aids contain an antihistamine, which tends to make many people drowsy. The majority of these products are actually ineffective and, like many other OTC products, very expensive.

Most people do in fact get the amount of sleep they need. Individuals calling themselves "insomniacs" tend to get as much sleep as people who consider themselves normal sleepers. The best advice for an individual with a self-diagnosed sleeping problem is to see a physician if the problem is particularly bothersome. An individual can also attempt to find out why he or she is having trouble sleeping. In many cases anxiety or difficulty in relaxing can be the cause; and if it is the cause, artificially inducing drowsiness through use of OTC sleep aids is not solving the problem.

Acne Medications

Acne is a problem mainly during the teenage years, but it may appear earlier and continue until middle age or later. Acne infections start around hair follicles that become plugged with shed inner skin cells mixed with sebum (a white, oily secretion) and bacteria. In cases of acne, the plug becomes an inflamed, deep pustule, or pimple, of

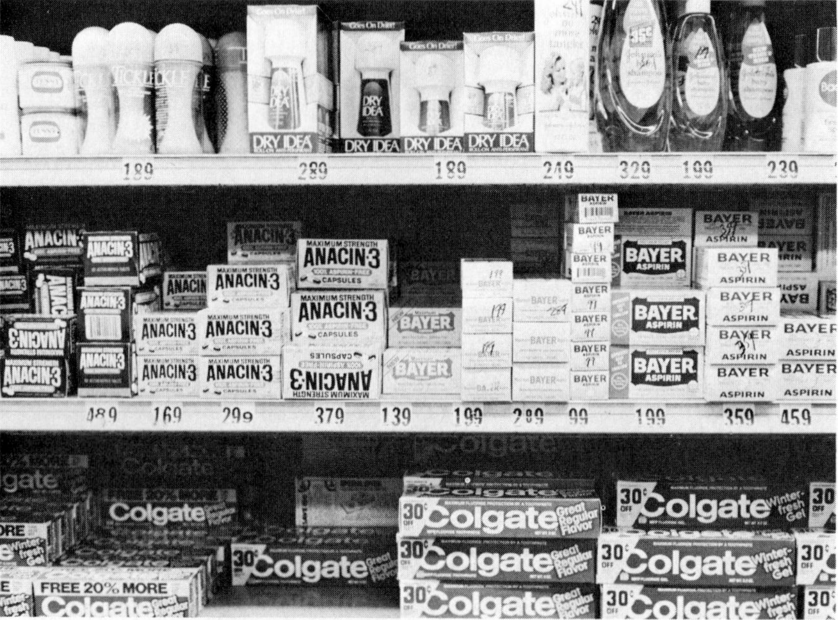

A wide variety of OTC drugs are available to the public. Consumers should be very careful about what medication they take and should remember to read labels carefully. (Photo by Marc P. Anderson)

which there are many. The amount of sebum produced is apparently related to the production of sex hormones: testosterone and progesterone stimulate the glands to activity; estrogen, in contrast, seems to slow their activity.

Most cases of acne respond to a cleansing of the skin and to the use of over-the-counter drugs containing sulfur, resorcinol, benzoyl peroxide, or salicylic acid. Because of individual skin sensitivity, however, these remedies must be experimented with to get the one most suitable. A druggist can be consulted for advice on the current products that appear to be most effective and that are most likely to suit a particular skin condition. Trust the druggist before you rely on advertisements, which may be deceptive or misleading. If an acne condition is obviously stubborn, consult a family physician, who will then determine whether the case warrants referral to a dermatologist.

Shampoos

For most people, a shampoo two or three times a week is adequate, but people can wash their hair as frequently as once a day without damage to their hair or scalp. People who have excessively oily hair or bad cases of dandruff—a mixture of dead skin and oil from sebaceous glands in the scalp—generally wash their hair frequently, often using dandruff-removing shampoos. Some of these products really do not help, however, and may even be harmful. When buying dandruff shampoo, look for the following ingredients, which may be helpful (in descending order): selenium sulfide, available only by prescription; zinc pyrithione; sulfur; salicylic acid; and tar. Washing with a mild soap shampoo is satisfactory for most people. The stronger detergent-type shampoos clean better but can also be too harsh, even with the addition of lanolin and other substances that help to soften their effect on the hair and scalp.

Suntan Lotions

A rich suntan continues to be a status symbol, although it is now known that, in addition to the pain and misery of sunburn, continued long exposure to the ultraviolet rays of the sun can produce skin cancer. According to the Federal Drug Administration, some 300,000 people have diagnosed cases of skin cancer every year, an increase of 100 percent in the past two decades. Fortunately, skin cancer is easily detected and treated, so nearly all patients are cured. People who expose themselves to the sun for long periods of time year after year may be lucky and escape skin cancer but develop a leathery, wrinkled skin, prematurely aged. The skin can be protected with sun-screen products available in drugstores, supermarkets, and other outlets. These lotions come in different degrees of strength, ranging from 15 (which gives the most protection) to 2 (which gives the least protection). The best sun-screening agents in lotions are benzophenone and para-aminobenzoic acid (PABA).

Prescription Drugs

A prescription drug is one dispensed by a pharmacist at the instruction of a doctor. Roughly 70 percent of all medicines manufactured in the United States are sold by prescription. Doctors, who write about 1.2 billion prescriptions a year, use mainly some 50 different drugs, with only roughly 200 drugs accounting for 65 percent of the sales. Nearly half of these have been in use for less than ten years. Many drugs can be purchased by their generic, or chemical, names at less cost than the same drugs sold under their brand names. However, drugs that are patented are available only under their brand names until the patents expire. This gives the company the opportunity to recover some of the money spent on research and development of the drug. The industry, for example, does extensive testing on more than 150,000 substances every year, but only 10 or 20 of these become new, useful, marketable medicines.

Prescription drug labels must bear the following information:

1. Name of the person for whom the prescription was written.
2. Name of the doctor who wrote the prescription.
3. Name of the drug.
4. Name of the pharmacy that dispensed the drug.
5. Precise instructions for the use of the drug.
6. An indication as to whether or not the drug can be refilled without an additional prescription from the doctor.

Generic drug A drug referred to by a chemical or nonproprietary name.

When a doctor prescribes a drug for you, do not hesitate to ask that the prescription be written **generically.** Doctors may routinely write prescriptions for brand-name drugs simply because those, rather than the generic names, are the names they are most familiar with. Just as we are exposed to advertisements for over-the-counter drugs, doctors see ads for prescription drugs in medical magazines. However, any doctor should have available a reference book which lists generic equivalents of brand-name drugs.

Of course, you must take prescription drugs only according to the dosage prescribed and be alert for possible side effects. You should also be certain that the doctor who prescribes a particular drug is aware of any other drugs you are taking. (For discussion of drug effects and the problem of drug abuse, see Chapter 11.)

Hospitals and Health Insurance

Evaluating Your Hospitals

If you should require hospital care, your choice of hospitals may be determined by which hospital your doctor is associated with. Nevertheless, it's a good idea to learn which of the hospitals convenient to you offers the best professional services and equipment at competitive prices. Three-fourths of the hospitals in the United States are *accredited,* that is, they conform to standards established by the Joint Commission on Accreditation of Hospitals. This does not mean that all of the others are substandard, however, for the accreditation is strictly voluntary.

The quality of emergency ward services in a particular hospital can sometimes be a matter of life or death to a seriously ill or injured person. And some hospitals have special facilities for the treatment of certain injuries — for example, burns or cardiovascular emergencies. Try to find out at which nearby hospital you would likely be best treated in the event of a particular medical emergency in the future, so that you can provide for going there if you have a choice.

Types of Hospitals

Voluntary hospitals Nonprofit hospitals.

About 50 percent of the nation's hospitals are **voluntary hospitals,** nonprofit organizations, run by and supported by patients' fees, insurance payments, private endowments, and contributions. They are typically guided by a board of trustees made up of a nongovernmental group of people. Sometimes, for example, they represent a particular religious sect.

Government (public) hospitals Hospitals funded by taxes and run by the government.

About 37 percent of all hospitals are supported wholly by taxes. They are referred to as **government,** or "public," **hospitals** and are owned and operated by the municipal, county, state, or federal government. Because of their funding, these hospitals provide services to those who might not be able to afford care in any other facility, and their bills are based on the patient's ability to pay. The budgets for operating hospitals of this sort fluctuate with the amounts of money made available from revenues, so the extent of the services also varies.

Private hospitals account for roughly 13 percent of those in the nation. They are owned and operated by individuals and corporations as profit-making ventures. Many are small, often with fewer than 50 beds. Some have been established by groups of doctors to serve needs in areas where no other hospitals exist, and they are operated on a break-even basis. As in other hospitals, the quality of service and the cost vary widely. They are subject to the fewest regulations and inspections, however, and because of their small size and more limited financing, they may lack equipment and services that are available in larger institutions.

Private hospitals Hospitals operated as profit-making ventures.

Your Rights as a Patient

Being in a hospital can be a distressing experience. Remember, however, that you have a right to courteous and professional treatment while hospitalized. To help patients become aware of the standards of hospital care they are entitled to and should insist upon, the American Hospital Association has published "A Patient's Bill of Rights." Among the rights listed are the right to considerate care; to obtaining complete and understandable information about the diagnosis, treatment, and prognosis of one's case; to be given any information necessary for giving informed consent to treatment; to refuse treatment; to have one's privacy respected and one's records kept confidential; to be informed of any proposed experimentation affecting one's treatment, and to refuse to participate in such research; to reasonable continuity in care; and to an explanation of one's bill.

Health Insurance

The high costs of medical attention and services make health insurance one of today's essentials, and more than 75 percent of Americans do have such insurance. Unfortunately, many people don't know what their insurance will or won't cover and buy insurance without carefully considering their needs and the options available. In choosing an individual policy, the consumer should seek the advice of a trusted insurance agent because of the wide range of coverages and fees available. In addition, the consumer should investigate before buying and examine several policies and their options.

The most common type of health insurance is **basic health insurance.** Typically, basic health insurance covers inpatient hospital care and such hospital-provided services as use of operating, delivery, and recovery rooms, drugs used in the hospital, and laboratory services. In addition, this type of insurance usually covers some outpatient

Basic health insurance Standard health insurance covering hospital-related services.

GROUP HEALTH INSURANCE CLAIM

Policy No.__________

PATIENT & INSURED (SUBSCRIBER) INFORMATION

1. PATIENT'S NAME (First name, middle initial, last name)
2. PATIENT'S DATE OF BIRTH
3. INSURED'S NAME (First name, middle initial, last name)
4. PATIENT'S ADDRESS (Street, city, state, ZIP code)
5. PATIENT'S SEX — MALE / FEMALE
6. INSURED'S I.D. No. or **MEDICARE No.** (include any letters)
7. PATIENT'S RELATIONSHIP TO INSURED — SELF / SPOUSE / CHILD / OTHER
8. INSURED'S GROUP NO. (Or Group Name)
9. OTHER HEALTH INSURANCE COVERAGE—Enter Name of Policyholder, Plan Name, Address and Policy or Medical Assistance Number
10. WAS CONDITION RELATED TO: A. PATIENT'S EMPLOYMENT — YES / NO; B. AN AUTO ACCIDENT — YES / NO
11. INSURED'S ADDRESS (Street, city, state, ZIP code)
12. PATIENT'S OR AUTHORIZED PERSON'S SIGNATURE — I Authorize the Release of any Medical information Necessary to Process this Claim and Request Payment of GUARDIAN Benefits Either to Myself or to the Party Who Accepts Assignment Below. SIGNED DATE
13. I AUTHORIZE PAYMENT OF MEDICAL BENEFITS TO UNDERSIGNED PHYSICIAN OR SUPPLIER FOR SERVICE DESCRIBED BELOW. SIGNED (Insured or Authorized Person)

PHYSICIAN OR SUPPLIER INFORMATION

14. DATE OF ILLNESS (FIRST SYMPTOM) OR INJURY (ACCIDENT) OR PREGNANCY (LMP)
15. DATE FIRST CONSULTED YOU FOR THIS CONDITION
16. HAS PATIENT EVER HAD SAME OR SIMILAR SYMPTOMS? YES / NO
17. DATE PATIENT ABLE TO RETURN TO WORK
18. DATES OF TOTAL DISABILITY — FROM / THROUGH; DATES OF PARTIAL DISABILITY — FROM / THROUGH
19. NAME OF REFERRING PHYSICIAN
20. FOR SERVICES RELATED TO HOSPITALIZATION GIVE HOSPITALIZATION DATES — ADMITTED / DISCHARGED
21. NAME & ADDRESS OF FACILITY WHERE SERVICES RENDERED (If other than home or office)
22. WAS LABORATORY WORK PERFORMED OUTSIDE YOUR OFFICE? YES / NO CHARGES:
23. DIAGNOSIS OR NATURE OF ILLNESS OR INJURY. RELATE DIAGNOSIS TO PROCEDURE IN COLUMN D BY REFERENCE TO NUMBERS 1,2,3, ETC. OR DX CODE
1.
2.
3.
4.

24. A DATE OF SERVICE	B* PLACE OF SERVICE	C FULLY DESCRIBE PROCEDURES, MEDICAL SERVICES OR SUPPLIES FURNISHED FOR EACH DATE GIVEN. PROCEDURE CODE (IDENTIFY:)	(EXPLAIN UNUSUAL SERVICES OR CIRCUMSTANCES)	D DIAGNOSIS CODE	E CHARGES	F

25. SIGNATURE OF PHYSICIAN OR SUPPLIER — SIGNED DATE
26. ACCEPT ASSIGNMENT — YES / NO
27. TOTAL CHARGE
28. AMOUNT PAID
29. BALANCE DUE
30. YOUR SOCIAL SECURITY NO.
31. PHYSICIAN'S OR SUPPLIER'S NAME, ADDRESS, ZIP CODE & TELEPHONE NO. — I.D. NO.
32. YOUR PATIENT'S ACCOUNT NO.
33. YOUR EMPLOYER I.D. NO.

*PLACE OF SERVICE CODES

1—(IH) —INPATIENT HOSPITAL
2—(OH)—OUTPATIENT HOSPITAL
3—(O) —DOCTOR'S OFFICE
4—(H)—PATIENT'S HOME
5— DAY CARE FACILITY (PSY)
6— NIGHT CARE FACILITY (PSY)
7—(NH) —NURSING HOME
8—(SNF)—SKILLED NURSING FACILITY
9— AMBULANCE
O—(OL)—OTHER LOCATIONS
A—(IL)—INDEPENDENT LABORATORY
B— OTHER MEDICAL-SURGICAL FACILITY

APPROVED BY AMA COUNCIL ON MEDICAL SERVICE 6-74

Health Insurance Form. (Photo by Paul Waldman)

care, including use of emergency rooms and outpatient diagnostic testing. Basic health insurance does, however, have maximum monetary amounts—which may be rather low—associated with each of the provisions of the policy. In case of a major illness, this type of insurance would not be nearly enough to cover all your medical expenses.

Major medical insurance Health insurance covering a wider variety of health services than basic coverage.

The second type of health insurance is called **major medical.** Major medical insurance is often held by individuals along with basic health insurance and is used to pay for lengthy illnesses and for services or supplies that are not covered under the basic health insurance policy. Some of these services include physician office visits for illness, out-of-hospital drugs that require a prescription, private duty nursing, and medical and surgical supplies prescribed by a physician.

It is important that prospective insurance buyers realize the limitations of both basic and major medical health insurance. Both insurances have waiting periods for certain preexisting conditions and deductible amounts that must be satisfied before the insurance can be used. Typically, these deductible amounts are $100–$200 per family member each year. Finally, individuals and families should realize that *comprehensive* health insurance coverage would include both basic health insurance and major medical. Why not respond to Self-Assessment Exercise 20.2 to determine if any deficiencies exist in your current health insurance coverage.

Health Maintenance Organizations (HMOs)

Health Maintenance Organization (HMO) A group plan in which prepaid premiums cover comprehensive medical care.

HMOs are growing in popularity across the United States. The advantage of the HMO concept is that once premiums are paid, the only other costs incurred by subscribers is the minimal (usually $3.00–$5.00) co-payment or processing fee to use the services. Regardless of the service provided—whether a simple office visit or surgery—the only cost that may be incurred in addition to the regular premiums is the co-payment. Premiums for belonging to an HMO are usually the same as those for private basic and major medical insurance, if not less.

Most HMOs offer a comprehensive health service, including dental and counseling services, as part of the subscriber benefits. One might ask, "How can HMOs function economically if they charge only as much as regular medical insurance but offer comprehensive health services for a minimal fee?" The answer is simple. If subscribers use HMO services only infrequently, expenses will be kept down. Therefore, many of the HMO efforts are directed at keeping subscribers healthy. Because of the low-cost care, subscribers are encouraged to come in early—before a minor condition becomes a serious one for the patient and a costly one to the HMO. In addition, many HMOs are offering health education programs to help their subscribers shape and maintain healthy life-styles.

HMOs employ rather large staffs, including MDs in all specialties and a support staff. Since in the case of the HMO the physician is salaried, the physician has what might be considered a regular work day. This is a very attractive working arrangement for many physicians who do not want to bother with all the problems associated with private practice.

The main advantage in belonging to an HMO is that the subscriber need not worry about medical expenses. With the cost of medical care so high, it is nice to know that regardless of the medical procedures needed, the costs will be minimal.

SELF-ASSESSMENT EXERCISE 20.2

How Good Is Your Health Insurance?

Directions: Check "Yes" or "No" for each of the following questions.

DOES YOUR HEALTH INSURANCE:

1. Have a reasonable deductible ($100–200/year)? ____ YES ____ NO
2. Cover the majority of inpatient hospital costs? ____ YES ____ NO
3. Cover outpatient services (e.g., emergency room visits, including physician fees)? ____ YES ____ NO
4. Cover physician expenses while in hospital? ____ YES ____ NO
5. Cover outpatient physician expenses? ____ YES ____ NO
6. Cover diagnostic procedures (e.g., lab, x-ray) done in physician's office? ____ YES ____ NO
7. Cover charges for second opinions? ____ YES ____ NO
8. Cover charges for psychological services? ____ YES ____ NO
9. Cover preexisting conditions after a reasonable waiting period? ____ YES ____ NO
10. Cover ambulance services? ____ YES ____ NO
11. Cover health education or health promotion services? ____ YES ____ NO
12. Cover prescription medication expenses after a certain reasonable limit has been reached? ____ YES ____ NO

Scoring: If you responded "No" to any of the above questions, it's time to reevaluate your health insurance. Be sure to talk with your insurance agent and find out how you can be covered on services you are presently lacking.

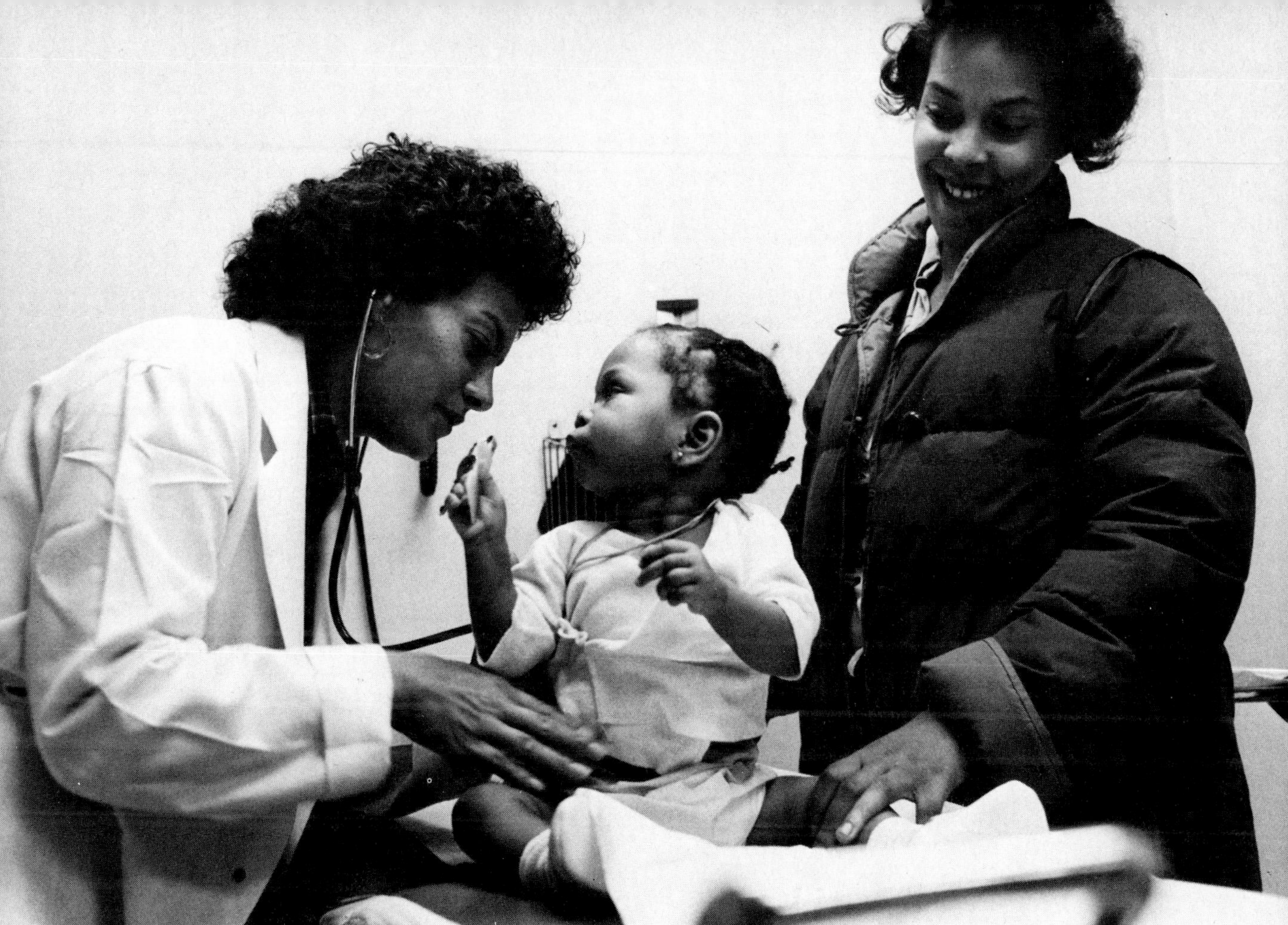

HMOs are becoming increasingly popular because as well as striving to keep their subscribers healthy, they provide low-cost care. (Photo © 1982 Catherine Ursillo)

The disadvantages of HMO membership include the following:

- limited choice of physicians
- time period delays in seeing specialists when needed
- elective surgeries are frowned upon by the HMO
- and for some people, especially the elderly, it is difficult getting transportation to the HMO, since the HMO usually has one medical building for a given area.

If one's primary concern with respect to seeking medical care is financial, then an HMO provides an excellent alternative. However, if one has a profound concern for such things as convenience, physician access, or choice of a physician, then private health insurance is a better choice.

Medicare and Medicaid

Two government plans also cover health maintenance. Medicare, administered through the Social Security Administration, provides coverage for hospitalization, limited posthospital care in a nursing home, and (under a separate, optional program) physicians' fees and other outpatient services. The hospitalization program is paid for out of Social Security. Those eligible for Medicare include persons 65 or older and disabled beneficiaries of Social Security; benefits are limited by deductibles, coinsurance provisions, and other factors. Medicaid, another government program, is designed to assist needy and low-income people. Requirements for eligibility vary from state to state. Benefits also vary from state to state, but they generally include hospital care and physicians' fees. Included in some states, too, are dental care, prescription drug costs, eyeglasses, clinic services, and rehabilitation costs. Both Medicare and Medicaid are subject to changes and revisions based on state and federal regulations.

Diagnostic Related Groups (DRG) A patient classifying system used by Medicare.

One such major change occurred in October 1983 when the Department of Health and Human Services imposed limits on what hospitals could charge Medicare. Under the new law the DHHS set fees for hospital treatments according to what are called **diagnostic related groups,** or **DRGs.** If, for example, the fee set by DHHS for the treatment for a cancer operation is $2,000 and the hospital charges $2,500, the hospital must absorb the difference in cost. If, however, the hospital charge is only $1,800, the hospital can keep the extra $200 set by DHHS. In order to keep medical costs from skyrocketing, as they have been in the past, the DHHS is also planning to instate a plan for "price controls" on physicians' fees as well as on hospital fees.

Medical Quackery

Nostrum Unproven "remedy" for illness.

Nostrums are unproven and generally unscientific, secret "remedies" for illnesses, and their purveyors are called quacks. It is unfortunate that some companies and individuals elect to thrive on a gullible public and often at the obvious expense of the consumer's health. The out-of-pocket money spent on quackery amounts to billions of dollars annually. On the other hand, it must be acknowledged that some quackery is practiced innocently in the sincere belief that the techniques or products offered really are beneficial. Whatever the intentions, however, purveying misinformation about health is medical quackery. Treatments for cancer and arthritis are the most common forms, but baldness, aging, and overweight also receive their share of attention from quacks.

"Miracle Treatments"

For Arthritis

Roughly 10 percent of Americans suffer some degree of discomfort or disability due to arthritis, and they spend hundreds of millions of dollars every year for relief from pain and for supposed "cures."

There really is no cure for arthritis, but at times the symptoms are less disturbing or may seem to have disappeared completely. It is during these periods of remission that a victim may believe a cure has been discovered.

Almost everything imaginable has been tried to give relief to arthritis sufferers, who are understandably attentive to any reported miraculous breakthroughs. Some desperate victims succumb to costly clinics where they are given heavy doses of drugs that do not help and that may be extremely harmful. Others buy massaging vibrators, copper bracelets, and an assortment of useless creams and lotions, or they submit to unusual diets, none of which at present has proved effective.

Aspirin, which is the primary ingredient in the over-the-counter drugs advertised as aiding arthritis victims, helps by alleviating pain and by suppressing inflammation. No matter what the claims say, plain aspirin works just as well as aspirin mixed with various other substances. Ointments — and there are many — induce a flow of blood to the skin and a feeling of warmth, which may give relief for a brief time. Never apply these "heat" ointments to mucous membranes, however, or put a heating pad over them to supply additional warmth. The result can be bad burns and blistering.

Since arthritis is the subject of constant research, help may be forthcoming, but the consumer should check the sources of any reported new remedies. If you have questions about the disease or its treatment, contact the nearest chapter of the Arthritis Foundation to get its opinion.

For Cancer

Probably the most feared of diseases, cancer is second only to heart disease as a cause of death among Americans. More than 50 million Americans now alive will develop cancer during their lifetime, but, on the basis of current statistics, more than 40 percent of these people can be expected to survive as long as five years after the disease is detected. Great strides are being made in treatment of these highly complex diseases, and many types of cancer are now curable if detected at an early stage.

"Miracle" treatments are a most sinister and dangerous form of quackery. Such nostrums can indeed be fatal when chosen by people who then forego professional treatment that might have saved their lives. Those trying to sell cancer remedies pull no punches in exploiting their merchandise, generally purported to be painless, inexpensive, and miraculous cures. Cancer victims, who are often willing to grasp at straws, are especially vulnerable to such claims. Among the most common remedies are certain salves and lotions that are supposed to "draw out" the cancer cells and kill them. A notorious example of quack treatment was that offered at the Hoxsey Cancer Clinic in Dallas, Texas, where patients were diagnosed and then prescribed

Hoxsey's special medicine — either a concoction of lactate pepsin and potassium iodide (the "pink" medicine) or a mixture of various types of roots, bark, and other ingredients (the "black" medicine). FDA investigations found no evidence of even one legitimate cure. Although the Hoxsey clinic was closed and its medicines removed from the market, the clinic was only one of many similar frauds, most of which are skillfully disguised behind a veneer of scientific knowledge and prestige.

The most recent fad in cancer cures is laetrile, also known as amygdalin and vitamin B_{17}, which is derived from apricot pits. Repeated and thorough tests with animals have demonstrated that laetrile has no effect on cancer cells, and recent trials on human patients, sponsored by the National Cancer Institute, found it had no therapeutic benefit. The substance nevertheless has an enthusiastic following among hopefuls, led on by promoters for whom the sale of laetrile represents a business in the millions of dollars.

Some clinics use simple but highly sophisticated-looking devices that give off vibrations and a variety of emanations that are reported to detect and eliminate cancer cells in the body. These are hoaxes. Diets reported to prevent and to cure cancers have also become a vogue. It is undeniably true that a good diet is a first step in the prevention of any illness and that there are literally hundreds of carcinogens in our environment, including some of our foods. But many of the diets touted for cancer prevention and cure are so specialized and unbalanced that they may actually be harmful.

People with cancer (or who suspect that they have it) should not stake their lives on unproven remedies or cures but should use the best possible methods known to cancer experts. Real breakthroughs by medical research will be well known and will not need crusading promotions. Testimonials from so-called cured patients cannot be relied upon, even though these people may genuinely believe what they say. Prescribed treatments are best, even if they do not appear to give immediate results. If a doctor gives up on a patient, then another doctor should be consulted.

Other Forms of Quackery

Balding, a sex-linked characteristic in men, is also subject to quackery. A few diseases also cause baldness, and even some women become bald, mainly as a result of endocrine imbalances. But when baldness is a family trait in men, it generally begins early in life and then proceeds inexorably. It is not the result of a bad case of dandruff, excessively oily hair, or any other readily identifiable and controllable cause. Yet men spend millions of dollars on useless hormones, lotions, ointments, and special massaging devices that are advertised either as stopping baldness or as surefire hair growers. Success has been attained with hair transplants if they are done by professionals, but most of the cures for baldness are a waste of money.

Fear of aging also makes people vulnerable to exploitation by medical quackery. Virtually all of us want to preserve our youthful looks and exuberance, and many people are willing to spend large sums of money in attempts to do so, buying quack medications parlayed as sure to remove wrinkles, brown spots on the skin, and other evidences of aging. Good diets maintain health and vitality, but consumers should avoid the advertised "youth restorers." Ponce de Leon's Fountain of Youth is still elusive, and while the normal life span has been increased greatly since the days of Ponce de Leon, there are at present no known miracle ways to stop or slow down the aging processes.

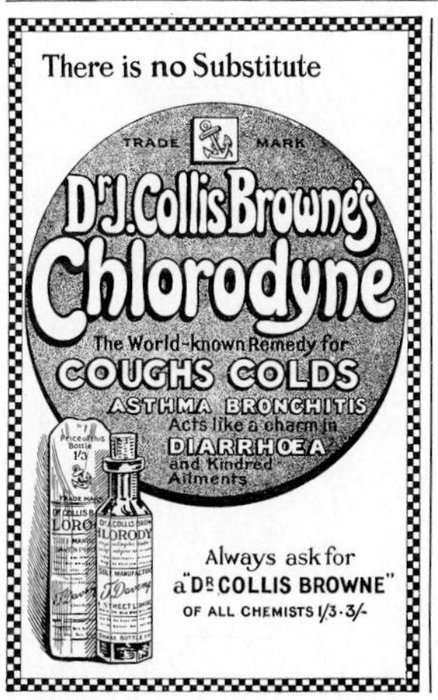

In the past, panaceas like this one were commonly used for all sorts of illnesses. (Photo from EKM-Nepenthe)

How to Recognize Quackery and What to Do

How can the consumer recognize quackery? No product is labeled as such, of course; so the consumer must simply be alert to the most common characteristics. Federal government sources suggest that the consumer ask the following questions about the product. If the answer is "yes" to any one of them, then quackery can be suspected.

1. Is the product or service being offered a "secret" remedy that is not available from any other source?
2. Does the sponsor claim to be battling the medical profession because they do not accept this wonderful discovery?
3. Is the remedy being sold from door to door by a self-styled "health adviser" or promoted in lectures from town to town?
4. Is the "miracle" drug, device, or diet being promoted in some primarily sensational magazine or tabloid newspaper, by a faith healer's group, or by some crusading organization of laymen?
5. Does the promoter expound the miracles that the product or service has performed for others?
6. Is the product or service good for a great variety of illnesses, whether real or fancied?

In addition, it is obvious that no one should accept diagnosis of an illness by mail and that all free trial packages of medication should be avoided unless they are of standard and properly labeled products. Do not believe testimonial letters that claim a product cures a disease or diseases that no other drug can. Secret devices and formulas are generally indications of quackery, as are attacks against the medical profession.

A consumer who suspects quackery should report the incident to the family doctor or the county medical society. The local Better Business Bureau can also be consulted for the reliability of the promoter if the sales are being negotiated locally. If such products come through the mail, the local post office should be informed as well as the Food and Drug Administration (at 5600 Fishers Lane, Rockville, Maryland 20852, if there is no local office). In reporting to the FDA, a

YOUR HEALTH TODAY

Propaganda Advertising Techniques

Technique	Typical Slogan
Bandwagon	"Everyone is doing it, so you should be doing it, too!"
Snob Appeal	"You'll be one of the privileged few to buy this product."
Testimony	"It worked for me, so it will work for you!"
False Image	"You'll be like (someone—usually a celebrity) if you use this product."
Rewards Appeal	"Not only will you get this product, but you will also receive free. . ."
Humor Appeal	Use of jokes or catchy songs to familiarize people with a product.
Just Plain Folks	"Used since the 1800s by good people like you."
Scientific Evidence	"Doctors recommend this product."
Nonverbal Appeal	Extensive use of pictures to sell a product.
Underdog Appeal	"We're number two, but we try harder."

consumer should state the problem clearly with all relevant details. Be able to specify where the product was obtained and precisely when the purchase was made. Keep whatever remains of the suspect product; it may be needed for examination.

Consumers should also be wary of many publications and of their advertisements. Just because something is in type does not mean it is accurate, nor do such words as "health" and "national" as part of the names of products or organization make them honest. Before accepting anything read in an article or an advertisement, check its authenticity with people or organizations that you are sure are professional and honest.

Examining Advertisements

Look critically at advertisements in magazines and newspapers, or examine those on television, and you will observe that the appeal is often made by playing on the consumer's emotions rather than on the basis of a full and accurate description of the product. Indeed, in order to persuade a consumer to buy certain products, such as cigarettes, an ad must downplay their obvious harmfulness to the consumer's health and focus instead on such qualities as the pleasure they may give and, perhaps subliminally, on their supposed contribution to the user's sex appeal. The techniques used to persuade people to buy a particular health product are called *propaganda advertising techniques.* The box on this page illustrates the various types of propaganda advertising techniques.

Subliminal advertising Advertising that appeals to consumers' subconscious.

The phrase **subliminal advertising** is applied to appeals in ads made so indirectly that they are unlikely to be consciously perceived by the consumer, though they may nevertheless affect the individual's subconscious. Superficially, the ad gives you various reasons to buy the product; but at the same time — without your awareness — it may be suggesting, for example, that the product will make you more attractive or successful.

To become more aware of the subliminal elements in ads you're exposed to, select a few to examine and ask yourself such questions as these: Why might this particular background have been chosen? Is it just a pretty picture, or might it mean something more to me or to other people? What about the people in the ads? Do I identify with them? If not, how do I react to them, and what sorts of people might identify with them? Do their poses and expressions suggest something in addition to what they're obviously doing or saying? Do any of the particular words in the ad have associations for me outside their apparent context?

Besides looking for the possible hidden message in an ad, you

What matters is Absorption
DOCTOR TESTED and Proven Effective
So be sure – for your health sake, ask for ESSENTIAL ORGANICS . . . the supplement that is proven effective by doctors.
Essential Organics
Look Slimmer Feel Better
Nature's Answer
Slendertone
the NATURAL way to lose weight
• No Caffeine • No Drugs
LOSE WEIGHT Naturally in 10 Days
"My wrinkles have nearly disappeared!"
Bee Pollen Cream
Your body deserves the best.
Health From The Sun
Why you should buy eyewear as carefully as you buy a fine watch.
THE FUTURE OF YOUR SKIN HAS JUST CHANGED.
MILLENIUM
Germaine Monteil knows 40 is Fabulous with Firming Action!
Our 46 year old model, Tish Hooker, is firm proof!

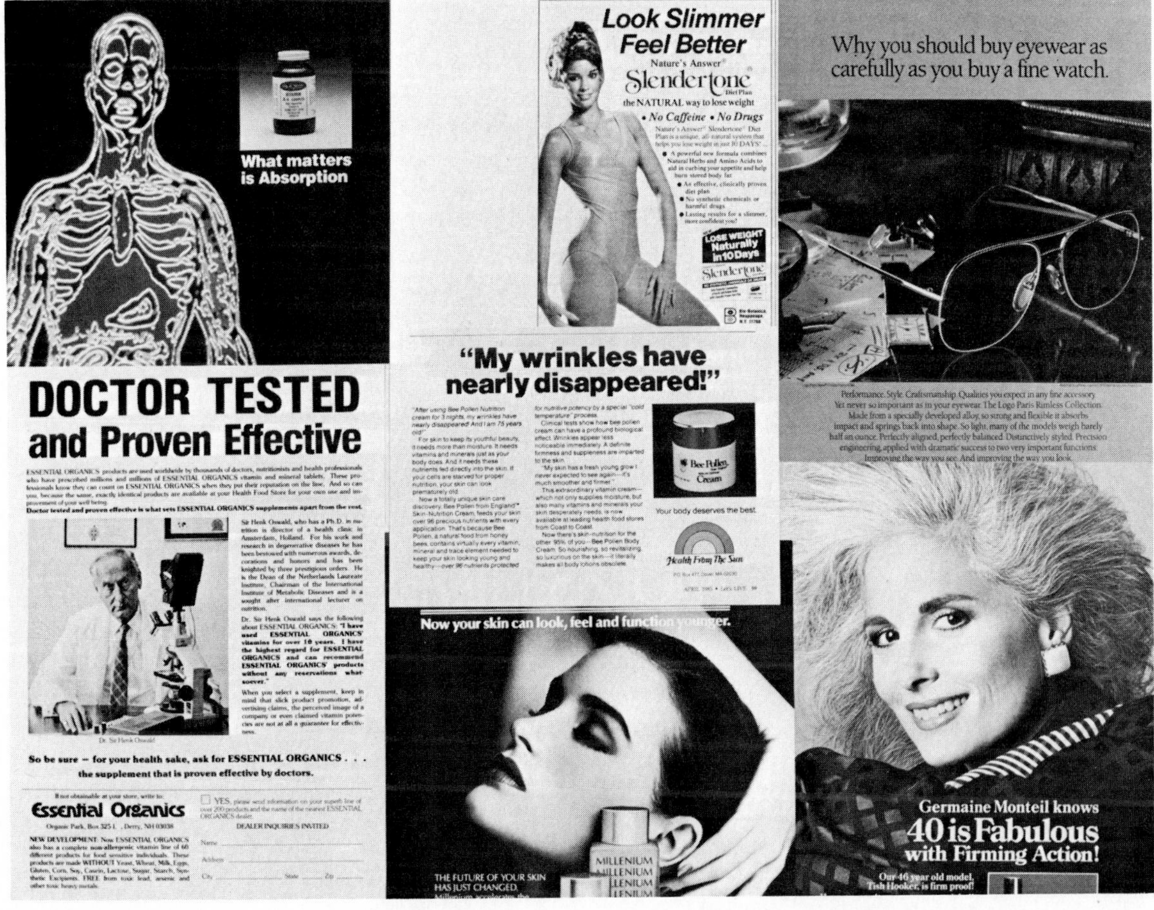

Examples of some advertising techniques used to get the consumer to buy various health and cosmetic products. (Photo by Paul Waldman)

should, of course, also question the direct claims being made. If supposedly scientific research is being cited as a reason for the superiority of a particular headache remedy, for example, is enough information given you to check on the accuracy of the claim? If not, you might well assume that the "nine out of ten doctors" referred to are entirely in the vivid imagination of the ad writer.

One important fact to keep in mind about an ad for any product is that the ad costs money and is ultimately paid for by consumers—including you, if you buy the product. That is one reason that, for example, a name-brand drug costs so much more than the identical drug sold generically. Unfortunately, the designers of advertising for many products that may affect your health and well-being are more interested in selling them by whatever means will be successful than in accurately informing the consumers about the qualities of the products.

Consumer Protection

In general, the likelihood of your being injured by a food or drug or other product you buy today is relatively remote in comparison with the past. Manufacturers of products and providers of services are required by law to adhere to high standards of safety, and considerable research is undertaken to determine just what constitutes safe use of a new drug or other product. If you purchase something like food that turns out to be contaminated, though, you may bring a complaint to the government agency charged with seeing that such products are made safe or removed from the marketplace.

Laws Aiding Consumers

Laws to protect the health and safety of consumers are not new. They date to the year 1202, when King John of England enacted a law prohibiting the adulteration of bread with ground-up peas, beans, and other such ingredients. In the United States the first general food law was enacted in Massachusetts in 1784, but really significant national laws did not come until much later. Following are some of the most important pieces of federal legislation that were finally passed:

1906—the first federal Food and Drug Act, prohibiting interstate commerce in misbranded and adulterated foods, drinks, and drugs. On the same day, the Congress also passed the Meat Inspection Act to help remedy unsanitary conditions prevailing in meat packing plants.

1912—the Sherley Amendment to the Food and Drug Act, prohibiting the labeling of medicines with false therapeutic claims with intent to defraud.

1938—the federal Food, Drug, and Cosmetic (FDC) Act, which

1. extended coverage of the 1906 act to cosmetics and therapeutic devices.
2. required government clearance before new drugs could be marketed.
3. eliminated the Sherley Amendment requirement of proving intent to defraud in drug mislabeling.
4. established tolerances for unavoidable poisonous substances.
5. authorized standards of identity, quality, and fill for food containers.
6. authorized factory inspections.
7. added the remedy of court injunction to previous remedies of seizure and prosecution.

1944—the Public Health Service Act, broadened many times since, which created the federal agency responsible for protecting and improving public health.

1951—the Durham-Humphrey Amendment, specifically requiring that drugs which cannot be used safely without medical supervision must be labeled for sale and dispensed only by prescription of a licensed medical practitioner.

1958—the Delaney Amendment, giving the FDA authority to ban the use of food additives known to be cancer-causing agents either in humans or in test animals.

1960—the Color Additive Amendment, allowing the FDA to establish the conditions of safe use for color additives in foods, drugs, and cosmetics and to require manufacturers to perform the necessary scientific investigations to establish safety.

1960—the Federal Hazardous Substances Labeling Act, requiring prominent warning labels on hazardous household chemical products.

1962—the Kefauver-Harris Amendments, assuring an even greater degree of safety and also strengthening the new drug clearance procedures. Drug manufacturers were required to prove to the FDA the effectiveness of their products before placing them on the market.

1965—the Drug Abuse Control Amendments, passed to deal with problems caused by the abuse of three groups of dangerous drugs—depressants, stimulants, and hallucinogens. This law allows the FDA to seize illegal supplies of controlled drugs, to serve warrants, to arrest violators, and to require all legal handlers to keep records of supplies and sales.

1966—the Fair Packaging and Labeling Act, requiring that consumer products in interstate commerce be honestly and informatively labeled. The FDA was given the power to enforce the provisions affecting foods, drugs, cosmetics, and medical devices.

1968—establishment of Radiation Control for Health and Safety, as a protection for the public from unnecessary exposure to radiation by such electronic products as color television sets, microwave ovens, and X-ray machines, based on standards established by the FDA.

1970—the Poison Prevention Packaging Act, enacted specifically to protect children from accidentally consuming toxic materials. Materials that are determined to be poisonous must be packaged so that children under the age of five find them difficult or impossible to open.

1976—the Medical Device Amendments, giving the FDA authority to check and demand the safety and effectiveness of devices before they are marketed, as well as afterward.

Enforcement Agencies

Agencies for protecting consumers exist at federal, state, and local levels. Some are government agencies; others are private, established and operated by citizen's groups. Following are some of the most important agencies, the functions of which include consumer protection.

Federal Agencies

Food and Drug Administration (FDA). The FDA is headed by a commissioner who controls seven bureaus plus the National Center for Toxological Research, and includes regional and district offices throughout the United States. Inspectors of the FDA periodically visit all kinds of food processing and storing establishments to check on the sanitary conditions and the procedures being followed. If violations are discovered and the firm is found guilty of the charges, the products are removed from the market, fines are imposed, and the violators may be jailed. Individuals can help in the enforcement of FDA laws by reporting suspected violations. The FDA requires that food be clean and safe to eat, which means also that it must not contain dangerous residues of chemical pesticides or other harmful substances. Manufacturers of all products used in producing or preparing food must pass FDA tests. Labels indicate what has been employed in the preparation or preservation of the food, and items listed on the label have passed the FDA inspection and requirements. FDA labeling regulations also require the precise and common name of the food or foods (in cases of combinations) on the package, exact amounts, the manufacturer's address, and other special information based on the product and its intended use. A label must not deceive or mislead a consumer. The FDA has similar control over drugs and cosmetics, veterinary medicines, household equipment, and other matters related to the health and safety of consumers.

Federal Trade Commission (FTC). The basic function of the Federal Trade Commission is to maintain free competitive enterprise and to prevent any stifling of the American economic system by monopolies or by unfair or deceptive trade practices. Its most direct service for the health consumer is the prevention of misrepresentations in the advertisement of foods, drugs, cosmetics, and devices. The FTC sponsors education programs to improve buyer awareness, to bring about more competition in markets, to prevent deception in packaging, advertising, or other selling methods, and to prevent price-fixing and other unfair business practices. The FTC investigates complaints from citizens or from officials in any case in which interstate commerce is involved, and violators may receive heavy fines or imprisonment if convicted. Other federal consumer protection agencies are listed in the box entitled "Important Consumer Protection Agencies."

State and Local Agencies

All states now have offices that provide information to consumers and handle complaints, referring them to the appropriate local, state, or federal agencies as necessary. Most states also have other consumer agencies that are duplicates of those at the federal level and can take action quickly. In some states the attorney general's office handles many matters concerning health and safety.

More than 300 local governments—in heavily populated counties and metropolitan areas—also have special divisions concerned with

YOUR HEALTH TODAY

Important Consumer Protection Agencies

United States Government

Food and Drug Administration (FDA)
Federal Trade Commission (FTC)
United States Postal Service (USPS)
United States Department of Agriculture (USDA)
Environmental Protection Agency (EPA)
Consumer Product Safety Commission (CPSC)

State and Local Agencies

Attorney General's Office
State Consumer Affairs Office

Private Agencies

American Medical Association
American Dental Association
American Osteopathic Association
American Cancer Society
American Heart Association
Arthritis Foundation
American Lung Association
Better Business Bureau

consumer health and safety. People who do not live in areas where such services are available might go to the Better Business Bureau, health department, or local prosecutor's office for advice.

Private Agencies

Hundreds of private organizations, many staffed primarily with volunteer workers, promote public health and safety, dispensing information and assistance to those in need. Among the best known of those with specific health concerns are the American Heart Association, the American Cancer Society, the American Lung Association, the March of Dimes, the Arthritis Foundation, and the American Diabetes Association. All of these and many more have branch offices in cities and towns throughout the nation. Besides those agencies that are basically concerned with health, there are a number of agencies that can be an important help to the consumer in various fields, including health.

One of these is the Better Business Bureau. With offices in hundreds of cities, the Better Business Bureau offers aid to consumers who have problems with purchases or services of various kinds. The Bureau insists on truth in advertising and on fair business practices and can be consulted for a rating on a company with which a consumer is considering doing business.

Public Citizen, Inc., headed by Ralph Nader, is an important consumer group that has been aggressively active in numerous well-publicized and effective programs in behalf of consumers. The organization does research, takes legal action, and also lobbies in Washington, D.C.

The Consumers Union of the United States, Inc., tests and compares products, publishing the results in a monthly magazine and a comprehensive annual buyer's guide. It also publishes many pamphlets and films and maintains a Washington, D.C., law firm that represents consumers in courts and in regulatory agencies. The Consumers Union does not print advertising in any of its various publications.

Personal Action

You are really your most important protection, for it is your personal health and safety that are at stake. When you make purchases, keep the sales slips and canceled checks. If you have a complaint on the basis of health, safety, or other reasons, go first to the place where you made your purchase. If you are not given satisfaction, write to the president of the company. To ensure attention and action, also send a copy of the letter to someone else in a high position in the company—the chairman of the board, advertising manager, or sales manager, for example—and indicate in or on your letter that you have done so. Keep a copy of the letter yourself, of course. If you do not get a satisfactory response, then send copies of your letter to the Better

Business Bureau, the consumer affairs office in your state, your state attorney general, and your senator and congressman; to consumer watchdog columnists who provide help via syndicated newspaper columns; and also to the most specifically applicable of the consumers' groups. If the product is from out of state, copies of your complaint should go to the FDA and FTC. Let the company know what you are doing.

If your complaint is legitimate, you will get action — probably more than you ever imagined. If the amount of money involved is small, you can sue and get reimbursement by going through a small claims court. The cost for its use is nominal. But most important, you are not only protecting yourself but also others who may buy and have trouble with the same product. Many problems can be avoided, of course, by becoming a careful and informed buyer. It is especially important to take extra precautions where health is involved.

Summary

Know where you will go for medical help before an emergency. Make sure the doctor you select has sound credentials. Your doctor should treat you courteously and with concern, answer your questions to your satisfaction, and not expose you to excessive treatments. A baseline physical is advisable upon seeing a new physician, and thereafter at appropriate intervals according to age. More frequent screenings should be done for specific health problems. Whenever a doctor or a dentist recommends a treatment that seems risky or extreme, you should get a second opinion. Controversial alternative systems of treatment include chiropractic, naturopathy, and acupuncture.

No prescriptions are necessary for over-the-counter drugs, which generally treat symptoms rather than cure illness. Though usually safe and effective, they may be harmful if used improperly. Prescription drugs must be dispensed at the instruction of a doctor. Don't hesitate to ask your physician to prescribe generic drugs when possible; these will cost you less than their brand-name equivalents.

Hospitals in the United States may be nonprofit organizations, government owned and operated, or profit-making and privately owned. Learn which hospitals near you offer the best professional services and equipment at competitive prices and where you would likely be best treated in the event of an emergency. When in the hospital you have a right to courteous and professional treatment and to specific rights enumerated by the American Hospital Association.

The principal forms of private health insurance are basic health insurance and medical. Insurance bought through a group usually is cheaper for the same coverage than when bought by an individual. Health maintenance organizations, systems providing comprehensive health care for prepaid premiums, are a popular alternative to traditional insurance. The U.S. government has established Medicare and Medicaid programs to help the aged and the poor. Consumers must be aware of the techniques used in advertisements that try to influence one's decision making. The techniques can be overt, as with propaganda techniques, or less noticeable, as with subliminal techniques.

Medical quackery is the purveying of misinformation about health, often in the form of "secret" remedies directed at the gullible. Among the most prevalent quack remedies are those aimed at arthritis and cancer patients. The most recent fad in cancer nostrums, laetrile, has not proven to be of any therapeutic value. You should suspect quackery when a product is offered as a secret remedy by someone who claims to be battling the medical profession, when it is promoted in sensational media or in crusading fashion, when it is said to bring about miraculous results, or when it is offered for a wide variety of illnesses.

Numerous consumer protection laws and government agencies have been established to maintain standards of safety in consumer products and are a source of redress if you should buy an unsafe product. Various private groups are also sources of information and help.

Review and Discussion

1. What factors should be considered in obtaining and evaluating medical care?
2. Describe the differences between an M.D. and a D.O.
3. List and describe types of alternative systems of healing.
4. Discuss the advantages and disadvantages of using different kinds of over-the-counter products.
5. Describe the various kinds of hospitals found in our health care delivery system.
6. Discuss the differences between basic health insurance and major medical.
7. What elements should you consider in choosing health insurance?
8. Describe some of the various types of medical quackery prevalent in the United States.
9. Describe the major types of propaganda advertising techniques.
10. What is subliminal advertising and why is it of concern?
11. List and describe some of the milestone laws concerning consumer protection.
12. List and describe the major national, state, and local consumer protection agencies and organizations.

Further Reading

Editors of Consumer Reports Books. *Health Quackery.* New York: Holt, Rinehart and Winston, 1981.
A careful discussion of the many forms of abuses in the consumer health field.

Editors of Consumer Report Books. *The Medicine Show.* New York: Consumers Union, 1980.
An informative examination of the major OTC products. Perhaps the most comprehensive guide to OTC products for the general public.

Gots, Ronald, and Arthur Kaufman. *The People's Hospital Book.* New York: Avon Books, 1981.
A practical guide to getting the best medical care from hospitals.

Graedon, Joe. *The People's Pharmacy—Two.* New York: Avon Books, 1980.
Valuable information on both over-the-counter and prescription drugs, with warnings about possible dangers.

Rosenfield, Isadore. *Second Opinions.* New York: Bantam Books, 1981.
A doctor's discussion of medical problems for which alternative treatments exist and a second opinion may be useful.

Shipley, Roger R., and Carolyn Plonsky. *Consumer Health.* New York: Harper & Row, Publishers, 1980.
A comprehensive examination of the major areas involved in consumer health.

Waller, Kal. *How To Recover Your Medical Expenses.* New York: Collier Books, 1981.
Explanations of Medicare benefits: what is covered and how to be reimbursed.

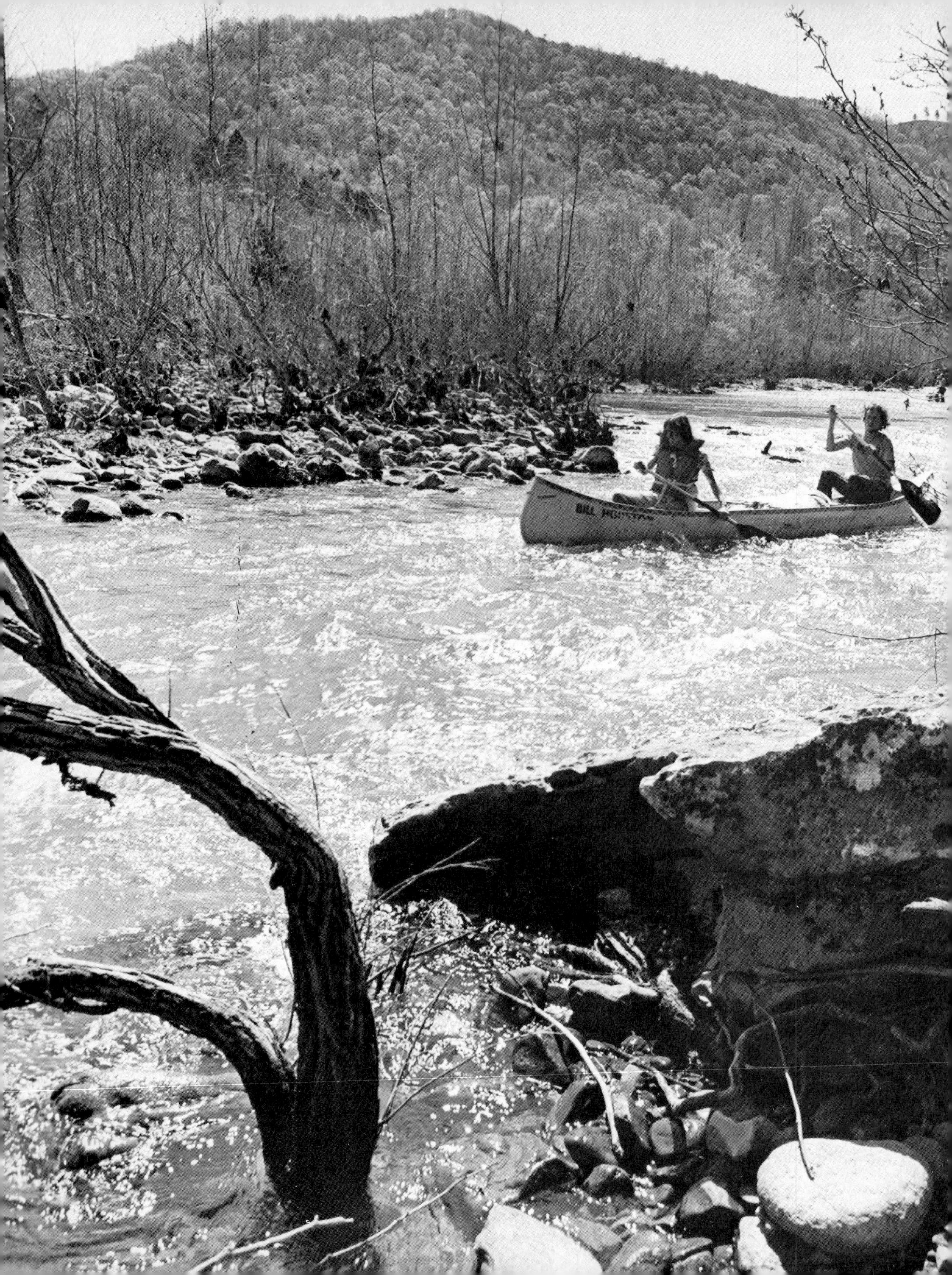
BILL

Chapter 21
Environmental Health

KEY POINTS

- ☐ There is a growing awareness of the importance of a healthy natural environment for human well-being.
- ☐ The earth's population is increasing dramatically, placing new demands on the environment.
- ☐ Air pollution, whose major constituents are carbon monoxide, hydrocarbons, nitrogen oxides, sulfur oxides, and particulates, remains a threat to health.
- ☐ Increasing demand for usable water has focused attention on the problem of water pollution.
- ☐ Noise pollution is now recognized as a serious health problem.
- ☐ The careful management of productive land is necessary if the nutritional needs of the world are to be met.
- ☐ Nuclear energy is an alternative to oil and coal, but serious questions have been raised about its safety.
- ☐ The solution of environmental problems will depend on a combination of individual action and public policy.

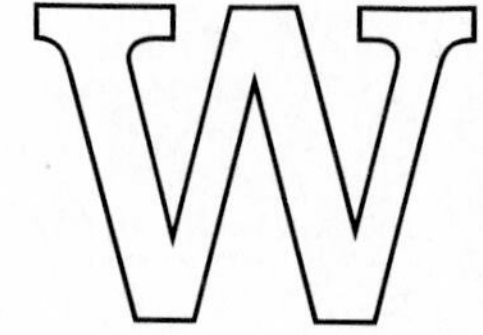

E SHARE the earth with some 4.5 billion other people and with countless billions of plants and animals. All of the people and other living things have similar essential needs — living space and a source of energy or food.

All living things affect their environment. Once people believed that the world was too vast and their powers too insignificant to leave lasting marks. Now they recognize that humans influence the world environment as other living beings cannot. They are learning that they must live as a part of nature, as one of the elements in a complex natural world.

In making "progress," people have made vast changes in the face of the earth. Resources are being depleted; the land, air, and waters are being polluted. Populations are increasing, bringing on greater needs, more wastes, and additional health problems.

Once people shared their everyday world mainly with relatives and a few neighbors just down the road, but now everyone in the world is in some way a neighbor. A resident of New York, Paris, London, or any other large city may be affected by how a farmer in Africa or Asia tills the soil and by whether that farmer has bad or bountiful crops. And the farmer, in turn, is affected by how the city dweller uses energy or disposes of wastes. Earth has indeed become just one world, with common problems and limited resources.

Conservationists, once thought of as people who planted trees, saved scenic views, and preserved endangered species of wildlife, are now charged with a task of enormous dimensions and importance — saving people. And they are not working alone. People now are seeing that it is no longer possible to run away from mistakes; they must be dealt with — and care taken not to repeat them.

World Population

About 250 million people inhabited the earth at the time of the birth of Christ. In the fewer than 2,000 years since then, the world population has multiplied rapidly. Shortly after 1800 it passed the billion mark. By 1930 it has jumped to 2 billion. By 1980 well over 4 billion people lived on earth, and by the year 2000 the world population is expected to reach nearly 6.5 billion.

For years, scientists have been watching this alarming population growth, and they have continually sounded warnings, most of which have gone unheeded. Thomas Robert Malthus, an English economist, pointed to this problem more than 150 years ago in his *Essay on the Principle of Population As It Affects the Future Improvement of Society.* He believed that the population was increasing faster than the supply of food and painted a gloomy picture of misery and starvation for the future.

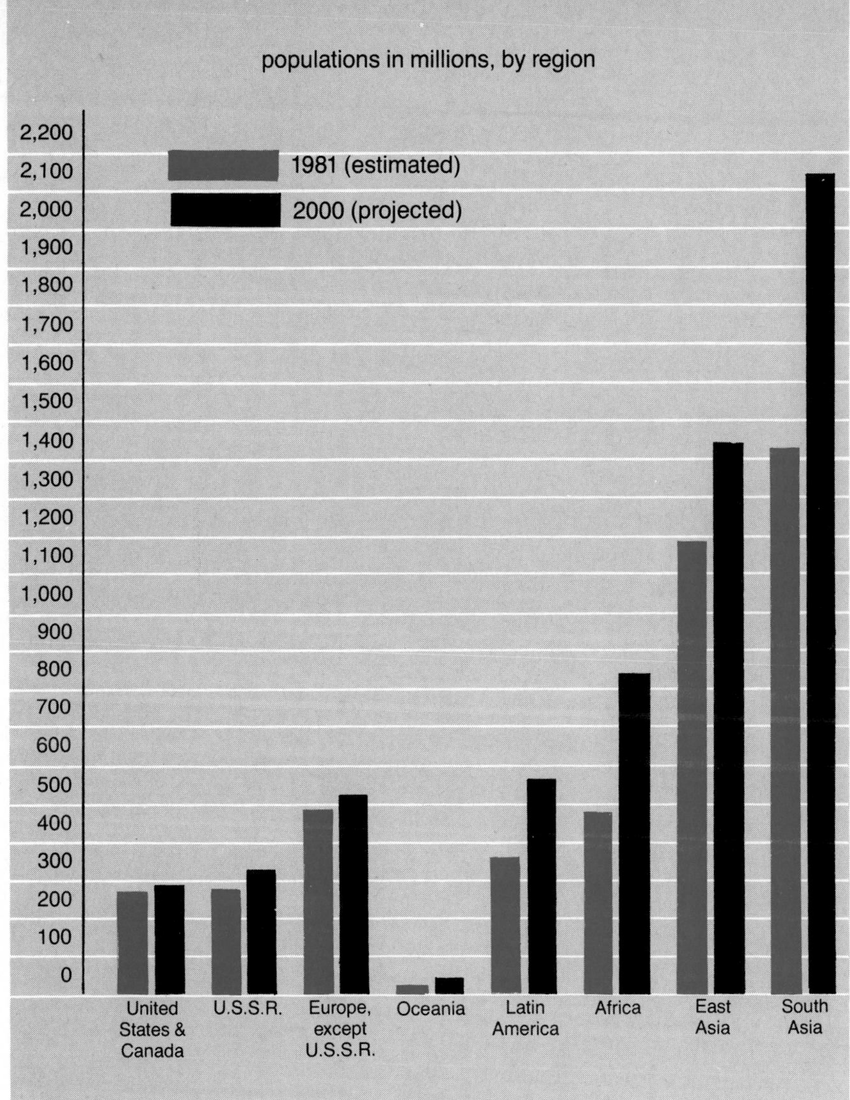

Figure 21-1. The World's Growing Population.
In the last decades of the twentieth century, population is expected to increase steadily in the developed regions of North America and Europe, and to continue expanding at rapid rates in other, generally less developed regions of the world. (Source: Based on estimates by the Population Reference Bureau.)

Can the world, in fact, support the further increases in population that will come during the last decades of this century and the early decades of the next century? Based on present conditions, some experts say it is highly questionable. Others maintain that we should move forward with confidence; they believe that survival will remain possible as a result of new discoveries in science and technology. Some say the earth has an absolute limit of about 10 billion people; others say it will be able to support substantially more — perhaps as many as 50 billion.

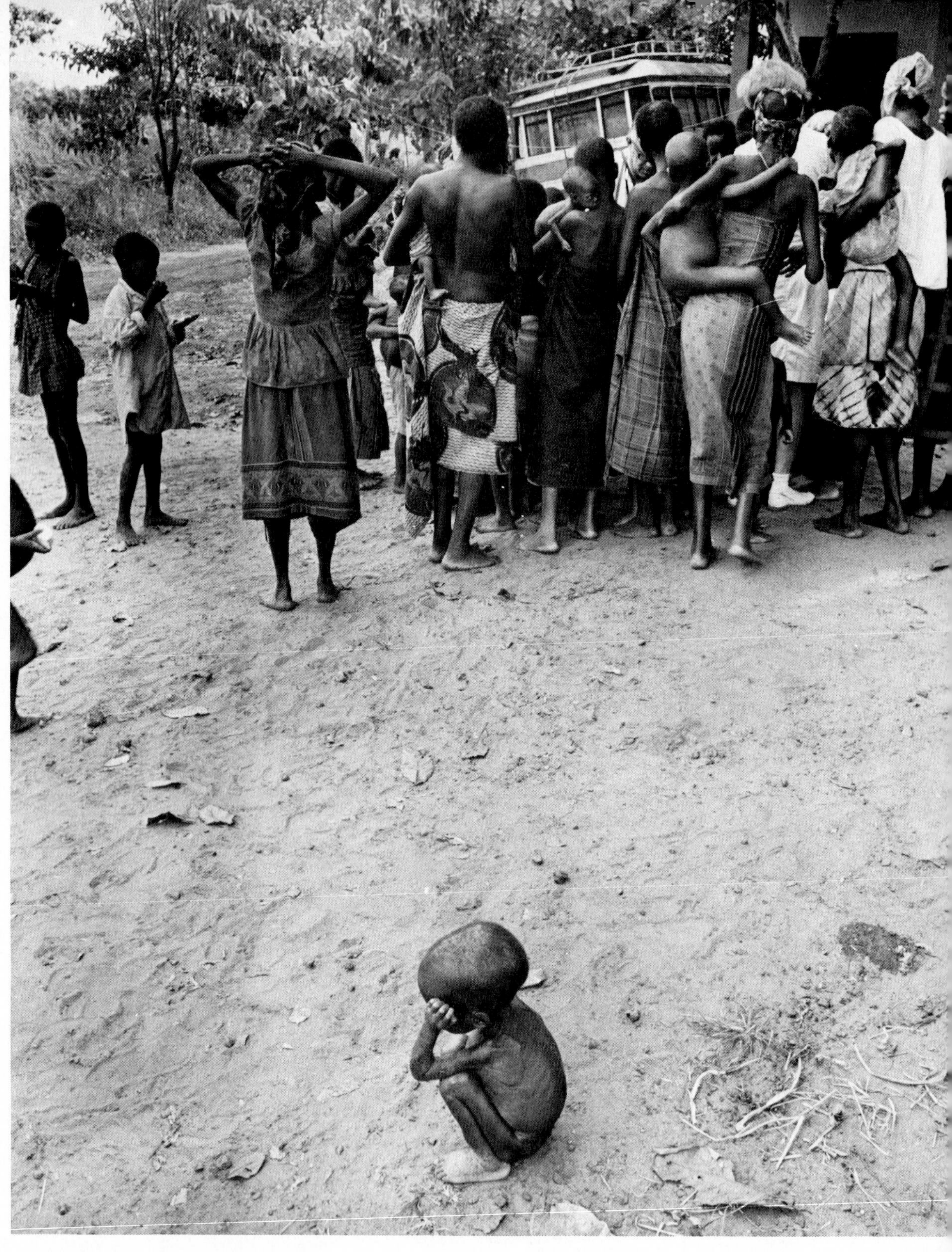

This Nigerian boy squatting on a dirt road is one of many suffering children who grow up in an unhealthy environment. (Photo by R. Farquharson/UNICEF)

Over the past centuries, human populations have been held in check by three factors: disease, famine, and war. Because of the human suffering involved, most societies, of course, do not regard these conditions as desirable, and people work to find ways of overcoming or avoiding them.

An obvious solution to the world population problem would be birth control. This is difficult because of the low level of education in many overpopulated countries and because moral issues are also involved. But the alternative is severe—misery and self-annihilation. New foods and greater agricultural productivity are also needed. Almost all of the land that can be put into efficient food production is being used now, and improved agricultural practices represent the major way to meet growing needs. Part of the answer may come from a more productive use of the sea, with its many potential food sources.

Of ultimate importance is the recognition and acceptance by people that the very existence of the human race is threatened, that the growth of population in future years could outstrip the available resources. People must learn how to live as a part of nature and at peace with one another.

United States Population

The United States is not immune to the population plague, although the high standard of living in this country makes it easy to overlook the growing and inevitable difficulties. With three out of four Americans now living in metropolitan areas, cities are outgrowing their capacities to accommodate more people and to provide quality living conditions. The result is more and more ghettos. Land for living space in these population centers is becoming scarce, and there are increasing problems in providing transportation in the cities and roads and highways to them. Recreational lands are being depleted.

As the population rises and the standard of living declines, the same nutritional difficulties that plague other nations will increase in the United States. Pollutants contribute to a whole new spectrum of health maladies. Added to them is the stress brought on by crowded living conditions. Many Americans are already experiencing degrees of discomfort, yet the United States, with only about 5 percent of the world population, uses a disproportionately large percentage of the world's resources—about 35 percent of those that are nonrenewable. Americans are also acquainted with the high demand for energy supplies and with the resulting soaring costs.

Population growth in the United States has fluctuated over the years, from the days when large families were fashionable in the early 1900s to the lows in the 1930s and 1940s. After World War II, there was a baby boom that reached its peak in the late 1950s; this was followed again by a general decline that reached a low in the 1970s, with births falling below the level needed to replace deaths.

Slight increases in birthrates came again in the 1980s, partly because many young people who were born during the baby boom after World War II were having families. The number of women of childbearing age will fall again after the mid-1980s, but at the turn of the century daughters born in the 1980s will be bearing children, causing an increase in birthrates even if fertility rates are low. Even in the United States, then, population growth will probably be a permanent problem.

What can be done? At all levels in educational systems, population growth and its impact on the nation and the world should be taught and made understandable. Courses in sex education should be made mandatory, and there should also be programs in birth control and family planning. Large-scale immigration, which can cause both social and health problems, should be monitored carefully, and policies for the future must be intelligently devised. It is not really a matter of how many people it is possible to accommodate at a mere survival level but rather of how many can be maintained without a serious deterioration of the quality of life.

Air Pollution

Air pollution can come from a volcano spewing fiery ashes and dust, darkening the sky for months or even years; from a forest fire that sends billows of smoke upward; from the legions of smokestacks of industries letting loose noxious fumes; or from bumper-to-bumper automobiles puffing out carbon monoxide and other poisonous exhausts.

Once it was believed that the atmosphere had unlimited capacity to purify itself of smoke, noxious fumes, and other wastes by means of the winds and the rains. No one worried about where the pollution was carried by the winds or about the fact that the rain falling from the sky carried pollutants back down to earth. Air pollution was ignored because the atmosphere seemed so vast that it could never be contaminated by human activities.

But now we know that the atmosphere can be contaminated. Many areas of the United States and other countries lie under an almost permanent haze. Tons of soot and other pollutants burden the skies over metropolitan areas and then spread. New York City, for example, incinerates roughly 200 tons of trash per square mile every day. Roughly a third of this is spewed back into the air as soot and ash.

The Major Air Pollutants

Air pollution is a major problem in modern industrial societies. If you live in or near a major metropolitan area, you may be especially aware of the problem; but even if you live high in the Sierras, or in the middle of a Kansas wheat field, you have probably experienced its effects in some degree. Almost nowhere is the air completely clear and clean.

The first human-caused air poullutants came from fires used for cooking and heating, wood initially and then later coal. There are still places on earth where fires of this sort form choking clouds when the smoke hangs close to the ground and fills entire valleys. But air pollution has changed in nature and in degree with the increases in population and the advances made by technology in modern times. The major pollutants are now carbon monoxide, hydrocarbons, nitrogen oxides, sulfur oxides, and particulates. There is also concern about the use of fluorocarbons in spray cans.

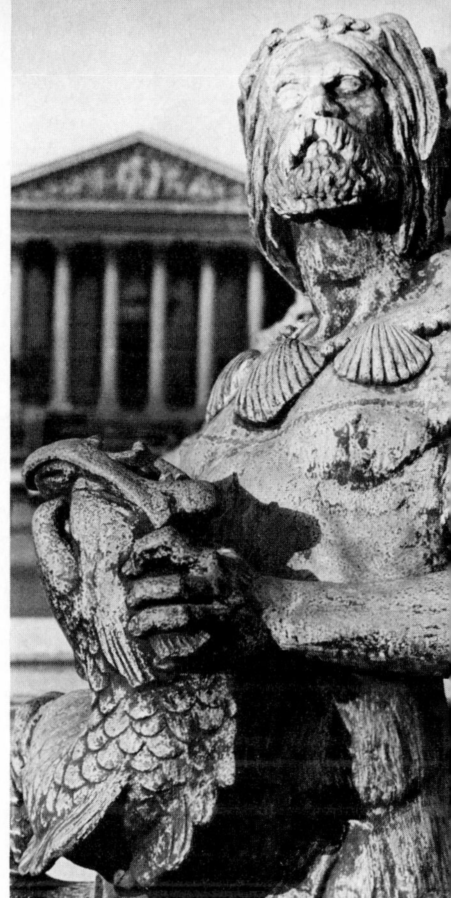

Air pollution in many major cities is gradually destroying valuable art and architecture. (Photo by J. C. Lozouet/Photo Trends)

Carbon Monoxide

Carbon monoxide is a by-product of some industrial processes, but the main nonnatural source of this air pollutant is the incomplete burning of fuels by engines. In urban areas where traffic is exceptionally heavy, engines account for about 99 percent of the carbon monoxide in the air. Fortunately, this gas rarely reaches dangerous levels, for the colorless, odorless, and tasteless carbon monoxide can be deadly. It unites with hemoglobin in the blood and thus reduces the amount of oxygen delivered to the cells. It also weakens heart contractions, reducing the amount of blood that is pumped through the body. A person who already has a heart problem or a respiratory illness can be affected by even small amounts of carbon monoxide. About half of all fatal poisonings in the United States are traceable to carbon monoxide; and because the gas is so difficult to detect, it may be responsible for even more damage and deaths than can be easily identified. Tobacco smoke is the second most common source of carbon monoxide, incidentally; as a result, smokers have reduced levels of oxygen in the blood. Headache and nausea are symptoms of carbon monoxide poisoning. In the United States, emission control devices and more efficient fuel-burning systems in automobiles have decreased carbon monoxide levels substantially.

Hydrocarbons and Nitrogen Oxides

Hydrocarbons, chemical compounds containing hydrogen and carbon, are usually the result of the incomplete combustion of petroleum products. In addition to releasing carbon monoxide into the atmosphere, automobiles account for most hydrocarbon emissions, though some are by-products of industry. Their direct effect on human health appears to be minimal, but in the presence of sunlight, hydrocarbons react with nitrogen oxides to form substances that are irritating to the respiratory tract and also cause the eyes to water.

Hydrocarbons Chemical compounds containing hydrogen and carbon that irritate the respiratory tract.

Nitrogen dioxide Dangerous chemical component of engine exhaust and tobacco smoke.

Nitric oxide A major cause of air pollution.

Two nitrogen oxides, **nitrogen dioxide** and **nitric oxide,** are major causes of air pollution and play a primary role in reactions with hydrocarbons. Nitrogen dioxide is the more dangerous; when present at high levels, which is rare, it produces the lung condition known as pulmonary edema and aggravates such respiratory ailments as chronic bronchitis and emphysema. Most nitrogen dioxide comes from the exhausts of engines; nitrogen dioxide is also one of the principal components of tobacco smoke.

Dioxin An extremely toxic by-product of several chemical products.

Another chemical compound that has been a source of much controversy is **dioxin.** For information regarding this chemical see the box entitled "Dioxin."

Sulphur Oxides and Acid Rain

Sulfur dioxide Pollutant that reacts to form acid rain.

Acid rain Pollutant high in sulfuric acid that is caused by industrial pollutin.

Sulfur dioxide and other sulfur oxides enter the atmosphere mainly from the burning of coal and oil, but they are also released from various industries. Wherever this pollutant is abundant, deaths from heart and lung diseases are also higher than the average. In the air, sulfur dioxide reacts chemically to form other compounds, and among them is sulfuric acid, responsible for the **acid rains** that plague many parts of the world today. The acid rains in Scandinavian countries are attributed to sulfur dioxide emissions from industries in England and western Europe, where industrial stacks were lifted higher to prevent the smoke and fumes from dropping locally. Similarly, the acid rains in New York are caused by sulfur dioxide emissions from industries in the Midwest.

In the past the burning of coal was the major contributor of sulfur dioxide to the atmosphere. A return to a greater use of coal in the coming years portends an increase in this pollutant, unless there are stringent regulations controlling emissions and effective enforcement of these rules.

Particulates

Particulates Minute solid particles in the air such as molds and allergens.

Pollen grains, spores of molds and other fungi, dusts of asbestos and other substances—all of the many kinds of tiny solid particles riding at least for a time in the air are called **particulates.** Some consist of organic matter. Others are inorganic, and still others are radioactive. The amount of particulate matter in the air varies greatly from time to time and from one place to another. Some bits of organic matter, for example, are the primary causes of hay fever and other seasonal allergies. Others, including the various metals, sulfates, and nitrates, can be serious health hazards, contributing to respiratory and other diseases. Some of the particulates are *carcinogens,* or cancer-causing agents. About 20 percent of the people in the United States live in areas where the particulates are in excess of the recommended standards.

Aerosols and Ozone

Ozone layer Atmospheric zone approximately twelve to twenty-one miles above the earth's surface.

The **ozone layer** is a zone of the atmosphere approximately 12 to 21 miles above the surface of the earth where the compound ozone is relatively common. It forms a protective shield, preventing the free

YOUR HEALTH TODAY

Dioxin

What is dioxin?

Dioxin is not one chemical. It is any of seventy-five chemicals in eight different families resulting from the combination of chlorine, hydrogen, and carbon. Dioxin is a by-product from the making of wood preservatives, plastics, insecticides, and herbicides.

Is it deadly?

Dioxin is considered by scientists to be one of the most toxic substances made by humans. It is 170,000 times more deadly than cyanide. The most deadly form of dioxin is TCDD or (2,3,7,8) tetrachlorodibenzo paradoxin.

Does it cause health problems?

While no human deaths have been linked to dioxin, it has been linked to a number of health problems.

- chloracne—a servere form of acne which may cause the skin to thicken and darken.
- liver disorders
- a decreased sex drive
- elevated cholesterol levels
- insomnia

Dioxin has been controversially linked to cancer and birth defects in humans.

Scientists do not know the smallest amount of dioxin necessary to make a person sick.

What is the extent of the problem?

Fish in rivers and lakes in Michigan and upstate New York have been found to be contaminated with dioxin.

Almost 3,000 rusting drums with high levels of dioxin have been found in the soil and streams for miles around a Jacksonville, Arkansas, waste dump.

High levels of dioxin have been found at the Hooker Chemical's dump sites in New York's Love Canal and Hyde Park.

High levels of dioxin in Times Beach, Missouri, forced the U.S. government to buy the town and relocate its 2,000 residents. There are at least twenty-six other sites in Missouri known to be contaminated, with almost three times that many suspected of being contaminated.

entry of large amounts of damaging ultraviolet rays from the sun. Destruction of the ozone layer could have a lethal effect on life on earth. A number of agents, including supersonic aircraft, have been suspected of reducing the amount of ozone. The most significant are the **fluorocarbons** that serve as propellants in the many types of aerosols, once widely used but now banned in most countries. High in the atmosphere the fluorocarbons break down into chlorine components that destroy the ozone. The U.S. National Academy of Sciences has suggested that a 7 percent decrease in the ozone in the ozone layer would result in a 14 percent increase in the incidence of skin cancer, already the most common of all forms of cancer.

Fluorocarbon Chemical agent that breaks down into ozone-destroying components.

At lower levels in the atmosphere, ozone itself becomes a pollutant. Produced by a chemical reaction between the nitrogen oxides and a number of different gases, such as gasoline vapors, chemical solvents, and the combustion by-products of fuels, it is a primary component in smogs. Ozone irritates the mucous membranes and reduces the ability of the lungs to function properly.

Temperature Inversions

Temperature inversion Layer of warm air trapping cooler, polluted air beneath it.

Air pollution problems are greatly aggravated when **temperature inversions** occur. Normally the warm air generated in urban areas rises and is spread out, or dissipated. However, in cases where the urban air is cooler than a layer of warmer air that has moved in over it forming a cap, the polluted air is trapped close to the ground.

On occason, inversions have been responsible for well-documented cases of air-pollution tragedies. In October 1948, for example, the city of Donora, Pennsylvania, experienced a windless calm for nearly a week while its steel, zinc, and other industries continued operating around the clock, pouring smoke and poisonous fumes into the air. Twenty deaths were directly and immediately attributed to the pollution. Most of the victims were older people who already had respiratory ailments. Thousands of people were hospitalized, and there is no way to determine how many died later as a result of those days of concentrated exposure to the poisonous air.

An inversion over London in 1952 was more tragic. More than 4,000 deaths were related directly to the stagnant polluted air that clung close to the ground in a dense fog. In New York City in 1963, 400 people died during a similar sort of heavy smog, and in 1969, an inversion held a layer of pollution over a 22-state area of the Midwest and Southeast for more than a week.

Fatalities resulting from minor inversions go virtually unnoticed. Deaths of 20 people in excess of the daily average in New York City do not command great attention. All major metropolitan areas, in fact, now monitor their air closely and keep their citizens informed of air-quality conditions. Many cities are taking positive steps toward improving air quality.

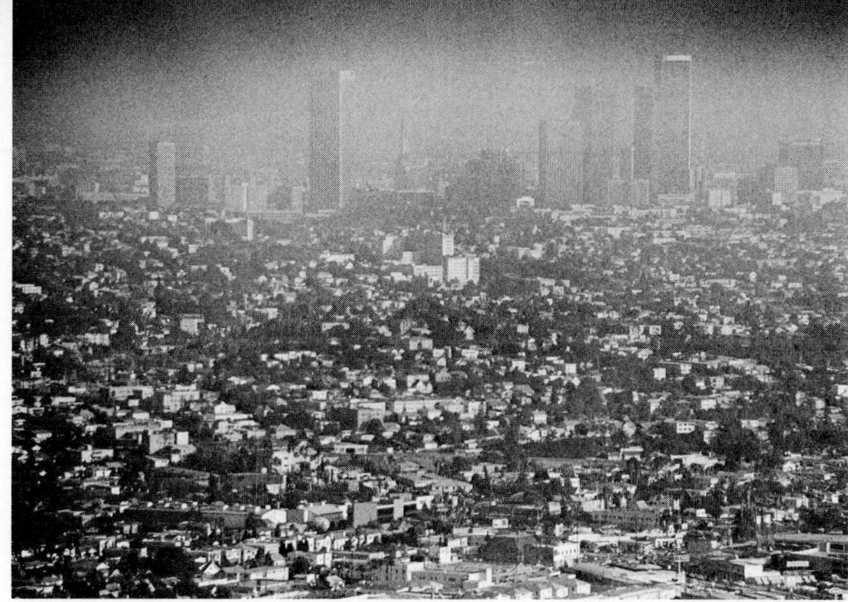

Thermal inversion is a big problem in major urban areas. Downtown Los Angeles is enveloped in smog when the warmer air above traps the pollution close to the ground. (Photo © Ellis Herwig 1980/Stock, Boston)

Effects of Air Pollution

Protection of health is the primary goal of air-pollution controls, of course, but polluted air also has economic effects of considerable dimension.

Damage to Plants. Air pollution damages plants as well as animals and thus has an effect on the quality and cost of foods. Plants take in air through their leaves and stems, and air that contains poisons damages the plants, even to the extent of killing them. Ponderosa pine forests, for example, have been killed by the drifting smogs from the heavily urbanized California coastal regions. Truck-farming operations in New Jersey and elsewhere in the East have been destroyed by pollutants from the nearby urban areas.

Damage to Animals. Livestock and pets are not exempt from the effects of air pollution. Dairy cows give less milk, and chickens lay fewer eggs. Heavy doses of fluorine from nearby phosphate industries crippled cattle in Florida a few years ago and forced dairymen and ranchers to abandon their lands.

In the case of both plants and animals, as with humans, the long-term effects are much more difficult to measure but may be responsible for slow growth, weakened conditions, and eventual deaths. Some pollutants may be concentrated in plant or animal tissues and, in the case of foods, later transmitted to humans.

Product Damage. Products are damaged by air pollutants, too. Clothes must be laundered or dry-cleaned more frequently. Soot and other kinds of airborne filth settle on windows, automobiles, outdoor furniture, and similar exposed items. Acid-type pollutants eat into paints and damage leather, plastics, and rubber. They also corrode metals and etch stone surfaces, eroding statues and walls of buildings. Damage from air pollution is estimated to cost every person in the United States more that $200 a year, not counting the cost resulting from health effects.

Health Considerations. Health factors understandably get the greatest attention. A person breathes in about 30 pounds of air every day and cannot screen out the pollutants. Resulting problems run the gamut from minor irritations to debilitating and fatal diseases. Any impurity in the air affects breathing and aggravates existing respiratory diseases, such as chronic bronchitis and asthma. Although tagging the specific causative agent is generally difficult, it is true that lung cancer is more prevalent in areas where air pollution is high. It is impossible to arrive at precise figures on health costs related to air pollution, but it is clear that air pollution is a major health hazard.

Legal Controls

Many laws to improve and protect environmental quality were passed in the 1960s, but the major legislation for air pollution came in 1970 with passage of the Federal Clean Air Act, amended and strengthened in 1977. This legislation has provided the guidelines for state control agencies and for industries. Air quality is now monitored at some 8,000 stations across the nation. By 1980 the reports were encouraging: levels of particulates had already been reduced by 32 percent, sulfur dioxide levels were down 67 percent, and carbon monoxide levels had been lowered by 36 percent. These figures indicate the sort of progress possible, and the biggest danger now is the possibility of relaxation, compounded by the probability of increased burning of coal in the immediate future.

Water Pollution

Only 1 percent of the water on earth is usable and fresh, and even this small amount is not evenly distributed. In some places on earth, there are surpluses; in others, water is scarce. But people and all plants and animals not adapted to life in the sea depend on this small amount of fresh water for survival. Until very recent times, most people in the United States took water for granted—as free, or nearly so, and certainly inexhaustible. But along with the burgeoning population have come critical water shortages.

How much water do you need? You can manage to survive if you have two or three quarts of water a day, but the kind of living to which most of us are now accustomed requires close to 100 gallons a day to provide for washing, flushing the toilet, and other purposes. Indirect uses—to irrigate crops for our food, generate electricity, and so forth—require hundreds of additional gallons per person. We use many times more water than any other resource in maintaining our standard of living.

Do we have enough fresh water? In the United States, about 650 billion gallons of water are available for use daily, but we are rapidly reaching that level of use. But even if an adequate supply of water can be maintained, we must be concerned about the quality of the water, whether for drinking, recreation, agriculture, industry, or fish and wildlife. The aesthetic value of having clean water in streams, lakes, and ponds must also not be overlooked.

Water Supplies

Earth's water is constantly on the move—from the land and sea into the air and then back gain. Some of the water that falls on the land runs off in streams, or it may be held in lakes or ponds. These, plus the oceans, constitute the earth's surface waters. From these bodies, or stationary reservoirs, water is evaporated, going back into the sky to form moisture-laden clouds that eventually lose their water again as rain or snow. But not all water goes through such a rapid circuit.

Some of the water soaks into the ground. This groundwater eventually returns to the atmosphere, too, but the cycling is much slower. Some of the ground water is used by plants in their growth and manufacture of foods. It is drawn into the plants by their roots and then

Figure 21-2. The Water Cycle.
The water cycle purifies water and redistributes it over the earth's surface, making fresh water available to land plants and animals.

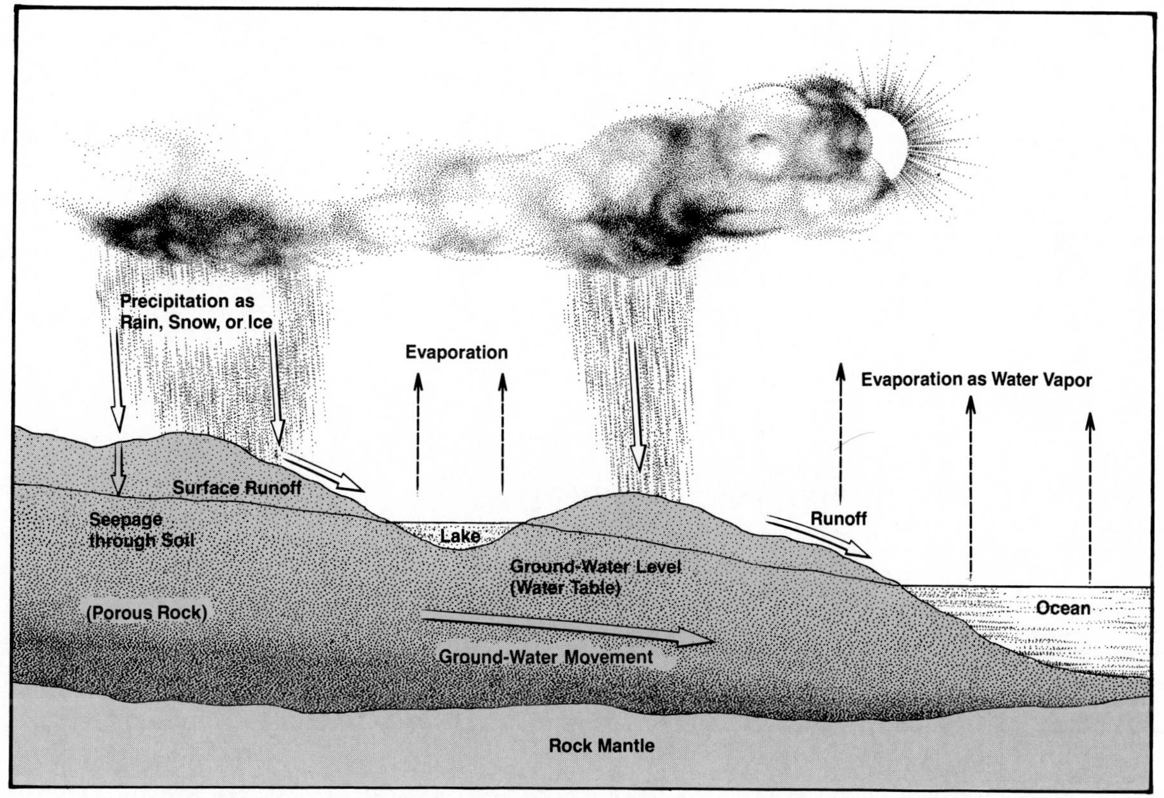

moves up the stems and leaves. Green plants over the earth's land surface thus move water steadily back into the atmosphere.

Water is returned to earth unevenly, however. Some land areas, such as the deserts of southwestern United States, get less than 6 inches of rain per year. Much of the humid southeastern United States gets more than 80 inches of rain every year, while parts of the rain forests of the Pacific Northwest record as much as 150 inches per year. A cloud forest in Hawaii gets more than 600 inches per year.

Groundwater is preferred for use by people. It has already been percolated through the soil and, in most cases, is purified by nature. But finding adequate groundwater sources for supplying large urban populations is difficult. Cities that do have good groundwater supplies benefit, because the cost of treatment is minimal, consisting mainly of removing excessive minerals. Most large cities, however, must use surface-water sources. New York City, Chicago, New Orleans, and many other cities draw their water from surface sources many miles away. These waters are lower in mineral content than are groundwaters, but they may also be high in pollutants; thus, treatment is necessary before they can be used for drinking or other uses.

Sewage Treatment

In the past, raw sewage and other wastes were dumped into streams, lakes, and ponds, and because the amount was small and did not include the very poisonous chemicals that are now so abundant, the water soon purified itself. Now, however, this is not possible, for the water must be recycled for use again almost immediately.

Sewage is typically given a primary treatment to remove solids, which are then destroyed by burning or are used for fertilizer. In some sytems, the treatment culminates at this phase, but most systems involve additional treatments. In the secondary treatment, the **effluent** (pollutants discharged into the water) from the primary stage is passed through a filter or an activated sludge aeration system. This further decreases the quantity of solids, but the effluent still contains a large amount of organic matter. If the sewage effluent is given only secondary treatment and the result is dumped into lakes or smaller bodies of water, it causes a great increase in the growth of algae and other plants, creating "blooms" that utilize all of the available oxygen and kill fish and other aquatic life.

Effluent Pollutant discharged into the water system.

The final stage of sewage treatment involves further reduction of the effluent with chemicals to get rid of the nitrogen and phosphorus that are the principal contributors to the growth of algae. When also treated with chlorine, passed through carbon filters, or given a similar final treatment, the water can be used for drinking or other purposes; the purification is complete.

Waterborne Diseases

Untreated human wastes discharged into waters are the most dangerous pollutants in terms of diseases. The disease organisms are discharged with the feces and then proliferate in the water, particularly if it contains other organic pollutants. The organisms are picked up by humans again when they swim in or drink the contaminated water.

Typhoid fever, dysenteries (some caused by one-celled animals, or protozoa; others by bacteria), and cholera are the major diseases transmitted by contaminated water. Others are gastroenteritis, poliomyelitis, and infectious hepatitis. Malaria and yellow fever are diseases transmitted by water-dwelling organisms, but the water in which these creatures live is not necessarily polluted. Some organisms, in fact, are even more sensitive to pollution than are humans. The filter-feeders, such as clams, are sometimes used as an indication of water purity. Where these animals cannot survive, we know that the water has indeed become unfit.

In developed countries, waterborne diseases have been brought under control by sanitation and by chemical treatment of water supplies. But in some instances, the chemical treatment may also cause problems.

People, plants, and animals all need fresh, nonpolluted water to survive. (© Frank Siteman 1980/EKM-Nepenthe)

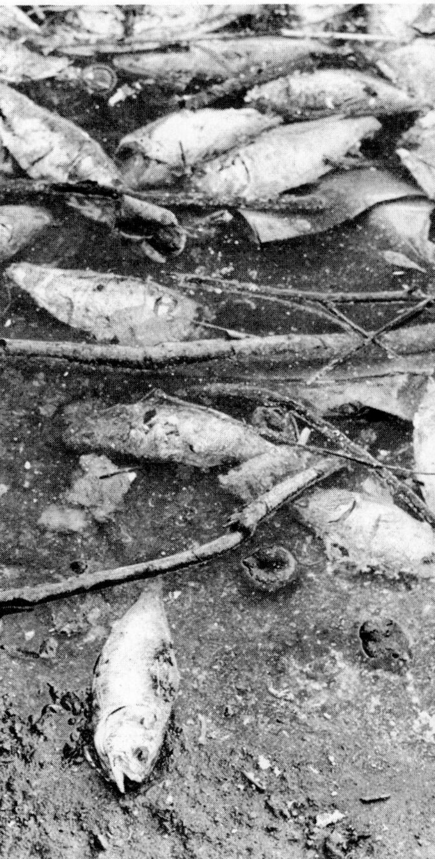

Sources of Water Pollution

Pollutants come from a wide range of sources. Surface waters are especially dangerous because of the traditional use of streams as sewers to carry away wastes. More than 700 chemical pollutants have been identified in surface waters. Of these, 22 have been identified by scientists of the National Academy of Sciences as carcinogens, and many of the others are known to be poisonous. Even some groundwater has also been polluted with toxic wastes. Much of it contains industrial solvents, which often occur in greater concentration in groundwaters than in surface waters.

Insecticides and Fertilizers

About half of all the water used in the United States is for irrigation of crops, but agriculture is also responsible for a large share of the pollution. Because the land is poorer than in the past, greater amounts of fertilizer must be used to produce bountiful crops. Millions of tons of insecticides are also put on croplands to help produce fruits, vegetables, and other products that are attractive and intact, though there is danger in some cases that they may carry poisonous residues. Both the fertilizers and insecticides wash from the soil and enter the water system. Fertilizers that get into ponds and lakes contribute to the rapid growth of algae. Chemicals from fertilizers and insecticides that get into water supplies become toxins and may eventually make their way into the foods of people or animals by way of the food chain.

The classic example is DDT, now banned, which was responsible for the near annihilation of both the brown pelican and the bald eagle. Both birds eat fish, and the fish were picking up small amounts of DDT in the waters where they lived. Eventually, the DDT reached damaging levels in the birds, causing the females to lay weak-shelled eggs that broke before they hatched. At the same time, DDT and similar residual insecticides began appearing in milk and threatening babies' lives.

Salt and Other Pollutants from City Streets

When it rains or when snow and ice melt, city streets are quickly drained of their excess water by sewer drainage systems. But these runoff waters carry with them whatever polluting substances have accumulated on the streets — from oil to various chemicals. One of the most damaging of these pollutants in recent years has been the salt spread on city streets in winter to help melt ice and snow for safe driving. The runoff in spring results in heavy salt concentrations that kill plants, destroy fish and other aquatic life, and invade drinking water, causing problems especially for people who require low sodium intakes because of hypertension, kidney diseases, or similar maladies. These rapid runoff waters that flood low-lying areas are dangerous also because of their spread of disease organisms.

Industrial Waste

Before regulations were imposed, industries used streams, lakes, and ponds for dumping their wastes. Some wastes, like those from slaughterhouses and food processing plants, were organic matter. Others were paints, oils, and other inorganic materials. Most of this indiscriminate dumping of wastes into waters has now been stopped by federal, state, and local laws, though some contaminants still get into the waters. Faced with a disposal problem, some industries dug wells thousands of feet deep and then pumped their wastes into them. But poisons seeping into groundwater supplies from these deep wells have become serious pollutants. Whenever contaminants other than those obviously and directly related to sewage or to agricultural practices are discovered, industry is immediately blamed because of past history and performance. However, many industries have been leaders in water purification programs, and they have also begun to police themselves. Industry needs clean water, too, for its survival.

Thermal Pollution

Nuclear power plants introduced a new kind of pollutant — heated water. The water is superheated when it is used to cool reactors, and when this hot water is discharged into the nearest natural body of water, it raises the temperature to a level that, in most areas, is beyond what can be tolerated by the native plants and animals. According to some estimates, as much as 20 percent of the water in the United States will be affected by this thermal pollution if nuclear power plants now in operation and those planned are all releasing heated water. Technologists are working on ways to put the heated water to productive use until it is cooled sufficiently for discharge. It may, for example, be utilized to heat greenhouses or even fields in which vegetables can be grown the year around. Or it may be used to heat living quarters for people in winter—and to operate air-conditioning systems in summer.

Lead and Mercury

Some specific water pollutants have drawn special attention in recent years; foremost among them are such heavy metals as lead and mercury. Like the insecticides, mercury may occur only in minute amounts in a single fish, but when fish are a major component of a diet, mercury accumulates in a person's body, reaching dangerous concentrations. The most dramatic cases of mercury poisoning to be recognized were in Japan in the early 1970s, when million of dollars in damages were paid to fishermen who were affected by mercury that had been released into waters by industry. Thousands claimed poisoning, and 45 deaths were documented as directly attributable to the mercury. Mercury poisoning affects the nervous system. It can cause blindness, insanity, paralysis—and eventually death. The incident in Japan precipitated investigations in many other parts of the world, where high mercury levels were also discovered in fish.

Lead has also been found in water supplies. When accumulated in the body to sufficient levels, it can cause severe damage to the nervous system, kidneys, liver, and reproductive organs.

Oil Leaks and Spills

Many of the more than half a million chemical compounds now used eventually find their way into the sea particularly in the coastal areas near population centers. Oil leaks and spills cause damage not only by polluting adjacent shores but also by killing fish and other marine life and by preventing the near-shore nursery grounds from being used. Rivers of creeping sludge from metropolitan areas such as New York

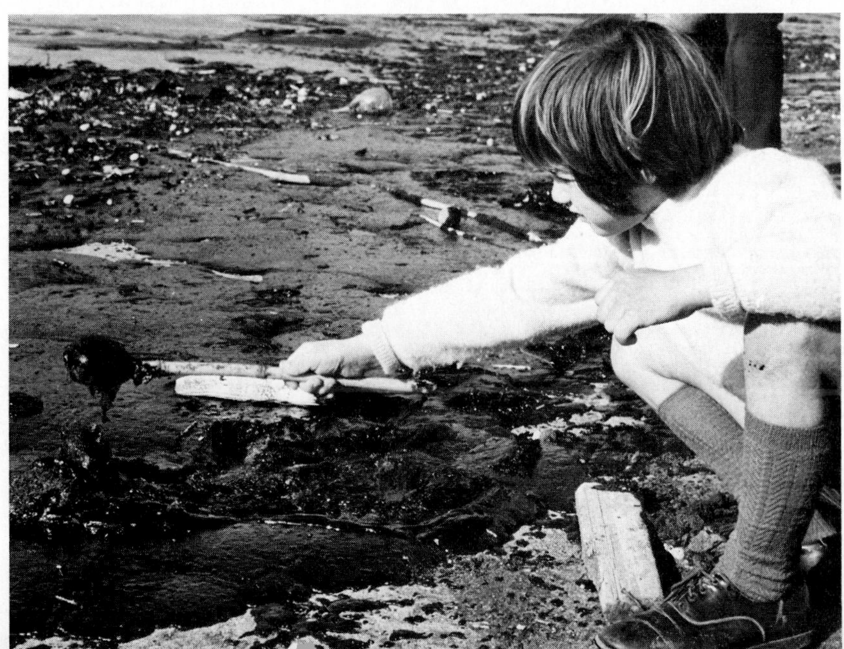

Oil slicks may occasionally intrigue children, but they kill marine life and interfere with the recreational uses of beaches. (Photo from United Press International)

City foul the ocean bottoms for hundreds of miles from their source. Some of this contamination is eventually returned to shore, and it can be found in seafoods.

Cleaning Up: Water Pollution Control

Cleaning up the nation's water and keeping it clean are enormous and seemingly impossible tasks. Hundreds of millions of tons of solid pollutants and billions of gallons of waste waters in various stages of treatment enter the water system every year. Since the publication of Rachel Carson's *Silent Spring,* which called attention in the 1960s to the dangers of water pollution, public pressure for strong regulations has continued to grow. Congress enacted a series of laws for control of water pollution—specifically, the Federal Water Pollution Control Act, the Safe Drinking Water Act, and the Clean Water Act of 1977. In addition, there are state, municipal, and local laws covering water and its purification. Existing laws do recognize the major problems and are amended appropriately when new circumstances are encountered. Administrating them is difficult, however.

No matter how it is accomplished, keeping waters pure enough to be usable has become expensive. Clean water in the future will undoubtedly account for a larger percentage of tax dollars and will also add to the cost of products from industry, but the investment in clean water contributes greatly to public health and should therefore be of concern to each of us. In the final section of this chapter, ways to deal with pollution control and other environmental issues are discussed.

Noise Pollution

In going about their daily work and play, people naturally make noise, but in recent years noises in some areas have reached high enough levels to be ranked as genuine health hazards. Noises are measured in decibels (for a sampling of sound readings, see Figure 21–3). Ordinary talk, for example, ranks at about 50 decibels and is not bothersome. But partial or complete deafness can result from prolonged exposure to sounds in the 80-decibel and higher ranges. Sounds at the 130-decibel level become painful. Even continued noises at the 60-decibel level can cause loss of sleep, fatigue, and emotional stress, which can lead to ulcers or similar disturbances. The noise produced by loud car stereos, or concerts, for example, can result in loss of sleep and temporary deafness. Hypertension is aggravated and perhaps even brought on by constant exposure to noise pollution. Work efficiency is reduced when workers are subjected to constant high noises. And noises are upsetting to wildlife, disturbing normal breeding cycles, feeding habits, and general life patterns.

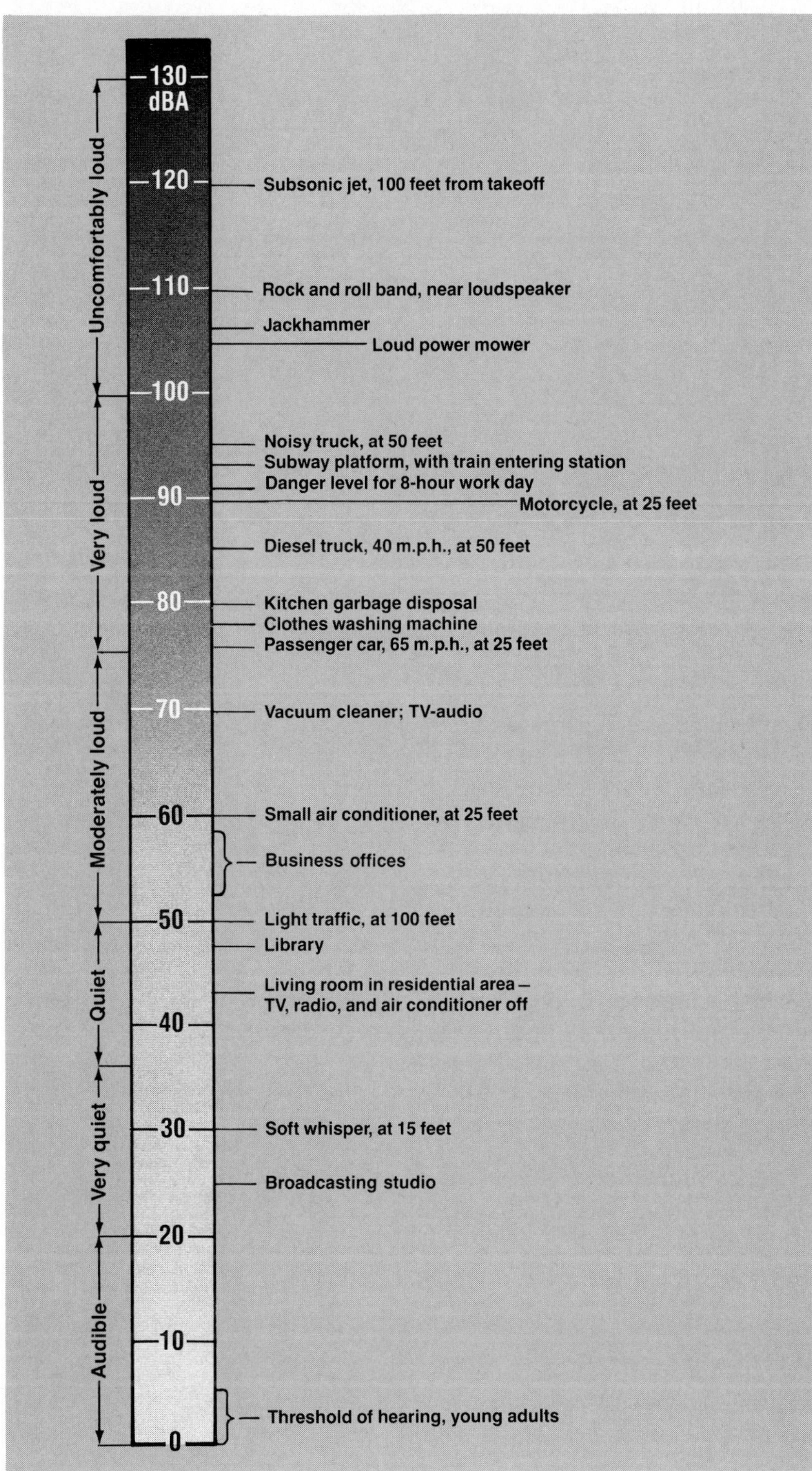

Figure 21-3. Noise Levels of Selected Sources.
The levels are measured in decibels on the A-scale (dBA) of a sound level meter. Note that individual noise sources often differ by 10 to 20 dBA from the values shown.

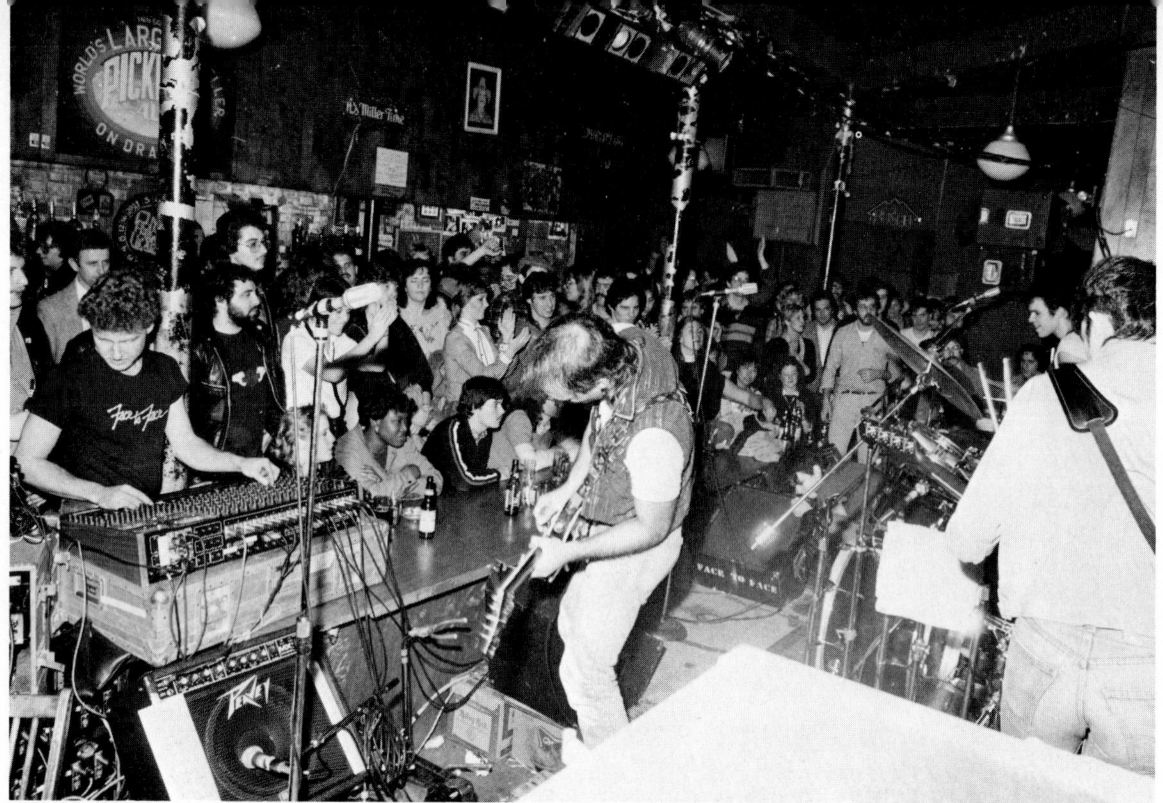

We don't often think of music as harmful. However, any loud noise can be disturbing and can result in impaired hearing. (Photo © Raimon/The Picture Cube)

Recognition of noise as a serious pollutant came in the 1960s, and officials have ever since been working on ways to reduce noise levels. New buildings are being soundproofed to protect those who live or work there. Buildings are shielded from the sounds of traffic on highways and freeways by mounds of dirt combined with the planting of trees and shrubs.

Ordinances in most cities require mufflers on vehicles, and manufacturers are designing "noiseless" products, such as cooking utensils that do not clang when bumped together. The airline industry, which drew the greatest criticism from the general public, has responded by designing quieter engines, by not allowing their aircraft to take off over highly populated areas, and by avoiding sonic booms. Sonic booms, or "breaking the sound barrier," have in the past caused millions of dollars in damage every day by shaking buildings and breaking windows—in addition to contributing to the general noise pollution. In industries where workers are exposed regularly to extremely high noise levels, special headgear and earplugs are provided to employees to block out the damaging sounds.

Some people are more easily affected by noises, but there is general agreement about the level at which noises become genuinely objectionable. As a group, citizens can voice their complaints. Some cities have a department of environmental protection that can be called to receive complaints regarding noise and other kinds of pollution. At present, noise control is primarily a responsibility of local governments, but there are national standards for permissible noise levels for many products, such as automobiles and airplanes.

Land Management

Only about a fourth of the earth's surface is land, and only about a fourth of this land is usable for crops, livestock, and living space for people. The remainder is deserts, mountains, cold polar regions, or other uninhabitable and unusable areas. In the past, land was generally used until its productivity was gone. Then it was abandoned, and new land was pioneered. Now nearly all of the most productive land has been inhabited and put to use—often in destructive ways.

In order to survive, however, people must learn how to use the land wisely and how to restore some lands that have become unproductive. To feed burgeoning populations, it is necessary also to increase food yields from existing areas by developing new kinds of crops, by utilizing new techniques, or by a combination of both. And more attention is being given to aquaculture, using both fresh and salt water, where yields per acre can be many times what comparable areas of land can produce. It is estimated, for instance, that the intensive production of clams on an underwater area the size of Long Island (in New York State) could yield as much seafood as is now obtained from all the world's oceans by present harvesting methods.

Worn-out lands can in most cases be restored to productivity, but the process is slow. In many places the land stripped of its protective natural vegetation has been permitted to erode, with wind and water carrying away rich topsoil that had been hundreds of thousands of years in the making. Much of this valuable soil now lies in the broad deltas at the mouths of rivers or on the bottoms of lakes or in the sea. Conservationists estimate that at one time the United States was losing about 8,000 acres of rich farmland every day as a result of agricultural practices that allowed erosion. An objective of planners today is the use of the land in ways that make slow and costly restoration unnecessary and that, in fact, continually improve the land's productivity.

Farming is not the only important use of the land, of course. Forests not only provide valuable timber but also protect the watersheds of streams, lakes, and reservoirs. Wetlands along coasts and in inland areas serve as the breeding and nursery grounds for fish and wildlife. Most of the seafoods harvested from continental shelves start life in these coastal waters, which are being constantly destroyed by pollutants and by drainage and development projects.

Our world consists of land, water, and air. Changes in the structure or condition of any one of these affects all the others. Land is thus one of the basic units of the environment. Well-managed soils can yield bountiful crops year after year; people fed from these soils are healthy and productive, too. The richest nations in the world are those located where the land is rich. No nation can afford land losses.

Nuclear Energy

World energy needs are soaring because of the increases in population, but a major energy source on which the world has become dependent—*petroleum*—is rapidly dwindling. Forecasts indicate that petroleum production will peak sometime between 1990 and 2010, with yields of about 100 million barrels per day. But by the year 2000, the more than 6.5 billion people then living in the world will be consuming energy at a rate equivalent to some 300 million barrels of petroleum every day. Alternate energy sources will have to be developed.

Coal and *natural gas* supplies are ample and will be utilized in greater amounts during the coming years. Their disadvantage is their air-polluting emissions—sulfur dioxide, carbon dioxide, nitrogen dioxide, and particulates. The United States has adopted strict standards for controlling the emissions resulting from the use of these fuels, but few other countries have done so. Air pollution from the use of these fuels will likely be a global problem before the end of this century.

Geothermal energy from inside the earth, *solar energy, ocean ther-*

Demonstrators (left) for and (right) against nuclear power. (Photo left © Steve Kagan 1980/ Photo Researchers, Inc.; photo right by Eric Roth/The Picture Cube)

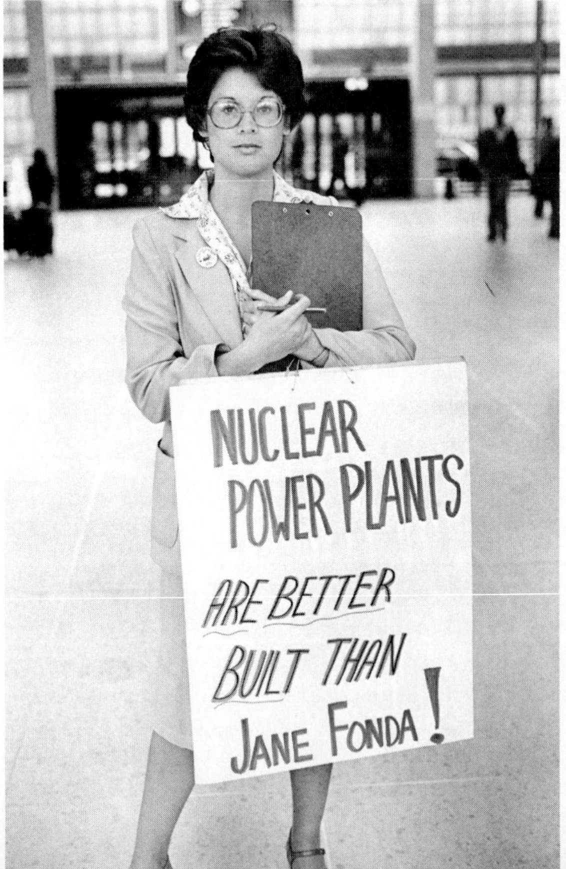

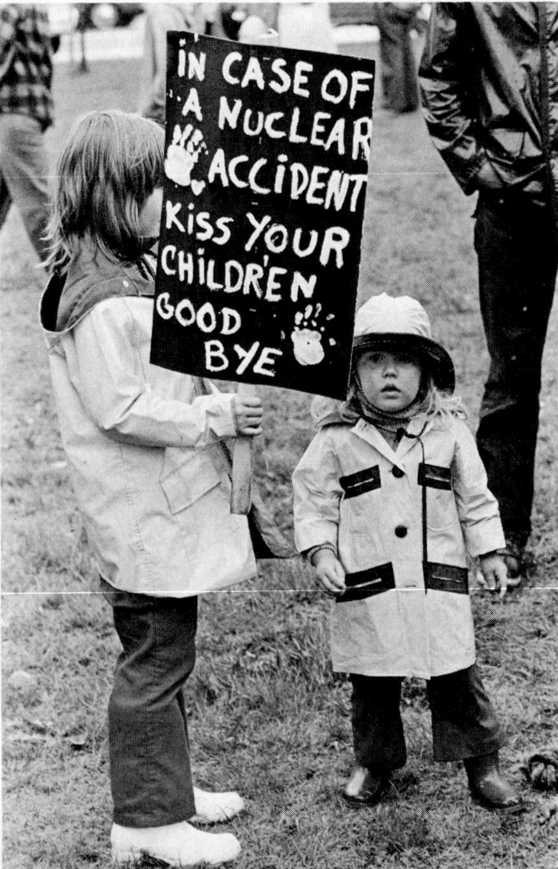

mal energy conversion—all of these are among the alternative energy sources being investigated and used now in limited amounts. At present, *hydroelectric power* and *nuclear energy* are the most productive non-fossil-fuel sources being exploited. However, the fuel used for nuclear fission reactors is limited. The world's known uranium sources, almost half of which are located in North America, will last roughly no longer than the oil and gas reserves. With a different technology—more specifically, the use of breeder reactors—the energy derived from a given amount of fuel might be increased by a hundred times, delaying the exhausting of the fuel. Research on different radioactive materials also continues.

Nuclear Pollution

Nuclear energy production does not pollute in the conventional sense—that is, no noxious fumes are emitted. (As mentioned before, however, nuclear power plants do produce large amounts of heated water that damage the environment if not sufficiently cooled before being released.) The greatest concerns are over the possible escape of radioactivity into the environment as a result of human error (as occurred at Three Mile Island in Pennsylvania in 1979), over the danger of the plants' being targeted by terrorists or saboteurs, and over the safe disposal of the toxic and highly radioactive waste materials, which pose possible threats to future generations as well as to people living today.

Radiation

Radiation is all around us constantly, of course. Light is radiant energy, and so is heat. But these kinds of radiation can be seen and felt, hence excesses can be avoided with normal care and attention. The dangerous kinds of radiation from radioactive materials cannot be sensed but can be devastating if received in large enough amounts. Radioactive materials can, for example, ionize at least some body tissues, splitting their molecules into electrically charged components. This sort of damage is irreversible.

If you would like to compare your radiation dose with the U.S. annual average, do Self-Assessment Exercise 21.1, "Your Radiation Dose Inventory."

Plutonium, one of the products of producing nuclear energy in breeder reactors, is a known cancer-causing agent and emits alpha particles. Plutonium will remain radioactive for thousands of years and is extremely poisonous—the inhalation of even a speck is fatal. While the breeder reactor is indeed a means of extending our limited uranium resources and deriving greater power per unit of fuel, these advantages may be offset by possible environmental hazards involved.

Fission vs. Fusion

Fission Splitting of atoms to create nuclear energy.

Fusion Merging of atoms for production of clean energy.

All of the nuclear energy currently produced is by **fission**—that is, by the disintegration or splitting of atoms. For decades, scientists have been working toward an opposite goal: the production of energy by **fusion** or the putting together of atoms. More specifically, this amounts to duplicating what the sun has been doing for aeons, for it is a fusion process that produces the sun's tremendous energy. The fuel for fusion will be forms of hydrogen, available in unlimited amounts from ordinary water, and the atoms will be combined to yield heavier and nonradioactive atoms. It would be an absolutely clean process. The problem? Fusion has already been accomplished at Princeton University and elsewhere, but the technology for containing the reactions on a large scale has not been developed. They occur at phenomenally high temperatures that will vaporize almost all known materials. If the process can be perfected and made economical, however, fusion might become the major source of energy in the next century. At present, it remains tantalizingly elusive.

Nuclear Energy Controls

Hundreds of nuclear power plants are now in operation. More are being built. There are regulations governing their construction and the safety measures that control their operation. But the regulations were made and are administered by people, the plants are operated by people—and people make mistakes. While the overall safety record of nuclear power plants has been excellent so far (despite the notoriety achieved by the incident at Three Mile Island), the fuel being dealt with is dangerous not only to people today but also to future generations. Because of these dangers, a very strong movement against the use of nuclear energy has arisen, and there are many books presenting the antinuclear position (including a popular book coauthored by Ralph Nader that is included in the list of suggested readings at the end of this chapter). At this time, the questions are important enough to generate great concern over expansion of this source of energy.

Responsibilities

Environmental health and safety are acknowledged global issues. No place in the world is completely isolated from all others. Even the air and waters of the remote polar regions have felt the impact of pollutants generated in the world's inhabited areas. On some of the problems, particularly health-related ones, nations have joined together to set standards and establish controls.

International Organizations

The *United Nations International Children's Emergency Fund (UNICEF)* is also primarily a health-oriented organization. UNICEF

SELF-ASSESSMENT EXERCISE 21.1

Your Radiation Dose Inventory

We live in a radioactive world—always have. Radiation is all about us as a part of our natural environment. It is measured in terms of millirems (mrems). The annual average dose per person is 180 mrems, but it is not uncommon for any of us to receive far more than that in a given year. This is not dangerous. As an example, exposure to 5,000 mrems a year is allowed for those who work with and around radioactive material.

	Common Sources of Radiation	Your Annual Dose (mrems)
WHERE YOU LIVE	**Location:** Cosmic radiation at *sea level*	26
	For your elevation in (feet) — add this number of mrem	______
	Elevation — mrem 1000-2 · 2000-5 · 3000-9 · 4000-15 · 5000-21 · 6000-29 · 7000-40 · 8000-53 · 9000-70 Elevation of some U.S. cities (in feet); Atlanta 1050; Chicago 595; Dallas 435; Denver 5280; Las Vegas 2000; Minneapolis 815; Pittsburgh 1200; St. Louis 455; Salt Lake City 4400; Spokane 1890. (Coastal cities are assumed to be zero, or sea level.)	
	Ground: U.S. average	26
	House Construction: For stone, concrete or masonry building, add 7	______
WHAT YOU EAT, DRINK AND BREATHE	**Food** **Water** — **U.S. Average** **Air**	24
	Weapons test fallout	4
HOW YOU LIVE	**X-ray and radiopharmaceutical diagnosis**	
	Number of chest x-rays × 10	______
	Number of lower gastrointestinal tract x-rays × 500	______
	Number of radiopharmaceutical examinations × 300	______
	(Average dose to total U.S. population — 92 mrem)	
	Jet Plane travel: For each 2500 miles add 1 mrem	______
	TV viewing: For each hour per day × 0.15	______
HOW CLOSE YOU LIVE TO A NUCLEAR PLANT	**At site boundary:** average number of hours per day × 0.2	______
	One mile away: average number of hours per day × 0.02	______
	Five miles away: average number of hours per day × 0.002	______
	Over 5 miles away: None	______
	Note: Maximum allowable dose determined by "as low as reasonably achievable" (ALARA) criteria established by the U.S. Nuclear Regulatory Commission. Experience shows that your actual dose is substantially less than these limits.	
	My total annual mrems dose	
	Compare your annual dose to the U.S. annual average of 180 mrems.	

One mrem per year is equal to: Increasing your diet by 4%.
Taking a 5-day vacation in the Sierra Nevada mountains.

*Based on the "BEIR Report-III"— National Academy of Sciences, Committee on Biological Effects of Ionizing Radiation. "The Effects of Populations of Exposure to Low Levels of Ionizing Radiation," National Academy of Sciences, Washington, D.C. 1980.

was established in 1946 to provide milk, drugs, and other much-needed items to children in European countries ravaged by World War II. Then in 1950, UNICEF received a mandate from its parent administrative organization to expand its scope and aim at improving the health and nutrition of children in all countries, recognizing young people as the most valuable of all world resources. UNICEF programs concentrate on the poorest children in the poorest areas of the poorest countries. The environment in which these children live is one of the agency's prime concerns.

The *World Health Organization (WHO)*, founded in 1948 as a division of the United Nations, assumed the responsibility for aiding people throughout the world in attaining the highest possible level of health. It serves as the directing and coordinating authority of international health, assisting its nearly 150 member nations and also pursuing programs it has initiated. One special subdivision of WHO is specifically concerned with environmental health issues on a global basis.

National Organizations

Environmental health is given attention also by the federal government. The *U.S. Public Health Service* was formed very early in the nation's history — in 1798 — but the scope of its authority and hence its effectiveness has been broadened over the years. It is charged with assuring the highest possible health level for every individual and family in the nation, and it assists other nations in attaining this goal.

The *Environmental Protection Agency (EPA)*, created in 1970 by the federal government, was established specifically to preserve a clean environment by monitoring, setting standards, and enforcing regulations. It also coordinates and supports the programs, research, and antipollution activities of state and local governments and private organizations. The EPA is the central agency providing the guidelines followed by state and local agencies that have comparable responsibilities. Some state and local regulatory agencies actually impose more stringent measures than the federal government, but they cannot do less than required by federal laws. Despite resistance by industry and delays by some state and local governments, the EPA has succeeded in bringing about substantial improvements in the nation's air and water quality over the years.

Industrial and Citizens' Groups

Industries and citizens' groups have also assumed responsibilities in regard to environmental health. Many industries, commonly targeted as the major contributors to environmental ills, have accepted responsibility for a cleaner environment and have turned their research toward investigating such problems as disposal of industrial wastes and the recycling of waste materials whenever possible. Though there are still problems with industries, their record in recent years has been one of steady improvement. Citizens' groups cover a broad spectrum of activities, ranging from traditional conservationism to the education of the public on environmental dangers.

The Individual

Ultimately, the responsibility lies with the individual who must support the programs to improve environmental health and safety and who must insist on their proper administration. Every citizen must exercise the right to vote and support politicians who are concerned with environmental issues. To keep informed, a citizen can become involved with such organizations as the Sierra Club, the Izaak Walton League, the National Wildlife Federation, or similar groups that focus attention on environmental matters.

Finally, personal life-styles are of utmost importance. Although many problems can be solved only on the national, or even global, scale, every person can make choices in daily life that will help protect the environment. These measures range from family planning to carpooling, from water conservation to recycling newspapers, from avoiding polluting products to reducing consumption of electricity. It is only through a combination of individual action and public policy that we will be able to meet the challenges of preserving a healthy environment.

Summary

In recent years there has been a growing awareness of the importance of the environment to human health and well-being. People are learning that their actions have a great impact on the complex interactions that support life on earth. Instead of seeing the environment as an inexhaustible source of resources that can withstand any amount of abuse, they are learning to see themselves as part of nature and as being responsible for the careful use of the earth's resources.

A major threat to human well-being is the rapid increase in the world's population, which places new demands on the environment. The population of the world, now approximately 4.5 billion, is expected to grow to about 6.5 billion by the year 2000. Populations are increasing most rapidly in the less developed countries, where economic resources are already severely strained. In the United States the rate of increase is much less, but population growth may still pose problems for the overall standard of living.

Despite improvement in some areas because of stricter laws, air pollution remains a significant threat to health. The principal air pollutants are carbon monoxide, hydrocarbons, nitrogen oxides, sulfur oxides, and particulates. There is also concern that fluorocarbons may reduce the amount of ozone in the ozone layer of the atmosphere, allowing too much ultraviolet light to reach the surface of the earth.

Ample supplies of water for consumption, irrigation, and industry are essential to our life-style, but pollution has affected many water sources. Groundwater is the preferred source for human consumption, but most large cities use surface water. Sources of water pollution include industrial chemicals, fertilizers, pesticides, and untreated sewage.

High noise levels are harmful to health, damaging hearing and producing stress. Noises are measured in decibels. At 60 decibels, noises become annoying, and sounds in the 130-decibel range are painful.

Erosion has led to the loss of much productive agricultural land. Sound agricultural practices can maintain soil and increase yields.

Increasing energy consumption has raised perplexing problems, particularly with regard to nuclear energy as an alternative to petroleum, coal, and natural gas. The principal concerns are the accidental escape of radioactivity, sabotage, and the safe handling of toxic and radioactive wastes.

Organizations and governmental bodies concerned with environmental health include the World Health Organization, UNICEF, and U.S. Public Health Service, the Environmental Protection Agency, and a wide range of citizens' groups. Individuals can change their life-styles to help preserve the environment, and it is hoped that by a combination of individual action and public policy the world will be able to support a healthy human population.

Review and Discussion

1. What are some of the problems with population control in developed and in developing countries?
2. What are the major air pollutants and how do they get into the atmosphere?
3. What is temperature inversion? How does it affect air quality?
4. What are three effects of air pollution?
5. Describe the water cycle. What is the difference between surface water and groundwater?
6. What are three sources of water pollution?
7. Discuss the effects that noise pollution has on human beings.
8. What are the major issues in the management of land resources?
9. What are the dangers associated with atomic energy?
10. Name several major environmental protection organizations and discuss their roles.

Further Reading

Carson, Rachel. *Silent Spring.* New York: Fawcett Books, 1978.
A pioneering work on the dangers of pesticides and a classic statement of concern for the environment, first published in 1962. (Paperback.)

Ehrlich, Paul R. *The Population Bomb.* New York: Ballantine Books, 1971.
An analysis of the implications of the population explosion and possible solutions. (Paperback.)

Nader, Ralph, and John Abbots. *The Menace of Atomic Energy.* New York: W. W. Norton & Company, Inc., 1979.
A presentation of the dangers associated with atomic energy. (Paperback.)

Schell, Jonathan. *The Fate of the Earth.* New York: Knopf, 1982.
Presents the perils of nuclear holocaust, nuclear arms, and global annihilation, as well as the deterrents to these threats.

Shakman, Robert. *Where You Live May Be a Hazard to Your Health.* Briarcliff Manor, N.Y.: Stein & Day Publishers, 1979.
A discussion of health and safety factors in 205 United States communities. (Paperback.)

U.S. Council on Environmental Quality and the U.S. Department of State. *Global 2000 Report to the President.* Washington, D.C.: U.S. Government Printing Office, 1981.
An official report on trends in many environmental areas.

U.S. Water Resources Council. *The Nation's Water Resources, 1975–2000. Vol. 1: Summary.* Washington, D.C.: U.S. Government Printing Office, 1978.
A comprehensive survey of present water supplies and the problems of meeting future needs for this vital resource.

Appendix
The Wellness Inventory

The Wellness Inventory was developed by John W. Travis, M.D., M.P.H., as a way for people to evaluate their total well-being. It assumes a holistic approach to health, insisting that well-being, or wellness, requires attention to the whole person, in a perspective that includes physical, mental, and social dimensions.

Wellness is not simply the absence of illness, and many different levels are possible. While traditional medicine concentrates on curing or alleviating disease, the wellness approach directs people beyond the point of a mere lack of illness and encourages them to improve their positive well-being in a variety of ways.

As Dr. Travis explains in his *Wellness Inventory* (Mill Valley, Cal.: Wellness Resource Center, 1977):

> Many people lack physical symptoms but are bored, depressed, tense, anxious, or generally unhappy with their lives. These emotional states often lead to physical disease through the lowering of the body's resistance. The same feelings can also lead to abuse of the body through smoking, drinking, and overeating. These behaviors are usually substitutes for other more basic human needs such as recognition from others, a stimulating environment, caring and affection from friends, and growth towards higher levels of self-awareness.
>
> Wellness is not a static state. It results when a person begins to see himself as a growing, changing person. High-level wellness means giving good care to your physical self, using your mind constructively, expressing your emotions effectively, being creatively involved with those around you, being concerned about your physical and psychological environment, and becoming aware of other levels of consciousness.

The self-assessment exercise that follows will help give you an idea of where you stand on the wellness scale. It will also help you reflect on some of the life-style choices that have an impact both on the prevention of illness and on the promotion of total well-being, or wellness.

INSTRUCTIONS

Put a check mark in the box following each statement that is true for you. Total up the number of marks for each section and transfer the results to the Interpretation section at the end of the test. An asterisk following a statement indicates that there is an explanatory footnote for that statement at the end of the items.

A. Productivity, Relaxation, Sleep

1. I usually enjoy my work. ☐
2. I seldom feel tired and rundown (except after strenuous work).* ☐
3. I fall asleep easily at bedtime. ☐
4. I usually get a full night's sleep. ☐
5. If awakened, it is usually easy for me to go to sleep again. ☐
6. I rarely bite or pick at my nails. ☐
7. Rather than worrying, I can temporarily shelve my problems and enjoy myself at times when I can do nothing about solving them immediately. ☐
8. I feel financially secure. ☐
9. I am content with my sexual life. ☐
10. I meditate in some way for 15 or 20 minutes at least once a day.* ☐

Total ________

B. Personal Care and Home Safety

11. I take steps to protect my living space from fire and safety hazards (such as unsafe wiring or volatile chemicals improperly stored). ☐
12. I have a dry chemical fire extinguisher in my kitchen and at least one other extinguisher elsewhere in my living quarters. (In a small apartment, a kitchen extinguisher alone is adequate.)* ☐
13. I regularly use dental floss and a soft toothbrush.* ☐
14. I smoke less than one pack of cigarettes or equivalent cigars or pipes *per week.* ☐
15. I don't smoke at all (if this statement is true, mark item above true as well). ☐
16. I keep an up-to-date record of my immunizations. ☐
17. I have fewer than three colds per year.* ☐
18. I minimize my exposure to sprays, chemical fumes, or exhaust gases.* ☐
19. I avoid extremely noisy areas (or wear protective earplugs).* ☐
20. I am aware of changes in my physical or mental state and seek professional advice about any that seem unusual. ☐

WOMEN

21. I check my breasts for unusual lumps once a month. ☐
22. I have a Pap test annually. ☐

MEN

23. If uncircumcised, I am aware of the special need for regular cleansing under my foreskin. ☐
24. If I am over 45, I have my prostate checked annually. ☐

Total ________

C. Nutritional Awareness

25. I eat at least one uncooked fruit or vegetable each day.* ☐
26. I have fewer than three alcoholic drinks (including beer) per week. ☐
27. I rarely take medications, including prescription drugs. ☐
28. I drink fewer than five soft drinks a week.* ☐
29. I avoid eating refined foods or foods with sugar added. ☐

30. I add little salt to my food.* ☐

31. I read the labels for the ingredients of the foods I buy. ☐

32. I add unprocessed bran to my diet to provide roughage.* ☐

33. I drink fewer than three cups of coffee or tea (except herbal teas) a day.* ☐

34. I have a good appetite and maintain a weight within 15 percent of my ideal weight. ☐

Total ______

D. Environmental Awareness

35. I use public transportation or car pools when possible. ☐

36. I turn off unneeded lights or appliances. ☐

37. I recycle papers, cans, glass, clothing, books, and organic waste (mark true if you do at least three of these). ☐

38. I set my thermostat at 68°F or lower in winter. ☐

39. I use air conditioning only when necessary and keep the thermostat at 76°F or higher. ☐

40. I am conscientious about wasted energy and materials. ☐

41. I use nonpolluting cleaning agents. ☐

42. My car gets at least 18 miles per gallon. (If you don't own a car, check this statement as true). ☐

43. I have storm windows and adequate insulation in attic and walls. (If you don't own your home or live in a mild climate, check this statement as true.) ☐

44. I have a humidifier for use in winter. (If you don't have central heating, check this statement as true.)* ☐

Total ______

E. Physical Activity

45. I climb stairs rather than ride elevators. ☐

46. My daily activities include at least moderate physical effort (such as rearing young children, gardening, scrubbing floors, or other work that involves being on my feet). ☐

47. My daily activities include vigorous physical effort (such as heavy construction work, farming, moving heavy objects by hand). ☐

48. I run at least 1 mile twice a week (or equivalent aerobic exercise).* ☐

49. I run at least 1 mile four times a week or equivalent (if this statement is true, mark the item above true as well).* ☐

50. I regularly walk or ride a bike for exercise. ☐

51. I participate in a strenuous sport at least once a week. ☐

52. I participate in a strenuous sport more than once a week (if this statement is true, mark the item above true as well). ☐

53. I do yoga or some form of stretching-limbering exercise for 15 to 20 minutes at least twice per week.* ☐

54. I do yoga or some form of stretching exercise for 15 or 20 minutes at least four times per week (if this statement is true, mark the item above true as well).* ☐

Total ______

F. Expression of Emotions and Feelings

55. I am frequently happy. ☐
56. I think it is O.K. to feel angry, afraid, joyful, or sad.* ☐
57. I do not deny my anger, fear, joy, or sadness, but instead find constructive ways to express these feelings most of the time.* ☐
58. I am able to say no to people without feeling guilty. ☐
59. It is easy for me to laugh. ☐
60. I like getting compliments and recognition from other people. ☐
61. I feel O.K. about crying, and allow myself to do so.* ☐
62. I listen to and think about constructive criticism, rather than reacting defensively. ☐
63. I would seek help from friends or professional counselors if needed. ☐
64. It is easy for me to give other people sincere compliments and recognition. ☐

Total ______

G. Community Involvement

65. I keep informed of local, national, and world events. ☐
66. I vote regularly. ☐
67. I take interest in community, national, and world events and work to support issues and people of my choice. (If this statement is true, mark both items above true as well.) ☐
68. When I am able, I contribute time or money to worthy causes. ☐
69. I make an attempt to know my neighbors and be on good terms with them. ☐
70. If I saw a crime being committed, I would call the police. ☐
71. If I saw a broken bottle lying in the road or on the sidewalk, I would remove it. ☐
72. When driving, I am considerate of pedestrians and other drivers. ☐
73. If I saw a car with faulty lights, leaking gasoline, or another dangerous condition, I would attempt to inform the driver. ☐
74. I am a member of one or more community organizations. ☐

Total ______

H. Creativity, Self-Expression

75. I enjoy expressing myself through art, dance, music, drama, sports, etc. ☐
76. I enjoy spending some time without planned or structured activities.* ☐
77. I usually meet several people a month whom I would like to get to know better. ☐
78. I enjoy touching other people.* ☐
79. I enjoy being touched by other people.* ☐
80. I have at least five close friends. ☐
81. At times I like to be alone. ☐
82. I like myself and look forward to the future. ☐
83. I look forward to living to be at least 75.* ☐
84. I find it easy to express concern, love, and warmth to those I care about. ☐

Total ______

I. Automobile Safety

If you don't own an automobile and ride less than 1,000 miles per year in one, enter 7 points as a total for this section and skip the individual items. (If you ride more than 1,000 miles per year but don't own a car, answer as many items as you can and show this copy to the car's owner.)

85. I never drink when I am going to be driving. ☐
86. I wear a lap safety belt at least 90 percent of the time that I ride in a car. ☐
87. I wear a shoulder/lap belt at least 90 percent of the time that I ride in a car. (If this statement is true, mark the item above true as well.)* ☐
88. I stay within 5 miles per hour of the speed limit. ☐
89. My car has head restraints on the front seats, and I keep them adjusted high enough to protect myself and passengers from whiplash injuries.* ☐
90. I frequently inspect my automobile tires, lights, etc., and have my car serviced regularly. ☐
91. I have disk brakes on my car.* ☐
92. I drive on belted radial tires.* ☐
93. I carry emergency flares or reflectors as well as a fire extinguisher in my car. ☐
94. I stop on yellow when a traffic light is changing. ☐
95. For every 10 miles per hour of speed, I maintain a car length's distance from the car ahead of me. ☐

Total ______

J. Parenting

If you don't have any responsibility for young children, enter 7 as a total for this section and skip the individual items. (If some of the items are not applicable because your children are no longer young, answer as you would if they were youngsters again.)

96. When riding in a car, I make certain that any child weighing under 50 pounds is secured in an approved safety harness similar to those sold by the major auto manufacturers.* ☐
97. When riding in a car, I make certain that any child weighing over 50 pounds is wearing an adult seat belt or shoulder harness.* ☐
98. When leaving a child, I make certain that the person in charge has the telephone numbers of my pediatrician or a hospital for emergency use. ☐
99. I don't let my children ride escalators in bare feet or tennis shoes.* ☐
100. I do not store cleaning products under the sink or in unlocked cabinets where a child could reach them. ☐
101. I have a lock on the medicine cabinet or other places where medicines are stored. ☐
102. I prepare my own baby food with a food grinder—and thus do not buy commercial baby foods.* ☐
103. I have sought information on parenting and raising children. ☐
104. I frequently touch or hold my children. ☐
105. I respect my child as an evolving, growing being. ☐

Total ______

Footnotes

These footnotes provide an opportunity to reflect on the significance of some practices that contribute to the achievement of total well-being, or wellness. The number or numbers before each footnote refer to the corresponding statement in the wellness test you have just completed.

2 Fatigue without apparent cause is not normal and usually indicates illness, stress, or denial of emotional expression.

10 Meditation greatly enhances one's sense of well-being.

12 Many injuries and much damage can be prevented by putting out fires when they first start. Dry chemical fire extinguishers are necessary for oil, grease, and electrical fires.

13 Regular flossing and using a good soft toothbrush with rounded-tip bristles prevent the premature loss of teeth. Be sure to learn the proper techniques from a dental hygienist or dentist.

17 If you have more than three colds a year, you may not be getting enough rest, eating a good diet, or meeting other energy needs properly.

18 All such toxins have a harmful effect on the liver and other tissues over long periods of time.

19 Very loud noises that leave your ears ringing can cause permanent hearing loss, which accumulates and is usually not noticeable until one reaches 40 or 50. Small cushioned earplugs (not the type designed for swimmers), wax earplugs, and acoustic earmuffs (which look like stereo headphones without wires) can often be purchased in sporting goods stores.

25 Fresh fruits and vegetables provide vitamins, minerals, trace nutrients, and roughage that are often lacking in modern diets.

28 Soft drinks are high in refined sugar, which provides only "empty" calories, and they usually replace foods having more nutritional value. Artificially sweetened soft drinks consumed in excess may have long-range consequences as yet not known. (Both types of soft drinks contain caffeine or other stimulants.)

30 Salting foods during cooking draws many vitamins out of the food and into the water, which is usually discarded. Use of heavily salted foods at the table may cause a strain on the kidneys and contribute to high blood pressure.

32 Wheat bran, usually removed in the commercial milling of wheat, is the single best source of dietary fiber available. The use of approximately two tablespoons per day (individual needs vary) may substantially reduce the risk of colon cancer, diverticulosis, heart disease, and other conditions related to refined food diets.

33 Coffee and tea (other than herbal teas) contain stimulants that, if abused, do not allow one's body to function normally.

44 Humidified heated air allows one to set the thermostat several degrees lower and still feel as warm as without humidification. It also helps prevent many respiratory ailments. Houseplants will require less watering, and be happier too.

48, 49 Vigorous aerobic exercise (such as running) must keep the heart rate at 150 beats per minute for 12 to 20 minutes to produce the "training effect." Less vigorous aerobic exercise (lower heart rate) must be maintained for much longer periods to produce the same benefit. The "training effect" is necessary to prepare the heart for meeting extra strain.

53, 54 Such exercise prevents stiffness of joints and musculoskeletal degeneration. It also promotes a greater feeling of well-being.

56 Basic emotions, if repressed, often cause anxiety, depression, irrational behavior, or physical disease. People can learn to feel and express their emotions, with a resulting improvement in their well-being. Some people, however, exaggerate emotions to control and manipulate others; this can be detrimental to well-being.

57 Learning ways to express these emotions constructively (so that all parties concerned feel better) leads to more satisfying relationships and problem solving.

61 Crying over a loss or sad event is an important discharge of emotional energy. It is, however, sometimes used as a manipulative tool or as a substitute expression of anger. Many males in particular have been erroneously taught that it is not O.K. to cry.

76 Spending time spontaneously without relying on an external structure can be self-renewing throughout adult life.

78, 79 Physical touch is important for the maintenance of life for young children and remains important throughout adult life.

83 With proper self-care, most individuals can reach this age in good health.

87 Shoulder/lap belts are much safer than lap belts alone. (Shoulder belts should never be worn without a lap belt.)

89 Whiplash injuries can be prevented by properly adjusted head restraints. These are required, in the United States, on the front seats of all autos made since 1968, but are often not raised high enough to protect passengers and driver.

91 Disk brakes provide considerably better braking power than conventional drum brakes.

92 For most cars, radial tires maintain firmer contact with the road and improve braking and handling better than bias-ply tires. They also have less rolling friction and give better gas mileage.

96, 97 Over 1,000 young children a year are killed in motor vehicle accidents in the United States. Many deaths could be prevented by keeping the child from flying about in a car crash. Most car seats do not provide enough protection—since government standards are low. Check consumer magazines for up-to-date information. Never use an adult seat belt for a child weighing under 50 pounds.

99 The bare feet of young children are often injured at the end of escalators. Wearing tennis shoes is equally dangerous, because the sturdy long laces get pulled into the mechanism and the thin canvas walls offer little protection.

102 Commercial baby foods contain high amounts of sugar, salt, modified starches, and preservatives which may adversely affect a baby's future eating habits and health. Federal legislation has been introduced to help correct this problem. Portable food grinders and blenders can be used to prepare for an infant the same food as eaten by the rest of the family. Individual servings can be packaged and frozen for future meals.

Interpretation. Add the subtotals for each section to find your total wellness score.

A. ☐ **Productivity, Relaxation, Sleep**

B. ☐ **Personal Care and Home Safety**

C. ☐ **Nutritional Awareness**

D. ☐ **Environmental Awareness**

E. ☐ **Physical Activity**

F. ☐ **Expression of Emotion and Feeling**

G. ☐ **Community Involvement**

H. ☐ **Creativity, Self-Expression**

I. ☐ **Automobile Safety**

J. ☐ **Parenting**

Total: ______________

Although the inventory cannot, by any means, offer a precise measurement of a person's wellness or health status, average scores tend to range from about 65 to 75 points.

Source: Copyright © 1981 by John W. Travis, M.D.; available in *The Wellness Resource Kit,* 42 Miller Avenue, Mill Valley, CA 94941.

Notes

Chapter 1

1. The Surgeon General of the United States, *Healthy People: The Surgeon General's Report on Health Promotion and Disease Prevention,* DHEW (PHS) Publication No. 79-55071 (Washington, D.C.: U.S. Government Printing Office, 1979), vii.

Chapter 2

1. National Association for Mental Health, *Mental Health is 1, 2, 3* (Arlington, Va.: The National Association, undated).

Chapter 3

1. Hans Selye, *The Stress of Life* (New York: McGraw-Hill, 1976), 10.
2. Thomas H. Holmes and Richard H. Rahe, "The Social Readjustment Scale," *Journal of Psychosomatic Research* 11 (1967):213–218.

Chapter 4

1. *The New Our Bodies, Ourselves,* published by and for women. The Boston Women's Health Collective Touchstone Book (New York: Simon & Schuster, Inc., 1984), 499.

Chapter 5

1. Zeller, Luria and Mitchel D. Rose, *Psychology of Human Sexuality* (New York: John Wiley, 1979), 26.
2. Shere Hite, *The Hite Report* (New York: Dell Publishing Co., 1976), 59–126.
3. Hite, *The Hite Report,* 62.
4. Linda Brower Meeks and Philip Heit, *Human Sexuality,* (Philadephia: W. B. Saunders Co., 1982), 125.
5. William H. Masters and Virgina E. Johnson, "Principles of the New Sex Therapy," *American Journal of Psychiatry,* 133:5 (May 1976):551.

Chapter 6

1. Betty Friedan, quoted in *Time,* Octover 12, 1981.
2. Melvin Zelnick and John F. Kantner, "Sexual Activity, Contraceptive Use, and Pregnancy Among Metropolitan Teenagers: 1971–1979," *Family Planning Perspectives* 12:5 (September/Octover 1980):230–237.
3. Zelnik and Kantner, "Sexual Activity," 237.
4. John H. Gagnon and Cathy S. Greenblatt, *Life Designs* (Glenview, Ill.: Scott, Foresman & Co., 1978), 140–141.
5. Ira L. Reiss, "Premarital Sexuality: Past, Present, and Future," in *Readings on the Family System,* ed. Ira L. Reiss (New York: Holt, Rinehart & Winston, 1972).
6. Talcott Parsons, *Essays in Sociological Theory* (Glencoe, Ill.: The Free Press, 1949), 187–189.
7. Kenneth L. Jones, Louis W. Shainberg, and Curtis O. Byer, *Health Science* (New York: Harper & Row, 1978), 453–455.
8. Quoted in William J. Lederer and Don D. Jackson, "The Eight Myths of Marriage," *New Woman,* September/October 1975, 60.

9. Lederer and Jackson, "The Eight Myths," 61.
10. John F. Cuber and Peggy B. Harroff, *Sex and the Significant Americans* (Baltimore: Penguin Books, 1965), 43–65.
11. Cuber and Harroff, *Significant Americans;* 52.

Chapter 9

1. J. Toohey, T. Dezelsky, and R. Kush. "A Ten Year Analysis of Non-medical Drug Use Behavior at Five American Universities," *Journal of School Health,* 51:1 (January 1981):51–55.
2. DHEW, *The Fourth Special Report,* 29.
3. DHEW, *The Third Special Report,* 54.
4. Thomas Pravet and Michael Affleck, *Alcohol and Behavior* (St. Louis: C. V. Mosby Company, 1980), 130.
5. DHEW, *The Third Special Report,* 63.
6. DHEW, *The Third Special Report,* 39–44.
7. DHEW, *The Third Special Report,* 65.

Chapter 10

1. C. Squier, "Smokeless Tobacco and Oral Cancer: A Cause for Concern?" *Cancer Journal for Clinicians* 34:5 (September/October 1984):242–247.

Chapter 11

1. Robert Byck, et al., "Cocaine: Chic, Costly, and What Else?" *Patient Care* 14 (September 15, 1980):136–138.

Chapter 13

1. O. Hays, M. F. Trulson, and F. J. Stare, "Suggested Revisions of the Basic Seven," *Journal of the American Dietetic Association* 31 (1955):1103–1107.

Chapter 17

1. Nancy Gutensohn and Philip Cole, "Science and the Citizen," *Scientific American,* April 1981.

Chapter 19

1. U.S. Department of Transportation, National Highway Traffic Safety Administration.

Chapter 20

1. Graduate Medical Education National Advisory Committee, *Summary Report of the Graduate Medical Education National Advisory Committee to the Secretary, Department of Health and Human Services,* Vol. 1 (Washington, D.C.: U.S. Government Printing Office, 1980), 99.

Glossary

Accident. A sequence of sudden, unplanned events that may result in personal injury or property damage.

Acid rain. A pollutant of streams and rivers, formed primarily by the reaction of sulfur and nitrogen with oxygen and water in the air to form sulfuric acid and nitric oxide.

Acidosis. An abnormal increase in the acidity of the blood and of body fluids.

Acupuncture. An ancient Far Eastern therapy based on the premise that needles inserted at the proper points on the body will relieve pain and restore the balance of health.

Adaptation. The body's attempt to maintain a state of balance, or homeostasis.

Addiction. Repeated compulsive use of a drug involving physical and psychological dependence.

Adipose tissue. An abnormal accumulation of fat in the body.

Adrenocorticotropic hormone (ACTH). A pituitary hormone that prepares the body for the fight-or-flee response.

Adrenalin. A popular name for the adrenal hormone epinephrine.

Adultery. Sexual intercourse between a married person and someone other than the spouse.

Aerobic exercise. Excercise designed to increase cardiorespiratory endurance.

Aerobic fitness. Ability of the body to continually meet its oxygen needs.

Ageism. The stereotyping of and discrimination against people because they are old.

Aging. The process of physical, mental, emotional, and social change that a person experiences throughout the life cycle.

AIDS (Acquired Immune Deficiency Syndrome). Condition characterized by the body's inability to fight off disease, resulting in the victim's susceptibility to a wide variety of rare diseases.

Alcoholic. A person who chronically drinks too much and cannot control how much he or she drinks.

Alcoholics Anonymous (AA). A rehabilitation program treating alcoholics who are motivated and willing to get help.

Aldosterone. A hormone secreted by the adrenal glands that facilitates retention of sodium, heightens muscle tone, aids adjustment to temperature change, and disperses wastes.

Alienation. A state of confusion in which nothing seems to make sense and the individual does not know exactly what he or she wants.

Allergen. An ordinarily harmless antigen that triggers an allergic attack.

Allergy. Hypersensitivity to a particular antigen.

Alzheimer's disease. A form of dementia characterized by memory lapses and periodic confusion.

Amenorrhea. The absence or abnormal cessation of menstruation.

Amino acids. A group of chemical compounds, some of which are the building blocks of protein.

Aminocentesis. The extraction and analysis of a small amount of amniotic fluid from the uterus, usually around the fourteenth to sixteenth week of pregnancy, to detect possible fetal abnormalities.

Amniotic sac. A sac filled with fluid that protects the embryo.

Anaerobic. The demand for oxygen exceeds the supply, resulting in oxygen debt.

Anaerobic exercises. Exercise designed specifically to develop speed, strength, and power.

Androgen. The male sex hormone responsible for stimulating the development of both the internal and external male genitals.

Androgyny. Having both masculine and feminine characteristics

Angina pectoris. Chest pain that begins beneath the breastbone and may spread to the left shoulder, arm, and jaw.

Ankylosis. A fusing of the joints, rendering them nonfunctional.

Anorexia nervosa. A psychological eating disorder leading to loss of appetite and malnutrition.

Antagonism. Drug used to counteract and reverse the symptoms of an overdose from a particular drug.

Antibiotics. Chemical substances produced by microorganisms that either destroy outright or interfere with the growth cycles of other microorganisms.

Anticonvulsant drug therapy. Use of drugs that prevent convulsions.

Antigens. Foreign proteins capable of producing an allergic reaction.

Anxiety. A feeling of fear and apprehension concerning the outcome of an event.

Areolae. The dark areas around the nipples of the breast.

Arrythmia. An irregularity of the heartbeat.

Arteriosclerosis. A condition wherein the arterial walls become hardened, thus causing the blood pressure to rise; also called hardening of the arteries.

Arthritis. Inflammation of the joints.

Asthma. Narrowing of the bronchioles.

Atherosclerosis. The most common form of arteriosclerosis, caused by the accumulation of cholesterol and fatty deposits on the inner surfaces of the arterial wall.

Athlete's foot. One of the best-known fungus infections. It is the common term for ringworm of the foot.

Autoimmune disorder. A malfunction that occurs when the immune system produces antibodies that attack the body's own tissues.

Bacteria. Single-celled plantlike organisms that reproduce asexually.

Bartholin's glands. Glands that create a genital scent and neutralize the vaginal environment.

Basic health insurance. Standard health insurance covering hospital-related service.

Benign tumor. A mass of relatively normal, specialized cells that grows within connective tissue and is restricted to a local area.

Bioecological stress. Stress arising from conditions in the environment that evoke a biological (physiological) response over which we can exert little, if any, control.

Bisexuality. The engagement in both homosexual and heterosexual behavior.

Blackout. A temporary form of amnesia caused by drinking.

Blood Alcohol Concentration (BAC). A measurement that indicates the amount of alcohol the body has absorbed.

Body composition. The comparative amounts of basic body tissue, muscle, bone, and fat.

Brachial artery. The main artery of the arm located on the inside of the arm.

Bronchitis. Lung disease that causes increases in the mucous secretions in the respiratory tract and an increase in the frequency of coughing.

Bronchodilator. A drug that opens up the air passageways to the lungs.

Bulbourethral (Cowper's) glands. Two pea-sized structures at the base of the penis, secreting a clear bit of fluid that appears on the tip of the penis during sexual arousal.

Bulemia. A psychological eating disorder involving the binge-purge syndrome, in which the individual exhibits an abnormal fear of becoming fat.

Burnout. Condition of complete overload in which the individual feels stretched to the limit.

Calorie. A unit of heat; specifically, the amount of heat needed to raise one gram of water one degree centigrade; also called a small calorie.

Carbohydrate. An essential nutrient comprised of sugar, starch, and fiber.

Carbon monoxide. A colorless, odorless, toxic gas that can reduce the blood's oxygen-carrying capability.

Carcinogen. Cancer-causing substance.

Carcinoma. The most common type of cancer, occurring in the body's surface tissue.

Cardiopulmonary resuscitation (CPR). An emergency revival technique used when heartbeat and respiration have stopped.

Cardiorespiratory endurance. The ability of the heart, lungs, and blood vessels to function efficiently during strenuous exercise or activity.

Cardiovascular system. Blood circulates continuously through this system, which consists of the heart and all the blood vessels leading to and from it.

Career counselor. An individual who is trained in helping people make career decisions (see also, guidance counselor).

Caries. Dental cavities, which are caused by bacteria living on the teeth as a gelatinous coating called plaque.

Celibacy. A life-style in which a person puts aside sexual fulfillment.

Cerebral embolism. An obstruction of a cerebral artery by a transported clot.

Cerebral hemorrhage. Seepage of blood into the brain as a result of a ruptured cerebral artery.

Cerebral thrombosis. The formation of a blood clot in a cerebral artery.

Cervix. The neck of the uterus, projecting into the vagina.

Cesarean section. A method of childbirth in which the baby is removed from the mother's body surgically, through an incision in the lower part of the abdominal wall and through the uterus.

Chemotherapy. The use of drugs or other chemicals to fight disease, particularly cancer.

Chiropractor. A professional who holds a Doctor of Chiropractic medical degree and treats spinal disorders.

Chlamydia. A recently recognized venereal disease that is similar to gonorrhea but twice as prevalent.

Cholesterol. A substance found in saturated fats vital for production of cortisone and sex hormones; its buildup can cause atherosclerosis.

Chromosomal abnormalities. Genetic disorders related to a defect in the structure of the chromosome or an abnormal number of chromosomes.

Chromosomes. Rod-shaped bodies that control individual heredity.

Cilia. Small hairlike projections in the respiratory system that help keep foreign material out of the lungs.

Circadian rhythm. The fixed pattern of changes in basic body processes during a twenty-four-hour period.

Clinical psychologist. A professional who diagnoses and treats behavior disorders but does not prescribe drugs; usually has a Ph.D. in clinical psychology.

Clitoris. A small organ of spongy erectile tissue located above the opening of the urethra; the most sensitive of all female genital organs.

Coenzyme. A substance working together with an enzyme so that the enzyme can complete its action.

Cohabitation. A man and a woman living together in a sexual relationship without being married.

Colostrum. Often referred to as early milk a usually a breast-fed baby's first nourishment; thin, yellow liquid that may drip from t mother's nipples during the last weeks of pre nancy.

Common cold. A viral infection of the upper re piratory tract.

Communicable diseases. Diseases that can b transmitted from person to person either direct or indirectly.

Complete protein. Foods containing all the e sential amino acids; usually animal proteins.

Corpus luteum. A temporary endocrine glan formed in the ovary after ovulation that pr duces estrogen and progesterone.

Crisis intervention counseling. Counseling ser vices established to focus on handling specifi and immediate problems confronting the indi vidual.

Cunnilingus. Oral stimulation of the female geni tals.

Cystic fibrosis. Genetic-related disorder involv ing exocrine glands.

Defense mechanism. Unconscious means of protecting oneself from stress.

Depressant. A drug that lowers nervous or functional activity by producing muscular relaxation.

Depression. A long-lasting, overwhelming feeling of sadness and lack of energy and motivation.

Desensitize. To gradually introduce allergens into the body to build up a tolerance and to alleviate allergic reactions.

Diabetes. Disease of the pancreas that prevents the body from utilizing sugars and starches to produce energy.

Diagnostic Related Groups (DRG). A patient classifying system currently used by Medicare.

Diastole. The second phase of the heartbeat, during which the heart fills with blood; as distinguished from systole.

Dioxin. Any of seventy-five chemicals in eight different families resulting from the combination of chlorine, hydrogen, and carbon; a by-product in the making of plastics, wood preservatives, and other chemical products.

Distilled spirits. Alcoholic beverages with high alcohol concentration; referred to as "hard" liquors.

Distress. The body's response to negative stressors.

Divorce. Legal dissolvement of a marriage.

ırgery (D.D.S.). Dentist; pro-
ıgnoses and treats disorders of
ıs.

dentistry (D.M.D.). Dentist; has pursued a different route of he doctor of dental surgery, known as dentists.

ic medicine (D.P.M.). Special-
seases and disorders of the feet,
ɪd premedical training plus four
ic medical college.

ne. Chromosomal abnormality
ɔy physical malformations and
mental retardation.

ıce that alters one or more body
ıding mood and behavior.

ıronically using a drug for a reason
as not intended.

Taking prescribed medication
lting a physician.

length of time of an exercise ses-
ıg warm-up, exercise, and cool-

. Difficult and painful menstrua-

Painful intercourse.

utants discharged into the water

ırt of the psyche that consciously
id's impulses and enables the indi-
apt to society's rules and inhibitions.

ıuct. The junction of the vasa defer-
ɪminal vesicles with the urethra.

ɔgram. A medical examination that
taching electrodes to different parts
to monitor heart functioning.

phlogram. A graphic tracing of the
al activity (electrical impulses) of the
.

he fertilized egg, which has been im-
the uterine wall, up until the eighth
evelopment.

Any response of the individual to posi-
ɪgative events or elements in the envi-

a. Chronic respiratory disease in
r sacs and some larger structures of the
their capacity to carry out respiratory
s.

ɪ. A feeling that results from a lack of
ɪial ties and friendships.

Endometrium. Uterine lining.

Engagement. The act of committing or pledging oneself to another for the purpose of marriage.

Epididymis. A tightly coiled duct that leads from the testicle to the vas deferens.

Epilepsy. Sudden discharge of electrical energy in the brain.

Epinephrine (adrenalin). A hormone secreted by the adrenal glands that acts as a potent stimulant to the circulatory system and gets the body ready to fight-or-flee.

Erectile dysfunction (impotence). The inability to attain or maintain an erection.

Essential amino acids. Nine indispensable amino acids (ten in children) that cannot be synthesized by the body and must therefore be ingested daily.

Essential fat. Temporary fat reserves that are drawn on to take care of normal body functions.

Essential hypertension. A consistent elevation of blood pressure with no known organic cause.

Essential nutrients. Those nutrients vital for proper body functions, consisting of carbohydrates, fats, proteins, vitamins, minerals, and water.

Estrogen. A female sex hormone produced by the ovaries, placenta, and adrenal cortex that stimulates secondary sex characteristics and acts on female organs during the menstrual cycle.

Ethanol (ethyl alcohol). The ingredient in alcoholic beverages that causes intoxication.

Eustress. The body's response to positive stressors; "good" stress.

Euthanasia. Easy, or good, death; the process of withdrawing life-support systems from an ill patient.

Excitement phase. The first phase of the sexual response cycle in humans.

Executor. A person appointed to see that the provisions of another individual's will are carried out.

Exercise physiologist. A person who specializes in the effects of exercise on the body.

Fallopian tubes. Extensions of the uterus which allow an egg to pass from the ovary to the uterus.

Family counseling. A therapy method in which all members of a family meet with a therapist to discuss a problem or problems common to all of them.

Family practitioner. A physician who specializes in the care of the entire family.

Fat. A concentrated, high-energy nutrient consisting of fatty acids and glycerol.

Fat-soluble vitamins. The vitamins that can be stored in the human body (vitamins A, D, E, and K); as distinguished from water-soluble vitamins.

Fellatio. Oral stimulation of the male's genitals.

Femoral artery. The main artery in the leg.

Fetal Alcohol Syndrome (FAS). Birth defects caused by alcohol consumption of the mother during pregnancy.

Fetus. A fertilized egg after the eighth week of development.

Fiber (roughage). Indigestible carbohydrates that make solid waste bulkier and softer, delay stomach emptying, and contribute to intestinal health.

Fight-or-flee. The body's response to any stressful situation, resulting from secretion of hormones into the bloodstream preparing the muscles to attack or run away.

Fission. A method of producing nuclear energy that involves the splitting of atoms.

Flexibility. The range of movement within a specified joint and its associated muscle groups.

Fluorocarbon. A chemical agent that, when released into the air, breaks down into chlorine components, which destroy the ozone.

Foreplay. Any act of touching or kissing that precedes intercourse.

Fornication. Sexual intercourse between unmarried consenting adults.

Free-floating anxiety. Generalized apprehension without a specific cause.

Frequency. The number of exercise sessions per week for an individual.

Frustration. A feeling of being trapped without an avenue of escape.

Fungi. Simple plants lacking chlorophyll, some of which are disease-causing organisms.

Fusion. The putting together of atoms.

Gender identity. The consistent awareness of maleness or femaleness.

Gene abnormality. A specific problem inherent in the DNA, which makes up the gene.

General Adaptation Syndrome (G.A.S.). A three-stage pattern of response to stressors, involving an alarm reaction, a resistance phase, and exhaustion.

Generic drug. A drug without a brand name, usually priced more cheaply than its brand-name equivalent.

Genital herpes. Also herpes II; the most common sexually transmitted disease, caused by transmission of a virus.

Genitals. The external sex organs.

Gerontology. The study of aging.

Glans penis. Highly sensitive conical head of the penis.

Glioma. Cancer of nerve tissue.

Glucose. A sugar that is both produced and used by the body.

Glycerol. A clear, colorless, syrupy liquid formed by the hydrolysis of fat.

Gonorrhea. A sexually transmitted disease that infects the mucous membrane of the urogenital tract.

Government hospitals (public hospitals). Hospitals that are supported wholly by taxes and are owned and operated by the municipal, county, state, or federal government.

Grand mal seizure. Type of epileptic seizure characterized by uncontrolled and sometimes violent muscle spasms.

Group counseling. A therapy method in which several people meet simultaneously with a therapist to discuss a problem or problems common to all of them.

Guidance counselor. An individual who is qualified to work with mild mental problems in a therapeutic setting.

Hallucinogen. A mind-altering drug used recreationally.

HDL (high-density lipoproteins). A protein molecule in the blood that combines with fat molecules.

Health Maintenance Organization (HMO). A group plan in which premiums are paid in advance for comprehensive medical care.

Heimlich maneuver. A technique used to expel foreign matter lodged in a choking victim's windpipe.

Hepatitis. An infection of the liver.

Herpes simplex (herpes I). A virus that is acquired through direct contact with the saliva of an infected individual and usually lies dormant in the body after an initial childhood infection; see genital herpes for herpes II.

Homeostasis. The state of and maintenance of bodily equilibrium with respect to various bodily functions and chemical composition of the tissues and fluids.

Homosexuality. Emotional or erotic attraction to and behavior with a member of the same sex.

Hospice. An institution that provides medical care and counseling for terminally ill patients and their families.

Hydrocarbons. Chemical compounds containing hydrogen and carbon, usually a result of the incomplete combustion of petroleum products and often an irritant to the respiratory tract.

Hydrogen cyanide. A gaseous component of smoke that can damage the lining of the respiratory system.

Hymen. A thin fold of membrane that surrounds the vaginal opening.

Hyperplasia. An increase in the number of fat or other cells; a cause of one form of obesity.

Hypertension. A condition of high blood pressure that usually results from arteriosclerosis, or plaque building along the arterial walls.

Hypertrophy. A condition wherein muscle fibers increase in size, thus resulting in increased strength; also, an abnormal increase in amounts of fat or other bulk in a stable number of cells; a cause of one form of obesity.

Hypnotics. Sleep-inducing drugs.

Hypoglycemia. A condition that occurs when blood levels of sugar fall too low.

Hypothermia. A lowering of the temperature inside the body.

Id. The basic part of the human psyche that is dominated by the pleasure principle and impulsive wishing.

Immunity. The body's ability to distinguish foreign matter from the self and to neutralize it; may be natural or acquired.

Immunosuppressive drugs. Drugs that block the production of antibodies.

Incomplete protein. Low-quality protein lacking some essential amino acids; usually plant protein.

Infection. Invasion of body tissue by a pathogen.

Infectious mononucleosis. A common viral disease, usually striking children and young adults, characterized by common viral infection symptoms as well as fatigue, swollen lymph glands, and a high count of abnormal lymphocytes.

Infidelity. Unfaithfulness in a relationship.

Influenza. A highly contagious infection of the respiratory tract characterized by sudden fever, coughing, headache, chills, and prostration.

Infradian rhythm. A biological cycle extending over days, weeks, or months, such as the female menstrual cycle.

Inhibition. Interference with the metabolism of a drug or displacement of a drug from its receptor sites.

Insulin. A hormone secreted by the pancreas that acts upon glucose so it can be used for energy production.

Insulin dependence. A condition in diabetes in which the pancreas produces insufficient insulin, requiring the victim to obtain a supply through injections.

Insulin shock. Serious condition that occurs when the blood sugar level falls too low because of excess insulin in the bloodstream.

Intensity. A measure of how hard the heart must work during exercise.

Intercourse (coitus). Sexual activity involving insertion of the penis in the vagina.

Interferon. A chemical released by body cells to combat viruses

Isokinetic. Sustaining maximal force throughout a range of motion.

Isometric. Putting resistance against an immovable object.

Isotonic. Lifting a movable object, such as a weight.

Jellnick model. A schematic that succinctly describes four phases involved in the development of an alcoholic.

Kilogram calorie. A unit of heat; specifically, the amount of heat needed to raise one kilogram of water one degree centigrade; used to measure the energy produced when food is oxidized in the body; also called a large calorie.

Labia majora. Two large folds of skin that contain sweat glands and hair follicles embedded in fatty tissue of the vagina.

Labia minora. Delicate folds of hairless skin located between the labia majora that are enriched with blood vessels and oil glands.

Lamaze method. A method of natural childbirth that enables women to remain alert during labor and delivery.

Leader nutrients. Basic nutrients that must be listed in labels specifying their amount in any food; they include protein, carbohydrates, fat, vitamins A and C, thiamin, riboflavin, niacin, calcium, and iron.

Lean body weight. Body weight consisting of the bones, muscles, connective tissue, and vital organs.

Legionnaires' disease. A family of infections that most seriously affect individuals with an immunity deficiency or underlying chronic disease.

Leukemia. Systemic cancer of the body or bone marrow.

Life-style factors. The day-to-day practices of the individual, including such things as cigarette smoking, regular exercise, eating nutritious foods, controlling stress and tension, misuse of alcohol or other drugs, and controlling one's weight.

Lightening. The fetus dropping into the pelvic cavity, relieving pressure on the mother's ribs and making breathing easier; usually occurs three or four weeks before labor begins and is experienced by women having a first child.

Living Will. A document indicating the signer's desire to die as quickly and painlessly as possible once he or she is diagnosed as terminally ill.

Loneliness. A feeling that arises from the perceived absence of a desired relationship.

Love (romantic). Strong emotional feelings for and attachment to another individual.

Lymphoma. Cancer of the lymphatic system.

Macrominerals. Minerals needed in the body in relatively large amounts, like calcium, phosphorus, potassium, sulfur, sodium, and magnesium.

Mainstream smoke. The smoke that is directly inhaled and exhaled by the smoker.

Major medical insurance. Health insurance that covers a wider variety of health services than basic health insurance.

Major tranquilizers. Class of drugs that are used in dealing with profound behavioral adjustment problems.

Malignant tumor. A tumor that multiplies rapidly, mutates frequently, and breaks away and invades other tissues, supplanting normal cells.

Marital rape. Tricking, pressuring, or physically forcing one's wife to have sexual relations.

Masturbation. The manipulation of one's own genitals.

Medical doctor (M.D.). A professional who has completed undergraduate school with premedical training, medical school, and an internship (general practitioner), plus a residency in some cases (specialist).

Megadose. An unusually large dosage, often of vitamins.

Melanoma. Cancer of the skin cells containing melanin (a dark pigment).

Menorrhagia. Profuse or prolonged menstrual bleeding.

Mental health. A state of being in which the individual feels comfortable about himself or herself and others and meets daily challenges with a minimum of unpleasant aftereffects.

Mental illness. A state of being in which the individual is not comfortable with himself or herself and others and does not seem able to meet the daily challenges of living.

Metabolism. The sum of all the chemical processes that occur in the body.

Metastasis. The spread of cancerous cells caused by the separation of parts of tumors or by the infiltration of malignant cells to other parts of the body.

Methadone maintenance. A drug-treatment program that substitutes an addictive but legal drug, methadone, for opiates.

Mineral. An inorganic element needed for basic body metabolism.

Minor tranquilizers. Drugs such as Valium and Miltown, commonly prescribed to relieve tension and anxiety.

Mons pubis. The most visible part of the female genitals, formed by a pad of fat located over the pubic bone.

Multiple sclerosis (MS). Neurological disorder characterized by progressive demyelination of neurons in the brain and spinal cord.

Muscular dystrophies. Group of inherited diseases that affect muscle tissue.

Muscular endurance. The ability of muscles to sustain force over time or repeatedly contract.

Mycosis. Infection caused by yeasts and molds.

Myelin sheath. Covering of an axon part of a nerve cell (neuron).

Myocardial infarction. A heart attack that results from oxygen deprivation of a portion of the heart muscle.

Myotonia. The delayed relaxation of a muscle following a contraction, as during sexual arousal.

Narcotics. Opiate derivatives used for pain relief.

Naturopathic doctor (N.D.). A practitioner who treats diseases or disorders with natural cures, such as herbs, vitamins, and spinal manipulation, and does not prescribe drugs.

Neoplasm. New growth of tumors resulting from the uncontrolled reproduction of abnormal cells.

Neuron. Nerve cell.

Nicotine. A substance present in tobacco smoke that affects the heart, blood vessels, kidneys, nervous system, and digestive tract.

Nitrates. Substances used in foods to retard bacterial growth.

Nitric oxide. A gas formed in part from nitrogen and oxygen when combustion takes place under higher temperature and high pressure.

Nitrites. Substances like nitrates that are used in foods to control bacterial growth.

Nitrogen dioxide. A compound produced by the oxidation of nitric oxide in the atmosphere; a major component of engine exhaust and tobacco smoke.

Nitrogen oxide. A pollutant found in smoke that is linked to lung disease.

Norepinephrine. A hormone known to reduce anxieties and bring about greater alertness.

Nostrum. Unproven remedy for illness, made from a secret formula.

Obesity. A condition wherein over 30 percent of total body weight is fat.

Open marriage. A marriage form that encourages growth, change, role flexibility, and open communication and that accepts sex outside the primary marital unit.

Organic foods. Foods grown with fertilizers and mulches consisting only of animal or vegetable matter, with no artificial chemical fertilizers.

Orgasm. The climax of sexual tension.

Orgasmic dysfunction. An inability to reach the orgasmic phase of the sexual response cycle.

Osteoarthritis. Milder form of arthritis usually found in people over fifty.

Osteopathic physician (D.O., or osteopath). Physician who has completed premedical and medical training and who specializes in manipulation, the manual application of pressure.

Osteoporosis. A disease involving bone loss plus easy breakage and slow healing of bones.

Ova. Germ cells, or eggs.

Ovaries. Two almond-sized and -shaped organs that are located in the lower abdominal cavity on either side of the pelvic region that produce the female sex hormones estrogen and progesterone plus small amounts of the male hormone androgen.

Overload. A stressful condition occurring when people receive more stimuli than their bodies and minds can process.

Overloading. Strength training wherein the muscles are forced to work harder than normal.

Over-the-counter (OTC) drug. Drug for which a prescription is not necessary.

Ovulation. The release of a mature ovum from the ovary.

Ozone layer. A zone of the atmosphere approximately twelve to twenty-one miles above the earth's surface.

Pap smear (Papanicolaou test). A laboratory test to detect cervical cancer by analyzing cells scraped from outside the cervix.

Parasitic worms. Largest of all pathogens, visible to the naked eye, which enter the human body through ingestion or contact with infected animals.

Particulates. Tiny solid particles, such as soot, fungi, and other substances, in the air.

Pastoral counselor. A member of the clergy specifically trained to work with mental health problems.

Pathogen. An organism that causes a communicable disease.

Penis. The male organ for copulation and urination.

Peridontal disease. Disease involving the gums; the major cause of tooth loss after age thirty-five.

Personality stress. Stress that arises from the way we perceive ourselves (self-concept) and our behaviors.

Petit mal seizure. Type of epileptic seizure characterized by a daydreaming appearance.

Petting. Any act of touching or kissing that excludes intercourse.

Pharmacological action. A drug's scientifically tested effects.

Phenylketonuria (PKU). Absence of an enzyme resulting in increased levels of phenylalanine in the blood.

Physical dependence. A state in which the body will undergo a withdrawal syndrome if the individual does not take a given drug.

Placebo. A pharmacologically inactive substance that is falsely expected by the user to act like a drug.

Placenta. The organ through which the fetus receives nourishment from, and empties waste matter into, the circulatory system of the mother.

Plaque. Deposits that form in the lining of the arteries or on the teeth.

Plateau phase. The second phase involved in the sexual response cycle wherein the circumference of the penis and the lubrication of the vagina increase.

Potentiation. An action in which the effect of two drugs given simultaneously is greater than the effect of the drugs given separately.

Premature ejaculation. The inability to postpone ejaculation.

Premenstrual Syndrome (PMS). A condition involving extreme discomfort and distress experienced by some women prior to each menstrual period; likely the result of an imbalance of estrogen and progesterone.

Preorgasmic ejaculation (love drop). A small amount of fluid, usually containing some sperm, that is involuntarily secreted from the penis during sexual arousal.

Prepared childbirth. A method of natural childbirth that requires expectant parents to attend a series of classes designed to reduce the fear and tension often associated with labor and delivery.

Pressure-point technique. A technique used to stop bleeding by manually applying pressure to key arteries.

Preventive health care. Actions taken by the individual to avoid getting ill; a conscientious attempt on the part of the individual to alter selected life-style factors that might be detrimental to personal well-being.

Private hospitals. Hospitals owned and operated as profit-making ventures.

Proctoscopy. Inspection of the rectum with a special instrument.

Progesterone. A hormone that prepares the uterus for the reception and development of the fertilized egg.

Prostate. Gland that surrounds the neck of the urinary bladder and the opening of the urethra in the male.

Protein. An essential nutrient that consists of various amino acids.

Protozoa. Single-celled organisms, some of which are parasitic and/or pathogenic.

Psychiatrist. A medical doctor who specializes in the diagnosis and treatment of mental disorders.

Psychoactive drugs. Drugs that affect primarily the nervous system and changes in mood and behavior.

Psychological dependence. Emotional attachment to a particular drug.

Psychologist. A professionally trained individual who helps persons understand and solve their own mental health problems.

Psychomotor seizure. Type of epileptic seizure characterized by involuntary muscle jerks.

Psychosocial stress. Stress that arises from faulty processing of the various stimuli we get from our social environment.

Psychosomatic relaxation. A relaxation technique that is initiated in the central nervous system, then spreads to the rest of the body.

Puberty. Physiological changes resulting in full sexual development.

Pulmonary circulation. The circulation of the blood from the heart to the lungs and back.

Radiation therapy. Treatment of cancer by bombarding cancer cells with X rays or other radiation.

Rape. Sexual penetration effected by force, duress, intimidation, or deception.

Recommended Dietary Allowances (RDAs). General guidelines for nutritional requirements according to age, weight, and sex.

Relaxation response. A method of relaxation used to reduce physiological responses and stress.

Resolution phase. The relaxation phase of the sexual response cycle.

Retarded ejaculation. The inability to ejaculate despite the achievement of an erection.

Rheumatic fever. An immune reaction, caused by strep throat or scarlet fever, attacking the heart and joints and causing chest pain.

Rheumatoid arthritis. Prolonged inflammation of the joints leading to their deformation.

Rickettsias. Pathogenic organisms, similar to bacteria, that have lost the ability to exist without a host.

Sarcoma. Cancer of the connective tissue.

Saturated fats. Fats usually from animal sources and often solid at room temperature; contain more cholesterol and triglycerides than unsaturated fats.

Scarlet fever. An infection in which the strep pathogen produces a toxin, causing nausea, vomiting, and high fever.

Scrotum. The pouch that contains the testicles.

Sedatives. Drugs that act as calming agents.

Self-actualization. The utilization of one's creative potential for self-fulfillment.

Self-help group. Group formed by persons with a shared concern to help the individual focus attention on solving a specific problem or group of problems.

Senescence. Biological deterioration associated with old age.

Set. Individual perceptions and expectations related to what a particular drug will do.

Set-point therapy. A theory of weight loss and gain maintaining that a person's body will "set" the percentage of body fat it will store; excess caloric intake will be burned off as metabolic heat, and caloric deficits will increase hunger.

Setting. Physical and social environment in which a drug is taken.

Sexually-transmitted diseases (STDs). All infections transmitted principally by sexual contact.

Sickle-cell anemia. Genetic disorder whereby red blood cells assume a sickle shape, which affects their oxygen-carrying capacity.

Sidestream smoke. The smoke that is generated by the tobacco-containing product (generally a cigarette) while it smolders in an ashtray or in a person's hand.

Singles scene. The mingling of unmarried people, with emphasis on sexuality and leisurely lifestyles.

Somatopsychic relaxation. A method of relaxation that begins in the periphery of the body's musculature and then spreads to the central nervous system.

Specific density. An individual's weight under water subtracted from the individual's weight on land; used to determine the percentage of fat in the individual's body.

Specificity. Exercises designed to work on a specific segment of fitness or a specific muscle group.

Sperm. Male reproductive cells capable of fertilizing the femal ovum.

Standard-sized drink. A serving containing about one-half ounce of ethanol (twelve ounces of beer, four ounces of wine, one ounce of distilled spirits).

Staphylococcal pneumonia. A serious infection caused by staph pathogens in the lungs.

Staphylococcus bacteria. Spherical, pathogenic bacteria appearing in irregular clusters.

Stimulant. A substance that stimulates the central nervous system, with one affect being the inability to fall asleep.

Storage fats. Excessive body reserves of fat.

Strength. The maximum amount of force muscles can apply in a single contraction.

Streptococcal sore throat (strep throat). An infection that reaches the acute stage after an incubation period of one to three days; symptoms include soreness and redness in the throat and, often, swollen tonsils.

Streptococcus bacteria. Spherical, chain-forming, pathogenic bacteria.

Stress. The range of responses of the body to demands made upon it.

Stressor. A physical, social, or psychological factor that triggers a stress response.

Stress test. A maximum exercise test to determine cardiorespiratory fitness.

Stroke (cerebrovascular accident). A blood clot that obstructs a vessel in the brain.

Subliminal advertising. Advertising that appeals to consumers' subconscious.

Sulfur dioxide. A gas formed primarily by the combination of fossil fuels.

Super ego. The basic part of the human psyche that evaluates the demands of the id and advises the ego on acceptable actions, thus essentially one's conscience.

Synergism. Augmentation of the activity of one substance by another substance.

Systemic circulation. The circulation of the blood from the heart through the body, excluding the lungs.

Systole. The first phase of the heartbeat, at which time the heart pumps the blood; as distinguished from diastole.

Syphilis. One of the most common sexually transmitted diseases, which may result in blindness, heart failure, brain damage, and even death.

Tar. The substance in cigarettes that contains most of the carcingoens.

Temperature inversion. A layer of warm air being capped by a layer of cooler air, resulting in polluted air being trapped close to the ground.

Terminal illness. An illness that cannot be cured, thus causing the death of the individual.

Testicles (testes). The sperm-producing organs.

Testosterone. The male sex hormone responsible for assuring that the male genital structures do not change into female genital structures.

Therapeutic community. Form of rehabilitation used with the overall goal of returning an addict to the outside world with the resources to make him or her drug-free.

Tolerance. A physical adaptation causing drugs to become less effective with repeated use.

Tourniquet. An apparatus used to stop the flow of blood from a wound when the blood loss is life-threatening.

Toxic Shock Syndrome. Acute bacterial infection associated with the continuous use of tampons during the menstrual period.

Trace elements. Chemical elements required in minute amounts for an organism's metabolism.

Trachea. Cylindrical tube in the respiratory system that conveys air to the lungs.

Transcendental meditation (TM). A method of stress reduction involving two twenty-minute periods of meditation a day; propounded by Maharishi Mahesh Yogi.

Trichomoniasis. A protozoal infection of the lower genitourinary tract.

Triglyceride. A true fat consisting of one molecule of glycerol and three molecules of fatty acids.

Tubal ligation. A form of female sterilization that involves cutting, tying, or otherwise closing the fallopian tubes.

Tuberculosis. A chronic disease usually affecting lung tissue, although all body tissue is susceptible; symptoms include coughing, fatigue, weight loss, and chest pain.

Tumescence. An enlargement of the vulva and clitoris in the female and the penis in the male as a result of an increase in the flow of blood to the respective areas.

Tumor. A mass of new tissue that serves no useful purpose; can be either malignant or benign.

Ultradian rhythm. Fixed patterns of changes in the basic life processes occuring in 90- to 100-minute cycles.

Underload (deprivational stress). The individual feels devoid of stimulation from a job, relationship, or the social environment.

Uniform Donor Card. A legal document specifying that upon death one wants his or her bodily organs to be donated for purposes such as medical transplants.

Unsaturated fats. Fats that occur primarily in vegetable oils and are liquid at room temperature.

Urethra. A tube that extends from the bladder to the external urethral opening; carries urine and ejaculate in the male.

Urethral opening. Opening of the urinary tract located just above the vaginal opening in the female.

U.S. Recommended Daily Allowances (U.S. RDAs). The legal standard for labeling the nutritional value and content of foods covering the needs of most healthy individuals.

Uterus. The womb.

Vagina. A thin-walled, muscular tube adapted to the reception of the semen during sexual intercourse.

Vaginal yeast infection. A fungus infection caused by the yeast Candida, a pathogenic invader transmitted during sexual intercourse.

Vaginismus. Strong, often painful contraction of the vagina.

Valley fever. A major fungal disease characterized by influenza-like symptoms that can affect the whole body.

Vas deferens. A cordlike structure that travels from the testicles to the abdominal cavity and serves as the storage place for sperm.

Vasectomy. A method of male sterilization in which the vasa deferentia are cut, tied, or otherwise closed.

Vasocongestion. The enlargement of the blood vessels, as occurs in the pelvic area during sexual arousal.

Vector. An organism, usually animal or insect, that transports pathogens either in or on its body.

Virus. A submicroscopic pathogen composed of a DNA or RNA core and a protein coating.

Vitamin. Organic compound needed in tiny amounts for normal metabolism.

Voluntary hospitals. Nonprofit hospitals.

Vulva. External female anatomy; includes the labia majora, labia minora, and the clitoris.

Water-soluble vitamin. A vitamin that is not stored in the body and is easily destroyed; as distinct from a fat-soluble vitamin.

Wellness. An ever-expanding experience of purposeful, enjoyable living; an experience that is created by the individual to maintain or improve health.

Withdrawal syndrome. Symptoms that occur when a drug to which the body has become adapted is no longer present in the body.

Index